D1218909

Medicinal Plants of the World

Medicinal Plants
of the
World

Chemical Constituents, Traditional and Modern Medicinal Uses

By

Ivan A. Ross

Humana Press ✳ Totowa, New Jersey

This publication is printed on acid-free paper. ∞
ANSI Z39.48-1984 (American Standards Institute)
Permanence of Paper for Printed Library Materials.

Cover illustration: *Catharanthus roseus* (*see* Chapter 8), *Psidium guajava* (*see* Chapter 24), *Mangifera indica* (*see* Chapter 17), *Momordica charantia* (*see* Chapter 19), *Jatropha curcas* (*see* Chapter 14), *Lantana camara* (*see* Chapter 15), and *Hibiscus rosa-sinensis* (*see* Chapter 12).

Cover design by Patricia F. Cleary.

For additional copies, pricing for bulk purchases, and/or information about other Humana titles, contact Humana at the above address or at any of the following numbers: Tel.: 973-256-1699; Fax: 973-256-8341; E-mail: humana@humanapr.com; or visit our Website: http://humanapress.com

Printed in the United States of America. 10 9 8 7 6 5 4 3 2

Library of Congress Cataloging in Publication Data

Medicinal plants of the world: chemical constituents, traditional, and modern medicinal uses/by Ivan A. Ross.
    p.   cm.
  Includes index.
  ISBN 0-89603-542-5 (alk. paper)
  1. Medicinal plants--Encyclopedias. I. Title.
RS164.R676   1999
615' .32--dc21   98-34758
              CIP

Preface

As a biologist with the US Food and Drug Administration I have been involved in toxicological research. On one occasion, while investigating herbal products sold in the United States as foods or food supplements, I realized that there was an abundance of information on plants that are commonly used as food and medicine. However, the material available was not compiled to optimally serve my interest. Most such books addressed the subject as folklore, and their information was not prepared as an educational resource on plant materials that are used as foods and food supplements by the general public. As a result, to obtain a fair knowledge of any specific plant, information from several books and journal articles had to be put together. It is this experience that guided me to compile *Medicinal Plants of the World*.

No current text describes the traditional medicinal uses, the chemical constituents, the pharmacological activities, and the clinical trials of those plants that are commonly used around the world as medicine. The objectives that guided the writing of this book were to create a reference for research scientists, phytochemists, toxicologists, physicians, pharmacists, and other health care providers; to integrate traditional and modern pharmacopoeias in order to develop a more efficient medicine; to build confidence and self-reliance in the use of medicinal plants; to revive an awareness of the importance of plants as sources of medicine; and to encourage their utilization and conservation.

Around the world, and even within countries, different names are used for the same plant, and different plants may be referred to by the same name. In an effort to familiarize readers with the International Code of Botanical Nomenclature system, the code's Latin binomial is used for each plant. The common names, together with the countries with which they are associated, are also listed. Color illustrations of the plants are provided to assist in their identification by those who are not familiar with the botanical name nor any of the common names. For the nonbotanist, the chapter on nomenclature and descriptive terminology, the botanical description, and the origin and distribution of each plant will be useful in the practical identification of the plants.

Since medical doctors are often reluctant to prescribe medicinal plants without supporting scientific data, the sections on pharmacological activities and clinical trials, as well as those on chemical constituents, constitute most useful references. These sections will also be of value to scientists with an interest in drug development. The section on traditional medicinal uses, listed by countries, will provide encouragement and build confidence and self-reliance in the traditional users of medicinal plants. Throughout, the book presents vital information that will find much use by students, practitioners, or researchers interested or engaged in the development, evaluation, or use of herbal medicines. The text presumes that the reader has had little to no experience or knowledge of medicinal plants. A bibliography of approximately 1600 references is presented for readers interested in more detailed information. It represents a diversity of disciplines that reflect the complexity of the field and the variety of interests in medicinal plants.

It is my hope that readers will find in *Medicinal Plants of the World* a wealth of practical ideas and theoretical information that will expose new horizons and little-known facts as well as their significant applications, thereby helping us become healthier people, better students, teachers, farmers, clinicians, researchers, and entrepreneurs.

Ivan A. Ross

Contents

List of Color Plates

Color plates appear as an insert following page 210.

1 | Nomenclature and Descriptive Terminology

For centuries, the only names of plants known by most lay people have been the common names. These common names are often simple, descriptive, and easy to pronounce and remember. These names may be words, phrases, and even sentences. Some favorites are *ram goat dash around* in Jamaica, and *piss a bed* in Guyana. However, there are disadvantages in using the common names, especially with intention of sharing information. Common names can be different from country to country, and even within a country. The same plant may be referred to by different names, and different plants may be referred to by the same name.

Common names are not decided upon by any logical system. Their origin can seldom be determined. During the First International Botanical Congress in Paris in 1867, the International Code of Botanical Nomenclature (ICBN) evolved. This system created a single valid universally recognized scientific name for each plant. Scientific names have thus facilitated the free transfer of ideas and information by botanists all over the world. The principle of this new system is that each plant be given a two element name or binomial. The two elements of the binomial that make up the scientific name are derived from the taxonomic hierarchy. The first element is called the genus and the second element is called the specific epithet; together, the genus and the specific epithet form the species name. The binomial, for accuracy, is followed by the abbreviation of the name of the person or persons who first applied that name to the plant. Most of the words that make up scientific names are derived from Latin or Greek, although there is no requirement that they must be. However, for technical purposes, the elements of the binomial are treated as Latin, no matter what their source. Most specific epithets indicate something characteristic about a species, such as growth pattern, habitat, season, shape of leaves, discoverer of the species, place of discovery, and type or color of flowers and fruit.

Our knowledge of the plants in our environment is far from complete. There are regions around the world, especially the tropical rain forest, where the plants have not been cataloged. This is a serious deficiency, considering the potential importance of the unknown species in terms of conservation, to establish natural preserves, and to locate and protect species that may provide germ plasm resources or that may possess medically useful chemical compounds. Without knowledge of the present botanical names of plants, it will be very diffi-

From: Medicinal Plants of the World By: Ivan A. Ross Humana Press Inc., Totowa, NJ

cult, if not impossible, to identify, classify, and assign new names to newly discovered species.

Because the identification and classification of plants is based somewhat on the details of their external features, a knowledge of the terminology of plant morphology is essential. Some commonly encountered terminology for descriptive plant taxonomy is illustrated in this chapter. Understanding these terms will help one to fully understand the botanical description of the plants.

Leaves are the most important plant organ in the identification and classification of a species. They are generally broad, flattened, and are borne at the nodes of a stem. Leaves are either simple—the blade is a single part—or compound—the blade is divided into smaller, blade-like parts (*see* Fig. 1). Just above the point of attachment of the leaf base or petiole, there is an axillary bud. A complete leaf is composed of the **blade**, the expanded flattened part; **petiole**, the supporting stalk, and **stipules**, appendages that, if present, may be leaf-like, scale-like, or tendrils. Any one of these parts of the leaf may be lacking or highly modified. The arrangement of the veins of the leaf blade is referred to as *venation*. The venation may be parallel or net. Net venation may be *palmate*, the main veins radiating from the point where they join the petiole, or *pinnate*, with one central vein or midrib that has lateral veins arising along its length and at angles from it. Leaves are generally arranged in one of three ways: *alternate*, having one leaf at each node, usually arranged in spirals around the stem; *opposite*, having leaves paired at each node on opposite sides of the stem; and ventricillate, or *whorled*, having three or more leaves at each node. The edge of a leaf is also referred to as the *margin*.

Some common types of leaves, stems, flowers, and fruits and shapes, characteristics, and arrangements are listed below:

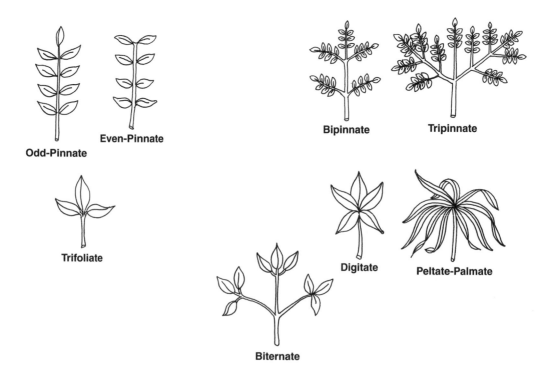

Odd-Pinnate   Even-Pinnate   Bipinnate   Tripinnate

Trifoliate   Biternate   Digitate   Peltate-Palmate

Fig. 1. Compound leaves.

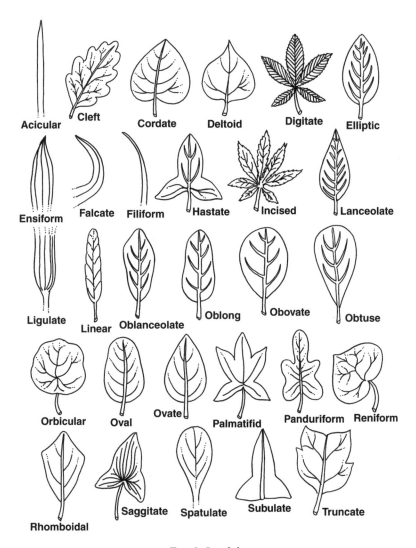

Fig. 2. Leaf shapes.

COMPOUND LEAVES *(Figure 1)*

Odd-pinnate　A pinnate leaf with a terminal leaflet, the number of leaflets being odd.
Even-pinnate　The condition in a compound leaf when an even number of leaflets is present, a terminal leaflet lacking.
Bipinnate　A leaf that is twice pinnately compound.
Tripinnate　Three times pinnately compound.
Trifoliate　Having three leaves.
Biternate　A ternate leaf in which the first order leaflets are themselves ternately compound.

Digitate　A compound leaf in which the leaflets arise from a single point at the end of the petiole; also referred to as *palmately compound*.
Peltate-Palmate　Attached to a supporting stalk at a point inside the margin, as in the petiole of a leaf of the stalk of certain cone scales.

LEAF SHAPES *(Figure 2)*

Acicular　Needle-like, round, or grooved in a cross-section.
Cordate　Heart-shaped.
Cuneate　Wedge-shaped, tapering toward the point of attachment.

Deltoid   Triangular.

Digitate   A compound leaf in which the leaflets arise from a single point at the end of the petiole; also referred to as *palmately compound*.

Elliptical   Having the shape of flattened circle, usually twice as long as broad.

Ensiform   Sword-shaped.

Falcate   Sickle-shaped.

Filiform   Thread-like.

Hastate   Arrowhead-shaped.

Incised   Cut deeply, sharply, and often irregularly into a leaf or petal margin.

Lanceolate   Lance-shaped, tapering from a broad base to the apex; much longer than wide.

Ligulate   Shaped like a strap or narrow band, as in a petal or the corolla.

Linear   Long and narrow with almost parallel sides.

Oblanceolate   Lanceolate, but with the broadest part near the apex.

Oblong   Much longer than broad, the sides being parallel.

Obovate   Ovate, but with the broadest part near the apex.

Obtuse   An apex formed by two lines which meet at more than a right angle.

Orbicular   Having a flat body with a circular outline.

Oval   Rounded at both ends, about twice as long as broad.

Ovate   Egg-shaped, with the broadest part toward the base.

Palmatifid   Lobed, cleft, parted, divided or compounded so that the sinuses or leaflets point to the apex of the petiole.

Panduriform   Fiddle-shaped.

Reniform   Kidney-shaped.

Rhomboidal   Parallelogram-shaped with opposing acute and obtuse angles.

Sagittate   Term describing basal lobes drawn into points on either side of the petiole.

Spatulate   Shaped like a spatula.

Subulate   Tapering from a broad base to a sharp point, awl shaped.

Truncate   A straight base or apex which appears to have been cut off.

LEAF MARGINS *(Figure 3)*

Ciliate   Having hairs on the margins.

Cleft   The condition in which the leaves are palmately or pinnately cut to about the midpoint.

Crenate   With low rounded or blunt teeth.

Crenulate   Having margins with very small rounded teeth; diminutive of *crenate*.

Dentate   Having sharp marginal teeth pointing outward.

Denticulate   Minutely toothed.

Entire   Smooth; devoid of any indentations, lobes, or teeth.

Incised   Cut deeply, sharply, and often irregularly into the leaf margin.

Lacerate   Torn or irregularly cleft.

Lobed   Divided into parts separated by rounded sinuses extending one-third to one-half the distance between the margin and the midrib.

Palmately Lobed   Like an open hand.

Parted   Cut or dissected almost to the midrib.

Pectinate   Parts are arranged like the teeth of a comb.

Pinnatisect   Cleft almost down to the midrib in a pinnate manner.

Serrate   Having marginal teeth pointing toward the apex.

Double-serrate   With small serration on larger serration.

Serrate   Minutely serrate.

Sinuate   Having a deeply wavy margin.

Spinose   With a spine at the top.

Undulate   Having a slightly wavy margin.

Bi-serrate   The condition in which serration are themselves serrate; also referred to as *doubly serrate*.

LEAF TIPS *(Figure 4)*

Acuminate   Tapering gradually to a prolonged point.

Acute   Ending in a point that is less than a right angle, but one that is not acuminate; distinct and sharp, but not drawn out.

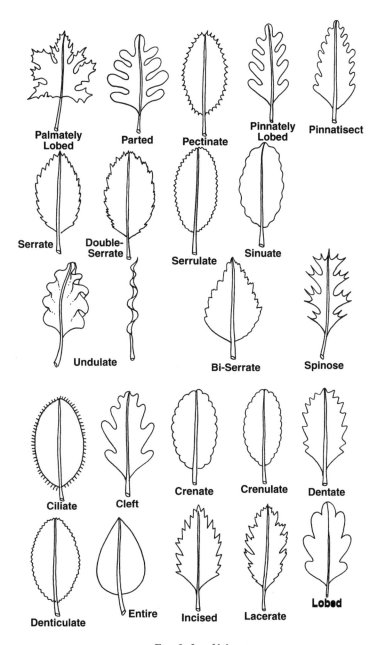

Fig. 3. Leaf Margins

Apiculate   A leaf apex which bears a short flexible point .

Aristate   With a bristle at the tip.

Caudate   Tailed.

Cirrhose   Tendril-like

Cleft   The condition in which the leaves are palmately or pinnately cut to about the midpoint.

Cuspidate   Tipped with a sharp and rigid point.

Emarginate   Callously notched and indented at the apex.

Mucronate   Abruptly tipped with a small point, projecting from the midrib.

Mucronulate   Having a sharp terminal point or spiny tip.

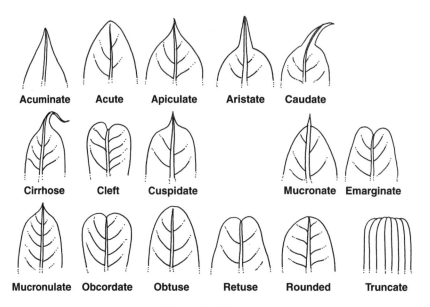

Fig. 4. Leaf tips.

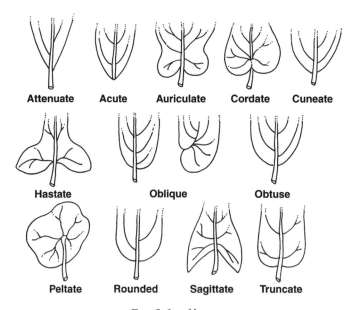

Fig. 5. Leaf bases.

Obcordate   The shape of an inverted heart.

Obtuse   An apex formed by two lines that meet at more than a right angle.

Retuse   With a shallow notch at a rounded apex.

Rounded   An apex that is gently curved.

Truncate   Cut squarely across at the apex.

LEAF BASES *(Figure 5)*

Attenuate   Characterized by a long gradual taper.

Acute   Ending in a point that is less than a right angle but one that is not acuminate; distinct and sharp, but not drawn out.

Auriculate   With ear-like appendages at the base.

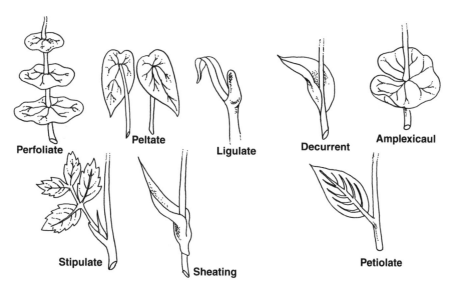

Fig. 6. Attachment to stem.

Cordate Heart-shaped, with a notch at the base.

Cuneate Wedge-shaped, gradually narrowed toward point of attachment.

Hastate Having the general shape of an arrowhead, but with the basal lobes turned outward at right angles.

Oblique Slanting or unequal-sided.

Obtuse With a blunt or rounded tip.

Peltate Attached to a supporting stalk at a point inside the margin.

Rounded With a broad arch.

Sagittate Basal lobes drawn into points on either side of the petiole.

Truncate Cut squarely across at the base.

ATTACHMENT TO STEM *(Figure 6)*

Amplexicaul Sessile with the base clasped around the stem.

Decurrent Leaf bases that extend downward and are adnate to a stem.

Ligulate Shaped like a strap or narrow band.

Peltate Attached to a supporting stalk at a point inside the margin.

Perfoliate The base surrounds the stem so that it appears that the stem penetrates the leaf.

Petiolate Having a petiole or leaf stalk.

Sessile Without a stalk; seated directly on the supporting structure.

Sheathing The enclosure of the stem by a sheath-like leaf

Stipulate Having stipules.

LEAF SURFACES

Papillate Having small pimple or nipple-like protuberances.

Pitted Having small cavities or depressions; also referred to as *punctate*.

Scurfy Covered with scales.

Uncinate Hooked.

Barbellate Hairs of barbs down the sides.

Glochidiate Having apical barbed hair or bristle.

Velutinous Velvety.

Tomentose With densely matted soft hairs; woolly in appearance.

Lanate Woolly, with long, intertwined, coiled hairs.

Floccose Covered with tufts of soft woolly hairs that are easily removed by rubbing.

Scabrous Rough to the tough.

Strigose Stiff hairs often appressed (i.e., pressed next to the stem) and pointing in one direction.

Glandular   Having glands or small secre-
tory structures.
Farinose   Covered with mealiness.
Hirsute   With long shaggy hairs, often stiff
or bristly to the touch
Hirtellous   Minutely hirsute.
Hispid   With stiff, rough hairs.
Echinate   With straight, often compara-
tively large, prick-like hairs.
Puberulent   Somewhat   or   minutely
pubescent.
Pubescent   Covered with short, soft hairs.
Pilose   With scattered long slender soft hairs.
Villous   Covered with long fine soft hairs.
Sericeous   With soft silky hairs, usually all
pointing in one direction.
Dolabriform   With forked hairs attached
at the middle.
Stellate   With star-shaped hairs.

   Flowers are highly modified shoots with
specialized appendages. Flowers may arise in
the axil of a leaf or, more often, in the axil of a
reduced leaf, which is called a bract. The
major components of the unmodified flower
are the **perianth, androecium,** and the **gynoecium.** The perianth is subdivided into the
calyx and the **corolla.** A group of **stamens,**
wherein the pollen is produced, is called the
androecium. The gynoecium consists of the
carpel, the innermost ovule-bearing part of
the flower. The arrangement of the flowers on
the plant is referred to as the inflorescence.
Some inflorescences are simple and readily
distinguishable, but others are complicated
and difficult to characterize. Some common
types of inflorescence are listed below.

TYPES OF INFLORESCENCE *(Figure 7)*
Solitary   With a single flower.
Axillary   Growing   out   of   the   angle
between the stem and the leaf stalk.
Terminal   Situated at the apex of a flowering stalk.
Axillary & Terminal   Growing out at the
axil, as in axillary and also at the apex of
the plant or the tip of the growing point.

Spike   An inflorescence with a single axis
and flowers without pedicels.
Spikelet   A small spike; the flowers inconspicuous and more or less hidden by bracts,
as in grasses and sedges.
Spadix   A thick or fleshy spike-like inflorescence with very small flowers that are massed
together and usually enclosed in a spathe.
Catkin   A soft spike or raceme of small
unisexual flowers, the inflorescence usually
falling as a unit.
Helicoid cyme   Formed like a spring or
snail shell.
Verticel   Flowers arranged in whorls at the
nodes.
Head   A dense cluster of stalkless flowers.
Raceme   An inflorescence with a single
axis and the flowers arranged along the
main axis on pedicels.
Umbel   An inflorescence of few to many
flowers on pedicels of approximately equal
length arising from the top of a peduncle.
Corymb   A broad inflorescence in which
the lower pedicels are successively elongate,
giving the inflorescence a flat-topped
appearance; indeterminate.
Dichasium   A terminal flower carried
between two roughly equally branches.
Panicle   A compound inflorescence in
which the main axis is branched one or
more times and may support spikes, racemes,
or corymbs.
Thyrse   A compound, compact panicle
with an indeterminate main axis and later-
ally determinate axes.
Compound umbel   A flower head in
which the flowers stems spring from a common point.
Raceme of umbels   An elongated inflorescence in which the umbels are inserted
along a rachis.
Corymbs of heads   A flat-topped flower
cluster in which the flower stalks emanate
from different parts of the main stem as different from **umbel** where they radiate from
a single point.

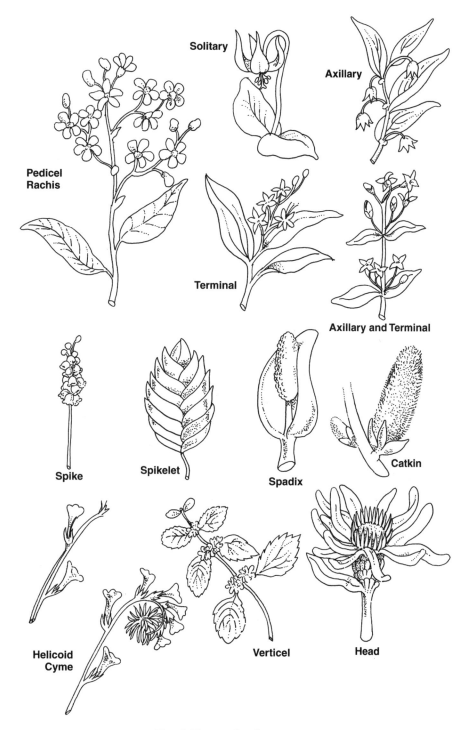

Fig. 7. Types of inflorescence.

Panicle of heads   A flower head with several branches, either opposite or alternate.

Panicle of spikelets   Panicle in which the branchlets terminate in spikelets rather than individual flowers, as in many grasses.

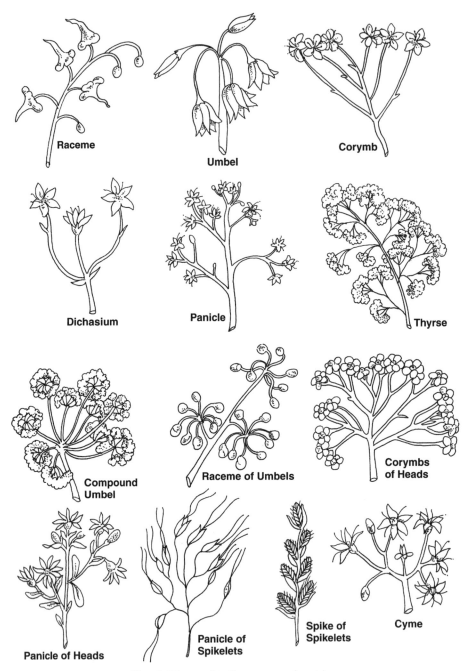

Fig. 7. Types of inflorescence (*con't*).

Spike of spikelets Spikelets are sessile along an unbranched rachis.

Cyme A broad more or less flat-topped inflorescence with the main axis terminating in a single flower that opens before the lateral flowers, determinate.

Fruits develop from ripened ovaries in the flower. Fruits may have other floral structures associated with them and normally contain seeds, which are ripened ovules. The seed germinates and produces a new plant. Many taxonomists restrict the use of the term

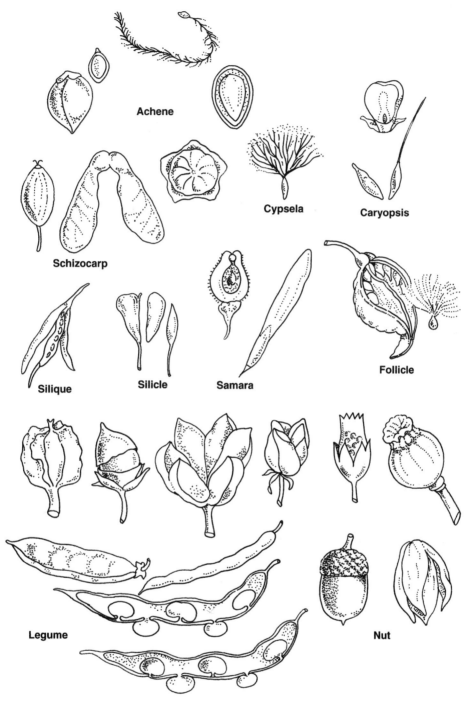

Fig. 8. Dry fruits.

"fruit" to the flowering plants and do not refer to the matured female reproductive structures in gymnosperms as fruits. The botanical definition is not very clear in common usage. Corn "seeds" is actually the fruit of this plant. Fruits such as squash, eggplant, and tomatoes are called vegetables. There are many kinds of fruits, some easy to classify,

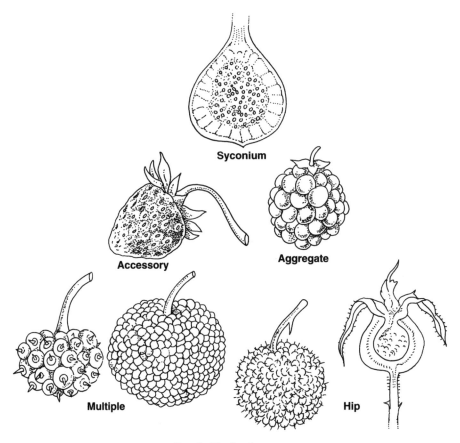

Fig. 9. Fleshy fruits.

and others more difficult. Two of the major groups of fruits are dry and fleshy. Some types of dry and fleshy fruits are listed below.

DRY FRUITS *(Figure 8)*

Achene   Seed and pericarp attached only at the funiculus, the seed usually tightly enclosed by the fruit wall, as in the sunflower.

Cypsela   An achene with an adnate calyx.

Casryopsis   Seed and pericarp completely fused, as in the grass family.

Schizocarp   The carpels separating from one another into one-seeded indehiscent segments.

Silique   The walls peeling away from a papery central partition.

Silicle   A silique that is not longer than it is wide.

Samara   A winged achene.

Follicle   A unicarpellate dehiscent dry fruit that opens along one suture.

Utricle   A small bladdery achene-like fruit with the seed loosely surrounded by the fruit wall, as in the pigweed.

Pyxis   Opening by a lid, as in the purslane.

Septicidal   A capsule that dehisces by means of openings along or within the septations.

Loculicidal   A capsule that dehisces by means of openings into locules, about midway between the partitions.

Denticidal   A capsule dehiscing by a series of teeth.

Poricidal   A capsule or anthler that opens by means of a pore or series of pores.

Legume   Unicarpellate, dehiscing along both sutures; the fruit type of the pea family.

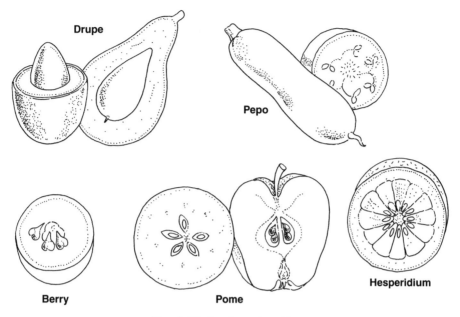

Fig. 9. Fleshy fruits *(con't)*.

Nut A dry hard indehiscent one-seeded fruit derived from a syncarpous gynoecium.

FLESHY FRUITS *(Figure 9)*

Drupe A fleshy indehiscent fruit, having its single seed enclosed in a stony endocarp.
Pepo A berry with a leathery rind; derived from an inferior ovary; use often restricted to the fruit of the Cucurbitaceae.
Berry A multiseeded indehiscent fruit in which the pericarp is fleshy throughout, as in the tomato.
Pome A fleshy indehiscent fruit derived from an inferior ovary surrounded by an adnate hypanthium, as in the apple.
Hesperidium A fleshy indehiscent fruit with conspicuous septations lined with succulent hairs; the fruit of the citrus group.

Accessory A false fruit, as in the strawberry, in which the bulk of the fleshy portion is derived from receptacle rather than gynoecium.
Aggregate A false fruit type in which the separate carpels of an apocarpous gynoecium collectively appear to form a fruit.
Syconium A vase-like structure with an opening at its apex and whose interior wall is lined with tiny flowers.
Multiple A type of false fruit in which several true fruits from separate flowers coalesce to produce a single structure that resembles a fruit, as in pineapple.
Hip Vase-like leathery hypanthium containing several seed-like achenes; the false fruit of the rose.

ABBREVIATIONS USED IN THE CHEMICAL CONSTITUENTS SECTION

Following the names of each chemical constituent is an abbreviation indicating the part of the plant in which the constituent is present; A number is then followed indicating the amount of that constituent present. This value is listed in either parts per million (ppm) or in percentage (%). Some of these values have a wide range; this is because the amount of the constituent is based on the dry weight as well the amount of moisture in the plant part in its natural state. The larger value is based on the dry weight and the smaller value on the natural moisture content of the part indicated. These values can also vary depending on such conditions as varieties, geographic location of production, method of production, maturity at harvesting, method of processing, and so forth.

Aer Aerial parts
An Anther
As Ash
Bd Bud
Bk Bark
Bu Bulb
Call Tiss Callus tissue
Cr Crown

Ct Coat
Cult Culture
Cx Calyx
Cy Cotyledon
Ct Coat
Em Embryo
EO Essential oil
Ep Epidermis
Fl Flower
Fr Fruit
Hu Hull
Gel Jell
Ju Juice
Lf Leaf
Lx Latex
Pe Peel
Pc Pericarp
Pl Plant
Pu Pulp
Pn Panicle
Pt Part
Pu Pulp
Rh Rhizome
Rt Root
Sd Seed
Sh Shoot
St Stem
Tr Trunk
Tu Tuber
Tw Twig

Ppm	% Conversion
10,000 ppm	1%
20,000 ppm	2%
30,000 ppm	3%
40,000 ppm	4%
50,000 ppm	5%
60,000 ppm	6%
70,000 ppm	7%
80,000 ppm	8%
90,000 ppm	9%
100,000 ppm	10%

2 | Abrus precatorius L.
Gaertn.

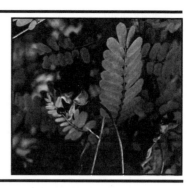

Common Names

Aainud-dik	India	Jequirity plant	Philippines
Aregllisse	West Indies	Jequirity	Taiwan
Benambo	Guinea-Bissau	Jequirity	India
Buck bean	Guyana	Jiquiriti	Brazil
Chanoti	Pakistan	Jumble bean	Virgin Islands
Chasm-I-kharosh	Pakistan	Jumble bean	Ivory Coast
Chirmu	Pakistan	Jumble bean	Virgin Islands
Chunhati	India	Kalyani	India
Crab's eye	Guam	Kikerewe	Tanzania
Crab's eye	India	Kolales halomtanto	Guam
Crab's eye	Nepal	Koonch	India
Crab's eye	USA	Krikpe	Ivory Coast
Crab's eye	Thailand	Kunni	India
Crab's stone	India	Laboma	Ivory Coast
Damabo	Ivory Coast	Latuwani	India
Gaungchi	India	Love bean	USA
Gchi	India	Lufyambo	East Africa
Ghongchi	India	Lyann legliz	Haiti
Ghumchi	India	Ma klam taanuu	Thailand
Ghun	India	Minimini	Mozambique
Goassien	Ivory Coast	Mishquina	Peru
Guinea pea	India	Miski miski	Peru
Gunch	India	Motipitipi	East Africa
Gunchi	Pakistan	Moudie-bi-titi	Ivory Coast
Gundumani	India	Mwanga-la-nyuki	East Africa
Gunja	India	Mwangaruchi	Tanzania
Guri-ginja	India	Namugolokoma	Mozambique
Gurivinda	India	Ndebie ni	Guinea
Gurje-tiga	India	Olho de pombo	Brazil
Habat al arus	Sudan	Olinda	India
Habat-elmlook	Sudan	Ombulu	East Africa
Indian licorice	India	Orututi	Tanzania
Indian licorice	Nigeria	Osito	East Africa
Jequiriti bean	Taiwan	Prayer bean	USA

From: Medicinal Plants of the World By: Ivan A. Ross Humana Press Inc., Totowa, NJ

Precatory bean	USA	Safed chirami	India
Rati gedi	Nepal	Saga	Indonesia
Rati	India	Saga saga	Philippines
Ratti	Pakistan	Sanga	Ivory Coast
Rosary bean	Pakistan	Sonkach	India
Rosary bean	USA	Sus	Egypt
Rosary pea	Egypt	Weglis	West Indies

BOTANICAL DESCRIPTION

A woody twinning plant of the LEGUMIN-OSAE family, with characteristic red and black seeds. The leaves are pinnate and glabrous, with many leaflets (12 or more) arranged in pairs. The leaflets are oblong, measuring 2.5-cm long and 1.5-cm wide. The plant bears orange-pink flowers, which occur as clusters in short racemes that are sometimes yellowish or reddish purple in color, small and typically pea-like. The plant produces short and stout brownish pods, which curl back on opening to reveal pendulous red and black seeds, four to six peas in a pod.

ORIGIN AND DISTRIBUTION

It grows wild in thickets, farms, and secondary clearings, and sometimes in hedges. It is most common in rather dry areas at low elevation throughout the tropics and subtropics.

TRADITIONAL MEDICINAL USES

Afghanistan. Dried seeds are taken orally as an aphrodisiac[K20642].

Brazil. Leaves and stem are said to be toxic when eaten by cattle[A05311]. Water extract of dried leaves and root is taken orally as a nerve tonic[K20642].

Cambodia. Hot water extract of seeds is taken orally for malaria[A06589].

Central Africa. Root is chewed as a snake bite remedy[A05825]. Seeds are taken orally by several Central African tribes for intestinal worms and as an oral contraceptive. The effect of a single dose (200 mg) is said to be effective for 13 menstrual cycles[A05825].

East Africa. Decoction of the aerial parts is taken orally for gonorrhea. A decoction of the plant plus three or four seed pods is taken. Fresh leaf juice is taken orally for gonorrhea, bilharziasis, stomach troubles, and as an antiemetic. Powdered leaves are applied to cuts and swellings. Decoction of leaves is taken orally for chest pains. For inflamed eyes, steam of boiling leaves is used. Water extract of dried seeds is applied to the eyes for purulent eye infections; the seeds are macerated in the water[T10828]. Fresh root is chewed as an aphrodisiac[A05825,A04594].

Egypt. Seeds are taken orally with honey as an aphrodisiac[T00687].

Guam. Seeds are reported to be toxic; half of one seed is reported as lethal. Seed coat must be broken to be toxic. Symptoms include acute gastroenteritis with vomiting, nausea, and diarrhea, followed by dehydration, convulsions, and death[A05675].

Guinea-Bissau. Leaf pulp is taken orally by men as an aphrodisiac and by women to facilitate childbirth. Seeds taken orally are considered an aphrodisiac and abortive[A00455].

Haiti. Decoction of leaves is taken orally for coughs and flu[T13846].

India. Hot water extract of dried leaves and roots are applied to the eye for eye diseases[T10064]. Hot water extract of root is taken orally as an emmenagogue[A00468]. Root brew is taken orally to produce abortion[A04300,A06589]. Hot water extract of seeds is taken orally as an antifertility agent[A00468], as an abortifacient[A04132], and to prevent conception[A04300]. Seeds are used as a poultice in the vagina in Ayurvedic and Unani medicine as an abortifacient. Seeds boiled in milk and drunk by males is used in Unani and Ayurvedic medicine as an aphrodisiac. It is claimed that the boiling destroys the toxic action of Abrin[A06589]. As birth control, one seed completely covered with Jaggary is swallowed during the menstrual period and is sufficient to prevent conception for one year[T16478]. Decoction of dried seeds is taken orally to induce abortion[K16006]. Hot water extract of dried seeds is taken orally as a sexual stimulant in the Unani system of medicine[T01655]. It is also taken for tuberculosis, painful swellings[T09394], and can also be used as an aphrodisiac and purgative[W03487]. Dried seed oil is taken orally as an abortifacient[W04510]. Plant juice is administered intravaginally to induce abortion[W00002].

Ivory Coast. Water extract of leaves and stem is taken orally by males as an aphrodisiac and by females to facilitate childbirth[A04941].

Jamaica. Decoction of dried leaves and root boiled in milk is used as a tonic[K20642].

Kenya. Fresh leaf juice is taken orally for coughs. Fresh leaves are taken orally for coughs[M25859].

Mozambique. Hot water extract of root is administered orally as an aphrodisiac[L01568].

Nepal. Seeds are taken orally as an aphrodisiac[A00020].

Nigeria. Hot water extract of fresh root is administered orally as an antimalarial and anticonvulsant[T06510].

Pakistan. Hot water extract of seeds is administered orally as an aphrodisiac. Seeds are used as a suppository for inducing abortion[A04580].

Sudan. Hot water extract of the plant is taken orally as an antifertility agent[T05013].

Taiwan. Decoction of dried root is taken orally to treat bronchitis and hepatitis[H16454].

Tanzania. Decoction of roots and leaf sap is taken orally for asthma and is also used as an aphrodisiac[T10828].

Thailand. Leaves crushed with oil is used as a poultice as an anti-inflammatory[T16711].

Virgin Islands. Extract of seeds is taken orally for coughs[W00903].

West Africa. Decoction of dried roots is taken orally as an antiemetic, for bilharziasis, tapeworms, gonorrhea, chest pains and is also used as an aphrodisiac. For snake bites, roots are chewed[T10828].

West Indies. Seeds are taken orally as an emetic, purgative, and anthelmintic[T00701].

CHEMICAL CONSTITUENTS
(ppm unless otherwise indicated)

(+)-Abrine, Pl
Abraline, Sd
Abrasine, Rt
Abrectorin, Sd
Abridin, Sd
Abrin, Sd
Abrisin, Pl
Abrulin, Sd
Abruquinone, Rt
Abrus agglutinin, Kr
Abrusgenic acid, Pl
Abrusgenic acid methyl ester, Pl
Abrusin, Sd
Abrusin-2'-0-apioside, Sd
Abruslactone, Rt; St;
Abrusoside, Lf 0.03%
Abrussic acid, Pl
Alanine, Sd
Alpha amyrin, Sd
Anthocyanins, Sd
Arabinose, St
Arachidic acid, Sd Ol
Arachidyl alcohol, Sd
Ash, Lf 1.7–8.1%
Behenic acid, Sd
Beta amyrin, Sd
Beta sitosterol, Sd
Brassicasterol, Sd
Calcium, Lf 1,266-2,660
Callistephin, Sd Ct
Campesterol, Sd
Carbohydrates, Lf 13.7-65.2%
Cholesterol, Sd
Choline, Sd
Chrysanthemin, Sd Ct
Cycloartenol, Sd
Cysteine, Sd
Cystine, Sd
Decan-1-ol, Sd
Delphin, Sd Ct
Delphinidin glycoside, Sd

Delphinidin, Pl
Docos-13-enoic acid, Sd
Docosadienoic acid, Sd Ol
Docosan-1-0l, Sd
Docosatetraenoic acid, Sd Ol
Docosatrienoic acid, Sd Ol
Docosenoic acid, Sd Ol
Dodecan-1-0l, Sd
Eicos-11-enoic acid, Sd
Eicosadienoic acid, Sd Ol
Eicosanoic acid, Sd Ol
Eicosatrienoic acid, Sd Ol
Elaidic alcohol, Sd
Fat, Sd 2.8%
Fiber, Lf 3.7–17.6%
Flucuronic acid, Sd
Galactose, St
Galacturonic acid, Sd
Gallic acid, Sd
Glutamic acid, Sd
Glutamine, Sd
Glycine, Sd
Glycyrrhizin, Lf 10%
Glycyrrhizin, Rt 1.25%
Hederagenin, Sd
Hemiphloin, Lf
Heneicosan-1-ol, Sd
Heneicosane,7,9,15-trimethyl, Sd
Heptacosan-1-ol, Sd
Heptadecan-1-ol, Sd
Hexacosan-1-ol, Sd
Hexadec-9-enoic acid, Sd
Hexadecan-1-ol, Sd
Hexadecenoic acid, Sd Ol
Hypahorine, Sd; Lf; Rt; St
Hypaphorine, Sd
Iso orientin, Sd
Iso leucine, Sd
Kaikassaponin III, Sd
Kilocalories, Lf 620-2,950
Lauric acid, Sd Ol
Lectin, Sd
Leucine, Sd
Lignoceric acid, Sd Ol
Linoleic acid, Sd Ol
Linolenic acid, Sd Ol
Luteolin, Sd
Lysine, Sd
Montanyl alcohol, Lf
Myricyl alcohol, Lf
Myristic acid, Sd Ol
N,N-Dimethyl tryptophan, Sd

N,N-Dimethyl-tryptophan-methocation
   methyl ester, Sd
N-Docosane, Sd
N-Dotriacontane, Sd
N-Eicosane, Sd
N-Heneicosane, Sd
N-Hentriacontane, Sd
N-Heptacosane, Sd
N-Heptadecane, Sd
N-Hexacosane, Sd
N-Hexadecane, Sd
N-Nonacosane, Sd
N-Nonadecane, Sd
N-Octacosane, Sd
N-Octadecane, Sd
N-Pentacosane, Sd
N-Pentatriacontane, Sd
N-Tetracosane, Sd
N-Tetratriacontane, Sd
N-Triacontane, Sd
N-Tricosane, Sd
N-Tritriacontane, Sd
Nonadecan-1-ol, Sd
Octacosan-1-ol, Sd
Octadeca-9,12-dienoic acid, Sd
Octadecadienoic acid, Sd Ol
Octadecatrienoic acid, Sd Ol
Octanoic acid, Sd
Oleic acid, Sd Ol
Orientin, Sd
P-Coumaroyl/galloyl glucodelphinidin, Pl
P-Sterone, Sd
Palmitic acid, Sd Ol
Pectin, Sd
Pelargonidin-3,5-diglucoside, Sd Ct
Pentacosan-1-ol, Sd
Pentacosanoic acid, Sd
Pentadecan-1-ol, Sd
Pentadecanoic acid, Sd Ol
Pentosans, Sd 9.2%
Phenylalanine, Sd
Phosphorus, Lf 650-3,095
Picatorine, Sd
Polygalacturonic acid, Sd
Polysaccharide, Rt
Precasine, Rt; Sd
Precatorine, Sd; Rt; Lf; St
Proline, Sd
Protein, Lf 5.6–26.7%
Protein, Sd 19.4%
Rhamnose, Sd
Serine, Sd

Sophoradiol, Sd
Sophoradiol-22-0-acetate, Sd
Squalene, Sd
Stearic acid, Sd
Stigamsterol, Sd
Tetracos-15-enoic acid, Sd
Tetracosan-1-ol, Sd
Tetradecan-1-ol, Sd
Tetradecanoic acid, Sd
Triacosan-1-ol, Sd
Tridecan-1-ol, Sd
Trigonelline, Sd; Lf; St; Rt
Tritriacontan-1-ol, Sd
Tyrosine, Sd
Undecan-1-ol, Sd
Ursolic acid, Sd
Valine, Sd
Water, Lf 79%
Xylose, St; Rt; Sd; Lf

PHARMACOLOGICAL ACTIVITIES AND CLINICAL TRIALS

Abortifacient effect. Chloroform/methanol extract of seeds, administered subcutaneously to rats at a dose of 50.0 mg/animal was inactive. Water extract of dried seeds, administered intragastrically to pregnant rats at a dose of 125.0 mg/kg was active[T16714]. Ethanol (95%) extract of seeds, when administered orally at a dose of 200.0 mg/kg was inactive on pregnant hamsters and active on pregnant rats[X00012]. Petroleum ether extract of seeds that was administered orally to rats was inactive[W01362].

Agglutinin activity. Water extract of fresh seeds in cell culture at a concentration of 2.0 microliters/ml was active on human lymphocytes[W04573].

Alkaline phosphatase inhibition. Petroleum ether extract of seed oil, administered orally, was active on the uterus of rats[T13678].

Analgesic activity. Ethanol/water (1:1) extract of the aerial parts, administered intraperitoneally to mice at a dose of 500.0 mg/kg was inactive vs tail pressure method[W00374].

Anthelmintic activity. Water extract of dried seeds produced weak activity on *Caenorhabditis elegans*. LC$_{50}$ 15.8 mg/ml[K21233].

Antibacterial activity. Ethanol/water (1:1) extract of the aerial parts at a concentration of 25.0 mcg/ml on agar plate was inactive on *Bacillus subtilis*, *Escherichia coli*, *Salmonella typhosa*, *Staphylococcus aureus* and *Agrobacterium tumefaciens*[W00374]. Ether extract of seeds on agar plate was active on *Staphylococcus aureus*. The ethanol (95%) extract was active on *Escherichia coli*, *Staphylococcus aureus*[A04908].

Anticonvulsant activity. Ethanol (70%) extract of fresh root, administered intraperitoneally to mice of both sexes at variable dosage levels was active vs metrazole-induced convulsions and inactive vs strychnine-induced convulsions[T06510]. Ethanol/water (1:1) extract of the aerial parts, administered to mice intraperitoneally at a dose of 500.0 mg/kg was inactive vs electroshock-induced convulsions[W00374].

Antidiarrheal activity. Chromatographic fraction of dried seeds, administered intragastrically to rats at a dose of 10.0 mg/kg was active vs castor oil-induced diarrhea[M29993].

Antiestrogenic effect. Ethanol (95%) extract of root, administered orally to mice at a dose of 10.0 mg/kg was active[A04238].

Antifertility effect. Chloroform/methanol extract of seeds, administered subcutaneously to female rats at a dose of 50.0 mg/animal was active[M31067]. Ethanol (80%) extract of seeds, administered orally and subcutaneously to female rats at a dose of 1.0 mg/animal was inactive[J05633]. Ethanol (95%) and water extracts of seeds administered orally to mice were inactive, petroleum ether extract was active[A02435]. Ethanol (95%), water and petroleum ether extracts of leaves administered orally to female mice were inactive[A02435]. Ethanol extract of seeds, administered intragastrically to male rats at a dose of 100.0 mg/kg for 60 days was active. There was a significant decrease in the number of pregnant females[M17846]. Ethanol/water (1:1) extract of dried seeds, administered by gastric intubation to male rats at a dose of 250.0 mg/kg was active. No pregnancies were reported for the 20 females paired with 10 males treated for 60 days; mating probably occurred in all cases, but this is not entirely clear. Pregnancies were again reported after withdrawal of treatment[T15892]. Hot water extract of dried plant, administered orally to human females at a dose of 0.28 gm/person was active. The extract was administered as a mixture of *Embelia ribes* (fruit), *Piper longum* (fruit), *Ferula assafoetida*, *Piper betele*, *Polianthes tuberosa* and *Abrus precatorius*. One dose was taken, starting from the second day of menstruation, twice daily for 20 days. Sexual intercourse was avoided during the dosing period. The treatment is claimed effective for four months. Biological activity has been patented[T02114]. Seed oil administered orally to female mice at a dose of 25.0 mg/animal, and to female mice and to rats at a dose 150.0 mg/animal were active. No control animal was used[A04238].

Antifungal activity. Ethanol/water (1:1) extract of the aerial parts at a concentration of 25.0 mcg/ml on agar plate was inactive on *Microsporum canis*, *Trichophyton mentagrophytes*, and *Aspergillus niger*[W00374].

Antigonadotropin effect. Ethanol (95%) extract of dried seeds, administered by gastric intubation to mice at a dose of 150.0 mg/kg, was active[T11438].

Anti-implantation effect. Chloroform/methanol (2:1) extract of seeds, administered subcutaneously to pregnant rats at a dose of 50.0 mg/animal was active[M31067]. Ethanol (95%) extract of root, administered orally to rats at a dose of 100.0 mg/kg was active[A04238]. Ethanol (95%) extract of seeds, administered orally to rats and hamsters at a dose of 200.0 mg/kg was inactive[X00012]. Water extract of seeds administered orally to rats was inactive, the petroleum ether extract was active[A02435]. Ethanol (95%), water and petroleum ether extracts of leaves administered orally to female rats were inactive[A02435].

Anti-inflammatory activity. Ethanol/water (1:1) extract of the aerial parts, administered orally to rats at a dose of 500.0 mg/kg was inactive vs carrageenin-induced pedal edema. Animals were dosed one hour before carrageenin injections[W00374].

Antispasmodic activity. Chromatographic fraction (a gel filtration fraction from a methanol-water (1:1) extract) of seeds, at a concentration of 0.2 mg/ml was active on the uterus of rats vs PGE-2-, ACh-, oxytocin- and epinephrine-induced contractions[T05949]. Ethanol (95%) extract of dried leaves at a concentration of 1.0 mg/ml was active on the phrenic nerve-diaphragm of rats vs nerve stimulation. The inhibition was potentiated by D-tubocurarine but reversed by physostigine. Results significant at $P < 0.001$ level. At a concentration of 4.0 mg/ml, the extract was also active vs direct muscle stimulation. At 1.0 mg/ml, it was active on toad rectus abdominus muscle vs ACh-induced contractions. Water and hot water extracts of dried leaves at concentrations of 6.72 mg/ml were inactive on phrenic nerve-diaphragm of rats vs nerve stimulation and direct muscle stimulation. At concentrations of 16.8 and 16.72 mg/ml, respectively, the extracts were inactive on toad rectus abdominus muscle vs ACh-induced contractions. Petroleum ether extract at concentrations of 19.2 and 48.0 mg/ml were inactive on rat phrenic nerve-diaphragm vs nerve stimulation and direct muscle stimulation and on toad rectus abdominus muscle vs ACh-induced contractions, respectively[T08109]. Ethanol/water (1:1) extract of the aerial parts was inactive on guinea pig ileum vs ACh- and histamine-induced spasms[W00374].

Antispermatogenic effect. Ethanol extract of seeds, administered intragastrically to male rats at a dose of 100.0 mg/kg for 60 days was inactive[M17846]. Ethanol/water (1:1) extract of dried seeds, administered by gastric intubation to rats at a dose of 250.0 mg/kg, was active. Although no significant histologic changes in the testes were reported, sperm concentration was reported to be significantly decreased in both cauda epididymis and testes after dosing for 60 days[T15892]. Sterol fraction of dried seeds administered intramuscularly to rats was active. Testicular lesions marked by the cessation of spermatogenesis and a significant reduction in the diameter of the seminiferous tubules were also noted[T03740].

Antitumor activity. Ethanol (95%) extract of dried leaves, administered intraperitoneally to mice at dose of 100.0 mg/kg was inactive on Sarcoma 180 (ASC)[M23643]. Water extract of seeds, administered intraperitoneally to mice at a dose of 5.0 mcg/kg was active on Sarcoma (Yoshida solid and ASC). A dose of 20.0 mcg/kg administered subcutaneously was inactive on Sarcoma (Yoshida ASC)[A03687]. Protein fraction of seeds administered intraperitoneally to rats was active on Sarcoma (Yoshida ASC)[A04246].

Antiviral activity. Ethanol/water (1:1) extract of the aerial parts at a concentration of 50.0 mcg/ml in cell culture was inactive on Ranikhet virus and Vaccinia virus[W00374]. Water and methanol extracts of dried seeds in cell culture were inactive on virus-HLTV-1. IC_{100} > 77.0 and > 40.0 mcg/ml, respectively, were observed. Activity was not observed below the cytotoxic doses[K21579].

Antiyeast activity. Dried seeds at a concentration of 1.0% on agar plate was active on *Cryptococcus neoformans*[W03711]. Ethanol/water (1:1) extract of the aerial parts at a concentration of 25.0 mcg/ml on agar plate was inactive on *Candida albicans* and *Crytococcus neoformans*[W00374].

CNS depressant activity. Ethanol (70%) extract of fresh root, administered intraperitoneally to mice of both sexes at variable dosage levels, was active[T06510].

Contraceptive and/or interceptive effect. Petroleum ether extract of seed oil, administered orally to rats was active[T13678].

Cytotoxic activity. Ethanol (95%) extract of dried stem in cell culture was inactive on CA-9KB. ED_{50} > 30.0 mcg/ml[T05943]. Water and methanol extracts of dried seeds in cell culture produced weak activity on cells MT-4. IC_{100} > 77.0, and >40.0 mcg/ml, respectively[K21579]. Water extract of seeds in cell culture produced strong activity on Sarcoma Yoshida ASC. ED_{50} 0.004 mcg/ml[A04780]. Water extract of seeds in cell culture was active on CA-9KB. ED_{50} < 20.0 mcg/ml[X00001]. Water extract of seeds was active on the testes of *Poecilocera picta*[A05153].

Death. Hot water extract of dried leaves, administered intravenously to chicken, was active at a dose of 20.0 mg/kg and caused spastic paralysis and death within 24 hours[T08109]. Seeds taken orally by male human adults were active. Twenty beans mixed with water in a blender and drunk produced death in two days. Symptoms included vomiting of blood, pain in eyes, and burning ears[A05858].

Diuretic activity. Ethanol/water (1:1) extract of the aerial parts, administered intraperitoneally to male rats at a dose of 250.0 mg/kg was inactive. Saline-loaded animals were used. Urine was collected for four hours postdrug[W00374].

Embryotoxic effect. Ethanol (95%) extract of seeds, administered orally to pregnant hamsters and rats at doses of 200.0 mg/kg was inactive[X00012]. Petroleum ether extract administered orally to rats at a dose of 150.0 mg/kg was inactive[W01362]. Water extract of dried seeds, administered intragastrically to pregnant rats at a dose of 125.0 mg/kg was inactive[K16006].

Estrous cycle disruption effect. Seeds administered orally to female rats at doses of 0.05, 0.5, and 5.0 mg/animal were inactive[L00302]. Chloroform/methanol (2:1) extract of seeds, administered subcutaneously to rats at a dose of 1.0 mg/animal, was active[J05633]. Seeds administered by gastric intubation to rats at doses of 10.0, 5.0, and 2.0 gm/kg were active; 80, 50, and 25%, respectively, of the rats depicted extensive leukocytic smears, but with no significant effect on uterine weight[T03902].

Hemagglutinin activity. Water extract of seeds was active on the red blood cells of ant (leafcutter), buffalo, cat, chicken, dog, duckling, guinea pig, horse, human adult (blood groups A, B, and O), lamb, mice, pigeon, rabbit, rat, and ox; weakly active on cow and ewe; and inactive on that of goat[A04910,A04913].

Hypoglycemic activity. Ethanol/water (1:1) extract of the aerial parts, administered orally to rats at a dose of 250.0 mg/kg was inactive. Less than a 30% drop in blood sugar level was observed[W00374].

Hypothermic activity. Ethanol/water (1:1) extract of the aerial parts, administered intraperitoneally to mice at a dose of 500.0 mg/kg, was inactive[W00374].

Inotropic effect positive. Hot water extract of dried entire plant at a concentration of 320.0 microliters was inactive on guinea pig atria[M29843].

Insect sterility induction. Petroleum ether extract of dried seeds applied externally at a concentration of 1.0 microliter was active on *Dysdercus cingulatus*. The extract was active in males alone. The saline extract produced weak activity in both males and females[M20390].

Insecticide activity. Acetone extract of dried root was inactive on *Culex quinquefasciatus*[A14266]. Acetone extract of dried stem at low concentration was inactive on *Culex quinquefasciatus*[A14266]. Seed at a concentration of 10.0% showed weak activity on *Musca domestica*. Less active than 0.25% DDT[A04839].

Intestinal fluid retention effect. Chromatographic fraction of dried seeds, administered intragastrically to rats at a dose of 10.0 mg/kg was active on the small intestine vs PGE_2-induced enteropooling. Effect assayed 30 minutes after oral dose of PGE_2[M29993].

Intestinal motility inhibition. Chromatographic fraction of dried seeds, administered intragastrically to rats at a dose of 10.0 mg/kg was active. Effect was not as great as that of an equal amount of atropine[M29993].

Luteal suppressant effect. Chloroform/methanol (2:1) extract of seeds, administered subcutaneously to rats at a dose of 50.0 mg/animal was active[M31067].

Mitogenic activity. Water extract of fresh seeds in cell culture at a concentration of 2.0 microliters/ml was inactive on human lymphocytes[W04573].

Mutagenic activity. Methanol (75%) extract of dried leaves at a concentration of 10.0 mg/ml on agar plate was inactive on *Salmonella typhimurium* TM677[M21299].

Neuromuscular blocking activity. Ethanol (95%) extract of dried leaves at a concentration of 0.5 mcg/ml was active on phrenic nerve-diaphragm[T08109].

Protease (HIV) inhibition. Water and methanol extracts of dried seeds were inactive. $IC_{50} > 500$ mcg/ml[K08273].

Reverse transcriptase inhibition. Water and methanol extracts of commercial sample of seeds in cell culture were inactive on virusavian myeloblastosis. $IC_{50} > 1000$ mg/ml[K08721].

Semen coagulation. Ethanol/water (1:1) extract of the aerial parts at a concentration of 2.0% was inactive on rat semen[W00374].

Smooth muscle stimulant activity. Chromatographic fraction (gel filtration 4–9 of a methanol-water (1:1) extract of seeds, at a concentration of 0.2 mg/ml was active on guinea pig ileum; a concentration of 0.5 mg/ml was active on the stomach of rats[T05949]. Seed oil at a concentration of 1.8 mcg/ml was active on the ileum of guinea pigs[T16531].

Spermicidal effect. Ethanol extract of seeds, administered intragastrically to male rats at a dose of 100.0 mg/kg for 60 days was active. Impaired sperm motility and structural abnormalities of sperm were observed. Sperm ATPase level was decreased[M17846]. Ethanol/water (1:1) extract of dried seeds was active on the sperm of rats. There was a decrease in motility when sperm were mixed with the extract. When administered by gastric intubation at a dose of 250.0 mg/kg, there was a large decrease in motility of sperm from the cauda epididymis of the rats given the extract for 60 days[T15892]. Ethanol/water (1:1) extract of the aerial parts at a concentration of 2.0% was inactive on the sperm of rats[W00374]. Methanol extract of dried seeds was active on the sperm of human adults. IC_{50} 2.29 mg/ml[T16555].

Taste aversion. Butanol extract at a concentration of 10.0 mg/ml, Ethanol (80%) extract at a concentration of 2.0 mg/ml, and water extract at a concentration of 10.0 mg/ml of dried leaves in the drinking water of gerbils were active. The ether and petroleum ether extracts at concentrations of 5.0 mg/ml were inactive[M23039].

Teratogenic activity. Water extract of dried seeds, administered intragastrically to pregnant rats at a dose of 125.0 mg/kg, was active[K16006,T16714].

Toxic effect (general). Seeds administered orally to horses at a dose of 15.0 gms was active. Tolerance developed when small, incrementally increased doses were given[A03648]. Seeds at a concentration of 0.5% of diet in chicken was active. Chicken were fed a mixture of *Abrus precatorius* seeds and *Cassia senna* fruit. Toxicity included catarrhal enteritis, hepatocellular necrosis, reduced weight, and anemia[K10577]. Ethanol (95%) extract of seeds, administered subcutaneously to male mice at a dose of 500.0 mg/kg, was active. One hundred percent mortality was observed within 48–49 hours[A04608]. Seeds administered orally to human adults were active. Severe gastroenteritis, multiple serosal hemorrhages, swelling and inflammation of the Peyer's patches, swelling and inflammation of retroperitoneal lymph nodes, focal necrosis in the liver and kidneys, retinal hemorrhages early in course of intoxication, nausea, vomiting, diarrhea, dehydration, convulsions, and collapse are possible symptoms. Symptoms may begin after delay of up to several days and may persist for as long as 10–11 days. Death in children has been reported from eating one or more seeds[A04250]. Two children who chewed seeds became

irrational, had tetany, flushing of skin, widely dilated pupils, and appeared to hallucinate. Treatment with neostigmine and barbiturates was successful[A05657]. Seeds, administered subcutaneously to male mice at a dose of 0.90 gm/kg, were active. Forty-four deaths were observed in 5–21 hours[A04608]. Seeds administered orally to cows at a dose of 0.09 gm/kg were active. One in 44 deaths was observed. Methanol (75%) extract of dried leaves administered intragastrically to mice at a dose of 2.0 gm/kg was inactive[M21299]. Leaf and stem administered to cows orally at a dose of 15.4 gm/kg was inactive[A05311]. Seeds in the ration of livestock was active. Nitrate poisoning was observed[K13618].

Toxicity assessment. Ethanol/water (1:1) extract of the aerial parts administered intraperitoneally to mice produced LD_{50} > 1.0 gm/kg[W00374]. Ethanol (95%) of dried leaves, administered intravenously to chicken produced LD_{50} 12 mg/kg[T08109]. Water extract of seeds, administered subcutaneously to female guinea pigs produced LD_{50} at <0.40 mg/kg[A04608]. When administered orally to guinea pigs, mice, rabbits, and rats LD_{50} 0.299 gm/kg, 6.638 gm/kg, 48.7 mg/kg and 2.711 gm/kg, respectively, were observed[A04245]. Toxicity of *Abrus* to goats has been evaluated. Doses of 2, 1, or 0.5 gm/kg/day by stomach tube caused death between days 2 and 5 for those given 2 or 1 gm/kg, and one goat that received 0.5 gm died on day 32, and the other was killed on day 33. The main signs of poisoning include inappetence, bloody diarrhea, dyspnea, dehydration, loss of condition, and recumbency.

Toxicity. Fatal incidents have been reported following ingestion of well-chewed seeds of *Abrus precatorius*. Because of its hard seed coat, it can pass through the gastrointestinal tract undigested and remain harmless. The unripe seed has a soft and easily broken seed coat and is thus more dangerous. It has been reported that poisoning has been experienced through a finger prick when stringing the seed. Symptoms may develop after a few hours to several days after ingestion. They include severe gastroenteritis with pronounced nausea and vomiting. Mydriasis will occur as well, as muscular weakness, tachycardia, cold sweat, and trembling. There is no known physiological antidote. The treatment is essentially symptomatic. Since there is a long latent period associated with abrin poisoning, little value can be placed on induction of emesis or gastric lavage; these measures are useful only if ingestion has just occurred. Bismuth trisilicate may be given during poisoning by *Abrus precatorius* to reduce the degree of gastrointestinal damage. If the emesis and/or diarrhea become excessive, replacement fluids and electrolytes are advocated. If hemorrhage occurs, blood transfusion may be necessary.

Uterine relaxation effect. Chromatographic fraction (a gel filtration fraction from a methanol/water [1:1] fraction) of seeds at a concentration of 1.1 mg/ml was active on the uterus of rats[T05949].

Uterine stimulant effect. Chromatographic fraction (gel filtration fractions 4–9 of a methanol/water [1:1] extract) of seeds at a concentration of 0.2 mg/ml was active on the uteri of pregnant and nonpregnant rats[T05949]. Ethanol (95%) extract of dried seed oil, administered intravenously to guinea pigs at a dose of 1000 mcg/ml produced weak activity[W04510]. Seed oil at a concentration of 3.6 mg was active on the uteri of guinea pigs and rats. The action was blocked by indomethacin but not by atropine[T16531]. Water extract of seeds was active on the uterus of guinea pig[A04132].

3 | Allium sativum L.

Gaertn.

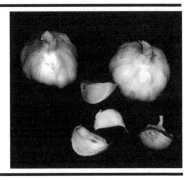

Common Names

Aglio	Italy	Kra thiam	Thailand
Aie	France	L'ail	West Indies
Ail	France	Lahsun	Fiji
Ail	Rodrigues Islands	Lahsun	India
Ail	Tunisia	Lai	Nicaragua
Ajo	Guatemala	Lai	West Indies
Ajo	Nicaragua	Lasan	Fiji
Ajo	Peru	Lasan	India
Akashneem	India	Lashun	India
Alubosa elewe	Nigeria	Lasun	Fiji
Banlasun	Nepal	Lasun	Nepal
Cebilhoums	France	Lasuna	India
Dasuan	China	Lay	Haiti
Dra thiam	Thailand	Lesun	Fiji
Garlic	Guyana	Majo	Mexico
Garlic	Brazil	Onion	India
Garlic	China	Poor man's treacle	Iran
Garlic	Cuba	Rashun	India
Garlic	Europe	Rason	India
Garlic	India	Sarimsak	Turkey
Garlic	Indonesia	Sarmisak	Turkey
Garlic	Iran	Seer	Iran
Garlic	Japan	Ta-suan	China
Garlic	Kuwait	Tellagaddalu	India
Garlic	Libya	Thom	Oman
Garlic	Mexico	Thoum	Jordan
Garlic	Nicaragua	Thum	Arabic countries
Garlic	Poland	Thum	Saudi Arabia
Garlic	Taiwan	Tum	Tunisia
Garlic	USA	Tuma	Morocco
Garlic	West Indies	Vellulli	India
Garlic clove	Nicaragua		

From: Medicinal Plants of the World *By: Ivan A. Ross Humana Press Inc., Totowa, NJ*

BOTANICAL DESCRIPTION

Garlic is an erect herb of the ALLIACEAE family, 30- to 60-cm tall. Bulb is on a disk-like stem, consisting of several segents (cloves), enclosed in a common membrane that is at the base of foliage leaves. Each clove consists of a protective cylindrical sheath and a small central bud. Leaf-blade is linear, flat, and solid, 1- to 2.5-cm wide, and 30- to 60-cm long, having an acute apex. Leaf sheaths form a pseudostem. Inflorescence are umbellate, having smooth scape, round, solid coiled at first; subtended by membranous, long-beaked spathe, splitting on one side and remaining attached to umbel. Small bulbils are produced in inflorescence; flowers are variable in number, and sometimes absent; they seldom open and may wither in bud. Flowers are on slender pedicels, consisting of perianth of six segents, about 4- to 6-mm long, pinkish; stamens: six, anthers exerted; ovary superior, trilocular. Fruit is a small loculicidal capsule. Seeds are seldom—if ever—produced.

ORIGIN AND DISTRIBUTION

Garlic is indigenous to Asia. It is now found worldwide as a cultivated crop, which is usually grown at high altitudes.

TRADITIONAL MEDICINAL USES

Arabic countries. Butanol extract of dried bulbs is inhaled in Unani medicine by fumigation by pregnant women as an abortifacient. The extract is used as an emmenagogue by fumigation inhalation and in the form of a pessary[T06813].

Argentina. Decoction of dried bulbs is taken orally against diarrhea and to treat respiratory and urinary tract infections[K17523].

Brazil. Hot water extract of fresh bulb is taken orally to treat hypertension or induce diuresis[T10632].

China. Hot water extract of the bulb is taken orally to treat high blood pressure and for amenorrhea[T05321].

East Asia. Hot water extract of bulb is taken orally as an aphrodisiac, anthelmintic, diuretic and for asthma[W02290].

England. Hot water extract of dried bulb is taken orally for diabetes[M22031].

Ethiopia. The bulb is chewed with leaves of Ruta and seeds of *Nigella sativa* as a remedy for stomachache[T05018].

Europe. Butanol extract of the bulb is taken orally to protect against atherosclerosis risk factors[T00911].

Fiji. Fresh bulb, together with dried *Ferula assafoetida* and sugar, is taken orally to cleanse the new mother. Bulb ground with ghee, and sugar is taken orally for dysentery. Fresh bulb juice warmed with coconut oil is dropped into the ear for earache[T10632].

Greece. Hot water extract of bulb is taken orally to protect against amoebae[A04939].

Guatemala. Hot water extract of dried bulb is used externally for ringworm, fungal diseases of the skin, and skin diseases and irritations, for leukorrhea, vaginitis, and infections of the skin and mucosa[T16068,M27151,T15445].

Haiti. Decoction of fresh bulb is taken orally for cutaneous infections; hot water extract is taken orally for malnutrition; the juice is taken orally for bronchitis, and butanol extract is taken orally for pneumonia[T13846].

India. Fresh bulb juice is taken orally as an abortifacient. Ten grams of *Momordica tuberosa* root, five grams of *Calotropis gigantea* stem bark, a few Brassica (species) seeds and a few cloves of *Allium sativum* are pounded together and the juice extracted. Two to three tablespoons of extract causes abortion within 12 hours. To relieve dysmenorrhea, paving the way for effective conception in future menstrual cycles, paste made of *Mucuna pruriens*, *Pygaeopremna herbacea*, *Tephrosia purpurea* & *Gardenia turgida* roots, plus a few cloves of *Allium sativum* is given orally. Twenty grams of the paste is given on the third day of menstruation[T09302]. Hot water extract of bulb is taken orally as an emmenagogue[A04132] and anthelmintic[W03487]. Ten grams of *Cocconia indica* leaves are pounded with 14 peppers and 14 pieces of bulb to make enough for nine pills and given one per day for nine days to treat rabies[K11282]. For scabies, *Piper betel* leaves are pounded with small quantities of sulfur, camphor, pepper, and garlic are roasted in sesame oil and applied to the skin. For leukorrhagia, garlic bulb is mixed with leaves of *Ziziphus mauritiana*, pepper, and salt and taken with buttermilk[K11282]. Hot water extract of dried bulb, mixed with an equal amount of honey is taken once a day for three days for whooping cough[T06479]. Hot water extract of dried seeds is taken orally as an emmenagogue[T14891]. Infusion of the entire plant along with sugar is drunk to treat fever[K11282].

Indonesia. Hot water extract of bulb in a mixture with wild herbs, the slough of a snake, and vinegar is taken orally as an abortifacient[K04296].

Italy. Fresh bulb is taken orally for gastronomic purposes[T16715]. Hot water extract of dried bulb is used externally for inflammations, as a cicatrizing agent, and to treat insect bites. The extract is taken orally as an anthelmintic, and hypotensive agent[T16715].

Jamaica. Hot water extract of bulb is taken orally as an emmenagogue[A03403].

Japan. Bulb is taken orally to treat hypertension[T05321]. Fresh bulb is taken orally as a food[K19968]. Water extract of fresh bulb is used externally to promote hair growth[T06579].

Kuwait. Bulb is taken orally to regulate menstruation[L02255].

Malaysia. Hot water extract of bulb is taken orally by females after childbirth[A06589].

Mexico. Decoction of dried bulb, *Allium cepa* and *Pimpinella anisum* are used orally for newborn infants[T08771]. Hot water extract of bulb is taken orally to induce abortion[A03593]. Hot infusion sweetened with honey is taken orally to aid expulsion of placenta[A04180]. Bulb crushed together with leaf of *Clematis dioica* is taken orally to treat catarrh[T08016]. A clove of garlic is inserted in the anus to reduce fever[W01266]. Hot water extract of fresh bulb is taken orally to speed labor, as an abortifacient, for rheumatism, and decoction is taken to facilitate birth process[T09672].

Nepal. Hot water extract of dried bulbs is taken orally as a sedative and for fever[T07944].

Nigeria. Dried entire plant soaked in juice of *Citrus aurantifolia* and a pinch of copper sulfate is given orally to children to treat convulsions. The mixture is left for four days in a bottle. Only a small quantity is to be given; excess results in vomiting or runny stool. To treat yellow fever, one to two handfuls of leaflets grounded with one small bulb of *Allium sativum* is taken orally with "Pap"[K08933]. Fresh bulb is taken orally as a tonic, an antirheumatic, an antipyretic, a hypotensive, and an analgesic[T06510].

Pakistan. Hot water extract of dried bulb is taken orally as a carminative, expectorant, and febrifuge[T09984].

Peru. Hot water extract of fresh bulb is taken orally as a vermifuge, febrifuge, diuretic, antiscorbutic, anti-inflammatory for respiratory pathways, for catarrh, arteriosclerosis, and externally used as an antiseptic and disinfectant[T15323].

Saudi Arabia. Hot water extract of dried bulb is taken orally as a diuretic, for diabetes, rheumatism, pyrexia, intestinal worms, colic, flatulence, menstrual suppression and mixed with sour milk for stomach pain[T10348]. Hot water extract of fresh bulb is taken orally for diabetes, rheumatism, pyrexia, intestinal worms, colic, flatulence, menstrual suppression, hepatitis, piles, dysentery, tuberculosis, rheumatism, colic, facial paralysis, hypertension, diabetes, bronchitis, and also used as an aphrodisiac[M23016].

South Africa. Bulb is taken orally as an aphrodisiac[A05825].

South Korea. Hot water extract of dried rhizome is taken orally as an abortifacient and emmenagogue[T10290].

Sweden. Fresh bulb is applied to excoriations and erosions resulting from scratching dry skin[M17640].

Thailand. Decoction of fresh bulb is taken orally as an anti-inflammatory, and the crushed bulb is used as a poultice on inflamed joints[T16711]. Hot water extract of dried bulb is used externally for treating wounds, toothache, and leprosy. It is taken orally for epilepsy and chest pain[P00123].

Tunisia. Hot water extract of dried bulb is taken orally as a hypotensive and vermifuge[T08514].

USA. Butanol extract of bulb is taken orally as an aphrodisiac. The preparation is said to contain "*Allium sativum*" (25%), "*Capsicum annuum*" (50%), "*Purus saccharum*" (25%). The propriety product is called "Pseudo love stimulant" and is used by both sexes[T00337]. Dried bulb is taken orally as an antihypertensive, vermifuge, and is also used against infection. Externally, the extract is used for treatment of sinusitis and coryza[M26697]. Fresh bulb is taken orally to treat infectious diseases, lung diseases, tuberculosis, as a blood purifier, and stimulant. The bulb applied to the feet is used against diarrhea and fever[W04177].

West Indies. Clove tea is used for intestinal worms. Hot water extract of the bulb is taken orally for hypertension and butanol extract is rubbed on the abdomen to facilitate parturition. Essential oil is taken orally as an antispasmodic, antimicrobial, diuretic, antiasthmatic, and emmenagogue[T00701].

Yugoslavia. Hot water extract of fresh bulb is taken orally for diabetes[T01919].

CHEMICAL CONSTITUENTS

(ppm unless otherwise indicated)

1-Hexanol, Bu
1-Methyl-2-(prop-2-enyl)-disulfane, Bu
1-Methyl-3-(prop-2-enyl)-trisulfane, Bu
2-Methylbenzaldehyde, Bu
2-Propen-1-ol, Bu 0.1-121
2-Propenyl L-cysteine sulfoxide, Bu
2-Propenyl-1-propenyl disulfide, EO
2-Vinyl-1,3-dithiene, Bu 2-29
3((S)-Allyl-sulfinyl)-1-alanine, Bu
3-Methyl-2-cyclopentene-1-thione, Bu
   0.16-1.6
3-Vinyl-1,2-dithiene, Bu 0.34-10.65
3-Vinyl-4(H)-1-2 dithiin, Bu

3(2-Propenyl-sulfinyl)-1-alanine, Bu
4-Methyl-5-vinylthiazole, Bu
5-Butyl cysteine sulfoxide, Bu
1,2-(Prop-2-enyl)-disulfane, Bu
1,2-Dimercaptocyclopentane, Bu
1,2-Epithiopropane, Bu 0.1-1.66
1,3-Dithiane, Bu 0.08-3
24-Methylene-cycloartenol, Pl
2,5-Dimethyl-tetrahydrothiophene, Bu 0.6
3,5-Diethyl-1,2,4-trithiolane, Bu 0.15-43
2,3,4-Trithiapentane, Bu
Acyl anthocyanin, Lf
Adenosine, Bu
Ajoene, Bu 411
Alanine, Bu 0.132–0.3168%
Allicin, Bu 0.15-2.78%
Alliin, Bu 0.5–1.3%
Alliinase, Bu 411
Allin, Bu
Allisatin, Pl
Allistatin-1, Bu
Allistatin-2, Bu
Allium fructan K-1, Bu
Allium fructan K-2, Bu
Allium fructan K-3, Bu
Allium fructan K-4, Bu
Allium fructan K-5, Bu
Allium fructan K-6, Bu
Allium fructan K-7, Bu
Allium fructan K-8, Bu
Allium lectin AS-1, Bu
Allium lectin AS-2, Bu
Allium sativum D-galactan, Bu
Allixin, Bu
Allyl methyl disulfide, EO
Allyl methyl sulfide, Bu, EO
Allyl methyl trisulfide, Bu; EO
Allyl trisulfide, Bu
Allyl disulfide, Bu
Allyl methyl disulfide, Bu
Allyl methyl disulfide, Bu
Allyl methyl trisulfide, Bu
Allyl propyl disulfide, Bu 36-316
Alpha-phellandrene, Bu
Alpha-prostaglandin-F-1, Bu
Alpha-prostaglandin-F-2, Nu
Alpha-tocopherol, Bu
Aluminum, Bu 52
Aniline, Bu Tr-10
Arachidonic acid, Bu
Arginine, Bu 0.634-1.5216%
Ascorbic acid, Bu 100-788

Ascorbic acid, Fl 440-3,793
Ascorbic acid, Lf 390-2,868
Ascorbic acid, Sh 420-1,883
Ash, Lf 1.0-7.4%
Ash, Sh 0.7-3.1%
Aspartic acid, Lf
Aspartic acid, Bu 0.489-1.1736%
Beta carotene, Bu 0-0.17
Beta carotene, Fl 0.6-5
Beta carotene, Lf 9-68
Beta carotene, Sh 2-9
Beta phellandrene, Bu
Beta sitosterol, Pl
Beta tocopherol, Bu
Biotin, Bu 22 mcg/g
Boron, Bu 3-6
Caffeic acid, Bu 20
Calcium oxalate, Bu
Calcium, Bu 180-4,947
Calcium, Fl 250-2,155
Calcium, Lf 580-4,265
Calcium, Sh 120-538
Calcium oxalate, Bu
Carbohydrates, Bu 27.4-85.1%
Carbohydrates, Fl 9.4-81.0%
Carbohydrates, Lf 9.5-69.9%
Carbohydrates, Sh 20.1-90.1%
Chlorogenic acid, Pl
Chlorophyll, Bu
Choline, Bu
Chromium, Bu 2.5-15
Cis-ajoene, Bu
Citral, Bu
Cobalt, Bu 0.5-100
Copper, Bu 4.8-9.7
Cycloalliin, Bu
Cysteine, Lf
Cysteine, Bu 650-1,560
Deoxy alliin, Bu
Desgalactotigonin, Rt 400
Desoxyribonuclease, Bu
Diallyl-disulfide, Bu 16-613
Diallyl heptasulfide, Bu
Diallyl hexasulfide, Bu
Diallyl pentasulfide, Bu
Diallyl sulfide, Bu 2-99
Diallyl tetrasulfide, Bu
Diallyl trisulfide, Bu 10-1,061
Digalactosyl diglyceride, Bu
Dimethyl ajoene, Bu
Dimethyl difuran, Bu 5-30
Dimethyl disulfide, Bu 0.6-2.5

Dimethyl sulfide, Bu, EO
Dimethyl trisulfide, Bu 0.8-19
Eicosapentaenoic acid, Bu
Eruboside B, Bu 13
Essential oils, Bu 600-3,600
Fat, Bu 0.2-1.2%
Fat, Fl 0.2-1.7%
Fat, Lf 0.5-3.7%
Fat, Sh 0.3-1.3%
Ferulic acid, Bu 27
Fiber, 1.7-7.6%
Fiber, Bu 0.7-3.9%
Fiber, Fl 0.8-6.9%
Fiber, Lf 1.8-13.2%
Foliacin, Bu 1
Fructose, Bu
Gamma glutamyl phenyl alanine, Bu
Gamma-L-glutamyl isoleucine, Bu
Gamma-L-glutamyl-L-leucine, Bu
Gamma-L-glutamyl-L-phenylalanine, Bu
Gamma-L-glutamyl-L-valine, Bu
Gamma-L-glutamyl-methionine, Bu
Gamma-L-glutamyl-S-(2-carboxy-1-Propyl)-
   cysteineglycine, Pl
Gamma-L-glutamyl-S-allyl-cysteine, Bu
Gamma-L-glutamyl-S-allyl-mercapto-cys-
   teine, Bu
Gamma-L-glutamyl-S-beta-carboxy-beta-
   Methyl-ethyl-cysteinyl-glycine, Bu
Gamma-L-glutamyl-S-methyl-L-cysteine-
   Sulfoxide, Bu
Gamma-L-glutamyl-S-propyl-L-cysteine, Bu
Geraniol, Bu
Germanium, Bu 754
Gibberellin-A-3, Bu
Gibberellin-A-7, Bu
Gibberellin-A-7, Bu
Gitonin, Rt 300
Glucose, Bu
Glutamic acid, Bu 0.805-1.932%
Glutathione, Bu
Glycerol sulfoquinovoside, Bu
Glycine, Bu 0.2–0.48%
Guanosine, Bu
Hexa-1,5-dienyl-trisulfide, Bu
Hexokinase, Bu
Histidine, Bu 0.113–0.2712%
Iodine, Bu
Iron, Bu 15–129; Fl 9–78; Lf 6–44; Sh 17–76
Isobutyl isothiocyanate, Bu 0.14–25
Isoleucine, Bu 0.217–0.521%
Kaempferol, Pl

Kilocalories, Bu 0.117–0.363%
Kilocalories, Fl 390–3,366
Kilocalories, Lf 440–3,240
Kilocalories, Sh 760–3,410
Leucine, Bu 3,050–7,392
Linalool, Bu
Linolenic acid, Pl
Lysine, Bu 0.273–0.655%
Magnesium, Bu 240–1,210
Manganese, Bu 5.4–15.3
Methionine, Bu 760–1,824
Methyl ajoene, Bu
Methyl allyl thiosulfinate, Bu
Methyl allyl disulfide, Bu 6–104
Methyl allyl sulfide, Bu 0.5–4.6
Methyl allyl trisulfide, Bu 6–279
Methyl propyl disulfide, Bu 0.03–0.66
Monogalactosyl diglyceride, Bu
Myrosinase, Bu
Niacin, Bu 4–17
Niacin, Fl 4–34
Niacin, Lf 6–44
Niacin, Sh 5–22
Nickel, Bu 1.5–1.7
Nicotinic acid, Bu 4.8
Oleanolic acid, Pl
Oleic acid, Pl
Ornithine, Lf
P-Coumaric acid, Bu 58
P-Hydroxybenzoic acid, Pl
Peroxidase, Bu
Phenylalanine, Bu 0.183–0.439%
Phloroglucinol, Pl
Phosphatidyl choline, Bu
Phosphatidyl ethanolamine, Bu, Lf
Phosphatidyl inositol, Bu
Phosphatidyl serine, Bu
Phosphorus, Bu 880–5,220
Phosphorus, Fl 460–3,966
Phosphorus, Lf 460–3,382
Phosphorus, Sh 520–2,332
Phytic acid, Pl
Potassium, Bu 0.373–1.367%
Potassium, Lf 0.326–2.397%
Potassium, Sh 0.273–1.224%
Proline, Bu 0.10–0.24%
Prop-2-enyl-disulfane, Bu
Propene, Bu 0.01–6
Propenethiol, Bu 1–41
Prostaglandin-A-1, Bu
Prostaglandin-A-2, Nu
Prostaglandin-B-1, Bu

Prostaglandin-B-2, Nu
Prostaglandin-E-1, Bu
Prostaglandin-E-2, Nu
Protein, Bu 3.5–17.9%
Protein, Fl 1.4–12.1%
Protein, Lf 2.6–19.1%
Protein, Sh 1.2–5.4%
Protodegalactotigonin, Bu 10
Protoeruboside-B, Bu 100
Pseudoscoridinine-A, Bu
Pseudoscoridinine-B, Bu
Quercetin, Bu 200
Quercetin-3-O-beta-D-glucoside, Pl
Raffinose, Bu
Riboflavin, Bu 0.5–3
Riboflavin, Fl 0.6–5.2
Riboflavin, Lf 1.4–10.3
Riboflavin, Sh 0.6–2.7
Rutin, Pl
S-(2-Carboxy-Propyl)-glutathione, Bu 92.5
S-Allo-mercapto cysteine, Bu 2
S-Allyl cysteine sulfoxide, Bu
S-allyl cysteine sulfoxide, Cal Tiss
S-Allyl cysteine, Bu 10
S-Allyl cysteine sulfoxide, Bu
S-Ethyl cysteine sulfoxide, Bu
S-Methyl cysteine sulfoxide, Bu; Cal Tiss
S-Methyl L-cysteine sulfoxide, Bu
S-Methyl cysteine, Bu
S-N-butyl cysteine sulfoxide, Bu
S-Propenyl cysteine, Bu
S-Propyl cysteine sulfoxide, Bu
Saponin, Bu
Sativoside-B-1, Bu 30
Sativoside-R-1, Rt 500
Sativoside-R-2, Rt 300
Scordine, Bu 250
Scordinin-A, Bu 3.9%
Scorodinin-A-1, Bu 67–30,000
Scorodinin-A-2, Bu 250–8,000
Scorodinin-B, Bu 800
Scorodinine-A-3, Bu 333
Scorodose, Bu
Selenium, Bu 16
Serine, Bu 1,900–4,560
Silicon, Tr; Bu
Sinapic acid, Pl 27
Sodium, Bu 158–559
Sodium, Lf 40–294
Stigamsterol, Pl
Succinic acid, Pl
Sucrose, Bu

Taurine, Pl
Thiamacornine, Bu
Thiamamidine, Bu
Thiamin, Bu 2–8
Thiamin, Fl 1.1–9.5
Thiamin, Lf 1.1–8.1
Thiamin, Sh 1.4–6.3
Threonine, Bu 1,570–3,768
Tin, Bu 6
Trans-1-propenyl methyl disulfide, Bu
Trans-ajoene, Bu 268
Trans-cis ajoene, Bu
Trans-S-(propen-1-yl)(+)cysteine sulfoxide, Bu
Trans-S-(propenyl-1-Yl)-cysteine-Disulfide, Bu
Tryptophan, Bu 660–1,584
Tyrosinase, Bu
Tyrosine, Bu 810–1,944
Uranium, Bu
Valine, Bu 2,910–6,984
Vitamin-U, Tr
Water, Bu 58.5–67.8%
Water, Fl 88.4%
Water, Lf 86.4%
Water, Sh 77.7%
Zinc, Bu Tr-15.3

PHARMACOLOGICAL ACTIVITIES AND CLINICAL TRIALS

Abortifacient effect. Ethanol (95%) extract of seeds at doses of 150.0 and 200.0 mg/kg, and petroleum ether extract at a dose of 100.0 mg/kg, administered orally to female rats were inactive[W01362].

Acetylcholinesterase inhibition. Essential oil of dried bulb was active on *Macaronesia fortunata* and *Musca domestica*[W04295].

Acid phosphatase inhibition. Butanol extract of dried bulb administered intragastrically to rats at a dose of 0.5 gm/kg was active vs isoprenaline-induced tissue necrosis of heart, liver, and pancreas[M20887].

ACTH-induction. Ethyl acetate, and Ethanol (95%) extracts of dried bulb, administered intramuscularly to rabbits at doses of 20.0 mg/animal daily for four days were active[W03437].

Adenosine deaminase inhibition. Fresh bulb and sap at concentrations of 10.0 mcg were inactive. Sap at a concentration of 10.0 microliters was active[T16590]. Water extract of dried bulb at a concentration of 10.0 mcg/ml in cell culture was active on aortic-endothelium[K21750].

Adherence inhibition (bacteria to host cells). Water extract of fresh bulb in cell culture, at a concentration of 0.4% was active on *Candida albicans*, adherence to buccal epithelial cells pre-incubated with compound, and 0.1% (adherence to buccal epithelial cells after oral rinse was measured). Concentration of 0.8% was inactive vs L-cysteine, mercaptoethanol or glutathione antagonistic effect[M22069].

Aflatoxin production inhibition. Water extract of fresh bulb at a concentration of 1.0 mg/ml was active on *Aspergillus flavus*. Aflatoxin B-1 production was inhibited 60.35%. The extract was also active when administered intragastrically to duckling at a dose of 2.5 mg vs aflatoxin B-1 hepatotoxicity. Enzyme was measured in serum[K08395].

AIDS therapeutic effect. Fresh bulb taken orally by human adults at variable dosage levels was active. Five grams of fresh bulb was taken daily for the first six weeks and 10 gm daily for the second six weeks. Diarrhea, genital herpes, candidiasis, and pansinusitus with recurrent fever improved in AIDS patients[M22066].

Alanine aminotransferase stimulation. Water extract of fresh bulb administered intragastrically to rat at variable dosage levels was inactive. Essential oil, administered intragastrically to rat at a dose of 0.067 mg/gm, was active[M23270].

Alanine aminotransferase inhibition. Seed essential oil, administered intragastrically to rat at a dose of 56.9 micromols was active[T16004].

Alkaline phosphatase stimulation. Butanol extract of dried bulb in the ration of rats at a dose of 6.7% of the diet was active vs cadmium toxicity[T08608]. Water extract of fresh bulb in the ration of rabbits at a dose of 1.0 gm/kg was active vs cholesterol-loaded animals[T16431].

Alkaline phosphatase inhibition. Essential oil, administered intragastrically to rat at a concentration of 0.067 mg/g was active. The rats were fasted for 24 hours[M23270].

Allergenic activity. Ethyl acetate, ethanol (95%), and water extracts of bulbs applied externally to human adults were active[T00609]. Butanol extract of fresh bulb applied externally to human adults was active. Garlic was used as a wet dressing for itchy dry skin and erosions caused by scratching. Afterwards, dermatitis became worse and spread. Upon corticosteroid treatment, the eczema disappeared. The patient had slight anemia, leukopenia, and elevated total serum IGE[M17640].

Alpha-amylase inhibition. Water extract of bulbs was active[T00171].

Aminolevulinic (delta) acid dehydrase inhibition. Water extract of dried bulb, at a concentration of 0.1 millimols was active on human blood[T12021].

Analgesic activity. Ethanol (70%) extract of fresh bulb administered intraperitoneally to mice of both sexes at variable dosage levels was active[T06510].

Angiotensin-converting enzyme inhibition. Lyophilized extract of fresh bulb at a concentration of 0.3 mg/ml was inactive. Lyophilized extract of fresh leaves, at a concentration of 0.3 mg/ml, was active. 30% inhibition was produced[T16651].

Anthelmintic activity. Butanol extract of dried bulbs, administered by gastric intubation to mice at a dose of 200.0 mg/kg on days 1–5, was active on *Aspiculurus tetraptera*[W04425]. Dried bulb administered by gastric intubation to ducks and geese infected with hymenolepis produced weak activity[W03448]. Essential oil, administered intragastrically to mice at a dose of 0.025 ml/kg on days 1–5 was inactive on *Aspiculurus tetraptera*[W04425]. Fresh bulb in the drinking water and hexane extracts were active on carp *Capillaria obsignata*, at a dose 200.0 mg/liter dosing twice daily on days 1–3[M18522]. Saline extract of fresh bulb at a

concentration of 5.0% was active on *Anisakis* species larvae[K23314].

Antiaging activity. Water extract of dried bulb in cell culture at a concentration of 100.0 mcg/ml increased the lifespan of leuk-P388(ARA-C) cells in cultures[K16939].

Antiallergenic activity. Water extract of fresh bulb in cell culture, at a concentration of 100.0 microliters/ml was active on leuk-RBL 2H3 vs biotinylated anti-DNP IGE/avidin-induced beta-hexosaminidase release[K19968].

Antiamebic activity. Essential oil in broth culture at a concentration of 2.0 microliters/ml was active on *Entamoeba histolytica*[K21149]. Fresh bulb juice in broth culture at a concentration of 25.0 mcg/ml was active on *Entameba histolytica*[M19268].

Antiarrhythmic activity. Dried bulb in the ration of rats at a concentration of 1.0% of the diet for 10 weeks decreased coronary artery ligation reperfusion-induced arrhythmias[K10232].

Antiascariasis activity. Ethanol (95%) extract of bulbs when applied externally, was active on earthworms. Paralysis occurred in 12 hours with death of 50% of the worms[J08904]. Water extract applied externally to earthworms at a concentration of 10.0 mg/ml produced strong activity[A05682].

Antiatherosclerotic activity. Butanol extract of dried bulb taken orally by human adults prevented the total rise in serum cholesterol, B-lipoprotein cholesterol, B-lipoprotein and serum triglycerides in patients with alimentary lipemia[T07883]. Dried bulb in the ration of castrated rams, at a concentration of 5% of the diet produced weak activity[K17621]. Water extract of fresh bulb in the ration of rabbits at a dose of 1.0 gm/kg was active vs cholesterol-loaded animals[T16431].

Antibacterial activity. Essential oil on agar plate was active on *Erwina amylovora*. MIC 112.5 mg/liter[M28770]. Amino acid fraction in cream form, and extract in ointment, essential oil in wound healing powder and essential oil in gel, of dried bulb on agar plate were active on *Escherichia coli*, *Klebsiella pneumonia*, *Proteus vulgaris*, and *Shigella sonnei*[P00110]. Ethanol (95%) extract was active on *Escherichia coli*, *Salmonella typhosa*, *Shigella sonnei*, and *Staphylococcus aureus*[P00047]. Water extract was active on *Bacillus mycoides*, *E. coli*, *Klebsiella pneumonia*, *Proteus vulgaris*, *Salmonella typhosa*, *Shigella sonnei*, and *Staphylococcus aureus*[P00036]. Aqueous high speed supernatant on agar plate at a concentration of 0.2 ml was active on *Escherichia coli*, *Proteus mirabilis*, *Proteus vulgaris*, *Pseudomonas aeruginosa*, *Staphylococcus aureus*, and *Klebsiella* species[T08945]. Bulb juice in broth culture was active on *Candida parapsilosis*. Thirty eight-milimeter zone of inhibition was produced[M01497]. Butanol, water and hot water extracts of fresh bulb on agar plate, at variable concentration was active on *Bacillus subtilis* H-17(Rec+), M-45(Rec-)[T07988]. Decoction of dried bulb on agar plate was active on *Pseudomonas aeruginosa*[K17523]. Hot water extract at a concentration of 62.5 mg/ml was active on *Staphylococcus aureus* and inactive on *Escherichia coli*[K14683]. Dried bulb on agar plate was active on *Xanthomonas campestris*[T13888]. Dried bulbs on agar plate at a concentration of 0.20 gm/plate produced strong activity on *Escherichia coli* and *Bacillus subtilis*[T10895]. Essential oil of dried bulb, administered intradermal to rabbit prevented Staphylococcal infections[W04034]. Essential oil of dried bulb, on agar plate was active on *Klebsiella pneumonia*, *Proteus vulgaris*, and *Pseudomonas aeruginosa*[P00110]. Fresh bulb juice on agar plate, undiluted, was active on *Bacillus subtilis*, *Pseudomonas aeruginosa*, and *Salmonella typhosa*[W04069]. Fresh bulb juice, undiluted on agar produced weak activity on *Streptococcus aureus* and *Escherichia coli*[W04024]. Fresh bulb and chloroform extract on agar plate were inactive on *Escherichia coli* and *Staphylococcus aureus*, MIC 7.5 and 6.0 mg/ml, respectively. Water extract at a concentration of 30.0 microliters/disk, on agar plate was active on *E. coli*, *Shigella dysenteriae 1*, *Shigella flexneri*, and *Shigella sonnei*. A dose of 1.5 ml/kg of fresh bulb, administered intra-gastrically to rabbit was active on *Shigella flexneri*[M26615]. Fresh bulb juice, undiluted on agar plate was active on *Proteus vulgaris*[W03630]. Fresh corn sap on agar plate was active on several gram negative organisms[T06881]. Fresh essential oil, undiluted on agar plate, was active on *Pseudomonas aeruginosa* and *Staphylococcus aureus*, and inactive on *Bacillus cereus* and *E. coli*[T06640]. Infusion of fresh bulb in broth culture was active on *Staphylococcus aureus* MIC 10.0 mcg/ml, *Clostridium paraputrificum* and *Propionibacter acnes* MIC 3.9 mg/ml, *Bacteroides vulgaris*, and *Bifidobacterium longum* MIC 7.8 mg/ml; inactive on *Clostridium perfringens*, *Bacteroides fragilis*, *Eubacterium limosum*, *Propionibacterium intermedium*, *Acinetobacter calcoaceticus*, and *Staphylococcus aureus* 25923 MIC 15.6 mg/ml, *Eubacterium nucleatum* and *E. lentum* MIC 31.3 mg/ml, *Bacteroides melaninogenicus*, and *Peptostreptococcus productus* MIC 62.5 mg/ml, *Citrobacter freundii* and *Serratia marcescens* MIC 625.0 mcg/ml, *Pseudomonas aeruginosa* and *Streptococcus faecalis* MIC >625 mcg/ml. The petroleum ether extract was inactive on *Clostridium paraputrificum* MIC 156.0 mcg/ml, *Bifidobacterium longum* MIC 312.0 mcg/ml, *Propionibacterium acnes* MIC 78.0 mcg/ml and *S. aureus* MIC 625 mcg/ml[M18532]. Leaf essential oil on agar plate was inactive on *Bacillus cereus*, *E. coli*, *Pseudomonas aeruginosa*, and *Staphylococcus aureus*[T14976]. Dried oleoresin in broth culture at a concentration of 5.0 gm/liter produced weak activity on *Staphylococcus aureus*[T15207]. Chloroform extract of dried bulb contained at least two active elements. One was chloroform soluble and had an antiseptic action, a slight tonic effect on isolated frog heart, a slight hypertensive effect on etherized cats, and a paralyzing effect on isolated rabbit intestine. The chloroform-insoluble fraction had no antiseptic effect, no action on isolated frog heart, a strongly hypotensive effect on etherized cats, and a tonic effect on isolated rabbit intestine[W03661]. Powdered dried bulb in broth culture at a concentration of 5.0 gm/liter was inactive on *Staphylococcus aureus*[T15207]. Tincture of dried bulb on agar plate, at a concentration of 30.0 microliters/disk (10 gm plant material in 100 ml ethanol) was active on *Escherichia coli, Pseudomonas aeruginosa*, and *Staphylococcus aureus*[T15445]. Water extract of bulb in broth culture at a concentration of 1.0% was active on *Clostridium perfringens*[T01900]. Water extract on agar plate was active on *Escherichia coli, Pasteurella multocida, Proteus* species, *Providencia* species, *Staphylococcus aureus, Streptococcus faecalis* and inactive on *Pseudomonas aeruginosa*. A dose of 1.0 ml/animal, administered orally to chicken caused a reduction in intestinal tract bacteria[N00016]. Water extract of bulb in broth culture was active on *Staphylococcus aureus*. The extract administered intraperitoneally to mice was inactive on *Staphylococcus aureus*. On agar plate, was active on *Erwinia carotovora* and *E. herbicola*[J02255]. Water extract of bulbs on agar plate at a concentration of 1–10 was active on *Escherichia coli*. Complete inhibition of several Enterotoxigenic strains of the test organisms was observed[T05764]. Water extract of dried bulbs on agar plate was active on *Streptococcus sanguis, Escherichia coli, Serratia marcescens, Lactobacillus odontolyticus, Streptococcus milleri, Streptococcus mutans*, weakly active on *Bacillus cereus, Enterobacter cloacae, Staphylococcus aureus, Streptococcus hominis* and inactive on *Pseudomonas aeruginosa*[T07185]. Water extract of fresh bulb was active on *E. coli* and *Micrococcus luteus*[K23492].

Anticardiotoxic effect. Water extract of aged bulb administered intraperitoneally to mice at a dose of 0.05 ml/animal six times weekly was active. Widening of GRS and lengthening of RR intervals induced by dox-

orubicin were diminished in treated animals. Doxorubicin-induced histologic changes were prevented by treatment[K17870].

Anticholinergic activity. Water extract of dried bulb was inactive on frog skeletal muscle and guinea pig small intestine vs ACh-induced contractions[P00078].

Anticlastogenic activity. Flower head juice, administered intragastrically to mice at a dose of 25.0 ml/kg, was active on bone marrow cells vs mitomycin C-, dimethylnitrosamine-, and tetracycline-induced micronuclei[K17562].

Anticonvulsant activity. Ethanol (70%) of fresh bulb, administered intraperitoneally to mice of both sexes at variable dosage levels, was active vs metrazole-induced convulsions and inactive vs strychnine-induced convulsions[T06510].

Anticrustacean activity. Ethanol (95%) extract of dried bulb was inactive on *Artemia salina*. The assay system was intended to predict for antitumor activity[K08041].

Anticytotoxic activity. Water extract of bulbs administered intragastrically to mice at a dose of 100.0 mg/kg was active vs arsenic-induced bone marrow cytotoxicity. Treatment with the extract reduced the chromosome breaks and cell damage induced by arsenic[K11174].

Antidiarrheal activity. Essential oil administered orally to mice at a concentration of 0.01 ml/gm was active vs castor oil-induced diarrhea[M16824].

Antiedema activity. Methanol extract of bulbs applied externally to mice at a dose of 2.0 mg/ear was active vs 12–0-tetradecanoylphorbol-13-acetate (TPA)-induced ear inflammation. Inhibition ratio (IR) was 32[K11173].

Antiestrogenic effect. Water extract of fresh bulb, administered intraperitoneally to female mice at a dose of 500.0 mg/day, was inactive[T16647].

Antifatigue activity. Ethanol (95%) extract of bulbs, administered intragastrically to mice at a dose of 125.0 mg/kg, was active. The dose had no effect after one session of rope climbing stress, but it prevented decline in performance, which was noted in controls after two weeks of repeated stress[M17484].

Antifilarial activity. Fresh bulb was active on *Setaria digitata*. LC$_{100}$ 600 ppm[M25236].

Antifungal activity (plant pathogens). Essential oil on agar plate was active on *Lenzites trabea, Lentinus lepideus* and *Polyporus versicolor*[A05942].

Antifungal activity. Bulb essential oil on agar plate, at a concentration of 10.0%/disk was active on *Geotrichum candidum, Candida lipolytica, Rhodotorula rubra, Saccharomyces cerevisiae,* and inactive on *Brettanomyces anomalus*. 1.0%/disk was active on *Kloeckera apiculata, Kluyveromyces fragilis, Pichia membranaefaciens,* and *Torulopsis glabrata.* Strong activity was produced on *Debaryomyces hansenii, Hansenula anomala, Lodderomyces elongisporus,* and *Metschnikowia pulcherrima*[T07904]. Bulb juice applied externally to rabbits at a concentration of 10% for 10 days after typical fungal-induced lesions appear was active on *Microsporum canis*[T05324]. Essential oil of dried bulb on agar plate was active on *Trichophyton rubrum*[P00110]. Essential oil of dried bulb, on agar plate was active on *Epidermophyton floccosum, Microsporum gypseum,* and *Trichophyton rubrum* (11% oil in gel was used). Water extract, 0.625% was active on *Trichoderma* species and *Trichophyton mentagrophytes;* 1.25% active on *Aspergillus niger* and *Epidermophyton floccosum;* inactive on *Aspergillus flavus, Basidiobolum meristosporus* strain T1, T2, T3, T4, T5, and T6, and *Trichophyton rubrum;* weak activity on *Aspergillus fumigatus, Curvularia* species, and *Fusarium* species[P00123]. Juice at a concentration of 0.25% was active on *Trichophyton mentagrophytes;* 0.5% was active on *Trichophyton rubrum*[P00145]. Two percent was active on *Alternaria alternata, Ceratocystis*

paradoxa, Fusarium solani, Geotrichum candidum, Melanconium fuligineum, Myrothecium roridum, Phytophthora species, *Phytium aphanidermatum, Rhizopus microsporus, Sclerotium rolfsii, Thanatephorus cucumeris, Tricholoma crassum, Ustilago maydis,* and *Volvariella volvacea;* 4.0% was active on *Colletotrichum denatium*[P00089]. 1.25% was active on *Microsporum gypseum* and *Trichophyton violaceum.* Two and one half percent active on *Epidermophyton floccosum, Microsporum canis, Trichophyton mentagrophytes,* and *Trichophyton rubrum*[P00052]. Essential oil on agar plate was active on *Botryotrichum keratinophilum, Malbranchea aurantiaca* and *Nannizzia incurvata*[M19606]. Ethanol/water (1:1) extract of dried bulbs on agar plate at concentrations of 417.0 and 500.0 mg/ml (expressed as dry weight of bulb) were active on *Penicillium digitatum,* and inactive on *Aspergillus fumigatus, Aspergillus niger, Botrytis cinerea, Rhizopus nigricans, Trichophyton mentagrophytes. Fusarium oxysporum* [T16238,T12725]. Fresh bulb on agar plate was inactive on *Trichophyton andouinii, T. mentagrophytes, T. rubrum, T. Schoenleini* and *T. tonsurans* MIC 1000 mcg/ml; *Aspergillus fumigatus* MIC 2000 mcg/ml and *Microsporum canis* MIC 500 mcg/ml[T16401]. Fresh bulb, undiluted on agar plate was active on *Nannizzia fulva, N. gypsea* and *N. incurvata*[T11589]. Water extract of the fresh bulb at a concentration of 1.0 mcg/ml inhibited growth in *Aspergillus flavus*[K08395]. The extract was active when applied externally at a dose of 20.0% twice daily for 15 days to a buffalo with dermatophytosis caused by *T. verrucosum;* twice daily for 10 days to a calf with dermatophutosis; twice daily for 10 days to a dog with dermatophytosis caused by *M. canis;* and twice daily for 10–20 days to six patients with dermatophytosis caused by *T. rubrum,* and *T. mentagrophytes*[T09441]. A concentration of 10.0% was active on *Trichoconiella padwickii*[M21140]. Fresh essential oil, undiluted on agar plate was inactive on

Penicillium cyclopium, *Trichoderma viride* and *Aspergillus aegyptiacus*[T06640]. Hot water extract of dried bulb in broth culture at a concentration of 1.0 ml was active on *Epidermophyton floccosum*, *Microsporum canis* and *Trichophyton mentagrophytes* vars. algodonosa and granulare[M27151]. Hot water extract of dried bulbs on agar plate at a concentration of 62.6 mg/ml was active on *Aspergillus niger*[T14683]. Leaf essential oil, on agar plate produced strong activity on *Aspergillus aegyptiacus*, *Penicillum cyclopium* and *Trichoderma viride*[T14976]. Water extract of bulbs on agar plate at a concentration of 5.0 mg/ml was active on *Fusarium oxysporum* F. Sp. Lycopersici[T16067]. Water extract of dried bulb in broth culture was active on *Fusarium moniliforme*. A decrease in nitrate and dimethylnitrosamine formation of the fungus was observed[T10838]. Water extract of fresh bulb at a concentration of 0.01 microliters/disk was equivocal on *Epidermophyton floccosum*; inactive on *Trichophyton soudanense*. Concentration of 6.67 mcg/disk was inactive on *Trichophyton erinacei* and *T. verrucosum*. The extract was active on *T. semii*, *Microsporum audouini*, *Trichophy-ton mentagrophytes*, *Microsporum canis*, *T. rubrum* and *T. violaceum*. IC_{50} 6.67 microliters/disk[K19555]. Water extract of fresh bulb on agar plate at a concentration of 5.0 mg/ml was active on *Epidermophyton floccosum*, *Microsporum audouini*, *M. canis*, *M. gypseum*, *Trichophyton concentricum*, and several plant pathogenic fungi[W03994]. Water extract of fresh leaves, on agar plate, at a concentration of 1:1 (one gram of dried leaves in 1.0 ml of water) was active on *Fusarium oxysporum*[K18143]. Strong activity was produced on *Ustilago maydis* and *U. nuda*[T08889]. Water extract of bulbs in broth culture was active on *Aspergillus fumigatus*, *Aspergillus flavus*, *Rhizopus rhizopodiformis*, *Aspergillus niger*, *Mucor pusillus*, and weak activity on *Rhizopus arrhizus*[N16937].

Antigout activity. Water extract of bulb, administered by gastric intubation to rats at a dose of 100.0 mg/kg was active. Daily dosing for 10 days to typhoid Bacillus-sheep RBC stimulated animals showed the antibody titer to be significantly inhibited[T06208].

Antihematopoetic activity. Dried bulb administered by gastric intubation to rats at a dose of 3.10 mg/kg was equivocal. There was a slight decrease in erythrocyte and hemoglobin levels in female rats, a much smaller decrease was seen in male rats. At a dose of 10.0 mg/kg, administered for three months, there was a slight decrease in erythrocyte and hemoglobin levels[T11284].

Antihepatotoxic activity. Butanol extract of bulbs administered intragastrically to mice at a dose of 100.0 mg/kg was active vs CCl_4-induced hepatotoxicity. Conjugated diene levels, thiobarbituric acid levels, hepatic triglycerides content and hepatic lipid content were decreased[T15338]. Essential oil of dried bulb in cell culture (rat liver cells) at concentrations of 0.01 and 1.0 mg/ml was active vs CCl_4-, and galactosamine-induced hepatotoxicity. Results significant at $P < 0.01$ and $P < 0.001$ levels respectively[T10949]. Ethanol (20%) extract of fresh bulb, administered by gastric intubation to mice at a dose of 100.0 mg/kg was inactive vs paracetamol- and carbon tetrachloride-induced hepatotoxicity[M24454]. Methanol-insoluble fraction of fresh bulb, turmeric, asafoetida, cumin, ellagic acid, and butylated hydroxy toluene and butylated hydroxy anisole, administered intragastrically to ducklings at a dose of 10.0 mg/animal was active vs aflatoxin B-1-induced hepatotoxicity[K17144].

Antihistamine activity. Water extract of dried bulb was active on guinea pig small intestine vs histamine-induced contractions[P00078].

Antihypercholesterolemic activity. Bulb in the ration of 16 weeks old male rats, at a concentrations of 2.0 and 4.0% of the diet were active in cholesterol-loaded and lard-fed animals. Results significant at $P < 0.05$ level[T05330]. Bulb in the ration of rabbits at variable concentrations, in a feeding study for 52–82 days was active vs cholesterol-loaded animals[A11518]. Bulb taken orally by human adults at variable dosage levels was active[T05321]. Bulb, administered by gastric intubation to dogs was active[T05542]. When administered orally to male human adults at a dose of 25.0 gm/person was active[T01895]. Butanol extract taken orally by human adults of both sexes at a dose of 1.35 gm/person daily for 100 days was active[T01671]. Butanol extract of fresh bulb taken orally by 10 healthy subjects below the age of 40. All were submitted to a 12-hour fast before receiving the test material. A fatty meal consisting of 100 gm butterfat on four slices of bread was given to each subject fresh as well as boiled garlic were administered in the study. Garlic appeared to prevent an increase in serum cholesterol statistical data in the report indicating significant results[T00877]. Water extract of fresh bulb in the ration of rabbit at a dose of 1.0 gm/kg was active[T16431]. Butanol extract of fresh bulb, administered by gastric intubation and in the ration of rats at concentrations of 2.0% of the diet for four weeks was active[T05762]; ethanol (95%) extract was inactive[T14340] vs cholesterol-loaded animals. Dried bulb in the ration of castrated rams at a concentration of 5.0% of the diet was active[K17621]. Essential oil, administered by gastric intubation to rabbits at variable dosage levels was active vs cholesterol-loaded animals[K19274]. In a randomized placebo-controlled double-blind study of the efficacy of garlic powder on cholesterol level, powdered bulbs was taken by 68 volunteers at a dose of 600.0 mg/person. Average cholesterol fell from 223 to 214 mg/dl[K19274]. Dried bulb in the ration of rats at a concentration of 2.0% of the diet was active vs high-fat diet-induced hypercholesterolemia[K16381]. Dried bulb taken orally at a dose of 198.0 mg/person, three doses in 34 human adults was inactive. A dose of 450.0 mg/person, three doses in 51 human adults was

inactive[T12166]. 600.0 mg/person for four weeks was active[M19432]. Dried bulb, taken orally by human adults twice daily for 15 days in a group of 10 hyperlipemic subjects, was active[T05482]. After garlic therapy of dried bulb (two capsules three times daily after meals for 12 weeks), serum cholesterol levels were brought down within the normal range in 26 out of 37 patients. The extract also lowered plasma fibrinogen levels, prolonged coagulation time and enhanced fibrinolytic activity in some of the patients[T05482]. Essential oil in the ration of male rabbit at doses of 0.25, 0.50, and 1.0 g/animal were active vs cholesterol fed animals[T00018]. Essential oil, administered by gastric intubation to rabbit at a dose of 250.0 mg/kg six days per week for 4–12 weeks, was active vs cholesterol-loaded animals[T09440]. Essential oil taken orally by human adults of both sexes, at a dose equivalent to 1.0 gm/kg of raw garlic daily for three months, was active[T01673]. Essential oil, administered by gastric intubation to rat at a dose of 100.0 mg/kg for 60 days was active. Results significant at $P < 0.01$ level vs ethanol-induced hyperglycemia[T09791]. When taken orally by human adults of both sexes at a dose of 0.25 mg/kg the dose was active. In a study with 62 patients with coronary heart disease with high serum cholesterol levels and 20 healthy individuals as a control group. Garlic oil was consumed daily for 10 months[T05071]. Ether extract of fresh bulb administered intragastrically to rat at a dose of 100.0 mg/kg was active vs streptozotocin-induced hyperglycemia. High-fat diet was used[T12374]. Fixed oil in the ration of male rats at a dose of 100.0 mg/kg was active. Simultaneous feeding of unsaturated oil from the plant material with a high-sucrose diet, significantly reduced serum and tissue cholesterol levels, and a small but significant tissue-protein reducing effect was also observed[T05323]. Freeze-dried bulb in the ration of female rats at concentrations of 0.5, 1.0, and 2.0% of the diet were active. Animals were fed a cholesterol-high diet for 6–8 weeks[T05157]. Essential oil, at a concentration of 0.13% of the diet of female rats was active vs cholesterol-loaded animals. Results significant at P < 0.001 level[T08228]. Fresh bulb in the ration of male rat at a concentration of 5.0% of the diet was active. Animals were fed a ration of 1% cholesterol plus 46.8% sucrose and the 5% garlic[T01894]. Powdered dried bulb taken orally by human adults of both sexes, at a dose of 900.0 mg/day was inactive in a double-blind, randomized crossover study on 30 subjects with mild to moderate hypercholesterolemia[K19779]. Water extract of fresh bulb, administered by gastric intubation to rabbits at a dose of 10.0 gm/animal (dry weight of plant) daily for five days, was active vs cholesterol-loaded animals[W03643].

Antihyperglycemic activity. Butanol extract of bulbs taken orally by human adults of both sexes at a dose of 1.35 gm/ person daily for 100 days was active[T01671]. Chloroform extract of bulbs administered orally to rabbits was active vs glucose-primed animals. Activity was 79.4% that of tolbutamide[K04655]. Decoction of fresh bulb, administered intragastrically to mice at a dose of 0.5 ml/animal was inactive vs alloxan-induced hyperglycemia. 25% aqueous extract was used. Maximal change in blood sugar was 6.2%[M22673]. Dried bulb taken orally by human adults at a dose of 350.0 mg/ person twice daily was inactive[M17987]. Ethanol (95%) extract of bulbs administered by gastric intubation to rabbits produced weak activity and petroleum ether extract was active vs alloxan- and epinephrine-induced hyperglycemia[T04535]. Ether extract of fresh bulb administered intragastrically to rat at a dose of 100.0 mg/kg was active vs streptozotocin-induced hyperglycemia[T12374]. Fresh bulb in the ration of male rat at a concentration of 5.0% of the diet was active. Animals were fed a ration of 1% cholesterol plus 46.8% sucrose and the 5% garlic. Sig-

nificant reduction of serum glucose but increased serum insulin and liver glycogen appeared to be associated with increase of insulin level[T01894]. Hot water extract of dried bulb, administered by gastric intubation to mice, at a dose of 0.5 ml (25% extract) was inactive vs alloxan-induced hyperglycemia[T10348]. Hot water extract of fresh bulb in the ration of mice at a dose of 6.25% of the diet was inactive vs streptozotocin-induced hyperglycemia[M24255]. Water extract of bulb administered orally to rats was active vs alloxan-treated animals. There was a 20% decrease in blood glucose[J06621]. Water extract of fresh bulb, administered intragastrically to rat at a dose of 0.07 gm/animal for 30 days was active vs inhibition of the formation of polyols in diabetic rat lens[M20202]. Fresh bulb juice, administered intragastrically to rabbit at a dose of 25.0 gm/animal (dry weight of plant material) was active vs glucose-induced hyperglycemia[A14332].

Antihyperlipemic activity. Bulb in the ration of 16 week-old male rats, at a concentrations of 2.0 and 4.0% of the diet were active in cholesterol-loaded and lard fed animals. Results significant at P < 0.05 level[T05330]. Bulb taken orally by male adults at a dose of 25.0 gm/person was active[T01895]. Dried bulb taken orally at a dose of 198.0 mg/person, three doses in 34 human adults was inactive. A dose of 450.0 mg/person, three doses in 51 human adults was inactive[T12166]; 600.0 mg/ person for four weeks was active[M19432]. Dried bulb taken orally by human adults twice daily for 15 days in a group of 10 hyperlipemic subjects was active[T05940]. Water extract of dried bulb administered orally to rabbits at a dose of 3.3 g/kg daily for two months was active on sucrose loaded animals (10 gm/kg/day). Statistical data indicated significant results[T02039]. Saponin fraction of dried bulbs taken orally by human adults at a dose of 50.0 gm/person was active[T15928]. Dried garlic preparations given to 30 patients of primary hyperlipoproteinemia orally at a dose of 700 mg/day was inactive. Serum cholesterol and triglycerides were not significantly reduced[T14960]. Essential oil, administered by gastric intubation to rabbit at a dose of 250.0 mg/kg six days per week for 4 to 12 weeks, was active vs cholesterol-loaded animals[T09440]. The essential oil taken orally by human adults of both sexes, at a dose equivalent to 1.0 gm/kg of raw garlic daily for three months, was active[T01673]. Essential oil, administered by gastric intubation to rat at a dose of 100.0 mg/kg for 60 days was active. The effects were measured in liver. Results significant at $P < 0.01$ level vs ethanol-induced hyperglycemia[T09341]. Fixed oil in the ration of male rats at a dose of 100.0 mg/kg was active. Simultaneous feeding of unsaturated oil from the plant material with a high sucrose diet significantly reduced serum and tissue lipids, and a small but significant tissue-protein reducing effect was also observed[T05323]. Fresh bulb in the ration of male rat at a concentration of 5.0% of the diet was active. Animals were fed a ration of 1% cholesterol plus 46.8% sucrose and the 5% garlic[T01894]. Pollen taken orally by human adults of both sexes at a dose of 900.0 mg/day was inactive in a double-blind, randomized crossover study on 30 subjects with mild to moderate hypercholesterolemia[K19779]. Water extract in the drinking water of rat, at a dose of 1.0 gm/ml, was active[T14158].

Antihypertensive activity. Bulb taken orally by human adults at variable dosage levels was active[T05321]. Bulbs, administered by gastric intubation to dogs and orally to human adults at variable concentrations was active[A11518]. Butanol extract of bulbs taken orally by human adults of both sexes at a dose of 1.35 gm/person daily for 100 days was active[T01671]. Dried bulbs taken orally by human adults at a dose of 2.4 gm/person produced decrease in diastolic pressure 5–14 hours after dosing in nine patients with essential hypertension[K13342]. Ethanol (95%) extract of bulb administered orally to 25 patients with hypertension was active[A00245]. Ethanol (95%) extract of fresh bulb in the ration of rats at a dose of 8.0 ml/animal was inactive. Extraction was made at 0°C; 4 ml of the extract was fed for three weeks, then salt was added and the dose increased to 8 ml. Salt did not affect blood pressure in the spontaneously hypertensive animals[M20655]. Fresh bulb taken orally by human adults was active. Analysis of random, controlled studies lasting at least four weeks, included 415 subjects showed significant decreases in both systolic and diastolic pressures[K16219].

Antihypertriglyceridemia effect. Bulb in the ration of rats at a dose of 2.0% of the diet was active vs high-fat diet induced hypertriglyceridemia[K16381]. Dried bulb taken orally by human adults at a dose of 900.0 mg/day was active. Twenty four volunteers with reduced HDL-cholesterol levels and hypertriglyceridemia were used in the six week study. Triglyceride levels were reduced up to 35% and HDL cholesterol levels increased[K10232]. Ether extract of fresh bulb administered intragastrically to rats at a dose of 100.0 mg/kg was active. High fat diet was used[T12374]. Outer skin fiber in the ration of male rats at a dose of 236.6 g/days was active[K19607]. Water extract of fresh bulb was active[M30030].

Antihypotensive activity. Water extract of fresh bulb, administered intravenously to rabbit at a dose of 500.0 mg/kg was active vs arachidonate-, and rattail-solubilized-collagen-induced thrombocytopenia, hypotension and increased TXB2 levels. The extract inhibits histopathological changes in lung and liver[K07929]. Intravenous infusion was also active vs arachidonate-induced hypotension[T16577].

Antihypothermic activity. Ethanol (95%) extract of bulbs administered intragastrically to mice at a dose of 250.0 gm/kg was active vs three weeks of cold stress[M17484].

Anti-inflammatory activity. Bulb taken orally by 30 patients with different rheumatic conditions was active[T05225]. Ethanol/water (1:1) extract of bulbs, administered intraperitoneally to rats was active vs carrageenin-induced pedal edema[A04819]. Water extract administered orally to rats at a dose of 2.0 gm/kg produced weak activity vs granuloma pouch and formalin-induced pedal edema[A04422]. Dried bulbs taken orally by human adults at variable dosage levels was active[T06320]. Ethanol (80%) extract of dried bulb, administered to male rats by gastric intubation, at a dose of 100.0 mg/kg was active vs carrageenin-induced pedal edema. 23% inhibition of edema was observed[M17807]. Seed oil, administered intragastrically to rat at a dose of 0.0025 ml/kg, was active vs formaldehyde-induced arthritis[T16004].

Anti-ischemic effect. Bulb in a preparation containing nicotinic acid, administered intragastrically to rats at a dose of 5.0 gm/kg daily for seven days, during the last two isoproterenol was also given. Isoproterenol-induced ischemic effects on the heart were prevented[M26052]. Powdered dried bulb in the ration of rats at a concentration of 1.0% of the diet for 10 days was reduced coronary artery ligation-induced infarct size[K10232].

Antimutagenic activity. Dried bulb on agar plate at a concentration of 12.5 mg/plate was active on *Salmonella typhimurium* TA100, vs aflatoxin B-1-induced mutagenesis. Metabolic activation was required for activity[T16254]. Fresh bulb in buffer, on agar plate, at a concentration of 14.75 mg/plate was inactive on *E. coli* WP2 TRP(-) induced by UV. Concentration of 7.38 mg/plate was active on *E. coli* WP2 TRP(-)UVR(-) and *E. coli* WP2 TRP(-). Methanol extract of fresh bulb on agar plate was active on *Salmonella typhimurium* TA98 and TA100[M31302]. Water extract of fresh bulb at a concentration of 0.8 microliters/ml was active on Hepatoma-AH109A vs gamma-ray-induced mutation. A concentration of 1.0 mg/plate was inactive on *Salmonella typhimurium*

TA100, vs 1,2-epoxy-3,3,3-trichloropropane-induced mutation. A concentration of 10.0 mcg/plate was inactive on *S. typhimurium* TA 100 vs sodium azide-induced mutation. A concentration of 100.0 mcg/plate was active on *S. typhimurium* TA 102 vs gamma-ray-induced mutation. Concentration of 3.0 mcg/plate was active on *S. typhimurium* TA 100 vs adriamycin-induced mutation. Concentration of 5.0 mcg/plate was inactive on *S. typhimurium* TA 100 and TA 98 vs 2-nitrofluorene-induced mutation. A concentration of 50.0 microliters/ml was active on *S. typhimurium* TA 102 vs cumene hydroperoxide-, T-butyl hydroperoxide-, hydrogen peroxide-, mitomycin C-, and streptomycin- induced mutations, and on TA 100 vs N-methyl-N- nitrosoguanidine-induced mutation[M20451].

Antimycobacterial activity. Bulb taken orally at variable dosage levels by a group of 55 patients was active on *Mycobacterium tuberculosis*[T05321]. Juice of the bulb on agar plate produced strong activity on *M. tuberculosis*[A03634]. Chloroform and water extracts of fresh bulb on agar plate at concentration of 1.0 mg/ml produced weak activity on *Mycobacterium avium*[K13895]. Dried bulb in broth culture was active on *Mycobacterium tuberculosis* and *Mycobacterium intracellular*, MIC 1.72 and 2.29 mg/ml respectively. No synergy between garlic extract and any of four antituberculosis drugs (Isonazid, streptomycin, ethambutal, and rifampin) was observed[T14828]. Essential oil of fresh bulb on agar plate, and when administered intraperitoneally to guinea pig was active on *Mycobacterium tuberculosis*[K12811]. Ethanol (95%) extract of bulbs on agar plate was inactive on *Mycobacterium tuberculosis*[W00143].

Antinematocidal activity. Water, and methanol extracts of dried bulbs on agar plate at a concentration of 10.0 mg/ml produced weak activity on *Toxacara canis*[M29965].

Antioxidant activity. Ethanol/water (1:1) extract of aged bulbs at a concentration of 0.15% produced 30.7% inhibition of low level chemiluminescence[K18314]. Fresh bulb at a concentration of 1.0% was active. The effect was seen at 120°F[K23506]. Hot water extract of aged bulbs at a concentration of 2.0 mg/ml was active vs hydrogen peroxide-induced LDH release and lipid peroxidation[K19194]. Powdered dried bulb was able to reduce radicals generated by Fenton reaction. Also had marked quenching effects on radicals present in cigarette smoke[K18618]. Resin of dried bulb at a concentration of 0.06% was inactive. Lard was used as a substrate in the antioxidant activity test[T09657]. Water extract of dried bulbs at a concentration of 10.0 mcg/ml was active against photo-induced, and superoxide radical mediated autoxidation of luminol. Photochemiluminescence method of detection was employed[K18619]. A concentration of 100.0 mcg/ml was active when tested in respect to the Cu^{2+}-iniated oxidation of low density lipoprotein. The extract showed dose-related oxidation-inhibiting effects[K19709].

Antiprotozoan activity. Fresh bulb juice, undiluted in broth culture was active on *Paramecium caudatum*[W03630].

Antispasmodic activity. Butanol extract of bulbs taken orally by 30 patients suffering from dyspepsia gave moderate to full relief in major symptoms, i.e., abdominal distension and discomfort, belching, and flatulence[T05141]. Water extract of bulbs at a concentration of 1.0 mg/ml was active on ureter[K15297]. Water extract of dried bulbs was active on guinea pig small intestine. The biological activity was highly dose-dependent vs ACh-, barium- and histamine-induced contractions[P00078].

Antispermatogenic effect. Dried bulbs, administered by gastric intubaion to male rats at a dose of 50.0 mg/animal daily for 45 and 70 days, caused spermatogenesis arrest at primary spermatocyte stage. The spermatogenesis arrest is claimed to be a secondary result of hypoglycemia-hypolipidemia[T05241]. Undiluted essential oil administered by

inhalation to male rats was inactive[W03098]. Water extract in the drinking water of mice at a dose of 100.0 mg/kg was inactive[T16647].

Antithiamine activity. Fresh bulb juice was active. The activity was heat stable[T08856].

Antithrombotic effect. Fresh bulb extract, administered intravenously to dogs at a dose of 1.0 ml/animal was active. Cyclic flow reductions in an artificially stenosed coronary artery were inhibited by administration of the extract. This is attributed to inhibition of cyclic thrombus formation/embolization. Epinephrine reversed this effect[T16537].

Antitoxic activity. Butanol extract of dried bulbs in the ration of rats at a dose of 6.7% of the diet was active vs cadmium toxicity[T08608]. Dried bulbs in the ration of rats at a concentration of 6.7% of the diet for 10 weeks was active vs methyl/mercury poisoning[T13208]. Dosing for 12 weeks lowered the effects of cadmium poisoning[T10469]. Butanol extract given for 12 weeks caused detoxication on phenylmercury poisoning[T10486]. Essential oil, administered by gastric intubation to rat at a dose of 100.0 mg/kg was active. The dose prevented the ethanol induced serum cholesterol and triglyceride rise, kidney and liver cholesterol accumulation, hepatic total lipid rise, and serum albumin reduction vs ethanol-induced hyperlipemia[T09341]. Fixed oil of fresh bulb, in the ration of rat at a concentration of 1.5% of the diet was active. The extract ameliorates pancreatic weight loss in animals on fructose and Cu-deficient diet[K08961]. Fresh bulb, administered intragastrically to mice at a dose of 100.0 mg/kg was active. The frequency of chromosomal aberrations was significantly lower in animals maintained on crude plant extract during exposure to sodium arsenite as compared to those treated with arsenite alone[K15986]. Ethanol (70%) extract of fresh bulb, administered intraperitoneally to mice at a dose of 50.0 mg/kg was active vs cyclophosphamide-induced toxicity. 77% ILS[T16322]. Butanol extract of dried bulb, administered by gastric intubation to rats at a dose of 0.25 gm/ kg was active on liver, pancreas, and heart vs isoprenaline-induced tissue necrosis[M20887].

Antitumor activity. Butanol extract of dried bulbs in the ration of mice at a dose of 0.6 gm/day was active on CA-Ehrlich-ascites. Results significant at $P < 0.001$ level[T08244]. Dried bulbs in the ration of mice was active on Sarcoma 180 (solid)[T05331]. Ethanol (95%) extract of bulb, administered intraperitoneally to rats at a dose of 50.0 mg/ kg, produced weak activity on Sarcoma III(MTK)[A05572]. Fresh bulb taken orally by human adults at variable dosage levels was active. Interviews with 564 patients with stomach cancer and 1131 controls revealed a significant reduction in gastric cancer risk with increasing consumption of *Allium sativum*[M18229]. Plant in the ration of female mice produced complete inhibition of spontaneous leukemia in C3H mice[A05467]. Water extract of bulbs administered intraperitoneally to mice at variable dosage levels produced weak activity on CA-Ehrlich-Ascites[A04440], and on tumor system[T05321]. Water extract of bulbs administered intravenously to mice was active on Sarcoma 180(ASC)[A03177]. Water extract of fresh bulb, administered intraperitoneally to mice at a dose of 50.0 mg/animal daily for five days was active on CA-Ehrlich ascites, 17% ILS and Dalton's lymphoma, 9.1% ILS. Intragastrically administration was active on CA-Erhlich ascites, 41% ILS[M23595].

Antitumor-promoting activity. Essential oil, applied externally to female mice at a dose of 1.0 mg/animal was active vs twice weekly 12-o-tetradecanoyl-phorbol-13-acetate-promotion (two weeks) followed by mezerein promotion (two weeks) followed by mezerein promotion (18 weeks). The dose given with second promoter gave 24% decrease in incidence of papilloma[M24720]. Ethyl acetate extract of fresh bulb in cell culture at a concentration of 100.0 mcg/ml was active on HELA cells, and a concentration

of 5.0 mg/animal, administered externally to mice was active vs 12-0-tetra-decanoyl-phorbol-13-acetate-induced tumor promotion[M20094]. The hot water extract in cell culture produced weak activity on RAJI cells vs phorbol myristate acetate-promoted expression of EB virus early antigen[K11079]. Fresh bulb applied externally at a dose of 0.1 ml/animal twice daily for 3 days every week before once per week application of DMBA, for 25 weeks. The incidence of tumors was decreased to 31.8% from 73.9% vs DMBA-induced carcinogenesis[M25494]. Water extract of fresh bulb applied externally to mice at a concentration of 200.0 microliters/animal was active vs DMBA and croton oil treatment[M23595]. Fresh bulb, in the ration of Syrian hamsters at a dose of 10.0% of the diet was active vs DMBA-induced carcinogenesis[M24837]. Hot water extract of fresh bulb applied externally to mice at a dose of 1.0 mg/animal was active. Phorbol myristate acetate followed by dose of compound 30 min later. This promotion regime is repeated three times weekly for 47–60 weeks vs DMBA-induced carcinogenesis[T16143].

Antitussive activity. Fresh bulb taken orally by human adults at variable dosage levels was active[A14981]. Lyophilized extract of dried bulb inhaled by children, at a dose of 1.0% was effective against respiratory tract diseases[T12684].

Antiulcer activity. Fresh bulb taken orally by human adults at variable dosage levels was active[A14981].

Antiviral activity. Commercial sample of bulbs in cell culture at a concentration of 0.15 mg/ml was active on Herpes Simplex 1 virus, Influenza virus B (Lee), and Coxsackie B1 virus, and HELA cells. Results significant at $P < 0.001$ level[T12680]. Dried bulb in cell culture was active on Cytomegalovirus[K11293]. Fresh bulb pulp in cell culture at a concentration of 1000 mg/ml produced weak activity on Herpes Simplex 1 and 2 viruses, Parainfluenza virus 3, Vaccina virus Elstree and Vesicular Stomatitis virus[K08754].

Antiyeast activity. Amino acid fraction of dried bulb in ream form, 11% essential oil in gel, essential oil in wound healing powder, Ethanol/Chloroform (25%) extract on agar plate, and water extract at a concentration of 0.313% in broth culture were active on *Candida albicans*[P00110,P00123]. Juice on agar plate at a concentration of 0.333% was active on *Candida guilliermondii, C. parapsilosis, C. tropicalis, C. albicans, C. stellatoidea,* and *C. krusei*[P00042]. A concentration of 2.0% was active on *Saccharomyces cerevisiae*[P00089]. Concentrations of 0.0625, 0.125, and 0.25% in broth culture were active on *Candida albicans*[P00145]. *Candida krusei, Candida tropicalis, Cryptococcus neoformans, Candida albicans, Candida parapsilosis, Candida stellatoidea, Cryptococcus albidus, Candida glabrata,* and *Candida guilliermondii*. A fresh extract of garlic administered orally to human volunteers at a dose of 10–25 ml/person produced weak activity. At intervals, serum and urine were collected and assayed for antifungal activity. The maximum tolerance dose of the extract was determined to be 25 ml. Larger amounts caused severe burning sensations in the stomach and esophagus, and vomiting. After oral ingestion of the extract, anticandidal and anticryptococcal activities were detected in undiluted serum 0.5 and 1 hour after ingestion. No activity was found at comparable times in the urine. It was concluded that oral garlic is of limited value in the therapy of human fungal infections[N16937]. Dried oleoresin on agar plate at a concentration of 500.0 ppm was active on *Debaryomyces hansenii* vs ascospore production and *Rhodotorula rubra* vs pseudomycelium production; inactive on *Candida lipolytica, Hansenula anomala, Lodderomyces elongisporus, Saccharomyces cerevisiae* and *Torulopsis glabrata* vs pseudomycelium and ascospore production. In broth culture, a concentration of 50.0 ppm was active on *Debaryomyces hansenii* and *Hansenula*

anomala, and at 500.0 ppm was active on *R. rubra* and *S. cerevisiae* vs biomass production. Inactive on *Candida lipolytica, Kloeckera apiculata, Lodderomyces elongisporus* and *Torulopsis glabrata* vs biomass production[T15123]. Essential oil of dried bulb on agar plate was active on *Candida albicans*[P00110]. Essential oil, undiluted on agar plate was active on *Candida albicans* and *C. monosa*[T01551]. Ethyl acetate extract of fresh bulb, on agar plate, was active on *Cryptococcus neoformans*. MIC 6.1 mcg/ml[K18841]. Water extract on agar plate, at a concentration of 5.0 mg/ml was active on *Candida parapsilosis, C. tropicalis* and inactive on *C. albicans*[M21145]. Water extract, administered intragastrically to mice at a dose of 0.5 ml/animal produced weak activity on *Cryptococcus neoformans*[M21145]. Fresh bulb juice, undiluted on agar plate was active on *Candida albicans*[W04024]. Fresh bulb on agar plate was inactive on *Candida stellatoide* MIC 1000 mcg/ml and *C. albicans* MIC 470.0 mcg/ml. Chloroform extract was inactive on *C. albicans* MIC > 6.0 mg/ml[T16401]. Water extract in broth culture was active on *C. pseudotropicalis, C. tropicalis* and *C. albicans* MIC 0.8 mg/ml[M17845]. Tincture of dried bulb on agar plate, at a concentration of 30.0 microliters/disk (10 gm plant material in 100 ml ethanol) was active on *Candida albicans*[T15445]. Methanol/water (1:1) extract of dried bulbs on agar plate, was active on *Candida albicans*[T16068]. Water extract of dried bulbs on agar plate produced weak activity on *Candida albicans* and *Saccharomyces cerevisiae*[T07185]. Water extract of fresh bulb in cell culture was active on *Candida albicans*, MIC 0.8 mg/ml[M22069]. Water extract of fresh bulb, undiluted, was active on *Candida albicans, C. guilliermondii, C. krushei, C. parapsilosis, C. stellatoidea,* and *C. tropicalis*[M17090]. Water extract, and chromatographic fraction of bulbs on agar plate was active on *Candida albicans*[M01499]. Undiluted bulb juice on agar plate was active on *Trichosporum capitatum,*

Candida pseudotropicalis, 39 mm zone of inhibition; *Candida rugosa, Candida stellatoidea, Candida tropicalis, Candida krusei*, 40 mm zone of inhibition; *Cryptococcus neoformans, Cryptococcus laurentii, Rhodotorula rubra, Trichosporon pullulans*, 37 mm zone of inhibition; *Cryptococcus terreus, Cryptococcus uniguttulatus, Candida albicans*, 36 mm zone of inhibition; *Candida guilliermondi, Candida tenuis*, 38 mm zone of inhibition, *Torulopsis glabrata*, 43 mm zone of inhibition; *Torulopsis candida, Torulopsis inconspicua*, 45 mm zone of inhibition[M01497]. Ethanol/water (1:1) extract of dried bulb on agar plate at a concentration of 417.0 and 500.0 mg/ml (expressed as dry weight of bulb) was inactive on *Candida albicans* and *Saccharomyces pastorianus*[T12725].

Arichidonate metabolism inhibition. Ethanol (95%) extract at a concentration of 40.0 mcg/ml and water extract at a concentration of 20.0 microliters, in cell culture, were active on platelets[M23138].

Ascaricidal activity. Ether, and ethanol (20%) extracts of bulb were active on *Ascaris lumbricoides*[W03633].

Aspartate aminotransferase induction. Essential oil administered intragastrically to rat at a dose of 0.067 mg/gm was active. Water extract of fresh bulb administered intragastrically to rats at a dose of 0.02 ml/gm was active[M23270].

ATP-ase (Na⁺/K⁺) inhibition. Aqueous (dialyzed) fraction of fresh bulbs, at a concentration of 0.49 units was active on the skin of toad. The extract was applied to the inner (serosal) surface of the skin. One unit of activity had the effect of one micromolar amiloride[M26051].

ATPase stimulation. Water extract of fresh bulb at a concentration of 5.0 mg/ml was active[T00032].

Bacterial stimulant activity. Dried oleoresin in broth culture was inactive on *Lactobacillus plantarum*. Fresh bulb in broth culture at a concentration of 1.0 gm/liter

was active on *Lactobacillus plantarum*. Powdered dried bulbs in broth culture, at a concentration of 5.0 gm/lites was active on *Lactobacillus plantarum*[T15207].

Barbiturate potentiation. Ethanol (95%) extract of bulb, administered intraperitoneally to male mice at a dose of 500.0 mg/kg was inactive[T01360].

Blood system effects. Butanol extract of fresh bulb, taken orally by human adults at a dose of 25.0 mg/day was active. An 87-year-old man presented with paralysis of the lower extremities. A spinal mass proved to be a spontaneous spinal epidural hematoma. The hematoma was removed and the patient recovered adequately. The hematoma was attributed to the man's high consumption of garlic (four cloves/day), as no other potential causes were found. Bleeding time during surgery was 11 minutes (three minutes normal) and prothrombin time was 12.3 seconds[M24904].

Blood viscosity decrease. Dried bulbs taken orally by 120 volunteers, with "probably increased thrombocyte aggregation", at a dose of 800.0 mg/person continued for four weeks in double-blind and placebo-controlled study. Plasma viscosity decreased by 3.2% vs control[T16354].

Body weight loss inhibition. Butanol extract of dried bulb administered intragastrically to rats at a dose of 1.0 gm/kg was active[M20887].

Bradycardia activity. Oven-dried bulb administered to dog by gastric intubation at a dose of 15.0 mg/kg was active. The action returned to normal after 15 minutes[T16338]. Water extract of dried leaves administered intravenously to cats and rats at a dose of 5–20 mg/kg produced weak activity[T09217].

Carcinogenesis inhibition. Dried bulb in the ration of rats at a concentration of 2.0% of the diet was active. Rats were fed the treatment diet for 20 weeks. The tumor incidence decreased from 85% to 40%, and the total number of tumors decreased from 41 to 18. In addition the binding of DMBA to DNA decreased significantly vs carcinogenesis induced by 7,12-dimethylbenz(a)anthracene[K08373]. Ethanol (20%) extract of six or seven dried cloves taken orally by 16 human adults daily for three months was inactive[K15055]. Essential oil, applied externally to mice at a dose of 0.01 mg/animal, was active vs phorbol myristate acetate induced carcinogenesis of mouse skin[T09455]. Ethanol (95%) extract of dried bulb in the drinking water of rats at a dose of 3.0 mg/ml for nine weeks was inactive. Hepatocarcinogenesis was induced by diethylnitrosamine[K15338]. Fresh bulb administered intragastrically to mice at a dose of 400.0 mg/kg, dosed two weeks before and four weeks following application of carcinogen, was active vs 3-methylcholanthrene-induced carcinogenesis in the uterine cervix[M22643]. Essential oil of fresh bulb applied externally to mice at a dose of 100.0 microliters/animal was active vs benzo(a)pyrene induced skin carcinogenesis. 10% garlic oil in acetone and croton oil was also applied[M19282]. Fresh bulb administered intragastrically to toad at a dose of 0.1 ml was active vs aflatoxin B1-induced carcinogenesis (lung and kidney). Garlic oil, 0.1 ml dissolved in 1 ml of corn oil, was administered for four months. The tumor incident decreased to 9%, which was originally 19% without the treatment. A dose of 20.0 mg/day was active vs aflatoxin B1-induced carcinogenesis (lung and kidney). Fresh garlic was administered for four months. The tumor incident decreased to 3% which was originally 19% without the garlic treatment[K15056]. Fresh bulb administered orally to hamsters at a dose of 0.5%/animal was active. The extract was painted on the mucosa three times/week for three weeks. Eleven weeks later, DMBA (0.5%) was painted for 10 weeks. Six weeks later, animals were sacrificed. Controls were painted with extract for 30 weeks. Mineral oil was used as vehicle for the extract vs DMBA-induced carcinogenesis[M24722]. Powdered fresh bulb in the ration of rat at a dose of 20.0 gm/kg was active. Tumor incidence was reduced from 84 to 56%. Tumor incidence in rats fed selenium enriched *Allium sativum* were reduced from 92 to 36% vs DMBA-induced carcinogenesis[K07155]. Water extract of fresh bulb administered by cheek pouch in mice was active vs 7,12-dimethylbenz(A)anthracene-induced carcinogenesis[M30049].

Cardiotonic activity. Chloroform extract of dried bulb contained at least two active elements. One was chloroform soluble, and had an antiseptic action, a slight tonic effect on isolated frog heart, a slight hypertensive effect on etherized cats and a paralyzing effect on isolated rabbit intestine. The chloroform-insoluble fraction had no antiseptic effect, no action on isolated frog heart, a strongly hypotensive effect on etherized cats and a tonic effect on isolated rabbit intestine[W03661].

Cardiotoxic activity. Essential oil of dried bulb, administered intragastrically to rats, at a dose of 2.0 gm/kg for 30 days was active. Animals were maintained on normal diet while given the essential oil, then observed for 30 days. ECG showed flattened T-wave and depressed ST segment during the dosing period. The changes persisted after garlic withdrawal, indicating possible permanent coronary ischemic damage in 8 of 10 animals[T15177]. Ether extract of dried bulb was active on frog heart. Effect is not reversed by norepinephrine and only partially reversed by caffeine of atropine[A12824].

Cardiovascular effects. Water extract of dried leaves, administered intravenously to cats and rats at a dose of 5–20 mg/kg, did not produced any appreciable alteration of ECG pattern[T09217].

Carminative activity. Dried bulb taken orally at a dose of 0.64 gm/person was active. In a series of 29 patients complaining of heaviness after eating, belching, gas colic, flatulence and nausea, two garlic tablets were given twice daily after lunch and dinner for a period of two weeks. A clinical investigation of dehydrated garlic showed this comparative to be highly effective for relief of heaviness after eating (epigastric and abdominal distress), belching, flatulence, gas colic, and nausea. Satisfactory therapeutic results were obtained in cases of flatulent dyspepsia, nervous dyspepsia and other gastric neuroses. Roentgenographically, a comparison of films with and without the medication showed that dehydrated garlic has a sedative effect on the stomach and intestines, relaxes spasms, retards hyperperistalis, and disperses accumulation of gas. It is believed that these studies explained the carminative action of garlic as caused by unidentified principles that have been designated as gastroenteric allichalcone. Since dehydrated garlic tablets are safe for long continued use, they may be indicated in a wide variety of functional disturbances of the stomach and intestines[W03626].

Carnithine acetyl-coenzyme A transferase induction. Methanol extract of fresh bulb in cell culture, at a concentration 0.5 mg/ml, was active on rat hepatocytes[M31064].

Catecholamine-releasing effect. Fixed oil of fresh bulb, administered intragastrically to rabbit was active vs cholesterol-fed animals[T15709].

Cell proliferation inhibition. Water extract of bulb in cell culture was active on Morris hematoma[T09455]. Water extract of dried bulbs in cell culture at a concentration of 100.0 mcg/ml was active on LEUK-P388(ARA-C). Cells transformed by SV-40 were more sensitive[K16939].

Choleretic activity. Water extract of fresh bulb in the ration of rats at a dose of 2% was active[T14340].

Cholesterol acyltransferase inhibition. Water extract of dried bulb in cell culture at a concentration of 1000 mcg/ml was active

on hepatocytes[M28525]. Water extract of fresh bulb at a dose of 1.0 g/kg in the ration of rabbit was active[T16431].

Cholesterol inhibition. Plant in the ration of rabbits was active[K03712]. Unripe fruit juice, administered orally to cholesterol fed male rabbits was active[K01311]. Water extract of dried bulb at a concentration of 20.0 microliters/insect was active on *Lohita grandis*[T11324].

Cholesterol level decrease. Dried garlic taken by human adults of both sexes, at a dose of 200.0 mg/person was active. Garlic-ginkgo combination tablets produced improvement in cholesterol, with no concurrent dietary or exercise changes[K19358].

Cholesterol synthesis inhibition. Chloroform, and chloroform/acetone extracts of fresh bulb, at concentrations of 166.0 mcg/ml were active on liver homogenates. Synthesis was inhibited 52.1 and 44.4% respectively[K07482]. Fresh bulb in cell culture was active on Hepatoma-HEP-G-2, IC_{50} 35.0 mcg/ml, and on rat hepatocytes, IC_{50} 90.0 mcg/ml. This inhibition was exerted at the level of hydroxymethylglutaryl-Co A reductase (HMG-Co A reductase) as indicated by direct enzymatic measurements and the absence of inhibition[K12841]. Water extract in cell culture was active on hepatocytes[M28525]. Water, methanol, and petroleum ether extracts of dried bulb at concentrations of 50.0 gm/liter were active on rat hepatocytes[K16381].

Cholesterol-7-Alpha-hydroxylase inhibition. Methanol extract of fresh bulb in the ration of pigs at a concentration of 3.15 gm/kg of diet for 29 days was active. Hepatic enzymes assayed and 40% inhibition was observed[M18549]. Water extract of bulbs in the ration of chicken of both sexes, at a concentration of 6.0% of the diet for three weeks was active[T06975]. Water extract of dried bulb in cell culture at a concentration of 1000 mcg/ml was active on hepatocytes[M28525].

Cholinesterase inhibition. Water extract of fresh bulb at a concentration of 5.0 mg/ml was active[T00032].

Chromosome aberration induced. Water extract of fresh bulb administered intragastrically to mice at a dose of 100.0 mg/kg daily for seven days was active on bone marrow[K11596]. Water extract of fresh bulb administered intragastrically to mice at a dose of 100.0 mg/kg was active on bone marrow cells vs sodium arsenite-, mitomycin- and cyclophosphamide-induced aberration[K11596].

Chronotropic effect negative. Water extract of fresh bulb, at a concentration of 0.1 mcg/kg was active on rat atria. When administered intravenously to dogs at a dose of 67.2 mg/kg, it was active[K11288].

Chronotrophic effect positive. Essential oil of dried bulbs, administered intragastrically to rats at a dose of 2.0 gm/kg was active during treatment and returned to normal after withdrawal. Animals maintained on normal diet were given essential oil for 30 days, then observed for 30 days[T15177]. Ethanol/water (1:1) extract of fresh bulb, administered by gastric intubation to rats at a dose of 40.0 ml/kg was inactive[T10632]. Fresh bulb juice, administered intravenously to rats at a dose of 0.5 ml/animal was active. There was a slight decrease in the P-R interval of the ECG[T08861].

Citrate lyase stimulation. Methanol extract of fresh bulb in the ration of pigs, at a concentration of 3.15 gm/kg of diet for 29 days was active. Hepatic enzymes were assayed[M18549].

CNS depressant activity. Ethanol (70%) extract of fresh bulb, administered intraperitoneally to mice of both sexes at variable dosage levels was active[T06510]. Ethanol (95%) extract of bulb administered intraperitoneally to male mice at a dose of 500.0 mg/kg was inactive[T01360].

Coagulant activity. Essential oil administered by gastric intubation to male rabbits at a dose of 1.0 g/kg for three months was active. Increased coagulation time was observed. Results significant at P < 0.001 level[M00151]. Water extract of fresh bulb was active[M30030].

Conditioned avoidance response increased. Ethanol (95%) extract of bulbs administered intragastrically to mice at a dose of 250.0 mg/kg was active vs alcohol-induced deficits in acquisition and performance of "step-through" test[M17484].

Corticosteroid type activity. Ethyl acetate extract of fresh bulb administered intramuscularly to rats daily for four days produced up to four times the normal 24 hour 17-keto steroid elimination[W04023].

Cyclo-oxygenase inhibition. Methanol extract of dried bulbs at variable concentrations was inactive vs ADP-, arachidonic acid-, epinephrine- and thrombin-induced aggregation[T07890]. Chloroform extract of bulbs administered to ewe at variable dosage levels produced weak activity on platelets[T05330]. Chloroform, and chloroform-acetone extracts of fresh bulb were active, IC_{50} 0.88 and 0.42 mcg/ml respectively[T16651]. Fresh bulb was active vs DMBA-induced carcinogenesis[T16143]. The ether-soluble fraction of methanol extract of fresh bulb at concentration 100.0 mcg/ml produced 50% inhibition on rat platelet, and the ether-insoluble fraction produced 5% inhibition[K12822].

Cytochrome B-5 reductase inhibition. Water extract of fresh bulb was active on liver microsomes[T16599].

Cytochrome C reductase inhibition. Methanol extract of fresh bulb in cell culture at a concentration of 1.0 mg/ml was inactive on rat hepatocytes[M31064].

Cytochrome oxidase induction. Essential oil of dried bulbs was inactive on *Macaronesia fortunata* and *Musca domestica*[W04295].

Cytochrome oxidase inhibition. Essential oil of dried bulbs was inactive on *Macaronesia fortunata* and *Musca domestica*[W04295].

Cytochrome P-450 inhibition. Water extract of fresh bulb was active on liver microsomes[T16599].

Cytotoxic activity. Acetone extract of dried bulb at a concentration of 5.0% by the cylinder plate method was equivocal on CA-Ehrlich-Ascites, 21 mm inhibition. Ether extract produced weak activity –40 mm inhibition; water extract, equivocal –20 mm inhibition; methanol extract, weak activity –40 mm inhibition[W03044]. Ethanol (90%) extract of dried bulb in cell culture at a concentration of 0.5 mg/ml was active on human lymphocytes; Vero cells ED_{50} 0.155 mg/ml; Chinese hamster ovary cells (CHO) ED_{50} 0.275 mg/ml; and Dalton's Lymphoma ED_{50} 0.5 mg/ml[M16771]. Ethanol (95%) extract of fresh bulb administered intragastrically to mice at a dose of 500.0 mg/kg produced weak activity. The animals were dosed for five days followed by sacrificing the animals and examination of marrow cells[M23016]. Fresh bulb at a concentration of 200.0 mg/ml was active on rat liver. On perfusion through a liver preparation, diallyl disulfide and allyl mercaptan were the metabolites of garlic extract. Allicin did not appear in perfusate unless the concentration of extract became toxic[K08304]. Fresh bulb pulp in cell culture at a concentration of 11.0 mg/ml was active on HELA cells, and 3.5 mg/ml active on VERO cells[K08754]. Protein fraction of dried bulbs in cell culture at a concentration of 10.0 mcg/ml was active on human lymphocytes; 5.0 mcg/ml active on LEUK-K562 and melanoma-M14, cytotoxicity was enhanced with IL-2[K14894]. Water extract of dried bulb in cell culture at a concentration of 500.0 mcg/ml produced weak activity on CA-Mammary-Microalveolar[M26592], and Fibroblast-Human-Lung-MRC-5[K11293]. Water extract of freeze-dried bulb in cell culture was inactive on LEUK-P815. Tumor toxic activity was evaluated by culturing mastocytoma P815 cells with macrophage cells and measuring the incorporation of 3H-thimidine radioactivity[M27208].

Death. Essential oil applied externally to mice at a dose of 10.0 mg/animal was active[T09455].

Dermatitis producing effect. Butanol extract of fresh bulb applied topically to human adults was active in 34 patients who developed contact dermatitis after exposure to Allium sativum[K10596]. Dried bulb taken orally by male human adults, in a double-blind oral provocation test to garlic tablets was active[K18264]. Fresh bulb applied externally to three males presented with bulbous eruptions on the arms and legs was active. On questioning two of the subjects revealed that they had repeatedly rubbed crushed garlic onto the affected areas in hopes of inducing dermatitis in order to elude their military assignments[T16165].

Desmutagenic activity. Aqueous high speed supernatant of fresh fruit juice, at a concentration of 0.5 ml/plate on agar plate was inactive on Salmonella typhimurium TA98 vs mutagenicity of L-tryptophan pyrolysis products. The assay was done in the presence of S9 mix[T12543].

Diuretic activity. Ethanol/water (1:1) extract of fresh bulb (five parts plant material in 100 parts ethanol/water) administered intragastrically to rats at a dose of 40.0 ml/kg was active[M17736]. Oven-dried bulb administered by gastric intubation to dog at a dose of 10.0 mg/kg was active[T16338]. Water extract of dried bulb administered intragastrically to rats at a dose of 5.0 gm/kg was inactive[M21416].

DNA repair induction. Water extract of fresh bulb, at a concentration of 20.0 microliters/ml was active[M20451].

DNA synthesis inhibition. Ethanol (90%) extract of dried bulb, at a concentration of 1.0 mg/ml was active[M16771].

DNA-binding inhibition. Dried bulb in the ration of rats at a concentration of 1.0%, water extract at a concentration of 0.75%, and ethanol (95%) extract at a concentration of 0.015% of the diet for two weeks prior to DMBA exposure were active vs dimethyl-bene[A]anthracene binding to mammary cell DNA[K13503].

Dopamine-beta-hydroxylase stimulation. Fixed oil of fresh bulb administered intragastrically to rabbit at a dose of 5.0 mg/kg was active[T15709].

Early antigen viral induction inhibition. Dried bulb in cell culture was active on Cytomegalovirus[K11293].

Embryotoxic effect. Ethanol (95%) extract of seeds at doses of 150.0 and 200.0 mg/kg, and petroleum ether extract at a dose of 100.0 mg/kg administered orally to female rats[W01362]; and a dose of 150.0 mg/kg administered by gastric intubation to pregnant rats were inactive[T05679].

Enzyme effects. Ethanol (95%) extract of dried bulbs administered by gastric intubation to male rats at a dose of 100.0 mg/kg for 25 days was active. Adipose tissue triglyceride lipase increased. Results significant at P < 0.01 level[T08094].

Estrogenic effect. Bulb juice administered orally to immature rats at a dose of 10.0 ml/kg produced weak activity[M00151]. Ethanol (95%) extract of dried bulb administered subcutaneously to ovariectomized rats at a dose of 2.0 mg/animal was active[W03436]. Water extract of fresh bulb administered intraperitoneally to female mice at a dose of 500.0 mg/day was inactive[T16647]. Water extract of bulbs administered subcutaneously to infant mice was active[W01848].

Ethanol elimination increased. Ethanol (95%) extract of bulbs administered intragastrically to mice at a dose of 125.0 mg/kg was active. Lowered blood alcohol levels relative to controls when administered simultaneously with alcohol, but not 30 minutes before alcohol[M17484].

Ethoxycoumarin deethylase inhibition. Water extract of fresh bulb was active on liver microsomes[T16599].

Fatty acid content decrease. Powdered dried bulb in the ration of rats, at a concentration of 1.0% of the diet for 10 weeks did not alter fatty acid composition of myocardial membrane[K10232].

Fatty acid synthase inhibition. Water extract of bulbs in the ration of chicken of both sexes, at a concentration of 6.0% of the diet for three weeks was active hepatocytes[T06975]. Water extract of dried bulb in cell culture at a concentration of 1000 mcg/ml was active on hepatocytes[M28525].

Fatty acid synthase stimulation. Methanol extract of fresh bulb in the ration of pigs at a concentration of 3.15 g/kg of the diet for 29 days was active. Hepatic enzymes were assayed[M18549].

Fatty acid synthesis inhibition. Water, methanol, and petroleum ether extracts of dried bulb at concentrations of 50.0 gm/liter were active on rat hepatocytes. If oleate was present, incorporation of labeled glycerol into triglycerides and phospholipids was not inhibited[K16381].

Fibrinolytic activity. Butanol extract of dried bulb taken orally by human adults was active in the blood of patients with alimentary lipemia. Juice in the ration of rabbits was active[T07883]. Dried bulb taken orally by human adults at a dose of 300.0 mg/person three times daily for two weeks to seven healthy males increased specific tissue plasminogen activator[K11043]. Dried bulb taken orally by human adults at a dose of 600.0 mg/person for four weeks was active[M19432]. Essential oil of bulb administered by gastric intubation to male rabbits at a dose of 1.0 gm/kg for three months caused a decrease in fibrinolytic activity. Results significant at P < 0.001 level[T08093]. Ether extract administered by gastric intubation to rats in a feeding study at doses of 2–4 gm crude garlic daily for three weeks was active[T05223]. Essential oil taken orally by human adults of both sexes at a dose equivalent to 1.0 g/kg of raw garlic daily for three months, was active[T01673]. The essential oil, taken orally, was also active in 30 patients with myocardial infarct and 10 normal (controls)[L02488]. Fresh bulb taken orally by human adults at a dose of 0.5 gm/kg was active. The study was conducted with 20 patients with ischemic heart disease. Fibrinolytic activity increased by 72% within six hours after administration and persisted for 12 hours[T06238]. Butanol extract of fresh bulb taken orally by human adults[T01193], and water extract in the ration of rabbit[T16431] at doses of 1.0 g/kg were active. Fried bulb taken orally by human adults at a dose of 0.5 gm/kg was active in 20 patients with ischemic heart disease. Fibrinolytic activity increased by 63% within six hours after administration and persisted for 12 hours[T06238]. Water extract of fresh bulb was active[M30030].

Food consumption reduction. Dried bulb, together with *Panax ginseng* and Vitamin B1 administered by gastric intubation to rats at a dose 10.0 ml/kg for three months was equivocal. Food consumption was lowered after 2–5 weeks, however, body weight gain was good[T11284].

Fungal stimulant. Butanol extract of fresh bulb on agar plate at variable concentration was inactive on *Bacillus subtilis* M-45 (Rec-)[T07988]. Dried bulb juice on agar plate at a concentration of 2.0% was active on *Absidia spinosa*, *Drechslera maydis*, *Pleurotus ostreatus* and *Sordaria fimicola*[P00089].

Gastric antisecretory activity. Dried bulb taken orally by human adults was inactive[W04661].

Gastric inhibitory polypeptide stimulation. Bulb in the ration of rabbits and rats was active vs cholesterol-loaded animals[T05226].

Gastric mucosal exfoliant activity. Water extract of fresh bulb administered to human adults by gastric intubation at a dose of 0.75 gm/person was active[M24843].

Gastric secretory stimulation. Dried bulb taken orally by human adults was inactive[W04661].

Genotoxicity activity. Bulbs administered by gastric intubation to mice at doses of 2.5 and 5.0 gm/kg were inactive on bone marrow cells[T07727].

Germ tube growth inhibition. Water extract of fresh bulb in cell culture at a concentra-

tion of 0.4 mg/ml was active on *Candida albicans*[M22069].

Glucose utilization stimulation. Protein fraction of bulb at a concentration of 100.0 mcg/ml was active on macrophages[T14866].

Glucose-6-Phosphate Dehydrogenase inhibition. Bulbs in the ration of four months old male rats at concentrations of 2.0 and 4.0% of the diet was active in cholesterol-loaded and lard fed animals. Results significant at P < 0.05 level[T05330]. Methanol extract of fresh bulb in the ration of pigs at a concentration of 3.15 gm/kg of the diet for 29 days was active. Hepatic enzymes were assayed[M18549]. Dried bulb in the ration of male rats at a concentration of 5.0% of the diet was active[K17621]. Fixed oil of fresh bulb in the ration of rats at a concentration of 1.5% of the diet was active. The extract ameliorated increased in enzyme activity seen in animals fed fructose and Cu-adequate diet[K08961].

Glucose-6-phosphate dehydrogenase stimulation. Butanol extract of dried bulb administered intragastrically to rats at a dose of 0.5 gm/kg was active on heart, liver and pancreas vs isoprenaline-induced tissue necrosis[M20887].

Glutamate dehydrogenase stimulation. Methanol extract of fresh bulb in cell culture at a concentration of 1.0 mg/ml was inactive on rat hepatocytes[M31064].

Glutamate oxaloacetate inhibition. Water extract of fresh bulb at a concentration of 10.0 mg/ml was active[T00032].

Glutamate oxaloacetate transaminase inhibition. Essential oil and ether extract of dried bulb administered by gastric intubation to rats at a dose of 5.0 mg/kg for three days was active vs galactosamine-induced toxicity[T10949].

Glutamate oxaloacetate transminase stimulation. Essential oil of dried bulb administered orally to rats at a dose of 5.0 mg/kg for three days produced weak activity. Ether extract was inactive[T10949].

Glutamate pyruvate inhibition. Water extract of fresh bulb at a concentration of 5.0 mg/ml was active[T00032].

Glutamate pyruvate transaminase inhibition. Essential oil and ether extract of dried bulb in cell culture, at a concentration of 1.0 mg/ml were inactive on rat hepatocytes. Essential oil administered by gastric intubation to rats at a dose of 5.0 mg/kg for three days was inactive. Ether extract administered orally at a dose of 5.0 mg/kg for three days was active vs galactosamine-induced toxicity[T10949].

Glutathione peroxidase inhibition. Lyophilized extract of fresh bulb in the ration of chicken, at a concentration of 2.0% of the diet was active[K07417].

Glutathione peroxidase stimulation. Butanol extract of dried bulbs at a concentration of 13.0 mcg/ml was active on rat liver microsomes. Juice administered by gastric intubation to rats at a dose of 5.0% of the diet for 25 days, was active in liver[T12183]. Dried bulbs in the ration of castrated rams, at a concentration of 5.0% of the diet was active[K17621].

Glutathione reductase stimulation. Dried bulbs in the ration of male rats at a concentration of 5.0% of the diet was active[K17621].

Glutathione transferase induction. Dried bulbs in the ration of male rats at a concentration of 5.0% of the diet was active[K17621].

Glutathione-S-transferase induction. Dried bulb in the ration of rats, at a concentration of 2.0% of the diet was active. Glutathione-D-transferase levels were 42% greater in rats fed the supplemented diet[K08373]. Dried bulb juice in the drinking water of rats at a dose of 5.0% of the diet for 25 days was active in liver[T12183].

Glutathione-S-transferase inhibition. Butanol extract of dried bulb at a concentration of 8.0 mcg/ml was active on rat liver microsomes[T12183].

GRAS status. Approved as generally recognized as a safe flavoring agent by the US Food and Drug Administration in 1976 (Sect. 582.10)[K00040].

Hair stimulant effect. Decoction of dried bulb in a mixture with *Polygonum multiflorum*, *Allium sativum*, *Zingiber officinale*, *Panax ginseng*, *Carthamus tinctorius*, *Platycodon grandiflorum*, *Biota orientalis*, *Ligusticum wallichii*, *Salvia miltiorrhiza*, *Angelica sinensis* and *Tetrapanax papyrifera* stimulate hair growth. The biological activity has been patented[K08554]. Decoction of fresh bulb together with extracts of *Polygonum multiflorum*, *Thuja orientalis*, *Zingiber officinale*, *Ligusticum wallichii*, *Salvia miltiorrhiza*, *Angelica sinensis*, *Carthamus tinctorius* and *Tetrapanax* species was active. The biological activity reported has been patented[K09587]. Fresh bulb juice applied topically to male mice at a concentration of 0.1 ml/liter was inactive[T06579].

Hematopoietic activity. Fixed oil of fresh bulb in the ration of rat at a concentration of 1.5% of the diet was active. The extract ameliorates decrease in hematocrit in animals on fructose and Cu-deficient diet[K08961].

Hepatotoxic activity. Dried bulb juice in the drinking water of rats at a dose of 5.0% of the diet for 25 days was inactive[T12183].

Histamine release inhibition. Ethanol (75%) extract of fixed oil in cell culture was active on human basophils. The biological activity has been patented[K21748].

HMG-CO-A inhibition. Water extract of bulbs in the ration of chicken of both sexes at a concentration of 6.0% of the diet for three weeks contained active hepatocytes[T06975].

HMG-CO-A reductase inhibition. Water extract of dried bulb in cell culture at a concentration of 50.0 mcg/ml was active on hepatocytes[M28525]. Methanol extract of fresh bulb in the ration of pigs at a concentration of 3.15 gm/kg of the diet for 29 days was active. Hepatic enzymes were assayed and 40% inhibition was observed[M18549].

Hypercholesterolemic activity. Bulb taken orally by human adults was active. Cholesterol levels were elevated in subjects on moderate or heavy amounts of onion,

50–100 gm, and garlic, 5–10 gm[K16146]. Dried bulb taken orally by human adults at a dose of 350.0 mg/person twice daily was inactive[M17987]. Essential oil of dried bulb administered intragastrically to rats at a dose of 2.0 gm/kg was active. Animals were maintained on normal diet and given essential oil for 30 days, then observed for 30 days. Cholesterol levels rose during garlic feeding and returned to normal after garlic withdrawal[T15177]. Ethanol (95%) extract of fresh bulb administered orally to male rabbits at a dose of 0.50 gm/animal for 16 weeks was active[T01904]. Fixed oil of fresh bulb in the ration of rat at a concentration of 1.5% of the diet was active. The extract was effective in animals fed fructose and Cu-deficient diet[K08961].

Hyperlipidemic activity. Dried bulb taken orally by human adults at a dose of 350.0 mg/person twice daily was inactive[P00123].

Hypertensive activity. Ethanol (95%) extract of bulbs administered to dogs and rats by injection at variable dosage levels were active[W03431]. Chloroform extract of dried bulbs administered intravenously to cats produced weak activity. The alcoholic extract contained at least two active elements. One was chloroform soluble and had an antiseptic action, a slight tonic effect on isolated frog heart, a slight hypertensive effect on etherized cats, and a paralyzing effect on isolated rabbit intestine. The chloroform-insoluble fraction had no antiseptic effect, no action on isolated frog heart, a strongly hypotensive effect on etherized cats and a tonic effect on isolated rabbit intestine[W03661].

Hypertriglyceridemia activity. Dried bulb taken orally by 24 human adults with reduced HDL cholesterol levels and hypertriglyceridemia, at a dose of 900.0 mg/day for six weeks, reduced triglyceride levels up to 35% and HDL cholesterol levels increased[K10150].

Hyperuremic activity. Essential oil administered intragastrically to rats after fasting

for 24 hours, at a dose of 0.067 mg/g was active[M23270]. Water extract of fresh bulb administered intragastrically to rats at variable dosage levels was active[T15939].

Hypocholesterolemic activity. Dried bulb administered by gastric intubation to male rats at a dose of 50.0 mg/animal daily for 70 days was active. Results significant at $P < 0.001$ level[T05241]. When administered for 45 days the dose was also active. Results significant at $P < 0.05$ level[T05241]. Dried bulb in the ration of rats at variable concentrations for 41 days was active[W04301]. Essential oil taken orally by human adults at a dose of 0.25 ml/person daily for 1–2 months was inactive[T06235]. Essential oil taken orally by human adults of both sexes, at a dose of 0.25 mg/kg was active. The study was conducted with 20 subjects having a normal serum cholesterol level. Garlic oil was consumed daily for 10 months[T05071]. Ether extract of bulbs administered by gastric intubation to rats in a feeding study at doses of 2–4 gm crude garlic daily for three days was inactive[T05223]. Water extract of bulbs taken orally by human adults at a dose of 0.5 ml/kg was active[L02154]. Fresh bulb taken orally by human adults at a dose of 4.0 ml/days was active[M23958]. Methanol extract of fresh bulb in the ration of pigs at a concentration of 3.15 gm/kg of the diet for 29 days was active. Serum total cholesterol plus LDL cholesterol decreased, and HDL cholesterol was anomalously high after 29 days of feeding[18549]. Lyophilized extract of fresh bulb in the ration of chicken at a concentration of 2.0% of the diet was active[K07417]. Powdered fresh bulb taken orally by human adults at a dose of 800.0 mg/day was active on 221 hypercholesterolemic patients given treatment for a total of 16 weeks. Serum cholesterol levels dropped 12%[M24883]. Water extract of bulbs in the ration of chicken of both sexes, at a concentration of 6.0% of the diet for three weeks was active[T06975]. Water extract of fresh bulb, taken orally by human adults with normal blood serum cholesterol levels, at a dose of 50.0 gm/person was inactive[T07866]. Fresh bulb taken orally by 25 healthy male adults (18–35 years), at a dose of 10.0 gm/person daily for two months, was active[T01426].

Hypoglycemic activity. Bulbs in the ration of 16-week-old male rats at concentrations of 2.0 and 4.0% of the diet was active in cholesterol-loaded and lard-fed animals. Results significant at $P < 0.05$ level[T05330]. Dried bulb administered by gastric intubation to male rats at a dose of 50.0 mg/animal for 45 and 70 days was active. Results significant at $P < 0.001$ level. Water extract of dried bulb administered orally to rabbits at a dose of 3.3 gm/kg daily for two months was active on sucrose-loaded animals (10 gm/kg/day). Statistical report indicated significant results[T02039]. Dried bulb taken orally by 120 human adults with "probably increased thrombocyte aggregation," at a dose of 800.0 mg/person for four weeks in a double-blind and placebo-controlled study was active. Average blood glucose fell by 11.6% vs control[T16354]. Essential oil taken orally by human adults at a dose of 0.25 ml/person daily for 1–2 months was inactive[T06235]. Essential oil administered intragastrically to rats was active[K10422]. Ethanol (95%) extract of bulbs administered by gastric intubation produced weak activity and petroleum ether extract was active[T04535]. Ether extract of bulbs administered by gastric intubation to rats in a feeding study at doses of 2–4 g crude garlic daily for three days was inactive[T05223].

Hypolipemic activity. Dried bulb administered by gastric intubation to male rats at a dose of 50.0 mg/animal for 45 was inactive, and active when administered for 70 days. Results significant at $P < 0.05$ level[T05241]. Dried bulb in the ration of rabbits prevented a rise in the levels of serum cholesterol for up to 60 days[T07883]. Essential oil administered by gastric intubation to rats at a dose of 100.0 mg/kg for 60 days was active.

The effects were measured in the liver. Results significant at $P < 0.01$ level vs ethanol-induced hyperlipemia[T09341]. Ethanol (95%) extract of dried bulbs administered by gastric intubation to male rats at a dose of 100.0 mg/kg for 25 days was active[T08094]. Fresh bulb taken orally by human adults at a dose of 4.0 ml/day was active[M23958]. Methanol extract of fresh bulb in the ration of pigs at a concentration of 3.15 gm/kg of diet was active[M18549].

Hypotensive activity. Dried bulb taken orally by 120 human adults with "probably increased thrombocyte aggregation," at a dose of 800.0 mg/person for four weeks in a double-blind and placebo-controlled study was active. Average diastolic pressure fell by 9.5% vs control[T16354]. Essential oil administered per rectum in human adults at a dose of 180.0 mg/person was active. The dose was given in conjunction with mistletoe, milfoil, horsetail, amylocaine, and chlorophyll. The biological activity has been patented[W04169]. Ethanol (95%) extract of bulbs administered to dogs and rabbits by injection at variable dosage levels were active[W03431]. Ethanol (95%), and water extracts of bulbs administered intravenously to dogs, guinea pigs, and rabbits were active[W03549]. Ethanol/water (1:1) extract of fresh bulb administered by gastric intubation to rats at a dose of 40.0 ml/kg was active. Results significant at $P < 0.05$ level[T10632]. Ether extract of dried bulb administered intravenously to rabbits at a dose of 4–8 ml/animal was active[A12824]. Chloroform extract of dried bulbs administered intravenously to cats was active. The alcoholic extract contained at least two active elements. One was chloroform soluble, and had an antiseptic action, a slight tonic effect on isolated frog heart, a slight hypertensive effect on etherized cats, and a paralyzing effect on isolated rabbit intestine. The chloroform-insoluble fraction had no antiseptic effect, no action on isolated frog heart, a strongly hypotensive effect on etherized cats and a tonic effect on isolated rabbit intestine[W03661]. Oven-dried bulb administered by gastric intubation to dog at a dose of 15.0 mg/kg was active. Gradual decrease was observed[T16338]. Water extract of dried leaves administered intravenously to cats and rats at a dose of 5–20 mg/kg produced weak activity[T09217]. Water extract of bulbs administered intravenously to cats at a dose of 0.05 gm/kg was active[A11518]. Water extract of fresh bulb administered intravenously to dog at a dose of 67.2 mg/kg was active[K11288].

Hypotriglyceridemia activity. Lyophilized extract of fresh bulb in the ration of chicken at a dose of 2.0% of the ration was inactive[K07417]. Powdered fresh bulb at a dose of 800.0 mg/days, taken orally by 219 hypertriglyceridemic patients given the treatment for a total of 16 weeks was active. Serum triglyceride levels fell a total of 17%[M24883]. Powdered fresh bulb in the ration of rat at a concentration of 0.8% of the diet was active[K22138].

Immunosuppressant activity. Hot water extract of bulbs administered intraperitoneally to rats was active[T04890]. Lyophilized extract of freeze dried bulb in the ration of mice at a concentration of 4.0% of the diet was active vs UVB-induced suppression of contact hypersensitivity to oxazolone and cis-urocainic acid (topical)-induced suppression of contact hypersensitivity to dinitrofluorobenzene[K15127].

Inotropic effect negative. Water extract of fresh bulb, at a concentration of 0.1 mcg/ml was active on rat atrium[K11288].

Inotropic effect positive. Essential oil of dried bulb administered intragastrically to rats at a dose of 2.0 g/kg was active and returned to normal after garlic withdrawal. Animals were maintained on normal diet and given the dose for 30 days[T15177]. Fresh bulb juice administered intravenously to rat at a dose of 0.1 ml/animal increased the amplitude of P wave and the ventricular complex QRS of ECG. The activity was highly dose-dependent[T08861].

Insect attractant activity. Butanol extract of fresh bulb, undiluted, produced weak activity of *Delia antiqua*[M13027].

Insecticide activity. Dried bulb at a concentration of 1.0% was active. One month after treatment, moisture, ash, fiber, fat, protein, and carbohydrate level remained unaffected[K14339]. A concentration of 2.0% produced weak activity on *Trogoderma granarium* in maize stored for six months. After six months, changes in nutritional composition were proportional to insect damage[K14339]. Essential oil of dried bulb was active on *Macaronesia fortunata* and *Musca domestica*[W04295]. Dried bulb was active on *Pericallia ricini* and *Spodoptera litura* larvae[K07325].

Insulin induction. Dried bulb taken orally by human adults at a dose of 350.0 mg/person twice daily was inactive[P00123]. Hot water extract of fresh bulb in the ration of mice at a dose of 6.25% of the diet was inactive vs streptozotocin-induced hyperglycemia[M24255].

Insulin level increase. Fixed oil of fresh bulb in the ration of rat at a concentration of 1.5% of the diet was active. The extract ameliorates decrease in insulin levels in animals fed fructose and Cu-deficient diet[K08961].

Insulin release inhibition. Essential oil administered intragastrically to rats was active[K10422].

Interleukin induction. Water extract of freeze-dried bulbs was inactive, IL-1 activity was measured by the IL-1 dependent growth of a T-helper cell line[M27208].

Interleukin-1 formation stimulation. Water extract of fresh bulb in cell culture at a concentration of 0.4 mg/ml was active on lymphocytes. Thiosulfonate fraction at a concentration of 1.6 mg/ml was inactive[K16143].

Interleukin-4 formation stimulation. Water extract of fresh bulb in cell culture at a concentration of 0.4 mg/ml was active on lymphocytes. Thiosulfonate fraction at a concentration of 1.6 mg/ml was active[K16143].

Intestinal motility inhibition. Essential oil administered orally to mouse at a dose of 0.01 ml/gm was active. Gastrointestinal transit of charcoal meal was reduced[M16824].

Lactate dehydrogenase stimulation. Essential oil administered intragastrically to rats at a concentration of 0.067 mg/gm, after fasting for 24 hours was active[M23270]. Water extract of fresh bulb administered intragastrically to rats at variable dosage levels was active[T15939].

Lactate dehydrogenase-X inhibition. Water extract of fresh bulb at a concentration of 10.0 mg/ml was active[T00032].

Larvicidal activity. Decoction of dried stem at a concentration of 100.0 ppm produced weak activity on *Aedes fluviatilis*[K11645]. Petroleum ether extract of essential oil at variable concentrations, was active on culex, pipensquinquefasciatus 1st instar larvae[W03556].

Lipase inhibition. Water extract of fresh bulb in the ration of rabbits at a dose of 1.0 gm/kg was active vs cholesterol-loaded animals[T16431].

Lipid metabolism effects. Fresh garlic taken orally by nine human adults with hyperlipidemia at a dose of 14 g/day for five months. The serum triglyceride levels were lowered and the high-density lipoprotein levels were increased[M15672]. Ethanol (95%) extract of fresh bulb in the ration of rats at a dose of 8.0 ml/animal was active. Extraction was made at 0°C. Four mililiters of the extract was fed for three weeks, then salt was added and the dose increased to 8 ml. Salt did not affect blood pressure in the spontaneously hypertensive animals. Linoleic acid increased and arachidonic acid decreases[M20655].

Lipid peroxide formation inhibition. Essential oil of dried bulb in cell culture at a concentration of 0.01 mg/ml was active on rat liver microsomes. Results significant at $P < 0.01$ level[T10949]. Ethanol (20%) extract of fresh bulb, at a concentration of 20.0 microcuries/ml was active. Formation of fluorescent substances was measured as an index of lipid peroxidation. At a concentration of 40.0 microcuries/ml strong activity was produced. Thiobarbituric acid assayed to determine peroxidation[M21918]. Hot water extract of fresh bulb produced weak activity vs T-butyl hydroperoxide/heme-induced luminol enhanced chemiluminescence[K11079]. Powdered fresh bulb at a concentration of 5.0 mg/ml inhibited lipid peroxidation by 45%[T16428]. Water extract of aged bulb administered intraperitoneally to mice at a dose of 0.05 ml/animal was active vs doxorubicin-induced lipid peroxidation[K17870]. Water extract of fresh bulb was active[T16599].

Lipid synthesis stimulation. Water extract of fresh bulb was active[M30030].

Lipoxygenase inhibition. Ether extract of fresh bulb in cell culture was active[M23059]. Methanol extract of dried bulbs at variable concentrations was inactive vs ADP-, arachidonic-, epinephrine-, and thrombin-induced aggregation[T07890]. Essential oil of fresh bulb was active. IC_{50} 15.0 mcg/ml[M21903]. The ether-insoluble fraction of methanol extract of fresh bulb at concentration 100.0 mcg/ml produced 44% inhibition on rat platelets and the ether-soluble fraction produced 5% inhibition[K12822]. Ethanol (75%) extract of fixed oil was active on guinea pig polymorphonuclear leukocytes. The biological activity has been patented[K21748]. Chloroform, and chloroform/acetone extracts of fresh bulb were active. IC_{50} 2.95 and 0.51 mcg/ml respectively[T16651].

Longevity prolongation. Ethanol (95%) extract of aged bulb in the ration of senescence accelerated mice(SAM P8) and senescence resistant strain(SAM R1), at a dose of 2.0% of the diet was active[K20475].

Macrophage cytotoxicity enhancement. Protein fraction of bulb at a concentration of 100.0 mcg/ml was active[T14866].

Malate Dehydrogenase inhibition. Bulbs in the ration of 16-weeks-old male rats at concentrations of 2.0 and 4.0% of the diet was active in cholesterol-loaded and lard fed animals. Results significant at P < 0.05 level[T05330].

Malic enzyme stimulation. Methanol extract of fresh bulb in the ration of pigs at a concentration of 3.15 gm/kg of the diet for 29 days was active. Hepatic enzymes were assayed[M18549].

Malondialdehyde inhibition. Water extract of fresh bulb at a concentration of 4.0% was active vs hydrogen peroxide-induced malondialdehyde formation[M20451].

Membrane fluidity increase. Ethanol (20%) extract of fresh bulb at a concentration of 20.0 mg/ml was active. Fluidity was measured by fluorescence anisotropy of DPH[M21918].

Memory retention improvement. Ethanol (95%) extract of aged bulb in the ration of senescence accelerated mice (SAM P8 and SAM R1) mice at a dose of 2.0% of the diet was active[K20475].

Miscellaneous effects. Fixed oil of fresh bulb administered subcutaneously to cat was active on spinal dorsal horn cells[K15234]. Fresh bulb taken orally by a total of 100 females and males in Helsinki were interviewed to evaluate beliefs, attitudes and norms concerning the consumption of garlic. In a subsequent postal questionnaire, the annoyance related to the smell of garlic, compared with other social odors, was also measured. The most frequent beliefs about garlic pertained to its good taste, unpleasant smell, and healthiness. Users and non-users showed distinctly different belief patterns. Sweat and alcohol were considered the most annoying social odors, and garlic and perfume/aftershave the least so. The Fishbein-Ajen model, in which individual beliefs and their evaluations as well as subjective norms were used as predictors, explained 30–35% of the variation of the reported consumption and intention to use garlic. The predictive power of the model rose 56–62%

when past behavior was included as a third independent variable. Although the predictive power of attitudes was greater than that of subjective norms, the latter were also significant predictors. Thus, use of garlic is a somewhat unusual form of food-related behavior in that it is controlled by both attitudes and normative factors[K14912]. Ginseng soaked in fresh bulb juice is used to facilitate the release of the active ingredients from the ginseng. The extract was free of bitter taste. The biological activity has been patented[N14330].

Mitogenic activity. Protein fraction of bulb at variable concentrations was active on mice splenocytes[T14866].

Mutagenic activity. Butanol extract of fresh bulb on agar plate at variable concentrations was inactive on *Bacillus subtilis* H-17(Rec+). Water and hot water extracts, at concentrations of 0.5 ml/disk on agar plate, were inactive on *B. subtilis* H-17(Rec+) and M-45(Rec-)[T07988]. Ethanol (95%) extract of dried bulb, at a concentration of 10.0 mg/plate, on agar plate was inactive on *Salmonella typhimurium* TA98 and TA102[K08041]. Ethanol (95%) extract of fresh bulb administered intragastrically to mice at a dose of 500.0 mg/kg daily for five days followed by sacrificing the animals and examination of marrow cells, was active[M23016]. Fresh bulb in buffer at concentrations of 14.75 and 7.38 mg/plate, on agar plate, were inactive on *E. coli* WP2 TRP(-) and *E. coli* WP2 TRP(-)UVR(-)[M21698]. Fresh bulb on agar plate, at a concentration of 1.2 mg/plate was active on *Salmonella typhimurium* TA1535 and TA1538, and inactive on TA98. A concentration of 2.4 mg/plate was active on *S. typhimurium* TA1537. Essential oil of fresh bulb at a concentration of 5.0 picoliters/plate was active on *Micrococcus flavus*[T16468]. Tincture of bulb on agar plate at a concentration of 160.0 microliters/disk was inactive on *Salmonella typhimurium* TA98 and TA100. Metabolic activation had no effect on the results[K19691]. Water extract of fresh bulb at a concentration of 100.0 mcg/ml was inactive on *S. typhimurium* TA102[M20451].

Natriuretic activity. Oven dried bulb administered by gastric intubation to dog at a dose of 10.0 mg/kg was active[T16338]. Water extract of dried bulb administered intragastrically to rats at a dose of 5.0 gm/kg was inactive[M21416].

Natural Killer Cell enhancement. Water extract of fresh bulb in cell culture at a concentration of 0.4 mg/ml was inactive on lymphocytes; thiosulfinate fraction at a concentration of 0.2 mg/ml was active[K16143]. Fresh bulb taken orally by human adults at variable dosage levels was active. Five grams were taken daily for the first six weeks and 10 g taken daily for the second six weeks. Diarrhea, genital herpes, candidiasis and pansinusitus with recurrent fever improved in AIDS patients[M22066].

Nitric oxide synthesis stimulation. Cell culture at a concentration of 25.0 mg/ml was active on placenta and platelets, the activity is highly dose-dependent. Bulb taken orally by human adults at a dose of 4.0 gm/person was active on platelets[K21731].

Norepinephrine level increase. Powdered fresh bulb in the ration of rats at a concentration of 0.8% of the diet was active. Interscapular brown adipose tissue was increased[K22138].

Oxidative phosphorylation inhibition. Essential oil of dried bulb was inactive on *Macaronesia fortunata* and *Musca domestica*[W04295].

Oxidative phosphorylation stimulation. Essential oil of dried bulb was inactive on *Macaronesia fortunata* and *Musca domestica*[W04295].

Peroxisomal fatty acyl-coenzyme A oxidase induction. Methanol extract of fresh bulb in cell culture, at a concentration of 0.5 mg/ml was active on rat hepatocytes[M31064].

Phagocytosis stimulation. Essential oil of dried bulb administered intradermal to mice was active[W04034]. Protein fraction of bulb administered intraperitoneally to mice at a dose of 5.0 mg/kg was active vs clearance of colloidal carbon[T14866].

Pharmacokinetic study. Essential oil administered per rectum in human adults, at a dose of 180 mg/person together with mistletoe, milfoil, horsetail, amylocaine and chlorophyll. The suppository was well absorbed through the rectal mucosa[W04169].

Phorbol ester antagonist. Essential oil applied externally to female mice at a dose of 5.0 mg/animal was active. The dose was applied 1 hour before application of 12-0-tetradecanoyl-phorbol-13-acetate. The rate of DNA synthesis 16 hours later was decreased by 55% vs DMBA-induced carcinogen-esis[M24720]. Fresh bulb was active vs phorbol myristate acetate-induced decrease in glutathione peroxidase, and stimulation of ornithine decarboxylase vs DMBA-induced carcinogenesis[T16143].

Phosphogluconate dehydrogenase stimulation. Methanol extract of fresh bulb in the ration of pig at a concentration of 3.15 gm/kg of diet for 29 days was active. Hepatic enzymes were assayed[M18549].

Phospholipase inhibition. Water extract of fresh bulb at a concentration of 20.0 microliters was active on cat platelets[M23138].

Plant germination inhibition. Water extract of dried leaves, at a concentration of 500.0 g/liter was active after six days exposure of *Cuscuta reflexa* seeds[M31053]. Water extract of dried stem at a concentration of 500.0 gm/liter was active on *Cuscuta reflexa* seeds after six days of exposure to the extract[M31053].

Plant growth inhibition. Water extract of dried leaves, at a concentration of 500.0 gm/liter was active after six days exposure of *Cuscuta reflexa* seedling. Length, weight and dry weight were measured[M31053]. Water extract of dried stem at a concentration of 500.0 gm/liter produced weak activity on *Cuscuta reflexa* after six days of exposure to the extract. Seedling length, weight and dry weight were measured[M31053].

Plant pollen tube elongation inhibition. Fresh tuber at a concentration of 0.4 gm/well was active vs *Camellia sinensis* pollen[T15031].

Plasminogen activation stimulation. Dried bulb taken orally by human adults at a dose of 600.0 mg/person for four weeks was active vs streptokinase activated plasminogen[M19432]. Essential oil, and water extract of fresh bulb were inactive[T06449].

Platelet adhesion inhibition. Essential oil at a concentration of 1:2 was active[T13301]. Essential oil of bulbs administered by gastric intubation to male rabbits at a dose of 1.0 gm/kg for three months was active. Results significant to P <0.001 level[T08093]. A concentration of 7.20% was active. When foreign material comes in contact with blood, protein is immediately adsorbed onto its surface. Thus, the effect of garlic oil vs controls of phosphoryl choline and stearic acid on protein adsorption onto polyether urethane urea was studied. In the presence of garlic oil, more albumin and less fibrinogen was adsorbed than in the presence of controls. Since platelets adhere to fibrinogen, this protein-adsorption phenomenon affected the results of the platelet-aggregation experiments[M18587]. Essential oil, at a concentration of 2.5 mcg was active on adult human platelets vs ADP-, collagen-, and epinephrine-induced aggregation[T07753].

Platelet aggregation inhibition. Alcohol extract of fresh bulb in cell culture at a concentration of 0.01% was active vs epinephrine-induced aggregation. 0.1% was active vs ADP-induced aggregation[K21731]. Butanol extract of fresh bulb taken orally by a patient who suffered a spontaneous spinal epidural hematoma, at a dose of 2000 mg/day was active[M26047]. Water extract of fresh bulbs in cell culture at a concentration of 0.01% was active vs ADP-, and epinephrine-induced aggregation[K21731]. Concentration of 10.0 microliters was active vs collagen-, epinephrine-, ADP-, and arachidonic acid-induced aggregation[M23139]. Con-

centration of 15.0 microliters was active vs ADP-, and arachidonic acid-induced aggregation[M22831]. Butanol extract of dried tuber, at a concentration of 11% was active on human platelets vs ADP-induced aggregation[M24277]. Chloroform extract of bulbs at variable dosage levels was active on rabbit and human adult platelets. Inhibition of platelet aggregation by blocking thromboxane synthesis[T01224]. Chloroform extract of fresh bulb at a concentration of 60.0 mcg/ml was active, 86.57% inhibition was observed vs PAF-induced aggregation and 99.89% inhibition vs ADP-induced aggregation. Chloroform/acetone extract was active with 24.70% inhibition vs PAF-induced aggregation and 35.55% inhibition vs ADP-induced inhibition[T16651]. Dried bulb taken orally by 120 human adults with "probably increased thrombocyte aggregation," at a dose of 800.0 mg/person for four weeks in a double-blind and placebo-controlled study was active[T16354]. Methanol extract at variable concentrations was active vs ADP-, arachidonic acid, epinephrine-, and thrombin-induced aggregation[T07890]. Powdered dried bulb taken orally by a 72-year-old man with platelet dysfunction was active[K23396]. Dried bulb taken orally by human adults at a dose of 300.0 mg/person three times daily for two weeks to seven healthy males was active vs ADP-, and collagen-induced aggregation[K11043]. Dried bulb taken orally by human adults at a dose of 600.0 mg/person for four weeks was inactive vs ADP- and collagen-induced aggregation[M19432]. A dose of 800.0 mg/day was active[K14305]. Essential oil at a concentration of 10.30 mcg/ml was active on adult human platelets vs ADP-induced aggregation. There was induction of a redistribution of the products of the lipoxygenase pathway. At a concentration of 30–60 mcg/ml there was complete suppression of the formation of all oxygenase products vs ADP-induced aggregation[T05159]. Essential oil produced weak activity on rabbit platelets vs ADP-induced platelet aggregation[T04067]. Ethanol/chloroform (25%) extract of fresh bulb was active vs epinephrine-induced aggregation[M30030]. Fixed oil was active vs arachidonic acid-induced aggregation[K21432].

Platelet aggregation inhibition. Fresh buds taken orally by human adults of both sexes, at a dose of 10.0 gm/person was active[T04069]. Water extract of bulbs in cell culture was active vs collagen-induced aggregation. IC_{50} 460.0 mcg/ml[T16663]. Water extract of fresh bulb at a concentration of 1.1% was active[M16831]. Water extract of fresh bulb at a concentration of 5.0 microliters was active vs ADP-, collagen, arachidonate-, calcium ionophore A23187, and epinephrine-induced platelet aggregation[M23138]. Water extract of fresh bulb was active vs ADP, or arachidonic acid-induced platelet aggregation[T03101]. Water extract of fresh bulb administered intravenously to rabbit at a dose of 500.0 mg/kg was active vs arachidonate-induced thrombocytopenia, hypotension and increased TXB2 levels. The extract inhibits histopathologic changes in lung and liver[K07929].

Platelet aggregation stimulation. Water extract of fresh bulb was active[M30030].

Platelet constituent release. Methanol extract of dried bulbs at variable concentrations was inactive. There was no degranulation, difference in ultrastructure, cell shape, distribution of granules or microtubule structures in the treated platelets when compared to controls[T07890].

Platelet stimulant. Water extract of fresh bulb administered by intravenous infusion to rabbit at a dose of 500.0 mg/kg was active vs arachidonate-induced platelet count decrease[T16577].

Pro-oxidant activity. Fresh bulb at a concentration of 1.0% was inactive. The effect was seen at 140°F. peroxides assayed in peanut oil[K23506].

Prostaglandin inhibition. Water extract of fresh bulb administered by intravenous infusion to rabbit at a dose of 500.0 mg/kg was active vs arachidonate, and collagen induced 6-keto-prostaglandin-F-alpha synthesis[T16577]. Water extract of fresh bulb in cell culture was active on platelets[M22831].

Prostaglandin synthesis inhibition. Water extract of bulbs at concentration of 12.5 mg/ml was active[K15297].

Prothrombin time decrease. Dried bulb taken orally by human adults at a dose of 198.0 mg/person, three doses in 34 subjects and a dose of 450.0 mg/person, three doses in 51 subjects were inactive[T12166]. Ether extract of bulbs administered by gastric intubation to rats in a feeding study at doses of 2–4 g crude garlic daily for three weeks was inactive[T05223].

Prothrombin time increase. Dried bulb taken orally by human adults at a dose of 198.0 mg/person, three doses in 34 subjects and a dose of 450.0 mg/person, three doses in 51 subjects were inactive[T12166]. Butanol extract of fresh bulb taken orally by human adults at a dose of 25.0 mg/day was active[M24904]. Essential oil administered intragastrically to rats at a dose of 50.0 mg/day was active vs streptozotocin-induced hyperglycemia[K11022].

Radical scavenging effect. Powdered fresh bulb, at a concentration of 90.0 mg/ml was active[T16428].

Salidiuretic effect. Water extract of dried bulb administered intragastrically to rats at a dose of 5.0 g/kg was inactive[M21416].

Sclerosing effect. Chloroform extract at a concentration of 138.0 mcg/ml, and ethanol (95%) extract at a concentration 53.0 mcg/ml of fresh bulb in cell culture was active on vein vs ADP-, epinephrine-, and arachidonic acid-induced aggregation[M23059].

Sensitization (skin). Powdered bulb applied topically to human adults at a concentration of 10.0% was inactive[K13524].

Smooth muscle relaxant activity. Ethanol (95%) extract of bulbs was active on rabbit intestine[W03431]. Ethanol (95%) extract of fresh bulb, at a concentration of 0.016 mg/ml was active on rat colon[M19330]. Ethanol/chloroform (25%) extract of fresh bulb at a concentration of 0.002 mg/ml was active on rat fundus (stomach) vs ACh-, and PGE-induced contractions[T08092]. Ether extract of dried bulb was active on rabbit intestine[A12824]. Fresh bulb juice at a concentration of 0.5 ml/unit was active on guinea pig ileum and rabbit jejunum juice in amounts of 0.005–0.5 ml inhibited ventricular contractions in rabbit[M29785]. Water extract of dried bulb, at a concentration of 0.04 g/ml was active on guinea pig's small intestine[P00078].

Smooth muscle stimulant activity. Ethanol (95%) extract of fresh bulb, at a concentration of 0.016 mg/ml was active on rat fundus (stomach)[M19330]. Fresh bulb juice, undiluted, was active on rabbit intestine[W03630]. Chloroform extract of dried bulb contained at least two active elements. One was chloroform soluble, and had an antiseptic action, a slight tonic effect on isolated frog heart, a slight hypertensive effect on etherized cats and a paralyzing effect on isolated rabbit intestine. The chloroform-insoluble fraction had no antiseptic effect, no action on isolated frog heart, a strongly hypotensive effect on etherized cats and a tonic effect on isolated rabbit intestine[W03661]. Water extract of dried bulb at a concentration of 0.04 g/ml was active on guinea pig small intestine. The effect was blocked by atropine and antihistamine[P00078].

Spasmogenic activity. Ether extract of dried bulb administered intravenously to rats at a dose of 20.0 ml/animal was active[A12824].

Spasmolytic activity. Fresh bulb juice at a concentration of 0.5 ml/units was active on guinea pig and rabbit aorta vs norepinephrine-induced contractions, and on rabbit trachealis muscle vs ACh- and histamine-induced contractions[M29785]. Water extract of fresh bulb was active on rat aorta vs norepinephrine-induced contractions. ED_{50} 5.28 mg/ml[K17872].

Spermicidal effect. Essential oil was active on guinea pig and rat sperm[W03098].

Spontaneous activity reduction. Water extract of dried bulbs, at a concentration of 20.0% was active on frog stomach[P00078].

Spontaneous activity stimulation. Ethanol (95%) extract of bulbs administered intragastrically to mice at a dose of 250.0 mg/kg was active. The extract inhibited decrease in spontaneous motor activity induced by oscillation stress[M17484].

Succinate dehydrogenase stimulation. Butanol extract of dried bulb administered intragastrically to rats at a dose of 0.5 gm/kg was active on heart, liver and pancreas vs isoprenaline-induced tissue necrosis[M20887].

Superoxide dismutase inhibition. Lyophilized extract of fresh bulb in the ration of chicken at a concentration of 2.0% of the ration was active. Cu-Zn superoxide dismutase activity was inhibited[K07417].

Superoxide inhibition. Lyophilized extract of fresh bulb in the ration of chicken at a concentration of 2.0% of the diet was active[K07417].

Sympathomimetic activity. Water extract of dried leaves, when administered intravenously to cats at a dose of 5–20 mg/kg had no effect on the contractile response of the cat nictating membrane evoked by preganglionic cervical sympathetic nerve stimulation[T09217].

Tachycardia activity. Ether extract of dried bulb administered intravenously to rabbits at a dose of 10.0 ml/animal was active[A12824].

Testosterone release stimulation. Ethanol (95%) extract of dried bulbs administered by gastric intubation to male rats at a dose of 100.0 mg/kg for 25 days was active. Results significant at $P < 0.001$ level[T08094].

Thrombin inhibition. Essential oil administered intragastrically to rats at a dose of

50.0 mg/day was active vs streptozotocin-induced hyperglycemia[K11022].

Thrombocytopenic activity. Ether extract of bulbs administered by gastric intubation to rats in a feeding study at doses of 2–4 gm crude garlic daily for three weeks was active[T05223].

Thromboplastin time increase. Essential oil administered intragastrically to rats at a dose of 50.0 mg/day was active vs streptozotocin-induced hyperglycemia. Kaolin activated partial thromboplastin time was assayed[K11022].

Thromboxane B-2 synthesis inhibition. Chloroform extract of bulbs at variable dosage levels was active on rabbit and human platelets vs incubation with labeled arachidonic acid. Inhibition of platelet aggregation by blocking thromboxane synthesis[T01224]. Ether, and water extracts of fresh bulb in cell culture was active on platelets[M23059]. Water extract of fresh bulb administered intravenously to rabbits at a dose of 500.0 mg/kg was active vs arachidonate-, and rat tail solubilized collagen-induced thrombocytopenia, hypotension and increased TXB2 levels and vs arachidonate- and collagen-induced thromboxane B-2 synthesis. The extract inhibits histopathological changes in lung and liver[T16577]. Water extract of fresh bulb in cell culture was active on platelets[M22831]. Water extract of fresh bulb was active[T03101].

Thyroxine level increase. Fixed oil of fresh bulb in the ration of rat, at a concentration of 1.5% of the diet was active. The extract ameliorated T_4 decrease in animals fed fructose and Cu-deficient diet[K08961].

Toxic effect (general). Butanol extract of fresh bulb taken orally by human adults was active. Two cases were reported of increased normalized ratio results previously stabilized to warfarin. Increases were attributed to ingestion of garlic products, since there were no other changes in medication and habits in either case. One patient had started taking garlic pearls, the other, garlic tablets, but in both cases, clotting times were roughly doubled. It was warned that this could be a potentially serious interaction[M27558]. Dried bulb juice in the drinking water of rats at a dose of 5.0% of the diet for 25 days was inactive[T12183]. Dried bulb taken orally by human adults at a dose of 350.0 mg/person twice daily was inactive[M17987]. Dried bulb, together with *Panax ginseng* and Vitamin B1 administered by gastric intubation to rats of both sexes at a dose of 10.0 ml/kg for up to three months was equivocal. Food consumption was decreased, but there was no change in body weight gain. Erythrocyte and hemoglobin levels were slightly low. There were no histopathological changes seen in the liver, stomach, pancreas, lung, heart, kidney, spleen, thymus, bone marrow, ovary, testis, thyroid, and adrenal. No other toxic symptoms were noted[T11284]. When administered by gastric intubation, dried bulb was inactive. Rats received from 0.3 to 10 ml/kg for three to six months. Body weight gain and urinary measurements were normal. There was a slight though inconsistent decrease in erythrocyte and hemoglobin levels, and slight enlargement of the spleen in high dose rats. There were no histopathological changes seen in the spleen, liver stomach, pancreas, lung, heart, kidney, thymus, ovary, testis, adrenal, of thyroid[T11283]. Essential oil of dried bulbs administered to rabbits at a dose of 0.755 ml/kg was active. The toxicity produced is described as "excito-stupefactive"[W04025]. Ethanol (95%) extract of dried bulbs administered by gastric intubation to rats at variable dosage levels was inactive[W03661]. Ether extract of bulbs administered by gastric intubation to rats in a feeding study at doses of 2–4 gm crude garlic daily for three weeks was inactive. No histopathological lesions of heart, kidney, adrenals, liver, spleen, or thyroid could be seen on autopsy[T05223]. Fresh bulb applied externally to a 17-month-old human infant was presented with burns on both feet derived from a garlic plaster, applied improperly. A mixture of more than 50% garlic cloves plus petroleum jelly had been applied to the feet for eight hours. Blisters were found on the dorsal surfaces of both feet, extending to the skin over the arches. There was a diffuse erythema around the blisters. Burns were diagnosed as second-degree burns and covered 4% of the body surface. The burns healed in two weeks with topical silver and sulfadiazine[M29073]. Butanol extract of fresh bulb, taken orally by human adults at a dose of 25.0 mg/day was active. An 87-year-old man presented with paralysis of the lowed extremities. A spinal mass proved to be a spontaneous spinal epidural hematoma. The hematoma was removed and the patient recovered adequately. The hematoma was attributed to the man's high consumption of garlic (four cloves/day), as no other potential causes were found. Bleeding time during surgery was 11 minutes (three minutes normal) and prothrombin time was 12.3 seconds[M24904]. Fresh bulb inhaled by three cases of occupational asthma and rhinitis was active[K14900]. Fresh bulb juice administered intravenously to rats at a dose of 1.0 ml/animal was inactive[T08861]. Seed oil administered intraperitoneally to rat at a dose of 0.5 ml/kg was inactive[T16004].

Toxicity assessment (quantitative). Dried bulb when administered by gastric intubation and subcutaneously to rats of both sexes $LD_{50} > 30.0$ ml/kg. When administered intraperitoneally to female rats LD_{50} 13.86 ml/kg and males LD_{50} 13.09 ml/kg[T11283,T11284]. Essential oil administered intragastrically to rats fasted for 24 hours, at a dose of 0.1 mg/g was active[T15939]. Water extract of fresh bulb administered intragastrically to rats LD_{50} 173.8 ml/kg[26615].

Tumor promoting effect. Hot water extract of fresh bulb applied externally to mice at a dose of 1.0 mg/animal was inactive. The dose was applied three times weekly for 49–60 weeks after tumor initiation vs DMBA-induced carcinogenesis[T16143].

Tumor promotion inhibition. Methanol extract of fresh root in cell culture, at a concentration of 200.0 mcg was inactive on EBV vs 12-0-hexadecanoylphorbol-13-acetate-induced EBV activation[T15279]. Water and methanol extracts of fresh sprouts, in cell culture at concentrations of 200.0 mcg produced weak activity on EBV vs 12-hexadecanoylphorbol-13-acetate-induced EBV activation[T15279].

Ulcerogenic activity. Ether extract of bulbs administered by gastric intubation to rats in a feeding study at doses of 2–4 gm crude garlic daily for three weeks was active[T05223].

Uterine stimulant effect. Ethanol (95%) extract of bulbs at a concentration of 2.0 mg was active on nonpregnant guinea pig uterus. There was an increase in tone and peristalsis. The same effect as 0.001 I.U. of pituitrin was produced. The extract was also active on the nonpregnant human uterus[A00096,A00097]. Ethanol (95%) extract of dried bulb at a concentration of 4–10 mg was active on nonpregnant guinea pig uterus[W03430]. Water extract of bulbs at a concentration of 50.0 mg/ml produced weak activity. The dose was equivalent to 0.003 IU of oxytocin[A04218]. Water extract of bulbs was active on the nonpregnant uterus and produced strong activity on the pregnant uterus of mice and rats[A05606].

Vasodilator activity. Dried bulb taken orally by human adults at a dose of 900.0 mg/person, in a randomized placebo-controlled double-blind crossover study showed significant increase in skin capillary perfusion five hours after administration[T16452]. Water extract of fresh bulb was active[M30030].

WBC stimulant. Fresh bulb juice administered intraperitoneally to mice increased neutrophil accumulation 82%. ED_{50} 0.07 ml/animal[K07106].

WBC-macrophage stimulant. Water extract of freeze-dried bulb, at a concentration of 20.0 mcg/ml was active. Nitrite formation was used as an index of the macrophage stimulating activity to screen effective foods[M27208].

Weight gain inhibition. Powdered fresh bulb in the ration of rats at a concentration of 0.8% of the diet was active[K22138].

Weight increase. Ethanol (95%) extract of bulbs administered intragastrically to mice at a dose of 250.0 mg/kg was active vs three weeks of cold stress. Weight gain was faster than in controls[M17484].

Wound healing acceleration. Plant applied externally to human adults was active. Perforated eardrums were healed in 18 cases[L01661].

4 | Aloe vera
(L.) Burm. f.

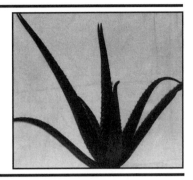

Common Names

'Awa'awa	Argentina	Ghrita kumari	India
Acibar	Argentina	Grahakanya	India
Aloe	Argentina	Guarka-patha	India
Aloe	Bimini	Gwar-patha	India
Aloe cactus	Cook Islands	Indi an aloe	Nepal
Aloe	Rodrigues Islands	Indian aloe	Nepal
Aloe	USA	Kathazhai	India
Aloe	Venezuela	Korphad	India
Aloes	Argentina	Kumari	India
Aloes	Trinidad	Kumaro	India
Aloes vrai	Tunisia	Kunvar pata	India
Aloes	West Indies	Kunwar	India
Alovis	West Indies	Laloi	Haiti
Barbadoes aloe	USA	Laloi	India
Barbados aloe	India	Laluwe	Trinidad
Barbados aloe	Nepal	Laluwe	West Indies
Barbados aloe	West Indies	Lo-hoei	Vietnam
Bitter aloes	Guyana	Lo-hoi	Vietnam
Bunga raja raja	Malaysia	Lou-houey	Vietnam
Chirukattali	India	Lu-chuy	Vietnam
Curacao aloe	West Indies	Manjikattali	India
Dickwar	India	Mediterranean aloe	West Indies
Gawar	India	Murr sbarr	Yunisia
Ghai kunwar	India	Musabar	India
Ghai kunwrar	India	Panini	India
Ghee-kanwar	India	Rapahoe	India
Gheekuar	India	Sabar	Saudi Arabia
Ghikanvar	India	Saber	Jordan
Ghikuar	Pakistan	Sabila	Canary Islands
Ghikumar	India	Sabila	Guatemala
Ghikumari	India	Sabila	Malaysia
Ghikwar	India	Sabila	Nicaragua
Ghiu kumari	Nepal	Sabila	Puerto Rico
Ghrit kumari	India	Sabilla	Cuba

From: Medicinal Plants of the World *By: Ivan A. Ross Humana Press Inc., Totowa, NJ*

Sabilla	West Indies	Tuna	Panama
Sabr	Saudi Arabia	Waan haang charakhe	Thailand
Saqal	Oman	Wan-hangchorakhe	Thailand
Savila	Mexico	Yaa dam	Thailand
Savila	Peru	Yadam	Thailand
Savilla	Bolivia	Zabila	Canary Islands
Semper vivum	West Indies	Zabila	Mexico
Siang-tan	Vietnam	Zabila	Panama
Sobbar	Jordan	Zabila	Venezuela

BOTANICAL DESCRIPTION

A short-stemmed succulent perennial herb of the LILIACEAE family, the succulent leaves are crowded on the top of their stems, spreading grayish green and glaucous; spotted when young, 20- to 50-cm long, 3- to 5-cm wide at the base, tapering gradually to the pointed tip, 1- to 2.5-cm thick; having spiny edges and bitter latex inside. Flowers are borne in cylindrical terminal racemes on central flower stalks, 5- to 100-cm high. The yellow perianth is divided into six lobes, about 2.5-cm long, with scattered bracts. Each flower has six protruding stamens and three-celled ovary with long style. Forms of the species vary in sizes of leaves and colors of flowers.

ORIGIN AND DISTRIBUTION

Aloe vera is native to North Africa, the Mediterranean region of southern Europe, and to the Canary Islands. It is now cultivated throughout the West Indies, tropical America, and the tropics in general.

TRADITIONAL MEDICINAL USES

Argentina. Hot water extract of leaves is taken orally to induce abortion and to facilitate menstruation[A05589].

Bimini. Leaf juice is used externally for skin irritations, cuts, boils, and sunburn[T00359].

Bolivia. Fresh leaf juice is used as an analgesic topically for burns and wounds. Orally, the juice is used as a laxative[T07560].

Brazil. Fresh leaf juice is taken orally as an anthelmintic and febrifuge. Infusion of dried root is taken orally to treat colic[T15975].

Canary Islands. Fresh fruit juice (unripe) is taken orally as an antiasthmatic and purgative[T15880]. Infusion of fresh leaf juice is taken orally as a laxative, for dental caries, and as a teniafuge[T10928].

China. Hot water extract of leaf juice is taken orally as an emmenagogue[K04768].

Cook Islands. Fresh sap in water is taken orally, regularly, to prevent high blood pressure, cancer and diabetes. Externally it is used to treat burns and cuts[K20471].

Cuba. Water extract of leaf pulp is taken as an emmenagogue[T11371].

Egypt. Fresh leaf juice administered intravaginally is used as a contraceptive before or after coitus. Data was obtained as a result of questioning 1200 puerperal women about their knowledge of birth control methods. 52.3% practiced a method, and 47.6% of these depend on indigenous methods and/or prolonged lactation[W02811].

England. Hot water extract of dried leaves with a mixture of *Zingiber officinale*, *Mentha pulegium* (essential oil), *Ipomoea purga*, *Glycyrrhiza glabra* and *Canella alba* is taken orally for amenorrhea[W03029].

Guatemala. Hot water extract of dried leaves is used externally for wounds, ulcers, bruises and sores, skin eruptions, erysipelas, dermatitis, inflammations, burns, abscesses, and furuncles, and scrofula[T15445].

Haiti. Hot water extract of dried leaves is taken orally both as a purgative and against diabetes and worms[T04647].

India. Decoction of dried leaves is taken orally to induce abortion[K16006], for sexual vitality,[T09486] and the dried leaf juice is taken as an emmenagogue[T14891]. Decoction of root is taken orally for venereal disease and externally it is used to treat wounds[M27166]. Fresh fruit juice (unripe) is taken orally as a laxative, cathartic, and for fevers[W03487]. Fresh leaves are crushed and applied locally for guinea worms[M28491]. Hot water extract of dried entire plant is taken orally as an emmenagogue, purgative, anthelmintic, stomachic, for liver enlargement, spleen enlargement, and piles. Hot water extract of fresh plant juice is taken orally for inflammation and amenorrhea[T15475]. The pulp of the plant is mixed together with salt and fermented sugar cane juice and taken orally to treat pain and inflammation of the body[K23156]. Hot water extract of leaf juice is taken orally as a cathartic; it should not be used by pregnant women[A00449]. Leaf pulp is taken orally regularly for 10 days to women to prevent conception[M23826]. Leaf juice is taken orally to treat viral jaundice. The juice is taken twice daily for three days[M27166].

Malaysia. Hot water extract of leaf juice is taken orally as a cholagogue and emmenagogue[A06589]. Hot water extract of leaves is taken orally as an emmenagogue[A00115].

Mexico. Fresh stem juice is taken orally for diabetes[K10686]. Infusion of dried leaves is taken orally to treat ulcers[K16948].

Nepal. Fresh leaf pulp is taken orally to relieve amenorrhea. 10–15 gm of leaf pulp is given with sugar or honey once a day[K23191]. Hot water extract of dried entire plant is taken orally as a purgative and to terminate pregnancy[T01728].

Panama. Fresh leaves crushed with egg white is taken orally as a laxative and demulcent. Sap is taken orally for stomach ulcers and externally for erysipelas and to treat swellings caused by injuries[T01287].

Peru. Hot water extract of fresh leaves is taken orally for asthma, as a purgative, and antivenin. Externally, the extract is used as an antiseptic for washing wounds[T15323].

Puerto Rico. Drink made from fresh leaf pulp plus fruit pulp of *Genipa americana* is a popular remedy for colds[T07825].

Saudi Arabia. Hot water extract of dried aerial parts is taken orally for liver complaints, piles, as an emetic, antipyretic, against tumors, for enlarged spleen, as a cooling agent, purgative, for diabetes, skin diseases and asthma[T15500]. Hot water extract of dried leaves is taken orally for functional sterility, amenorrhea, piles, thermal burns, constipation, flatulence, intestinal worms, diabetes, to treat functional sterility, amenorrhea, to treat constipation, and piles. Externally the extract is used for burns[T10348].

South Korea. Hot water extract of whole dried plant is taken orally as a contraceptive, an abortifacient, and emmenagogue. Use of the extract is contraindicated during pregnancy[T10290].

Switzerland. Hot water extract of leaves is taken orally as an abortifacient[A00386].

Taiwan. Decoction of dried leaves is taken orally to treat hepatitis[M29355].

Thailand. Fresh leaf juice is used on burns[T11371]. Hot water extract of dried resin is taken orally as a cathartic[W03804].

Trinidad. Gum is taken orally as an abortifacient[K03665].

Tunisia. Hot water extract of dried leaves is taken orally for diabetes and to treat problems of venous circulation. Externally, the extract is used for eczema[T08514].

USA. Fresh leaf juice is taken orally for stomach ulcers and used externally to heal wounds[W02962]. Fluid extract of leaf juice is taken orally as an emmenagogue[A05642]. Hot water extract of dried leaves is taken orally as a cathartic[W03671]. Hot water extract of gum is taken orally as an emmenagogue to promote and stimulate menstruation[W01317]. Water extract of leaves is used externally for insect bites, myopathies, arthritis, topical ulcers, and other skin conditions[J02536]. Hot water extract is taken orally to increase menstrual flow; the extract should be avoided during pregnancy[M00554].

Venezuela. Bitter latex is taken orally as a laxative[A05449]. Hot water extract of leaves is taken orally as an emmenagogue[J10140].

Vietnam. Sap is taken orally as an emmenagogue[A04942].

West Indies. Gum is taken orally as an abortifacient[T00701]. Leaf juice is taken orally as an emmenagogue, anthelmintic and purgative[A05150]. Yellow latex from the epidermis is taken orally to prevent syphilis, as a purgative, to improve appetite, for intestinal worms, and to promote menstrual flow. Externally, split leaves are applied to wounds[T00701].

CHEMICAL CONSTITUENTS

(ppm unless otherwise indicated)

1-1-2-triphenyl cyclopropane, Gel
1-1-bis-(2-hydroxy-3-5-dimethyl-phenyl)-2-methyl propane, Gel
2(3H) benzothiazolone, Gel
2-Methyl-2-phytyl-6-chromanol, Pl
3-3'-bis para methane, Gel
4-4-dimethyl-3-(2-4-5-trimethoxy-phenyl)pentanoic acid ethyl ester, Gel
7-Hydroxy-chromone, Pl
7-Hydroxyaloin, Pl
8-Methyl-tocol, Pl
8-oleic acid methyl ester, Gel
9-propanoyl-methoxy-methyl phenanthrene, Gel
12-methyl tridecanoic acid methyl ester, Gel
13-methyl pentadecanoic acid methyl ester, Gel
14-methyl pentadecanoic acid methyl ester, Gel
15-methyl hexadecanoic acid, Gel
16-methyl heptadecanoic acid methyl ester, Gel
1,8-Dihydroxyanthracene, Pl
Acemannan, Lf
Alanine, Lf
Albumin, Lf 1-5
Aleosone, Pl
Aliinase, Lf
Alocutin A, Pl
Aloe emodin, Lf
Aloe polypeptides, Lf
Aloe vera compound LM, Lf 47.5%

Aloe vera compound HM, Lf 7.5%
Aloe emodin anthranol, Pl
Aloeferon, Lf Gel
Aloenin, Pl
Aloesin, Lf
Aloesone, Pl
Aloetic acid, Pl
Aloetin, Pl
Aloetinic acid, Pl
Aloin A,7-hydroxy-6'-0-para-coumaroyl, Lf
Aloin B,7-hydroxy-6'-0-para-coumaroyl, Lf
Aloin, Lf
Aloinose, Pl
Aloinoside-A, Pl
Aloins, Pl 27-30%
Alpha cellulose, Pl
Aluminum, Lf 22
Amylase, Lf 0-20
Anthracene, Pl
Anthranol, Lf
Anthraquinone glycoside, Pl
Anthraquinones, Pl
Anthrol, Pl
Apoise, Pl
Arabinan, Pl
Arabinose, Lf
Arachidic acid methyl ester, Gel
Arachidonic acid, Aer
Arginine, Lf
Ascorbic acid, Lf 6,260
Asparagine, Lf
Aspartic acid, Lf
Barbaloin, Pl 4.24%
Behenic acid methyl ester, Gel
Benzaldehyde,4-hydroxy-3-5-di-tert-butyl, Gel
Benzylacetone, Pl
Beta barbaloin, Lf
Beta carotene, 7.2.mg/g
Beta sitosterol, Lf
Calcium oxalate, Lf
Calcium, Lf 190-4,600
Campesterol, Lf
Carbohydrates, Lf 89.6%
Casanthranol-I, Pl
Casanthranol-II, Pl
Catalase, Pl
Chloride, Lf 10-110
Cholesterol, Lf 40-120
Choline, Pl
Choline salicyclate, Pl
Chromium, Pl, Lf

Chrysamminic acid, Pl
Chrysazin, Lf
Chrysophanic acid, Lf
Chrysophanic acid, Pl
Chrysophanol, Pl
Chrysophanol glycoside, Pl
Cinnamic acid, Pl
Cobalt, Tr, Lf
Coniferyl alcohol, Pl
Coumarin, Pl
Creatinine, Lf 1-15
Cycloeicosane, Gel
Cysteine, Lf
Cystine, Lf Ju
D-Freidooleanan-3-one, Gel
D-Galactan, Pl
D-Galactose, Lf
D-Galactouronic acid, Pl
D-Glucitol, Pl
D-glucose, Lf
D-mannose, Lf
Decyl cyclohexane, Gel
Dehydro abietal, Gel
Dehydro abietic acid methyl ester, Gel
Di-(2-ethylhexyl)phthalate, Pl
Dibutyl phthalate, Gel
Diheptyl phthalate, Gel
Dioctyl phthalate, Gel
DNA, Rt
Dodecyl benzene, Gel
Emodin, Pl
Fat, Lf 8,000
Fiber, Lf 17.7%
Folic acid, Lf 27-200
Formic acid, Pl
Fructose, Lf; St; EO
Galactan (aloe vera), Lf Pu
Galactose, Lf
Globulin, Lf 0-2
Gluco-galacto mannan (aloe vera), Lf
Glucomannan (aloe vera), Lf Pu
Glucosamine, Pl
Glucose, Lf 280-1,030
Glutamic acid, Lf
Glutamine, Lf
Glycerol, Pl
Glycine, Lf
Hecogenin, Pl
Heneicosanoic acid methyl ester, Gel
Heptadec-1-ene, Gel
Hexauronic acid, Pl
Histidine, Lf

Homonataloin, Pl
Hydrocinnamic acid, Pl
Hydroxy proline, Lf Ju
Hydroxymethylanthraquinone, Pl
Iron, Lf 30-300
Iso citric acid, Lf
Iso-leucine, Lf
Isobarbaloin, Pl
Kilocalories, Lf 2,800
L-Asparagine, Pl
Lauric acid methyl ester, Gel
Lauric acid, Gel
Leucine, Lf
Lignin, Pl
Linoleic acid ethyl ester, Gel
Linoleic acid, Gel
Lipase, Lf 0-16
Lupeol, Lf
Lysine, Lf
Lysophosphatidyl inositol, Aer
M-Protocatechuic aldehyde, Pl
Magnesium, Lf 930
Manganese, Lf 6
Mannose, Lf
Margaric acid methyl ester, Gel
Margaric acid, Gel
Monooctyl phthalate, Gel
Mucilage (aloe vera), Lf
Mucilage, Pl
Mucopolysaccharides, Pl
Myristic acid methyl ester, Gel
Myristic acid, Gel
N-docosane, Gel
N-eicosane, Gel
N-heneicosane, Gel
N-heptadecane, Gel
N-hexadecane, Gel
N-nonadecane, Gel
N-octadecane, Gel
Nataloin, Pl
Niacin, Lf 64
Niacinamide, Pl
Nonadec-1-ene, Gel
Nonadec-trans-5-ene, Gel
Octadec-1-ene, Gel
Octadec-7-enoic acid, Gel
Octadeca-10-13-dienoic acid methyl ester, Gel
Octadeca-6-9-dienoic acid methyl ester, Gel
Octadeca-9-12-dienoic acid methyl ester, Gel
Oleic acid ethyl ester, Gel
Oleic acid methyl ester, Gel
Oleic acid, Aer

Oligosaccharide (aloe vera), Lf Pu
Oxidase, Pl
P-Coumaric acid, Pl
P-Methoxy-hydrocinnamic acid, Pl
P-Methoxybenzylacetone, Pl
Palmitic acid ethyl ester, Gel
Palmitic acid methyl ester, Gel
Palmitic acid, Gel
Palmitoleic acid methyl ester, Gel
Palmitoleic acid, Gel
Para coumaric acid, Lf
Pectic acid, Pl
Pentadecanoic acid, Gel
Phisphatidyl inositol, Aer
Phosphatidic acid, Aer
Phosphatidyl choline, Aer
Phosphatidyl ethanolamine, Aer
Phosphatidyl serine, Aer
Phosphorus, Lf 6-940
Phytosterols, Pl
Polyphenols, Pl
Polysaccharide (aloe vera), Lf
Polyuronide, Pl
Potassium, Lf 100-850
Proeinase, Pl
Proline, Lf
Protein, Lf Ju 2.5%
Pteroylglutamic acid, Pl
Purine, Lf 1-56
Quinone, Pl
Resin, Pl
Resitannols, Pl
Rhamnose, Lf
Rhein, Pl
Riboflavin, Tr, Lf
Sapogenin, Pl
Saponins, Pl
Selenium, Lf 23
Serine, Lf
Silicon, Lf 22
Sodium, Lf 40-510
Spingomyelin, Aer
Stearic acid ethyl ester, Gel
Stearic acid, Gel
Stigmasterol, Aer
Sulfoquinovosyl diglyceride, Aer
Tetradecyl benzene, Gel
Thiamin, Lf 0.8
Threitol, Pl
Threonine, Lf
Tin, Lf 11
Tricosanoic acid methyl ester, Gel

Tridecyl benzene, Gel
Trihydroxymethylanthraquinone, Pl
Triolein, Aer
Tyrosine, Lf
Undecyl cyclohexane, Gel
Urea, Lf 10
Uronic acid, Pl
Valine, Lf
Water, Pl 99.5%
Xylose, Lf
Zinc, Lf 11-770

PHARMACOLOGICAL ACTIVITIES AND CLINICAL TRIALS

Abortifacient effect. Ethanol (95%), water, and petroleum ether extracts of fresh leaves administered orally to female rats at doses of 150.0, 150.0, and 100.0 mg/kg, respectively, were inactive[W01362].

Adjuvant activity. Aqueous (dialyzed) fraction of freeze-dried leaf juice administered intraperitoneally to mice at variable dosage levels was active[M21549].

Alkalinizing activity. Undiluted fresh leaf juice applied externally on female adults with dermatitis caused by X-ray treatment was active[W02241].

Analgesic activity. Ethanol (95%) extract of aerial parts administered intragastrically to mice at a dose of 500.0 mg/kg was active vs hot plate method[M21425]. Fresh leaf gel at a concentration of 0.125% formulated into a toothpaste that also contained sodium fluoride was equivocal. Alleviation of root pain was not significantly greater in treatment group vs controls[K18704]. Fresh leaf pulp when used externally on patients with chronic and acute athletic injuries three times per week for three weeks was active[M21051]. Water extract of dried leaf juice administered intraperitoneally to rats at a dose of 250.0 mg/kg was active vs tail flick response to radiant heat[T07815]. Water extract of fresh leaf juice administered subcutaneously to mice at a dose of 100.0 mg/kg was active. Decolorizing *Aloe vera* extract was given daily for seven days to normal and diabetic test groups. Treated normal group showed a doubling of the time to pain response relative to untreated diabetics (13.7 vs 10.7 seconds) vs carrageenin-induced pedal edema and hot plate method[M19504].

Anesthetic activity (local). Undiluted fresh leaf juice was active as an analgesic for insect stings on human adults. The biological activity has been patented[T01428].

Anti-asthmatic activity. Fresh leaf extract administered orally to human adults was active[T15461].

Antibacterial activity. Chromatographic fraction of fresh leaves on agar plate was active on *Bacillus subtilis*[T15169]. Decoction of dried fruit on agar plate produced weak activity on *Streptococcus mutans*. MIC 62.5 mg/ml[M22285]. Dried entire plant juice on agar plate was active on *Proteus vulgaris* and *Pseudomonas aeruginosa*[T09032]. Ethanol (95%) and water extracts of leaves on agar plate were inactive on *Escherichia coli* and *staphylococcus aureus*[A15179]. Fresh leaf juice at a concentration of 1:50 on agar plate was active on *Streptococcus pyogenes*, *Corynebacterium xerosis* and *Staphylococcus aureus*; and inactive on *Escherichia coli* and *Salmonella schottmuelleri*. The activity was lost quickly as the juice darkens in color. Whole leaf minus the juice, the leaf mesophyll, and leaf epidermis was devoid of activity[W00353]. Tincture of dried leaves, at a concentration of 30.0 ml/disk (10 gm of leaves in 100 ml ethanol) on agar plate was inactive on *Escherichia coli*, *Pseudomonas aeruginosa*, and *Staphylococcus aureus*[T15445]. Undiluted fresh leaf juice in broth culture was active on *Bacillus subtilis*, *Enterobacter* species, *Escherichia coli*, *Serratia marcescens*, *Staphylococcus aureus*, *Streptococcus agalactiae*, *Streptococcus pyogenes*, and inactive on *Klebsiella* species[T01708].

Antiburn effect. Dried entire plant juice, applied externally to guinea pigs, was active vs experimental burn[T09032]. Fresh undiluted leaf juice applied externally to human adults of both sexes was active. Three cases of burn caused by hot water and two cases of severe sunburn were treated[T01740]. Undiluted fresh leaf juice applied externally to human adults of both sexes with X-ray-induced ulcers was active[W02242]. Undiluted fresh leaf juice applied topically to X-ray-induced, acute third degree burns was active[W02112]. Undiluted leaf gel applied externally was inactive. Twelve volunteers received UVB irradiation from a light pen at two sites on each arm. Aloe leaf gel was applied to two sites on one arm. Blood flow and redness of irradiated areas did not differ from controls at six and 24 hours post-burn[M25705]. Water extract of dried leaves, applied externally to third degree burns induced by X-rays on rats at a concentration of 10.0% was active. The inner rind of the leaf was dried before being extracted[W02112].

Anticomplement activity. Aqueous (dialyzed) fraction of freeze-dried leaf juice at a concentration of 300.0 mg/ml was active on human serum. Inhibition of alternate pathway complement activity. Effect resulting from depletion of complement factor 3[M21549]. Water extract and polysaccharide fraction of leaves were active in human serum[T14987]. Water extract of fresh leaves at variable concentrations was active[H04248].

Anticrustacean activity. Ethanol (95%) extract of dried plant juice was inactive on *Artemia salina*, the assay system was intended to predict for antitumor activity[K08041].

Antifertility effect. Ethanol (95%) and petroleum ether extracts of leaves administered orally to female mice were active. Positive data was reported, but they are of questionable significance to fertility regulation. Water extract was inactive. Ethanol (95%), water, and petroleum ether extracts of root administered orally to female mice were inactive[A02435].

Antifungal activity. Anthraquinone fraction of fresh leaf juice on agar plate was active on *Trichophyton mentagrophytes*[K18822]. Dried juice from entire plant, applied externally to human adults, was active in treating trichophytiasis[T09032].

Antihypercholesterolemic activity. Hot water extract of dried leaf juice administered intragastrically to rats at a dose of 0.5 gm/kg for seven days was active. The effect was tested by a mixture of *Nigella sativa*, *Commiphora*, *Ferula assafoetida*, *Aloe vera*, and *Boswellia serrata* vs streptozotocin-induced hyperglycemia[M20731].

Antihyperglycemic activity. Twenty-five percent aqueous extract of decoction and hot water extract of dried leaves administered intragastrically to mice at a dose of 0.5 ml/animal was inactive vs alloxan-induced hyperglycemia[T10348]. Chromatographic fraction of a commercial sample of leaves administered intraperitoneally to mice at a dose of 5.0 mg/kg daily for four days was active vs alloxan-induced hyperglycemia. Leaf exudate administered intragastrically to mice at a dose of 500.0 mg/kg was inactive. When administered twice a day for four days, the exudate was active vs alloxan-induced hyperglycemia[M22720]. Fresh leaf gel administered intragastrically to male rats at a dose of 2.0 ml/kg was inactive. The gel did not lower blood glucose in alloxan treated rats, blood glucose rose with treatment[K19856]. Fresh sap administered intragastrically to mice at a dose of 1.0 gm/kg was active vs alloxan-induced hyperglycemia[M22020]. When administered orally to five diabetic patients for 4–14 weeks, the sap was active[M22020]. Hot water extract of dried leaf juice administered intragastrically to rats at a dose of 0.5 gm/kg for seven days, was active. The effect was tested by a mixture of *Nigella sativa*, *Commiphora*, *Ferula assafoetida*, *Aloe vera*, and *Boswellia serrata* vs streptozotocin-induced hyperglycemia[M20731].

Anti-implantation effect. Ethanol (95%) and petroleum ether extracts of leaves administered orally to female rats were active. Positive data was reported, but they are of questionable significance to fertility regula-

tion. Water extract was inactive[A02435]. Ethanol (95%) extract of leaf pulp administered orally to female rats at a dose of 100.0 mg/kg was inactive[A04512]. Ethanol (95%), water, and petroleum ether extracts of root administered orally to female mice were inactive[A02435].

Anti-inflammatory activity. Water extract of fresh leaf juice, applied externally to mice at a concentration of 1.0% was active. Decolorized *Aloe vera* extract was applied to the ear 30 minutes after the application of croton oil. The extract reduced ear swelling by 67% relative to controls[M19503]. The extract was also active in rats vs mustard-induced pedal edema. Inhibition of edema was greater with RNA and vitamin C added[M17603]. When administered subcutaneously to rats at a dose of 10.0 mg/kg the extract was active. Decolorized *Aloe vera* extract was given one day before induction of edema by plantar injection of 2% mustard solution. A 60% reduction of edema was seen in treated diabetic animals relative to untreated diabetics vs carrageenin-induced pedal edema. A dose of 400 mg/kg was inactive vs cotton pellet granuloma[M17603]. Ethanol (95%) extract of fresh leaf juice, applied externally on mice was active vs croton oil-induced edema and carrageenin-induced pedal edema[K18822]. Ethanol/water (1:1) extract of leaf juice used externally on mice at a concentration of 5.0% was active vs croton oil-induced edema[A00433]. Fresh leaf gel administered intraperitoneally to male rats at a dose of 2.0 ml/kg was active vs carrageenin-induced pedal edema[K18667]. Fresh leaf juice administered by means of injection to 50 patients with first-third stage of parodontosis yielded a satisfactory effect only in the first and second stages of the disease. The content of calcium elevated in the blood serum in parodontosis normalizes in the treatment with Aloe extract[W03275]. Fresh leaf juice applied externally to female mice at a dose of 5.0% was active vs croton oil-induced edema[M23281]. The decolorized extract at a concentration of 1.0% was active vs croton oil-induced edema[M25704]. When administered subcutaneously to rats at a dose of 25.0 mg/kg the extract was active vs mustard-induced pedal edema, 46% decrease in paw volume; when combined with 1.0 mg/kg hydrocortisone, 66% decrease in paw volume; 86% inhibition of edema for combination with 0.1% hydrocortisone vs croton oil-induced edema[M25704]. Ethanol/water (1:1) extract of fresh leaves administered subcutaneously to mice at a dose of 150.0 mg/kg was active vs croton oil-induced edema[T16496]. Fresh leaf pulp administered via drinking water and intragastrically to rats at doses of 100.0 mg/kg were active vs croton oil-induced ear swelling. A time study showed that food grade *Aloe vera* administration reduced swelling to a large degree when used over a 21-day period as opposed to 7 or 14 days. Decolorized *Aloe vera* was inactive when administered through the drinking water as well as intragastrically. A dose of 150.0 mg/kg administered subcutaneously to rats was active vs gelatin-, kaolin-, albumin-, carrageenin-, dextran-, and mustard-induced pedal edema[M23680]. Leaf juice injected into mice at a dose of 10.0% was active. Inflammation was introduced by administration of air under the skin producing a pouch followed by administration of 1% carrageenan directly into the seven-day-old air pouch, which produced an inflammation characterized by an increase in mast cells and wall vascularity. After administration of the extract vascularity was reduced by 50% and the number of mast cells was decreased by 48%[M31110]. Water extract of dried leaves administered subcutaneously to male mice at a dose of 20.0 mg/kg was active[M23710]. Water extract of fresh leaf gel (undiluted) was active when applied externally on human adults[T16559]. Fresh leaf gel, applied externally on mice at a dose of 300.0 mg/kg was active[K15034].

Antileukopenic activity. Dried entire plant juice was active vs cobalt-60 or X-ray radiation[T09032].

Antimycobacterial activity. Ethanol (95%) and water extracts of fresh leaves in broth culture was active on *Mycobacterium tuberculosis*[A15139]. Ethanol (95%) and water extracts of leaves on agar plate were inactive on *Mycobacterium tuberculosis*[A15179]. Ethyl acetate extract of dried leaves on agar plate was active on *Mycobacterium tuberculosis*[A15166].

Antipyretic activity. Ethanol (95%) extract of aerial parts administered intragastrically to mice at a dose of 500.0 mg/kg was active vs yeast-induced pyrexia[M21425].

Antitumor activity. Acid/water extract of dried leaves administered subcutaneously to mice of both sexes at a dose of 0.005 gm/kg and dried-leaf administered as a powdered suspension at a dose of 1.0 gm/kg were inactive on Sarcoma 37[W03671]. Dried juice from the entire plant administered intraperitoneally to mice was active on CA-Ehrlich-Ascites and Sarcoma 180 (solid)[T09032]. Leaf gel of dried gland (ink) administered intraperitoneally to male mice at doses of 10.0 and 50.0 mg/kg were inactive on Sarcoma 180 (solid). The relative change in the tumor weight was not statistically significant[K18060].

Antiulcer activity. Aqueous slurry (homogenate) of dried exudate administered by gastric intubation to rats at doses of 0.5 and 1 gm/kg was inactive vs Phenylbutazone-, cysteamine- and reserpine-induce ulcers; the 500.0 mg/kg dose was inactive vs stress-induced ulcers. Aqueous slurry (homogenate) of fresh leaves administered by gastric intubation to rats at a dose of 1.0 gm/kg was inactive vs phenylbutazone-, and cysteamine-induced ulcers; a dose of 0.5 gm/kg was inactive vs aspirin-, reserpine-, and stress-induced (restraint) ulcers[T12102]. Fresh leaf gel administered intragastrically to male rats at a dose of 2.0 ml/kg was inactive. The gel did not prevent ethanol-induced of cold-restraint gastric ulcers. Also, neither prenor post-treatment accelerated healing of ulcers[K19856]. Fresh leaf pulp juice administered intragastrically to rats at a dose of 2.0 ml/animal daily for seven days after induction of lesions was active vs stress-induced (restraint) ulcers and aspirin-induced ulcers[T06533]. Blended fresh leaf pulp administered orally to rats at a dose of 2.0 ml/animal twice daily for six days was active. Ulcer reduction of 50% relative to control was observed vs aspirin-induced ulcers[T02648]. Water extract of leaf pulp administered orally to rats at a dose of 4.0 ml/animal was active. Gastric ulcers was produced by forced immobilization. The effect was both prophylactic and therapeutic[J08942].

Antiviral activity (plant pathogens). Ethanol (95%) extract of dried leaves in cell culture was active on distortion ringspot, mild mosaic and ringspot viruses[W00025].

Antiviral activity. Anthraquinone fraction of fresh leaf juice in cell culture was active on herpes simplex virus (HSV) 1[K18822]. Methanol extract of dried leaves applied externally was active on HSV 1 and 2. The biological activity reported has been patented[T13636].

Antiyeast activity. Ethanol (60%) extract of dried leaves on agar plate was inactive on *Candida albicans*[M31296]. Tincture (extract of 10 gm leaves in 100 ml ethanol) at a concentration of 30 microliters/disk on agar plate was inactive[T15445]. Undiluted fresh leaf juice in broth culture was active on *Candida albicans*[T01708].

Arachidonate metabolism inhibition. Anthraquinone fraction of fresh leaf juice was active on calf skin[K18822].

ATP-ase (Na⁺/K⁺) inhibition. Anthraquinone fraction of fresh leaf juice increases permeability across colonic mucosa[K18822].

Bradykinin antagonist activity. Exudate of fresh leaf juice was active[K18822].

Bronchodilator activity. Hot water extract of dried leaves administered intravenously to guinea pigs at a dose of 1.5 ml/animal was inactive[M29843].

Cardiac depressant activity. Tincture of leaf juice produced weak activity in rabbit heart perfusion[A00433].

Cell attachment enhancement effect. Fresh leaf homogenates in cell culture was active vs human embryonic-lung cells and inactive vs CA-ME-180[T15275]. Fresh leaves was active on human lung cells and CA-cervical-squamous cells[W02965]. Leaf homogenates in cell culture was active on CA-ME-180 and human embryonic lung cells[T15275]. Leaf juice (commercial sample) was active on CA-cervical-squamous and human-lung cells[T13461]. Fresh leaf homogenates in cell culture was active vs human embryonic lung cells and inactive vs CA-ME-180[T15275]. Fresh leaves was active on human lung cells and CA-cervical-squamous cells[T13641].

Cell proliferation stimulation. Water extract of fresh leaf gel in cell culture, at a concentration of 0.162 mcg/ml was active on pheochromocytoma-rat-PC12 cells. A concentration of 0.325 mcg/ml was active on human fibroblast lung-HEL. The was seen only in long-term culture[K21357].

Cell transformation inhibition. Freeze-dried gel in cell culture was active on C3H-10T1/2 cells vs methylcholantrene-induced transformation[K16977].

CNS depressant activity. Hot water extract of leaves administered intraperitoneally to rabbits at a dose of 10.0 mg/kg was active[T07129].

Conditioned taste aversion. Frozen stem and leaves administered intragastrically to rats at a dose of 925.0 mg/kg was inactive. Administration of test substance was temporally paired with introduction of sodium saccharin solution. Consumption of saccharin solution two days after test was used to estimate aversiveness of test substance[T13641].

Cosmetic activity. A mixture of *Aloe vera*, *Mentha piperita* extract, and allantoin was active when applied externally on human adults. The biological activity has been patented[M20293].

Cytotoxic activity. Ethanol/water (1:1) extract of leaves in cell culture was inactive on CA-9KB. ED_{50} >20.0 mcg/ml[A04741]. Ethanol/water (1:1) extract of the entire plant in cell culture was inactive on CA-9KB. ED_{50} >20.0 mcg/ml[A03335]. Leaf gel of dried gland (ink), in cell culture produced weak activity on human colorectal cancer cell line SNU-C2A, IC_{50} 5.0 mg/ml and human SNU-1 cells IC_{50} 5.25 mg/ml[K18060].

Death. Ethanol (95%) extract of the aerial parts administered intragastrically to mice at a dose of 3.0 gm/kg was inactive[M21425].

DNA synthesis inhibition. Chromatographic fraction of fresh leaf gel in broth culture was active on *Bacillus subtilis*[T15169].

Embryotoxic effect. Benzene, water, petroleum ether, and ethanol (95%) extract of leaves administered orally to pregnant rats at doses of 100.0 mg/kg were active. Fifty, 85, 37, and 85% reduction in fertility, respectively, was observed. Chloroform extract was equivocal, 28% reduction in fertility[T00214]. Ethanol/water (1:1) extract administered orally to female rats at a dose of 200.0 mg/kg was active[W01378]. Ethanol (95%) extract of leaf pulp administered orally to female rats at a dose of 100.0 mg/kg was inactive[A04512]. Ethanol (95%), water, and petroleum ether extracts of fresh leaves administered orally to female rats at doses of 150.0, 150.0, and 100.0 mg/kg respectively were inactive[W01362]. Ethanol/water (1:1) extract of dried leaves at a dose of 150.0 mg/kg, water extract at a dose of 125.0 mg/kg and benzene extract at a dose of 100.0 mg/kg administered by gastric intubation to pregnant rats were inactive[T05679]. Water extract of dried entire plant administered intragastrically to pregnant rats at a dose of 125.0 mg/kg was equivocal[M19981].

Emollient effect. Undiluted leaf juice applied externally on human adults was active[L02050].

Estrogenic effect. Leaf juice administered orally to immature rats at a dose of 10.0 ml/kg, produced weak activity[M00151].

Glucose-6-phosphate dehydrogenase inhibition. Anthraquinone fraction of fresh leaf juice was active[K18822].

Hair conditioner. Water extract of dried leaves applied externally on human adults at a concentration of 86.6% was active[K07487].

Hair loss inhibition. Fresh leaf gel applied externally to human adults at a concentration of 6.8 ml/day was active. Biological activity has been patented[K15683].

Hair loss stimulant effect. Fresh leaf gel applied externally to human adults at a concentration of 6.8 ml/day was active. Biological activity has been patented[K15683]. Fresh leaf juice applied undiluted externally to human adults was active. There was improvement of hair in patients with alopecia areata[W02968].

Hemagglutinin activity. A commercial sample of leaf juice was active[T13461]. Chromatographic fraction of fresh leaf gel was active on human red blood cells[K23067]. Fresh leaf homogenates was active[T15275]. Leaf homogenate was active[T15275].

Histamine release inhibition. Water extract of dried leaves was active on mast cells of rats. IC_{50} 0.14 mg/ml vs antigen-induced histamine release and IC_{50} 0.92 mg/ml vs compound 48/80-induced histamine release[K18681].

Hypoglycemic activity. Fresh sap administered intragastrically to mice at a dose of 1.0 gm/day for five days was active[M22020]. Fresh stem juice administered intragastrically to rabbits at a dose of 4.0 ml/kg was active. Glucose levels were decreased 27.9%[K10686]. Polysaccharide fraction of dried whole plant was active on mice[M10008]. Polysaccharide fraction of fresh leaves administered intraperitoneally to mice at a dose of 100.0 mg/kg was active[M13204]. Polysaccharide fraction of fresh leaves administered intraperitoneally to mice at a dose of 100.0 mg/kg was active[T15461]. Polysaccharide fraction of fresh leaves administered intraperitoneally to mice at a dose of 100.0 mg/kg was active[M13204].

Hypolipemic activity. Hot water extract of dried leaf juice administered intragastrically to rats at a dose of 0.5 gm/kg for seven days, was active. The effect was tested by a mixture of *Nigella sativa*, *Commiphora*, *Ferula assa-foetida*, *Aloe vera*, and *Boswellia serrata* vs streptozotocin-induced hyperglycemia[M20731].

Hypotensive activity. Tincture of leaf juice administered intravenously to rabbits was inactive[A00433].

Immunostimulant activity. Lyophilized extract of leaves applied externally on mice at a concentration of 1.67% was active vs UV irradiation-induced suppression of contact hypersensitivity[T16948].

Irritant activity. Water extract of dried leaves applied externally on guinea pigs in a six week cutaneous irritation study at a concentration of 5.0% was inactive[T07202].

Lectin activity. Chromatographic fraction of fresh leaf gel was active. The fraction bind to alpha-D-glucose and mannose sites[K23067].

Leukocyte migration inhibition. Decolorized extract of fresh leaves administered subcutaneously to rats at a dose of 25.0 mg/kg was active vs mustard-induced pedal edema, resulting in 64% reduction in migration and 84% reduction of migration for combination with 0.1 mg/kg hydrocortisone[M25704].

Mitogenic activity. Chromatographic fraction of fresh leaf gel was active[K23067].

Molluscicidal activity. Aqueous slurry (homogenate) of fresh entire plant was inactive on *Lymnaea columella* and *L. cubensis*. LD_{100} >1000 ppm[T04621].

Mutagenic activity. Ethanol (95%) extract of dried plant juice on agar plate at a concentration of 10.0 mg/plate was inactive on *Salmonella typhimurium* TA98 and weak activity on *Salmonella typhimurium* TA102[K08041]

Ovulation inhibition effect. Ethanol/water (1:1) extract of leaves administered orally to female rabbits at a dose of 100.0 mg/kg was equivocal vs copper acetate-induced ovulation[W01378].

Oxygen radical inhibition. Water extract of fresh leaf juice in cell culture was active on polymorphonuclear leukocytes vs PMA-stimulated release. The effect antagonized by Ca^{2+} ionophore[K18822].

Peptidyl transferase inhibition. Dried leaves at a concentration of 10.0 mg was active[M23597].

Phagocytosis inhibition. Aqueous (dialyzed) fraction of fresh leaves at a concentration of 0.5 mg/ml was inactive on polymorphonuclear leukocytes. Phagocytosis and intracellular killing of *Staphylococcus aureus* and *Candida albicans* was not inhibited[T16120].

Phagocytosis stimulation. Fresh leaf juice at a concentration of 4.0 mg/ml was active[T15461].

Phorbol ester antagonist. Aqueous (dialyzed) fraction of fresh leaves at a concentration of 0.5 mg/ml was active on *Polymorphonuclear leukocytes* vs phorbol myristate acetate activation. Low M-R gel-extract-constituents were examined, and oxygen uptake and oxygen and hydrogen peroxide release were inhibited[T16120].

Plant germination inhibition. Water extract of dried leaves at a concentration of 500.0 gm/liter produced strong activity on *Cuscuta reflexa* seeds after six days of exposure to the extract. Water extract of dried stem at a concentration of 500.0 gm/liter was active on *Cuscuta reflexa* seeds after six days of exposure to the extract[M31053].

Plant growth inhibitor. Water extract of dried leaves at a concentration of 500.0 gm/liter was active on *Cuscuta reflexa* seedlings length, weight, and dry weight were measured after six days of exposure to the extract. Water extract of dried stem at a concentration of 500.0 gm/liter was active on *Cuscuta reflexa* seedlings after six days exposure to the extract. Seedling length, weight, and dry weight were measured[M31053].

Polymorphonuclear leukocyte activation inhibition. Water extract of fresh leaves at variable concentrations was active[H04248].

Protein kinase inhibition. Polysaccharide fraction of fresh leaves was active[M16086].

Protein synthesis inhibition. Chromatographic fraction of fresh leaf gel in broth culture was active on *Bacillus subtilis*[T15169]. Dried leaves at a concentration of 1.0 mg were active. Incorporation of leucine into protein was inhibited, as well as were elongation factors EF-1 and EF-2[M23597].

Skin pigmentation effect. Water extract of leaf gel, applied externally, undiluted to human adults was active. A preparation containing extract of given plant was patch-tested on skin exposed to UVA radiation for 30–180 seconds. Areas treated with preparation showed pigmentation for more than one year after treatment[M31028].

Smooth muscle stimulant activity. Tincture of leaf juice was active on rabbit intestine and produced weak activity on the bladder[A00433].

Stability study. Fresh leaf gel could be stabilized with algal polysaccharides of xanthum gum[K08099].

Teratogenic activity. Water extract of dried entire plant administered intragastrically to pregnant rats at a dose of 125.0 mg/kg was active[M19981]. Water extract of dried leaves administered intragastrically to pregnant rats at a dose of 125.0 mg/kg was active[K16006].

Toxic effect (general). Ethanol (95%) of dried aerial parts in the drinking water of mice, at a dose of 100.0 mg/kg for three months was active. Toxic signs included alopecia, degeneration and putrefaction of the sex organs, sperm damage, and decrease RBC levels. When the extract was administered intragastrically at a concentration of 3.0 gm/kg to mice, it was inactive[T15500]. Frozen leaf and stem administered intragastrically to rats at a dose of 925.0 mg/kg was inactive. Administration of test substance was temporally paired with introduction of sodium saccharin solution. Consumption of saccharin solution two days after test was used to estimate aversiveness of test substance, which is related to its toxicity[T13641].

Toxicity assessment (quantitative). Ethanol/water (1:1) extract of dried leaves administered intraperitoneally to mice produced LD_{50} >1.0 gm/kg[A04741]. Ethanol/water (50%) extract of the entire plant administered intraperitoneally to mice to mice produced LD_{50} 250.0 mg/kg. The maximum tolerated dose was 100.0 mg/kg[A03335].

Uterine stimulant effect. Tincture of leaf juice was active on the non-pregnant uterus of rabbits. Stimulation of amplitude of contraction with tonic contraction and loss of rhythmic contraction was observed[A00433]. Water extract of leaves at a concentration of 250.0 mg/liter was active on guinea pig uterus[A04132].

Wound healing acceleration. Ethanol (95%) extract of fresh leaf gel when used externally on guinea pigs at a concentration of 5.0% was active. Partial thickness burn healing assessed. Similar effect seen in use of antithromboxane U38485, lipid peroxidation inhibitor U75412E and xanthine oxidase inhibitor U4285E[K11195]. A concentration of 5.0% applied externally to human adults was active on intra-arterial drug use-induced injury, frostbite injuries, and partial thickness burns. When applied externally to rabbits at a concentration of 5.0%, the extract was active alone and in combination with methimazole improved tissue survival in intra-arterial drug abuse in rabbit ear model. The extract was not as effective against frostbite injury as methylprednisolone or acetylsalicyclic acid. In rats at 5.0% concentration the extract, alone and in combination with methimazole improved tissue survival in electrical injury model[K11195]. Ethanol/water (1:1) extract of fresh leaves administered subcutaneously to mice at a dose of 150.0 mg/kg was active[T16496]. Fresh leaf homogenates in cell culture was active on CA-ME-180 and human embryonic lung cells[T15275]. Fresh leaves applied topically to human adults were active. Eighteen derm-abrasion patients with acne vulgaris were included in the study[T16100]. Fresh leaf juice applied topically at a concentration of 25.0% and in the drinking water at a dose of 100.0 mg/kg were active. Both groups were dosed daily for two months, the wound healing (6-mm punch biopsy wounds) was significantly faster than the untreated control[T16135]. Fresh leaf juice, applied topically to human adults at a concentration of 40.0%, was active in several cases of Roentgen ray dermatitis[W02967]. Undiluted leaf juice was active in on case of radiation ulcers of the tongue, floor of the mouth, and mandible resulting from intraoral radium therapy and external deep X-ray therapy[W02965]. Fresh leaf gel administered intragastrically to male rats at a dose of 2.0 ml/kg was active[K18667]. Fresh leaf juice applied to wounds induced with sterile sandpaper in tips of the fingers of human adults, at a concentration of 50.0% in the form of an ointment using petroleum as a base was active[W02963]. Juice administered subcutaneously to mice at a dose of 300.0 mg/kg was active. The juice blocked 100% of the wound healing suppression of hydrocortisone acetate[K18084]. When applied, undiluted from 1–4 weeks externally on cats, dogs, and horses for a variety inflammatory conditions, the juice was active[T04658]. A case of Roentgen ray dermatitis with ulceration in human adult was treated with undiluted fresh leaf juice with positive results. External application produced weak activity on surgically induced skin wounds[W02960]; active on rabbits and rats vs dermatitis produced by 14,000 Rep of beta radiation and on rabbit on 28,000 Rep of beta radiation[W02966]. The juice, when applied for 14 days, was equivocal on rats vs third degree Roentgen radiation[W02961]. Leaf pulp application externally on human adults at a concentration of 20.0% was active. Epidermal cell prolifera-

tion was 168% of untreated skin[W02968]. Ophthalmic application of undiluted fresh leaf juice was active on rabbits. Traumatic corneal ulcers were produced in 30 animals, and the juice was used as eye drops three times daily[T00876]. Increase rate of wound healing in patients with chronic leg ulcers and improved skin conditions in human patients with acne vulgaris, seborrheic alopecia, and alopecia areata was observed[W02968]. Water extract of fresh leaves applied externally to human adults of both sexes was active[T03940]. Fresh leaf pulp applied externally to patients with chronic and acute injuries three times per week for three weeks was active[M21051]. Leaf gel cream was applied to frost-bitten rabbit ears. Recovery of tissue was enhanced. Effect was increased by co-administration of pentoxyphylline[K23796]. Leaf juice, applied externally on female human adults undiluted, was active. One patient with roentgen dermatitis when treated with fresh leaf juice, itching and burning subsided in 24 hours. After five weeks, there was complete regeneration of skin, new hair growth, complete restoration of sensation, and lack of scar tissue[W00341]. After treatment of Roentgen ray ulcers in a 40-year-old man by daily application of fresh leaf juice, healing began 4–6 weeks after initiation of treatment, with no pain relief for 2–3 weeks after start of treatment. In the treatment of Roentgen ray dermatitis in a 46-year-old man, pain subsided 48 hours following initiation of treatment. Epithelization started in 48–72 hours after start of treatment[W00344]. Leaf juice, applied externally on rabbits at a concentration of 30%, was active. When ointment was applied twice daily on experimentally-induced thermal burns on the back of rabbits, the lesions healed in two weeks without gross evidence of scarring[W00343]. Undiluted leaf juice was active on human adults[T14664]. Water extract of fresh leaf gel (undiluted), when applied externally, was active. The treatment was found to promote fibroblast generation, fibrocytic activity, and collagen proliferation in patients who have undergone nasal surgery[T16559]. The leaf gel administered subcutaneously to mice at a dose of 300.0 mg/kg was active[K15034]. Water extract of fresh leaf juice administered subcutaneously to mice at a dose of 1.0 mg/kg was active. The decolorized extract was used. A 6-mm circular piece of skin was removed from both sides of bodies of normal and diabetic rats. Test groups were dosed daily for seven days. Treated diabetic animals showed a wound reduction of 47% after seven days, relative to a 35% reduction in untreated normal controls and 28% for untreated diabetic controls vs carrageenin-induced pedal edema[M19504]. Water extract administered subcutaneously to mice at a dose of 10.0 mg/kg was active. Wound healing was more rapid when decolorized Aloe (e.g. with anthraquinone removed) was used. When administered subcutaneously to rats, Aloe powder (anthraquinone fraction present) was more effective than Aloe powder combined with RNA and vitamin C[M17603]. Water extract of fresh leaves applied topically to human adults at a concentration of 0.5% was active. The biological activity reported has been patented[M30273]. Water extract of leaves, applied undiluted externally on human adults following dental surgery, was active[J09755]. Water extract when applied externally on guinea pig was active vs burn injury[K18822]. On human adults, the juice speeded laparotomy wounds healing by secondary intention[K18822].

5 | Annona muricata

L.

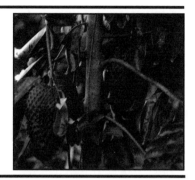

Common Names

Anyigli	Togo	Quanabana	Nicaragua
Apele	Togo	Saput	Nicaragua
Apple leaf	West Indies	Sarifa	Nicaragua
Beleda	Borneo	Seremaia	Nicaragua
Corosol	West Indies	Sorsaca	Curacao
Corossol	Dominica	Sour sop	Dominican Republic
Corossol	Rodrigues Islands	Sour sop	Guyana
Custard apple	Rodrigues Islands	Sour sop	Puerto Rico
Dian	Borneo	Sour sop tree	USA
Guanabana	Barbados	Sour-sop	Jamaica
Guanabana	Cuba	Soursop	Barbados
Guanabana	Dominican Republic	Soursop	Dominica
Guanabana	Panama	Soursop	Guam
Guanabana	Puerto Rico	Soursop	Jamaica
Katara ara tara	Cook Islands	Soursop	Nicaragua
Korosol	Haiti	Soursop	Virgin Islands
Kowosol	West Indies	Soursop	West Indies
Laguana	Guam	Soursop leaf	West Indies
Pumo	Nicaragua	Sowasap	Nicaragua
Puntar waithia	Nicaragua	Ualapana	Dominica

BOTANICAL DESCRIPTION

This small tree of the ANNONACEAE family is 5- to 7-meters in height. The leaves are oblong-obovate to oblong, 2- to 15-cm long, pointed at both ends, smooth, shiny, usually with petioles 5-cm long. Flowers are large and solitary, yellowish or greenish yellow in color. Three outer petals broadly ovate with heart-shaped base, inner three also large elliptical and rounded. The fruit ovoid, 18-cm long or more, is covered with scattered spine-like structures. The pulp is soft white, and rather fibrous and fleshy, with an agreeable sour flavor.

ORIGIN AND DISTRIBUTION

Native of tropical America, it is now commonly cultivated worldwide.

TRADITIONAL MEDICINAL USES

Barbados. Hot water extract of dried leaves is taken orally as a sedative[T05032].

From: Medicinal Plants of the World By: Ivan A. Ross Humana Press Inc., Totowa, NJ

Brazil. Hot water extract of fresh leaves is taken orally as an analgesic[M18488].

Cook Islands. Decoction of dried leaves is used externally to treat rashes and skin diseases and skin infections. Patient is bathed in the cool green solution obtained by boiling the leaves in water. The decoction is taken orally to treat indigestion[K20471]. Crushed leaves produce a scent that is inhaled for dizziness and fainting spells.

Curacao. Hot water extract of leaves is taken orally for gall bladder trouble. The extract is taken orally with *Citrus aurantium* every morning to relieve nervousness. The extract is also taken orally for easy childbirth[A05332].

Dominica. Fruit, when eaten by women, is believed to induce lactation[W01267]. Hot water extract of leaves is taken as a tea by women in labor[W01267].

Guam. Hot water extract of leaves is used as a tea for asthma sufferers[A01962].

Guatemala. Hot water extract of dried leaves is used in a poultice for ringworm[M27151].

Haiti. Decoction of dried leaves is taken orally for grippe, coughs, and asthenia. Fresh fruit juice is taken orally for asthenia[T13846].

India. Hot water extract of dried leaves is taken orally as an antiphlogistic[A05825].

Jamaica. Hot water extract of dried parts is used as bush tea[W04546]. Infusion of hot water extract of leaves is used as an antispasmodic; beverage is prepared as a lactagogue. The heart of the fruit is given to children orally, as a remedy for worms. Fruit taken on an empty stomach as a cure for intermittent fevers, and as a diuretic[W01316].

Mexico. Decoction of dried bark is taken orally to treat diarrhea[K19153]. Fruit is used as a food[T15121].

Nigeria. Fresh fruit juice is taken orally as an antipyretic; applied externally it is an astringent[T06510]. Hot water extract of dried stem is taken orally to treat arthritis[T05549].

Panama. Decoction of the plant is used as an anthelmintic. Piscicidal activity is reported[T01287]. Hot water extract of the bark is taken orally to treat diarrhea. Pulp is taken orally to treat stomach ulcers[T01287]. The leaves are also used alone or with leaves of calabash and sapodilla to make a tea used as a sedative.

Togo. Decoction of dried leaves is taken orally for malaria[M23556].

Trinidad. Hot water extract of dried leaves is taken orally to lower high blood pressure and as a galactagogue[T05032].

Virgin Islands. Water extract of leaves is used externally as a "cooling agent;" taken orally, excess of three leaves will make one drowsy[W00903].

West Indies. Decoction of hot water extract of leaves is taken orally to ease delivery; tea is used for hypertension; tea with castor oil for worms; tea with *Stachytarpheta jamaicensis* and *Chenopodium ambrosioides* used for worms; the extract is taken orally for diarrhea and as a lactagogue. Fruit is eaten or applied externally as a poultice on the breast to induce lactation[T00701].

CHEMICAL CONSTITUENTS
(ppm unless otherwise indicated)

2-4-Cis, iso-annonacin, Lf
2-4-Trans, iso-annonacin, Lf
4-Deoxy-howiicin B, Sd
Acetaldehyde, Fr
Aluminum, Fr 5
Amylcaproate, Pl
Amyloid, Pl
Annomonicin, Sd 56.5
Annomontacin, Sd 60.3
Annomuricine A, Lf 4
Annomuricine B, Lf 3.5
Annomuricine C, Lf 4
Annonacin A, Lf
Annonacin, Sd 1.0%; Lf
Annonacin-10-0ne, Sd 13.6
Annonacinone, Sd 0.007-1.07%
Annonain, Pl
Anomuricine, Rt; Bk; Lf
Anomurine, Rt; Bk; Lf
Anoniine, Pl

Anonol, Lf
Arginine, Pu
Ascorbic acid, Fr 0.019-0.154%
Ash, Fr 0.50-3.80%
Atherospermine, St Bk
Atherosperminine, Rt; Bk; Lf
Beta sitosterol, Lf; Sd Ol
Beta carotene, Fr 0.6
Boron, Fr 3
Caffeic acid, Pl
Calcium, Fr 0.014-0.260%
Campesterol, Sd Ol
Caproic acid methyl ester, Fr
Caprylic acid methyl ester, Fr
Carbohydrate, Fr 8.9-14.9%
Cellobiose, Pl
Cholesterol, Pl
Citric acid, Pl
Citrulline, Pu
Coclaurine, Rt; Bk; Lf
Copper, Fr 1.6
Corepoxtlone, Sd 6.2
Coreximine(+), Rt
Coreximine(-), Bk; Lf
Corossolin, Sd 0.0029-1.01%
Corossolone, Sd 0.0004-1.02
D-Sucrose, Fr
Deacetyl uvaricin, Sd
Dextrose, Pl
Diepoxy muricanin, St Bk
Epomuricenin A, Sd 27.8
Epomuricenin B, Sd 27.8
Epoxy murin A, St Bk
Epoxy murin B, St Bk
Ethanol, Fr
Fat, Sd 21.1%
Fiber, Fr 0.6-6.5%
Fixed oil, Sd 23.86%
Folic acid, Pl
Fructose, Pl
Galactomannan, Pl
Gamma amino butyric acid, Pu
Gentisic acid, Lf
Geranyl caproate, Pl
Gigantetrocin A, Sd 18.1
Gigantetrocin B, Sd 13.6
Gigantetrocin, Sd 22.1
Gigantetronenin, Lf
Glucose, Lf
Goniothalamicin, Sd 5.9-166
HCN, Pl
Hex-trans-2-en-1-ol, Fr

Howiicin A, Sd
Howiicin B, Sd
Howiicin F, Sd
Howiicin G, Sd
Iron, Fr 5-33
Iso-annonacin, Sd 27.7
Iso-annonacin-10-one, Sd 11.3
Isocitric acid, Pl
Kilocalories, Fr 0.059-0.355%
Lignoceric acid, Lf
Linoleic acid, Sd Ol; Lf
Lysine, Fr 0.060-0.318%
Magnesium, Fr 0.021-0.240%
Malic acid, Pl
Manganese, Fr 2.7
Mericyl alcohol, Pl
Methanol, Fr
Methionine, Fr 70-370
Methyl-hexanoate, Pl
Montanacin, Sd 249
Muricatacin, Sd
Muricatetrocin A, Sd; Lf
Muricatetrocin B, Sd; Lf
Muricatocin A, Lf 4.5
Muricatocin B, Lf 4
Muricatocin C, Lf
Muricine, Bk
Muricinine, Bk
Murisolin, Sd 6-93
Myricyl alcohol, Lf
Myristic acid, Pl
Neo, iso-annonacin-10-one, Sd
Niacin, Fr 9-77
Nitrogen, Fr 0.27%
Oleic acid, Sd Ol, Lf
Ornithine, Pu
P-Coumaric acid, Pl
Palmitic acid, Sd Ol
Pantothenic acid, Fr 2.5-13
Paraffin, Pl
Phosphorous, Fr 0.021-0.340%
Potassium chloride, Lf
Potassium, Fr 0.255-3.600%
Procyanidin, Pl
Protein, Sd 21.43%
Resin, Pl
Reticuline(+), Rt; Bk; Lf
Reticuline, St Bk
Riboflavin, Fr 0.5-6
Rolliniastatin 1, Sd
Rolliniastatin 2, Sd
Scyllitol, Pl

SFA, Sd 6.2%
Sodium, Fr 0.0065- 0.1035%
Solamin, Sd 3.6-11.6; St Bk;
Stearic acid, Lf; Sd Ol
Stepharine, Pl
Stigmasterol, Sd Ol
Sulfur, Fr 0.021-0.270%
Tannin, Lf
Thiamin, Fr 0.7-4.8
Tryptophan, Fr 110-585
UFA, Sd 15.9%
Vitamin B6, Fr 0.6-3
Water, Fr 81.16-83.2%
Xylosyl cellulose, Pl
Zinc, Fr 4

PHARMACOLOGICAL ACTIVITIES AND CLINICAL TRIALS

Analgesic activity. Ethanol/water (1:1) extract of fresh leaves administered intra-gastrically to mice at a dose of 1.0 gm/kg was inactive vs writhing and tail flick tests[M18488].

Anti-amebic activity. Ethanol (95%) extract of dried bark was active on *Entamoeba histolytica*. MIC 63.0 mcg/ml[K19153].

Antibacterial activity. Acetone extract of dried leaves on agar plate was active on *Escherichia coli, Pseudomonas aeruginosa, Salmonella B, Salmonella newport, Salmonella typhosa, Serratia marcescens, Shigella flexneri, Staphylococcus albus, Staphylococcus aureus,* and inactive on *Sarcina lutea*. The ethanol (95%) extract was inactive on *E. coli, P. aeruginosa, Salmonella B, S. newport, S. typhosa, S. lutea, S. marcescens, S. flexneri, S. flexneri 3A, S. Albus,* and *S. aureus*. The water extract was active on *E. coli, P. aeruginosa, S. flexneri,* and inactive on *Salmonella B, S. newport, S. typhosa, Sarcina lutea, Serratia marcescens, S. flexneri, S. albus,* and *S. aureus*[K09159]. Ethanol (95%) extract of dried bark at a concentration of 10.0 mcg/disk, on agar plate was active on *Escherichia coli* and *Micrococcus luteus*. At a concentration of 5.0 mcg/disk, the extract was active on *Bacillus subtilis*[K19153]. Acetone extract of dried stem on agar plate was active on *Escherichia coli, Salmonella B, Salmonella newport, Salmonella typhosa, Shigella flexneri,* and *Shigella flexneri 3A;* inactive on *Pseudomonas aeruginosa, Sarcina lutea, Serratia marcescens, Staphylococcus albus,* and *Staphylococcus aureus*. Ethanol (95%) extract was inactive on *Pseudomonas aeruginosa, Salmonella B, Salmonella newport, Salmonella typhosa, Sarcina lutea, Serratia marcescens, Shigella flexneri, Shigella flexneri 3A, Staphylococcus albus,* and *Staphylococcus aureus*. Water extract was active on *Escherichia coli, Pseudomonas aeruginosa, salmonella newport, Salmonella typhosa,* and *Shigella flexneri;* inactive on *Salmonella B, Sarcina lutea, Serratia marcescens, Shigella flexneri 3A, Staphylococcus albus,* and *Staphylococcus aureus*[K09159]. Ethanol (95%) extract of dried root bark at a concentration of 2–3 mcg/plate on agar plate was active on *Bacillus subtilis* and *Staphylococcus albus* and inactive on *Klebsiella pneumoniae* and *Pseudomonas aeruginosa*. Ethanol (95%) extract of dried seeds at a concentration of 2–3 mcg/liter on agar plate was active on *Bacillus subtilis* and *Staphylococcus albus* and inactive on *Klebsiella pneumoniae* and *Pseudomonas aeruginosa*. Ethanol (95%) extract of dried stem bark on agar plate at a concentration of 2–3 mg/plate was active on *Bacillus subtilis* and *Staphylococcus albus* and inactive on *Klebsiella pneumoniae* and *Pseudomonas aeruginosa*[K15021].

Anticonvulsant activity. Ethanol (95%) extract of fresh fruit at variable dosages administered intraperitoneally to mice of both sexes was inactive vs strychnine and metrazole-induced convulsions[T06510].

Anticrustacean activity. Ethanol (95%) extract of dried leaves was active on *Artemia salina* larvae. LC_{50} 0.17 mg/ml[H16272]. Hexane extract of dried seeds was active on *Artemia salina* LD_{50} 30.0 ppm and LC_{50} 0.8 ppm[H06944]. Methanol extract was also active LD_{50} 5.0 ppm on adults[H14312] and 40.0 mg/liter on larvae[M28527]. Methanol/water (1:1) extract produced strong activity LD_{50} 0.8 ppm[H12985].

Antifungal activity. Acetone, Ethanol (95%), and water extracts of dried leaves at a concentration of 50.0% on agar plate was inactive on *Neurospora crassa*[T08589]. Ethanol (95%) extract of bark at a concentration of 5.0 mcg/disc, on agar plate was active on *Penicillum oxalicum* and on *Cladosporium cucumerinum* at a concentration of 7.0 mcg/disk[K19153]. Hot water extract of dried leaves at a concentration of 1.0 ml in broth culture was inactive on *Epidermophyton floccosum*, *Microsporum canis*, *Microsporum gypseum*, *Trichophyton mentagrophytes* vars. algodonosa, and granulare, *Trichophyton rubrum*[M27151]. Acetone, water, and ethanol (95%) extracts of dried stem, at concentrations of 50% on agar plate were inactive on *Neurospora crassa*[T08589].

Antihepatotoxic activity. Decoction of dried leaves at a concentration of 1.0 mg/plate in cell culture produced weak activity on hepatocytes; measured by leakage of LDH and ASAT. It reduced the leakage of ASAT[K23019].

Antimalarial activity. Chloroform extract of wood administered subcutaneously to chicken at a dose of 118.0 mg/kg and water extract administered orally at a dose of 3.675 gm/kg were inactive on *Plasmodium gallinaceum*[A00785]. Ethanol (95%) extract of dried leaves produced weak activity on *Plasmodium falciparum* W-2 IC_{50} 20.0 mcg/ml and inactive on *Plasmodium falciparum* D-6 [K16971].

Antiparasitic activity. Methanol extract of dried seeds, in broth culture was active on *Nippostrongylus brasiliense* LD_{50} 20.0 mg/liter, *Molinema dessetae* LD_{50} 6.0 mg/liter, *Trichomonas vaginalis* MIC 30.0 mg/liter, inactive on *Entamoeba histolytica* MIC >100 mg/liter[M28527].

Cardiac depressant activity. Water extract of bark was active on the heart of rabbits[A04104].

Cytotoxic activity. Ethanol (95%) extract of leaves on cell culture was active on CA-9KB. ED_{50} <20.0 mcg/ml. Ethanol (95%) extract of stem in cell culture was active on CA-9KB. ED_{50} <20.0 mcg/ml[X00001].

Hypertensive activity. Ethanol (95%) and water extracts of leaves and stem administered intravenously to dogs at doses of 0.1 ml/kg were active[A03360].

Hypotensive activity. Hot water extract of dried leaves, at a dose of 1.0 ml/animal administered intravenously to rats was active. Blood pressure fell by more than 30%[M29843].

Inotropic effect positive. Hot water extract of dried leaves at a concentration of 320.0 microliters was inactive on guinea pig atria[M29843].

Insecticidal activity. Ethanol (95%) extract of leaves at a concentration of 5.0% produced weak activity on *Macrosiphoniella sanborni*. Ethanol (95%) extract of dried seeds at a concentration of 5.0% was inactive on *Macrosiphoniella sanborni*. Ethanol (95%) extract of root at a concentration of 5.0% produced weak activity on *Macrosiphoniella sanborni*. Ethanol (95%) extract of seeds at a concentration of 5.0% was active on *Callosobruchus chinensisi*[M25852] and strongly active on *Macrosiphoniella sanbornii*[W00220].

Larvicidal activity. Water extract of dried leaves and stem at a concentration of 0.03 gm of fresh plant material per ml of water was inactive on *Culex quinquefasciatus*[M19731].

Lipid peroxidation formation inhibition. Decoction of dried leaves at a concentration of 1.0 mg/plate in cell culture was inactive on hepatocytes. Monitored by production of malonaldehyde[K23019].

Molluscicidal activity. Aqueous slurry (homogenate) of fresh entire plant (fruits, leaves and roots) was inactive on *Lymnaea columella* and *Lymnaea cubensis*. LD_{100} >1 M ppm[T04621].

Radical scavenging effect. Decoction of dried leaves, at a concentration of 250.0 mg/liter was inactive. Measured by decoloration of diphenylpicryl hydroxyl radical solution. 16% decoloration[K23019].

Smooth muscle relaxant activity. Ethanol (95%) and water extracts of leaves and stem, at concentrations of 3.3 ml/liter were active on rabbit duodenum[A03360].

Spasmogenic activity. Ethanol (95%) and water extracts of leaves and stem, at a concentration of 0.033 ml/liter was active on guinea pigs ileum[A03360].

Toxicity assessment (quantitative). Water extract of leaves and stem administered intraperitoneally to mice produced a minimum toxic dose of 1.0 ml/animal[A03360].

Uterine stimulant effect. Ethanol (95%) and water extracts of leaves and stem, at a concentration of 0.033 ml/liter was active on the uterus of rats[A03360].

Vasodilator activity. Ethanol (95%) extract of leaves and stem at a concentration of 0.033 ml/liter was active on the isolated hind quarter of rats[A03360].

6 | Carica papaya

L.

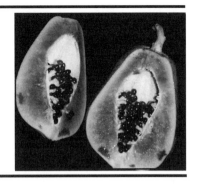

Common Names

Aanabahe-hindi	India	Jhad-chibhadi	India
Ababau	Nicaragua	Karumusa	India
Amita	India	Karutha kapalam	India
Badie	Ivory Coast	Kath	India
Bake	Ivory Coast	Kunam-paran popo	Admiralty Islands
Bedon-al-babo	Guinea-Bissau	Lesi	Admiralty Islands
Bepaia	Guinea-Bissau	Lesi tangata	Tonga
Boppai	India	Lo hong phle	Vietnam
Boppaya	India	Mak hung	Vietnam
Buah betek	Malaysia	Malako	Thailand
Buah ketela	Malaysia	Mama	Angola
Buah papaya	Malaysia	Mamioko	Bougainville
Budibaga	Senegal	Mamoeiro	Paraguay
Bumpapa	Senegal	Mande	Ghana
Bupapay	Senegal	Mande	Senegal
Chibda	India	Manjan	Borneo
Chichihualxochitl	Mexico	Melon tree	India
Chirbhita	India	Melon tree	Nigeria
Common papaw	India	Mewa	Nepal
Du du	Vietnam	Mikana	Hawaii
Ebabayo	Tanzania	Mokka	Japan
Ehi	Tanzania	Mupapawe	Venda
Eranda-kakadi	India	Nita	Cook Islands
Esi	India	O rabana	Senegal
Fafy	Oman	Ojo-mgbimgbi	Nigeria
Fakai	Sierra Leone	Olesi	Nigeria
Fakai laa	Sierre Leone	Omita	India
Fruta bomba	Cuba	Ommal	India
Fruto bomba	Cuba	Pace	Guinea-Bissau
Goppe	India	Papae	Guinea-Bissau
Gwanda	Nigeria	Papai	India
I'ita	Nigeria	Papai	West Indies
Ibepe	Nigeria	Papaia	Guinea-Bissau
Ipi	Papua-New Guinea	Papapa	Fiji

From: Medicinal Plants of the World *By: Ivan A. Ross Humana Press Inc., Totowa, NJ*

Papaw	Guyana	Papeya	India
Papaw	Jamaica	Papia	Senegal
Papaw	Malaysia	Papita	Fiji
Papaw	USA	Papita	India
Papaw	West Indies	Papitha	India
Papay	Haiti	Papoia	Guinea-Bissau
Papay	India	Parimi	India
Papaya	India	Parindakaya	India
Papaya	Brazil	Paupau	India
Papaya	Fiji	Paw paw	Nigeria
Papaya	Gold Coast	Pawpaw	East Africa
Papaya	Guatemala	Pawpaw	England
Papaya	India	Pawpaw	Fiji
Papaya	Indonesia	Pawpaw	India
Papaya	Japan	Papaw	Malaysia
Papaya	Malaysia	Pawpaw	Oman
Papaya	Nepal	Pawpaw	Papua-New Guinea
Papaya	Papua-New Guinea	Pawpaw	Philippines
Papaya	Peru	Poi poi	Kenya
Papaya	Tanzania	Popai	India
Papaya	USA	Poyam	Admiralty Islands
Papaya tree	India	Puppai	India
Papaye	Guadeloupe	Tree melon	India
Papaye	Rodrigues Islands	Tuunuk	Nicaragua
Papayer	Ivory Coast	Twas	Nicaragua
Papayer	Vietnam	Ulmak	Nicaragua
Papayer	Zaire	Vatakumba	India
Papayi	Guadeloupe	Vatre	Ivory Coast
Papayo	Mexico	Vi nita	Ivory Coast
Papayu	India	Wayoye	Papua
Papeeta	Pakistan	Weleti	Papua
Papeta	India	Wi	Papua

BOTANICAL DESCRIPTION

This is a perennial, herbaceous plant of the CARICACEAE family, with copious milky latex reaching to as high as 10 meters. The stem is about 25-cm thick, simple or branched above the middle and roughened with leaf scars. Leaves, clustered around the apex of the stem and branches, have nearly cylindrical stalks, 25- to 100-cm long; the leaf blade has 7 to 11 main lobes and some secondary irregular pointed lobes and prominent veins; leaf surface is yellow-green to dark-green above and paler beneath. Usually male and female flowers are borne on separate plants, but hermaphrodite flow-ers often occur, and a male plant may con-vert to a female after being beheaded. Flow-ers emerge singly or in clusters from the main stem among the lower leaves, the fe-male short-stalked, the male with drooping peduncles 25- to 100-cm long. Corolla is 1.25- to 2.5-cm long, with five oblong re-curved white petals. Fruit is extremely vari-able in form and size; it may be nearly round, pear-shaped, oval, or oblong; that of the wild plants may be as small as an egg, whereas in cultivation, the fruit ranges from 10-cm to 60-cm in length and up to 20-cm thick. Its skin is smooth, relatively thin, and deep-yellow to orange when the fruit is ripe.

Flesh is succulent, yellow to orange or salmon-red, sweet and more or less musky. The central cavity is lined with a dryish pulpy membrane to which adhere numerous black rough peppery seeds, each with a glistening transparent gelatinous coating.

ORIGIN AND DISTRIBUTION

It is believed that papaya originated in Southern Mexico and Central America, though it was cultivated as far south as Lima, Peru, in pre-Spanish times. Today, papaya is grown in all tropical and subtropical countries as a commercial crop.

TRADITIONAL MEDICINAL USES

Admiralty Islands. Fresh leaf sap is applied to skin with Siponia eruptions twice daily. The treatment is repeated in five days, if needed. Fresh soft bark is scraped onto a leaf and heated over a fire. The soft material is rubbed onto a new cut to promote healing[T07369].

Bougainville. Fresh leaves are squeezed to a pulp and plastered onto cuts or wounds to promote healing[T05034].

Brazil. Latex is taken orally as an anthelmintic[A06732]. Unripe fruit is applied to the skin for ringworm and dermatitis. Ripe fruit is eaten for constipation[T00359].

Cook Islands. Fresh seeds are eaten whole as a treatment for intestinal worms[T09553]. Fresh unripe fruit is used externally to treat cuts and sores, skin infections[K20471]. For boils and carbuncles, the unripe fruit is grated, mixed with coconut oil, and rubbed in affected part[T09553].

Cuba. Unripe fruit is eaten for hypertension[A05591].

East Africa. Hot water extract of leaves is taken orally as an anthelmintic[T01420]. Hot water extract of dried roots is taken orally for syphilis and as an anthelmintic[A05825]. Hot water extract of latex is taken orally as an anthelmintic. Hot water extract of roots is taken orally as an anthelmintic. Hot water extract of seeds is taken orally as an anthelmintic[T01420]. Unripe fruit juice is taken orally as an abortifacient[A04281].

Ecuador. Hot water extract of fresh fruit is taken orally as a contraceptive[T15375].

Fiji. Fresh sap is used externally for ringworm. Ground dried leaves is taken with salt for coughs. Fresh ripe fruit pulp is taken orally for indigestion, as an appetizer, and for diarrhea and dysentery[T10632].

Ghana. Hot water extract of seeds is taken orally as an abortifacient. Latex is used as an abortifacient[T01420]. Root blended with salt and triturated with water is used as a douche to induce abortion[A00708]. Hot water extract of root is taken orally as an abortifacient[T01420].

Gold Coast. Hot water extract of root is taken orally as an abortifacient[A00115].

Guadeloupe. Seeds are eaten as a vermifuge[T07660].

Guinea-Bissau. Decoction of hot water extract is taken orally as an abortive. Unripe fruits are crushed and part of the pulp is used to massage the breasts as an emmenagogue; the remaining part is mixed with water and boiled with vapors being placed on the woman's breasts. After cooling, the decoction is administered orally in divided doses throughout the day[A00455].

Guinea. Decoction of hot water extract of leaves is taken orally to provoke abortion. Decoction of hot water extract of unripe fruit is taken orally to provoke milk secretion. Latex of unripe fruits is massaged over the breasts to provoke milk secretion. Seeds are eaten to induce abortion[A00708].

Haiti. Fresh fruit juice is taken orally for hypertension. Fresh latex is taken orally for toothache. Water extract of dried root is taken orally for urethritis[T13846].

Hawaii. Unripe fruit is claimed to be beneficial in producing lactation. The fruit is washed, cut into cubes, and boiled as for a soup. The broth is taken by new mothers. Within a few days, stinging sensations in the breasts begin, and the breasts then fill up with milk[W00534]. Water extract of unripe fruit is taken orally for asthma[K18991].

India. A mixture of *Carica papaya* root and *Ferula narthex* resin is used to induce abortion. The root of *Carica papaya* with girth able to penetrate the vagina and about 8- to 10-in long is obtained. At one end, an incision a half an inch deep in the shape of a cross is made in such a way that the root does not break into separate portions. In these cuts, the *Ferula marthex* resin is put, better if somewhat crushed and refined. The vagina is penetrated with the portion containing the *Ferula marthex* to go deep inside and most probably to touch the os uteri. Penetration and maintaining the root in this way daily for 7–8 hours in the vagina is said to result in abortion, even in a fetus 3–4-month-old[T06787]. Decoction of inner stem-bark is taken orally twice daily for dental caries[M27166]. Dried seeds eaten by pregnant women will produce abortion and is a powerful emmenagogue[A05825]. Powdered seeds is taken orally as an anthelmintic[M22542]. Hot water extract of seeds is taken orally as an anti-inflammatory and analgesic[T15475]. Fresh fruit is eaten as an abortifacient. Tender fruits are used in different forms. To expel intestinal worms, ripe fruits are eaten[T08282]. Fruit is taken orally as an emmenagogue[A04132]and abortifacient[A04610]. Pregnant women are strictly prohibited from eating papaya during pregnancy for fear of inducing labor. Some tribal people believe that papaya has a powerful antifertility property[T00706]. Hot water extract of flowers is taken orally as a heart tonic. Hot water extract of leaves is taken orally as a febrifuge and heart tonic[T01420]. Hot water extract of ripe-dried fruit is taken orally as an emmenagogue[T14891]. Hot water extract of ripe fresh fruit is said to be astringent to the bowels, an aphrodisiac, and is used for biliousness[T15475]. Unripe fresh fruit is taken orally for abortion. Ripe fruits are taken orally as a diuretic and to treat flatulence[K11282]. Latex

is taken orally for indigestion, abdominal colic, hemorrhoids, worms, and for liver and spleen enlargement[T15475]. To treat worms, leaf extract and latex of raw fruit are taken orally[K08933]. Hot water extract of root is taken orally as an abortifacient and to treat yaws[T01420]. Latex is applied to the os uteri for inducing abortion[A00115]. Latex is taken orally as an anthelmintic[T03054]. Plant juice taken orally is said to be a powerful anthelmintic, applied to the os uteri, it produces abortion[W00002]. Seeds are taken orally as a powerful emmenagogue, an abortifacient when mixed with *Zingiber officinale* and honey[A00115]. Unripe fruit is eaten for gastric disorders. Young fruit is eaten together with the young seeds to cause abortion[T07374]. Unripe fruit juice, taken orally is claimed to a powerful galactagogue, emmenagogue, and abortifacient. Application to the os uteri is believed to interrupt pregnancy[T00213]. Young fresh leaves are made into a fine paste and taken orally for a week at doses of 5–6 gm, for severe jaundice[M29106].

Indonesia. Seed and flesh of fruit are eaten to promote abortion[K04296].

Ivory Coast. Decoction of hot water extract of leaves is taken orally in case of difficult delivery; if the decoction is drunk, it can cause abortion; externally it is used as a galactagogue[A04941]. Fresh leaves are used externally as a hemostatic[T15327].

Jamaica. Fresh latex is used externally in the treatment of ringworm[W01316].

Kenya. Decoction of dried root is taken orally for venereal diseases. *Carica papaya* and *Carissa edulis* and other species are combined[M25859].

Malawi. Water extract of dried root is taken orally to cure yellow fever[M23819].

Malaysia. Fresh unripe fruit juice is taken orally as an emmenagogue. Hot water extract of flowers is taken orally as an emmenagogue[T01420]. Hot water extract of roots is taken orally as an abortifacient[T01420]. Latex is applied to the os uteri to induce abortion[A00115]. The latex is taken orally as an abortifacient[A03602,A04587]. Seeds are taken orally to induce abortion in early pregnancy[A03602]. Hot water extract of seeds is taken orally as an abortifacient and emmenagogue[T01420]. Unripe fruit is considered dangerous for pregnant women[A03602]. Unripe fruit is considered dangerous to be eaten by women during pregnancy[A04587].

Mexico. Fresh latex is taken orally to treat constipation. The exudation is taken as a purgative[K16948]. Fresh unripe fruit juice is taken orally as an emmenagogue[T01420]. Hot water extract of latex is applied externally to skin rash. Orally, it is taken for ulcers and as a digestive[J01414]. Hot water extract of seeds is taken orally as an emmenagogue[T01420]. Water[A00115] and hot water[T01420] extracts of flowers are taken orally as emmenagogue.

Mozambique. Hot water extract of leaves is taken orally as a febrifuge[A04941].

Myanmar. Unripe fruit is eaten as an abortifacient[A04277].

Nigeria. Dried leaves cooked with *Musa sapientum* in equal proportions is taken orally or as a bath to treat body infections; the leaf extract is taken with salt, orally, to treat yellow fever, and the infusion prepared from leaves is taken orally to treat stomach-ache. Fresh fruit is eaten as a treatment for beri-beri[K08933]. Hot water extract of fresh leaves is taken orally as a purgative, anti-pyretic, analgesic, and anthelmintic. Hot water extract of fresh root is taken orally as an anthelmintic, antipyretic, and analgesic. Fruit is eaten for nausea, as a carminative, for yaws, as an antipyretic, purgative, and for dysentery[T06510].

Panama. Fruit juice is taken orally for diarrhea and dysentery. Toasted and powdered seeds mixed with honey is taken orally, one teaspoon, followed by a laxative (castor oil) as an anthelmintic[T01287].

Papua-New Guinea. Dried seeds of a ripe fruit are chewed for cough and stomach-ache[K18559]. Fresh sap from any part of the plant mixed with lime is rubbed into *Tinea imbrication* and other skin eruptions[K18142,T09033].

Paraguay. Dried seeds are eaten as a vermifuge[K18765].

Peru. Hot water extract of dried fruit is taken orally for gall bladder and liver conditions and for disorders of fat digestion and dyspepsia. Hot water extract of dried leaves is taken orally for gallbladder and liver conditions, and for disorders of fat digestion and dyspepsia[T15323].

Senegal. Decoction of dried fruit and citrus species is taken orally for venereal diseases[M24038]. Decoction of young leaves is taken orally as an abortifacient, for blennorrhagia, and for yellow fever. Hot water extract of dried root is taken orally for gonorrhea and venereal disease, yellow fever, toothache, and dysentery. Hot water extract of dried seeds is taken orally for fungal infections of the skin. Hot water extract of fresh latex is used externally for sores. Hot water extract of unripe fruit is taken orally for coughs, and externally for sores[M21947]. Seeds are taken orally as an abortifacient and emmenagogue[A04296].

Sierra Leone. Old yellowish leaves are rubbed in a calabash and water added, the liquid is taken orally to stimulate labor[T08806]. Decoction of dried leaves is taken orally for yellow fever[T09679].

Tanzania. Hot water extract of dried root is taken orally as an anthelmintic[T03389]. Hot water extract of fresh leaves is taken orally for gonorrhea[T10354].

Thailand. Hot water extract of dried root is used as a diuretic[W03804].

Tonga. Dried stem scrapings are used to prepare an infusion that is taken orally to remedy failure of lactation[T08685].

Vanuatu. Unripe fruit is taken to induce abortion. Four small unripe fruits is eaten together with four tablets of nivaquine and the juice of two limes[K18109].

Venda. Decoction of dried root of *Carica papaya*, *Terminalia sericea*, *Parinari curatellifolia*, and *Citrus limon* is used. One tablespoonful of the decoction is taken orally[T08732].

Vietnam. Unripe fruit is eaten as an abortive[A04766].

West Africa. Hot water extract of dried root is taken orally as an abortifacient[A05825].

West Indies. Hot water extract of flowers is taken orally as an emmenagogue. Hot water extract of fresh unripe fruit is taken orally as an emmenagogue[T01420]. Hot water extract of seeds is taken orally as an emmenagogue[T01420]. Latex of milk from incisions in stem is taken orally as a diuretic. It is said that "it burns but it makes the urine flow"[L01534]. Unripe fruit juice and hot water extract is taken orally for hypertension[T00701].

CHEMICAL CONSTITUENTS

(ppm unless otherwise indicated)

(E)-beta-ocimene, Fr
(Z)- beta-ocimene, Fr
2-6-Dimethyl-3-7-diene-2-6-diol, Fr EO
2-6-Dimethyl-oct-7-ene-2-3-6-triol, Fr EO
2-6-Dimethyl-octa-1-7-diene-3-6-diol, Fr EO
2-6-Dimethyl-octa-cis-2-7-diene-1-6-diol, Fr Eo
2-6-Dimethyl-octa-trans-2-7-diene-1-6-diol, Fr EO
2-Methyl-butan-1-al
3-Methyl-butyl-benzoate, Fr
4-Hydroxy-4-methyl-pentan-2-one, Fr
4-Terpineol, Fr
5-Dehydro-avenasterol, Sd oil
5-Hydroxytryptamine
6-7-epoxy linalool, Fr EO
6-Methylkept-5-en-2-one, Fr
7-Dehydro-avenasterol, Sd oil
24-Methylene cycloartenol, Sd oil
5,6-Monoepoxi-beta carotene, Fr
Acetyl-hexosamide, Lx
Alanine, Fr 140-1,253
Alkaloid, Lf 1,300-1,500
Alpha linolenic acid, Fr 250-2,238
Alpha terpinene, Fr

Alpha tocopherol, Lf
Alpha-phellandrene, Fr
Amyl iso-acetate, Fr
Amyl-acetate, Fr
Arachidic acid, Sd oil 0.5-1.0%
Arginine, Fr 100-895
Ascorbic acid, Fr 330-5,732; Lf 1,400-6,222
Ash, Fr 0.58-5.73%; Lf 2.2-15.4%; Sd 8.8%
Aspartic acid, Fr 490-4,387
Behenic acid, Sd oil 1.6%
Benzaldehyde, Fr 0.3 mg/mg
Benzyl alcohol, Fr 0.2 mg/kg
Benzyl glucosinolate, Fr
Benzyl-iso-thiocyanate, Sd 0.2-0.5%
Benzyl-isothiocyanate, Fr
Benzylsenevol, Sd
Beta carotene, Fr 10-123
Beta sitosterol, Lf; Sd ; Fl; Fr
Beta-beta carotene, Lf 116-514
Beta-beta carotene-3-diol, Lf
Beta-epsilon carotene, Lf
Beta-phellandrene, Fr
Beta-pseudo carotene, Lf
Boron, Fr 5-15
But-2-enoic acid benzyl ester, Fr 0.1 mg/kg
But-2-enoic acid methyl ester, Fr 0.3 mg/kg
Butanedione, Fr
Butanoic acid methyl ester, Fr 46.7 mg/kg
Butanoic acid, Fr pu 1.2
Butyl-acetate, Fr
Butyl-alcohol, Fr
Butyl-benzoate, Fr
Butyl-hexanoate, Fr
Caffeic acid, Lf
Calcium, Fr 100-2,729; Lf 0.344-2.380%
Callose, Lx
Campesterol, Sd oil
Caoutchouc, Lx 4.5%
Caproic acid, Fr
Carbohydrates, Fr 9.5-99.1%; Lf 11.3-55.6%; Sd 15.5%
Carica papaya alkaloid(C-11-H-14-N-2-0), Lf 2.8
Carica papaya amylase, Fr
Carica papaya anticoagulant, Fr Lx
Carica papaya polysaccharide P-1, Lx
Carica papaya polysaccharide PP-11, Lx
Carica papaya polysaccharide, Lx
Caricacin,

Caricin, Sd
Carpaine, Lf 1,000-1,500; Sd; Fr; Bk, Rt
Carpasamine, Sd 0.35%
Carposide, Lf
Caryophyllene, Fr
Cholesterol, Sd oil
Choline, Lf 0.02%
Chrysanthemexanthin, Fr
Chymopapain A, Lx
Chymopapain, Lx
Chymopapain-B, Lx
Cis-beta ocimene, Fr 0.4 mcg/kg
Cis-linalool oxide, Fr 7.1 mcg/kg
Citric acid, Fr
Copper, Fr 0.1-5
Cotinine, Lf 27.8
Cryptoxanthin monoepoxide, Fr peel
Cryptoxanthin, Fr peel
Cycloartanol, Sd oil
Cyclobranol, Sd oil
D-galactose, Fr
D-galacturonic acid, Fr
Decanal, Fr
Dehydrocarpaine 1, Lf
Dehydrocarpaine 11, Lf
Dehydrocarpamines, Pl
Delta octalactone, Fr 0.1 mg/kg
Delta-5-stigmasterol, Sd oil
Essential oil, Sd 900
Epsilon carotene, Fr peel
Ethanol, Fr
Ethyl acetate, Fr
Ethyl alcohol, Fr
Ethyl benzoate, Fr
Ethyl butyrate, Fr
Ethyl octanoate, Fr
Fat, Fr 0.098-2.2%; Lf 0.8-13.6%; Lx 2.4; Sd 25.3%
Fatty acids, Sd oil
Fiber, Fr 0.696-7.554%; Lf 1.8-14.5%; Sd 17%
Fixed oil (Carica papaya), Sd
Flavonols, Lf 0-2,000
Fructose, Fr; Lf; Tr Bk
Galactose, Tr Bk
Gamma carotene, Fr
Gamma terpinene, Fr
Gamma -octalactone, Fr
Gentisic acid, Lf
Geranyl acetone, Fr
Germacrene-D, Fr
Glucotropaelin, Pl

Glutamic acid, Fr
Glycine, Fr 180-1,611
Heptan-2-one, Fr
Heptanal, Fr
Hex-2-enoic acid methyl ester, Fr
Hexadecenoic acid, Sd oil 0.8%
Hexanal, Fr
Hexanoic acid methyl ester, 0.1 mcg/kg
Hexyl acetate, Fr
Hexyl alcohol, Fr
Histidine, Fr 50-448
Iron, Fr 0.8-38; Lf 8-38
Iso-butyl acetate, Fr
Iso-butyl-alcohol, Fr
Iso-propyl alcohol, Fr
Isoamyl acetate, Fr
Isoleucine, Fr 80-716
Kilocalories, Fr 390-3,491; Lf 740
Kryptoflavin, Fr
Kryptoxanthin, Fr
Lauric acid, Fr 10-90; Sd
Leucine, Fr 160-1,432
Lignoceric acid, Sd oil
Linalool oxide-A, Fr
Linalool oxide-B, Fr
Linalool, Fr 0.3 mcg/kg
Linoleic acid, Fr 60-537; Fl; Lf; Sd 5,389
Lycopene, Fr
Lysine, Fr 250-2,238
Lysozyme, Lx
Magnesium, Fr 82-1,058
Malic acid, Fr
Malic acid, Lx 4,400
Manganese, Fr 0.1-1.1
Methanol, Fr
Methionine, Fr 20-179
Methyl acetate, Fr
Methyl cyclohexane, Fr 4.5 mcg/kg
Methyl hexanoate, Fr
Methyl nicotinate, Fr
Methyl octanoate, Fr
Methyl salicyclate, Fr
Methyl thiocyanate, Fr
Methylgeranate, Fr
MUFA, Fr 380-3,402
Mutatochrom, Fr
Myosmine, Lf 1.4
Myrcene, Fr
Myristic acid, Fr 70-62; Sd; Lf
Myristoleic acid Fl
Myrosin, Sd
N-butanol, Fr

N-docosane, Sd oil
N-dodecane, Sd oil
N-dotriacontane, Sd oil
N-Eicosane, Sd oil
N-heneicosane, Sd oil
N-hentriacontane, Sd oil
N-heptadecane, Sd oil
N-hexacosane, Sd oil
N-hexadecane, Sd oil
N-N-dimethylformamide, Fr 0.1%
N-nonacosane, Sd oil
N-nonadecane, Sd oil
N-octacosane, Sd oil
N-octadecane, Sd oil
N-pentacosane, Sd oil
N-pentadecane, Sd oil
N-tetracosane, Sd oil
N-tetradecane, Sd oil
N-triacontane, Sd oil
N-tricosane, Sd oil
N-tridecane, Sd oil
N-tritriacontane, Sd oil
Neoxanthin, Fr
Niacin, Fr 3-33; Lf 21-93
Nicotine, Lf 0.01028%
Nonanal, Fr
Octadecadienoic acid, Sd oil
Octadecenoic acid, Sd oil
Octan-3-ol, Fr
Octanal, Fr
Octanoic acid methyl ester, Fr 0.2 mg/kg
Octanoic acid, Fr
Oleic acid, Fr 180-1,611; Sd oil 75.0%; Sd
    19.35-20.24%; Lf; Fl
Ortho-xylene, Fr
Palmitic acid, Fr 320-2,865, Lf, Fl
Palmitic acid, Sd 2.879-3.011%; Sd oil
    18.0%
Palmitoleic acid, Fr 200-1,790, Fl
Pantothenic acid, Fr 2-19
Papain, Fr; Fr Lx 5.1-8.4%; St Lx 13.5%
Papaya peptidase A, Lx
Papaya peptidase B, Lx
Papaya polysaccharide II, Fr
Papaya proteinase omega, Lx
Pectin (Carica papaya), Fr (unripe)
Pentadecane, Fr
Pentan-2,4-Dione, Fr
Phenyl acetonitrile, Fr
Phenylalanine, Fr 90-806
Phosphatidyl glycerol, Lf
Phosphorus, Fr 45-1,260

Phosphorus, Lf 1,420-6,311
Phytoene, Fr
Phytofluene, Fr
Potassium, Fr 0.2294-2.5469%
Potassium, Lf 0.6520-2.8978%
Proline, Fr 100-895
Prop-2-yl-butyrate, Fr
Propyl acetate, Fr
Propyl alcohol, Fr
Protease (Carica papaya), Call Tiss
Protease, Call Tiss
Protein, Fr 0.5-5.737%
Protein, Sd 40.0%; Lf 20.90%
Proteinase, Lx
Prunasin, Lf
Pseudo-carpaine, Lf 0.01%
Pseudo-pseudo carotene, Lf
PUFA, Fr 310-2,775
Pyridine, Fr
Resin, Lx 2.8%
Riboflavin, Fr 0.3-3; Lf 5-21
Serine, Fr 150-1,343
SFA, Fr 430-3,850
Sodium, Fr 26-554; Lf 160-711
Squalene, Sd oil
Stearic acid, Fr 20-179; Sd oil 5.0%; Lf
Stearic acid, Sd 1.265-1.328%; Fl
Stigmasterol, Sd oil
Styrene, Fr 0.1%
Sucrose, Fr; Trunk Bk; Lf
Sulfoquinovosyl-diacyl glycerol, Lf
Sulfur, Fr 300-900
Tannins, Lf 0.5-0.6%
Tartaric acid, Fr
Terpinolene, Fr
Tetraphyllin B, Lf
Thiamin, Fr 0.2-2.6; Lf 1-4
Threonine, Fr 110-985
Toluene, Fr
Trans-linalool oxide, Fr 0.7 mg/kg
Triacetin, Fr
Tricosanoic acid, Sd oil
Tryptophan, Fr 80-716
Tyrosine, Fr 50-448
Valine, Fr 100-895
Violaxanthin, Fr; Lf
Vitamin B6, Fr 0.2-1.7
Water, Fr 86.5-91.8%; Lx 75%
Water, Lf 69.7-70.3%
Xylitol, Trunk Bk
Zeaxanthin, Fr
Zinc, Fr 1.8-5.4

PHARMACOLOGICAL ACTIVITIES AND CLINICAL TRIALS

Abortifacient effect. Extract of ripe dried fruit was active. Percentage effectiveness in studies reviewed was 100%[T14891]. Fruit in the ration of pregnant rats at a dose of 300.0 gm/kg was equivocal. Saponifiable fraction of unripe fruit in the ration of pregnant rats, at a dose of 300.0 g/kg was active. Seeds in the ration of pregnant rats at a dose of 300.0 gm/kg was inactive[T00213].

Allergenic activity. Water extract of pollen administered intradermal to human adults of both sexes, at a concentration of 1:50 was active[W02402].

Analgesic activity. Ethanol (100%) extract of dried leaves administered intraperitoneally to rats at a dose of 20.0 mg/kg was active[T16133]. Ethanol (95%) extract of dried seeds was inactive[T07645]. Ethanol/water (1:1) extract of the aerial parts administered intraperitoneally to mice at a dose of 500.0 mg/kg was inactive vs tail pressure method[W00374].

Anthelmintic activity. Ethanol (95%) extract of dried seeds administered to chicken, was active on *Ascaridia galli*[T07645]. Ethanol (95%) extract of fruit juice at a concentration of 0.11 ml produced weak activity on *Ascaridia galli*[K03520]. Ethanol (95%) extract of latex from the stem, at a concentration of 7.5 mg/ml produced weak activity on *Ascaridia galli*[M22633]. Ethanol (95%) extract of seeds at a concentration of 25.0 mg/ml was active on *Ascaridia galli*[K03520].

Antiandrogenic effect. Dried seeds administered by gastric intubation to rats at a dose of 20.0 mg/animal was inactive[T02688].

Antiascariasis activity. Water extract of leaves, at a concentration of 10.0 mg/ml was active on earthworms. Water extract of seeds at a concentration of 10.0 mg/ml produced strong activity on earthworms[A05682].

Antibacterial activity. Acetone extract of dried leaves, on agar plate was active on *Pseudomonas aeruginosa*, *Salmonella newport*, *Sarcina lutea*, *Serratia marcescens* and *Shigella flexneri* 3A. Inactive on *Escherichia coli*, *Propionibacterium acnes*, *Salmonella typhosa*, *Shigella flexneri*, *Staphylococcus albus*, and *Staphylococcus aureus*. The ethanol (95%) extract was active on *Escherichia coli*, *Propionibacterium acnes*, *Pseudomonas aeruginosa*, and *Salmonella newport*. Inactive on *Salmonella typhosa*, *Sarcina lutea*, *Serratia marcescens*, *Shigella flexneri*, *Shigella flexneri* 3A, *Staphylococcus albus*, and *Staphylococcus aureus*. Water extract was active on *Escherichia coli*, *Propionibacterium acnes*, *Pseudomonas aeruginosa*, *Salmonella newport*, *Sarcina lutea*, *Serratia marcescens*, *Shigella flexneri* and *Staphylococcus aureus*. Inactive on *Salmonella typhosa*, *Shigella flexneri* 3A, and *Staphylococcus albus*[K09163]. Ethanol (95%) extract of dried fruit, on agar plate, undiluted was active on *Escherichia coli* and *Staphylococcus aureus*[W03693]. Ethanol (95%) extract of dried leaves, undiluted on agar plate, was inactive on *Escherichia coli* and *Staphylococcus aureus*[W03693]. Ethanol (95%) extract of dried root, on agar plate undiluted, was active on *Escherichia coli* and *Staphylococcus aureus*[W03693]. Methanol extract of dried root at a concentration of 1.0% on agar plate was equivocal on *Escherichia coli* and inactive on *Staphylococcus aureus*[T03389]. Ethanol (95%) extract of dried seeds, undiluted on agar plate, was active on *Escherichia coli* and *Staphylococcus aureus*[W03693]. Ethanol (95%) extract of latex, on agar plate, undiluted was inactive on *Escherichia coli* and *Staphylococcus aureus*[W03693]. Ethanol/water (1:1) extract of aerial parts on agar plate at a concentration of 25.0 mg/ml was inactive on *Bacillus subtilis*, *Escherichia coli*, *Salmonella typhosa*, *Staphylococcus aureus*, and *Agrobacterium tumefaciens*[W00374]. Juice of unripe, dried fruit, on agar plate, was active on *Bacillus subtilis*, MIC 500.0 mcg/ml, zone of thinning 15.0; *Enterobacter cloacae*, MIC 500.0 mcg/ml, zone of thinning 13.0; *Escherichia coli*, MIC 500.0 mcg/ml, zone of thinning 13.5; *Klebsiella pneumoniae*, MIC 500.0 mcg/ml, zone of thinning 10.5; *Proteus vulgaris*, MIC 500.0 mcg/ml, zone of thinning 5.0; *Pseudomonas aeruginosa*, MIC 500.0 mcg/ml, zone of thinning 9.5; *Salmonella typhi*, MIC 500.0 mg/ml, zone of thinning 8.0; *Staphylococcus aureus*, MIC 500.0 mg/ml, zone of thinning 10.5[K14611]. Protein fraction of fresh leaves, on agar plate at a concentration of 2.0 mg/ml was active on *Bacillus cereus*, *Escherichia coli*, *Pseudomonas aeruginosa*, *Shigella flexneri*, and *Staphylococcus aureus*; inactive on *Streptococcus faecalis*, and weak activity on *Proteus vulgaris* and *Salmonella typhimurium*[T06395]. Protein fraction of fresh, ripe seeds, on agar plate at a concentration of 2.0 mg/ml was active on *Bacillus cereus*, *Escherichia coli*, *Pseudomonas aeruginosa* and *Shigella flexneri*. Inactive on *Streptococcus faecalis*, and weak activity on *Proteus vulgaris* and *Salmonella typhimurium*[T06395]. Acetone extract of dried stem on agar plate was active on *Escherichia coli*, *Propionibacterium acnes*, *Pseudomonas aeruginosa*, *Salmonella typhosa*, *Sarcina lutea*, *Serratia marcescens*, *Shigella flexneri*, *Shigella flexneri 3A*, and *Staphylococcus aureus* and inactive on *Salmonella newport* and *Staphylococcus albus*. Ethanol (95%) extract was active on *Escherichia coli*, *Propionibacterium acnes*, *Pseudomonas aeruginosa*, *Salmonella newport*, *Shigella flexneri*, *Shigella flexneri 3A*, and *Staphylococcus albus*. Inactive on *Salmonella typhosa*, *Sarcina lutea*, *Serratia marcescens* and *Staphylococcus aureus*. Water extract was active on *Escherichia coli*, *Propionibacterium acnes*, *Pseudomonas aeruginosa*, *Salmonella newport*, *Sarcina lutea*, *Serratia marcescens*, *Shigella flexneri*, *Shigella flexneri 3A*, and *Staphylococcus albus*. Inactive on *Salmonella typhosa* and *Staphylococcus aureus*[K09163]. Protein fraction of ripe-fresh endocarp tissue, on agar plate, at a concentration of 2.0 mg/ml was active on *Bacillus cereus*, *Escherichia coli*, *Pseudomonas aeruginosa*, *Shigella flexneri*, and *Staphylococ-*

cus aureus; inactive on *Streptococcus faecalis*; and weak activity on *Proteus vulgaris* and *Salmonella typhimurium*[T06395]. Protein fraction of ripe-fresh epicarp, on agar plate, at a concentration of 2.0 mg/ml was active on *Bacillus cereus*, *Escherichia coli*, *Pseudomonas aeruginosa*, *Shigella flexneri*, and *Staphylococcus aureus*; inactive on *Streptococcus faecalis*; and weak activity on *Proteus vulgaris* and *Salmonella typhimurium*[T06395]. Water extract of fresh bark at a concentration of 1.0% on agar plate was inactive on *Neisseria gonorrhea*[T10354]. Water extract of fresh latex, on agar plate, at a concentration of 335.0 units/ml was active on *Micrococcus leisodeikticus*[W02043]. Water extract of fresh root, on agar plate at a concentration of 1.0% was inactive on *Neisseria gonorrhea*[T10354].

Anticlastogenic activity. Fruit and seed juice administered intraperitoneally to mice at a dose of 50.0 ml/kg was active on marrow cells vs tetracycline-, mitomycin-, and dimethylnitrosamine-induced micronuclei[K17561].

Anticoagulant activity. Fresh leaf at a concentration of 50% was active on human whole-blood[T15327].

Anticonvulsant activity. Ethanol (100%) extract of dried leaves administered intraperitoneally to rats at a dose of 100.0 mg/kg was active vs maximal electroshock-induced convulsions. A dose of 20.0 mg/kg was active vs pentylenetetrazole-induced seizures[T16133]. Ethanol (70%) extract of fresh root administered intraperitoneally to mice of both sexes, at a dose of 100.0 mg/kg was equivocal vs strychnine-induced convulsions, 20% protection was observed. Weak activity was observed vs metrazole-induced convulsions, 30% protection[T06510]. Ethanol/water (1:1) extract of aerial parts administered intraperitoneally to mice at a dose of 500.0 mg/kg was inactive vs electroshock-induced convulsions[W00374].

Antiedema activity. Methanol extract of fruit applied onto the ear of mice at a dose of 2.0 mg/ear was active vs 12-0-tetradecanoylphorbol-13-acetate(TPA)-induced ear inflammation. Inhibition ratio (IR) was 5[K11173].

Antiestrogenic effect. Seeds administered orally to mice at a dose of 1.5 g/kg was active[A04351].

Antifertility effect. Dried seeds administered by gastric intubation to male rats at a dose of 20.0 mg/animal was active[T02688]. Acetone and water extracts of dried leaves, on agar plate at a concentration of 50% was inactive on *Neurospora crassa;* ethanol (95%) extract was active[T08589]. Acetone/water (50:50) extract of fresh latex, on agar plate was inactive on *Microsporum gypseum* and *Trichophyton mentagrophytes*[M21482]. Ethanol (100%) extract of fresh leaves at a concentration of 10.0%, ethanol/acetone (50%) extract at a concentration of 50.0%, ethanol/water (1:1) at a concentration of 1.0%, and water extract at a concentration of 1.0%, on agar plate were active on *Neurospora crassa*[T07844]. Ethanol/water (1:1) extract of aerial parts, on agar plate at a concentration of 25.0 mcg/ml was inactive on *Microsporum canis, Trichophyton mentagrophytes* and *Aspergillus niger*[W00374]. Methanol extract of unripe fruit, on agar plate, at a concentration of 0.03% was inactive on *Trichophyton mentagrophytes*[T06031].

Antihepatotoxic activity. Water extract of trunkbark administered orally to male rats at a dose of 500.0 mg/kg was active vs jaundice induced by intraperitoneal injection of *Brenania brieyi* fruit saponin fraction[M01377].

Anti-implantation effect. Ethanol (95%) extract of unripe fruit administered orally to rats at a dose of 500.0 mg/kg produced weak activity[A04511]. Ethanol (95%), petroleum ether, and water extracts of seeds administered orally to pregnant rats were inactive[J05751]. Petroleum ether extract of seeds administered orally to rats at a dose of 500.0 mg/kg was active. Pregnancy was prevented in 60% of the rats. No activity was observed at lower doses[J08538]. Unripe, dried fruit pulp administered intraperitoneally to rats was active[T14891]. Ethanol/water (1:1) extract of aerial parts administered orally to male rats at a dose of 500.0 mg/kg was inactive vs carrageenin-induced pedal edema. Animals were dosed one hour before carrageenin injections[W00374].

Antimalarial activity. Chloroform and water extracts of flowers administered orally to chicken at doses of 166.0 mg/kg, and 3.72 gm/kg respectively, were inactive on *Plasmodium gallinaceum*[A00785].

Antimycobacterial activity. Water extract of fresh leaves (one part of fresh weight of leaves to three parts of water), on agar plate, produced weak activity on *Mycobacterium tuberculosis*[W01074].

Antioxidant activity. Juice of unripe, dried fruit at concentrations of 25.0 and 58.0 mg/ml was active. Superoxide radicals were generated using the hypoxanthine-xanthine oxidase system[K14611].

Antisickling activity. Water extract of unripe, fresh fruit was active on RBC[T14020].

Antispasmodic activity. Ethanol/water (1:1) extract of aerial parts was inactive on the ileum of guinea pigs vs ACh- and histamine-induced spasms[W00374].

Antispermatogenic effect. Dried seeds administered by gastric intubation to male rats at a dose of 20.0 mg/animal daily for eight weeks was inactive. Animals were mated with adult females of proven fertility and at estrus following treatment[T02688].

Antitumor activity. Ethanol (95%) extract of dried leaves administered intraperitoneally to mice at a dose of 100.0 mg/kg was inactive on Sarcoma 180(ASC)[M23643].

Antiulcer activity. Fresh fruit latex administered by gastric intubation to rats at a dose of 0.75 gm/kg twice daily for six days, was inactive vs aspirin-, prednisolone-, and stress-induced ulcers (water immersion). Fresh latex administered by gastric intubation to rats at a dose of 0.75 gm/kg, twice daily for six days, was active vs stress-(water-immersion), and prednisolone-induced ulcers. The treatment was inactive vs aspirin-induced ulcers. Fresh seeds administered by gastric intubation to rats at a dose of 0.75 gm/kg, twice daily for six days was inactive vs aspirin-, prednisolone-, and stress-induced (water immersion) ulcers. Fresh unripe fruit administered by gastric intubation to rats at a dose of 0.75 gm/kg, twice daily for six days was active vs stress-induced ulcers (water-immersion); and inactive vs aspirin-, and prednisolone-induced ulcers[T06809].

Antiviral activity. Ethanol (80%) extract of freeze-dried leaves, in cell culture at variable concentrations was equivocal on Coxsackie B2 virus vs Plaque-inhibition; inactive on Adenovirus, Herpes virus type 1, measles virus, polio virus and Semlicki-forest virus vs plaque inhibition[T06435]. Ethanol (95%) extract of leaves, in cell culture was active on distortion ringspot virus, mild mosaic virus and ringspot virus[W00025]. Latex in cell culture was active on Tobacco mosaic virus[A04618].

Antiyeast activity. Ethanol/water (1:1) extract of aerial parts at a concentration of 25.0 mcg/ml was inactive on *Candida albicans* and *Cryptococcus neoformans*[W00374]. Fresh latex on agar plate was active on *Candida albicans*. LC_{100} 138.0 mcg/ml[K07404]. Fresh latex, at a concentration of 10.0% on agar plate, was active on *Candida albicans*, *Candida guilliermondii* and *Candida tropicalis*[T04064]. Methanol extract of unripe fruit, on agar plate, at a concentration of 0.03% was inactive on *Candida albicans*[T06031]. Water extract of dried root, on agar plate was active on *Candida albicans* using hole-plate diffusion method and produced weak activity in broth culture using test-tube dilution method. Chloroform and methanol extracts were inactive on agar plate using hole-plate diffusion method, and in broth culture using test-tube dilution method. Petroleum ether extract was active on agar plate using hole-plate diffusion method, and in broth culture using test-tube dilution method[T10823].

Ascaricidal activity. Fruit latex administered orally to dogs at a dose of 1.50 ml/kg was active on *Ascaris lumbrcoides*[A05123].

Cardiac depressant activity. Hot water extract of fruit taken orally by human adults at a dose of 0.02 gm/person was active[A05591].

Chronotropic effect positive. Ethanol (100%) extract of dried leaves administered intraperitoneally to rats at a dose of 200.0 mg/kg was active[T16133].

Detoxifying effect (non-immunologic). Methanol extract of dried leaves at a concentration of 100.0 ppm was inactive on *Bulinus globosus*[T04176].

Diuretic activity. Ethanol/water (1:1) extract of aerial parts administered intraperitoneally to male rats at a dose of 250.0 mg/kg was inactive on saline-loaded animals. Urine was collected for four hours post-drug[W00374].

Embryotoxic effect. Fruit in the ration of pregnant rats at a dose of 300.0 gm/kg was equivocal[T00213]. Water and petroleum ether extract of seeds administered orally to pregnant rats were active[J05751]. Seeds in the ration of pregnant rats at a dose of 300.0 gm/kg was inactive[T00213].

Fish poison. Water extract of fresh bark was inactive[T14676].

Gastric antisecretory activity. Fresh latex administered by gastric intubation to rats at a dose of 0.75 gm/kg, twice daily for six days, was active vs histamine-induced ulcers[T06809].

Gastric secretory stimulation. Fruit juice taken orally by human adults was inactive[A05197].

Hemagglutinin activity. Water extract of dried seeds was active on human RBC. No specificity for any particular blood group was observed[W03791].

Hypoglycemic activity. Ethanol/water (1:1) extract of aerial parts administered orally to rats at a dose of 250.0 mg/kg was inactive. Less than 30% drop in blood sugar level was observed[W00374]. Fruit administered orally to rabbits was inactive[A05423].

Hypotensive activity. Ethanol (95%) extract of seeds administered intravenously to dogs was active. Respiration was also depressed[A05126].

Hypothermic activity. Ethanol/water (1:1) extract of aerial parts administered intraperitoneally to mice at a dose of 500.0 mg/kg was inactive[W00374].

Inflammation induction. Fresh latex injected into rats at a dose of 0.25% was active vs aspirin, prednisolone, levamisole, and boswellic acid anti-inflammatory treatment. The dose was inactive vs piroxicam, ibuprofen, and chloroquine phosphate anti-inflammatory treatment[K08278].

Insecticide activity. Ethanol (95%) extract of dried seeds, at a concentration of 50.0 mg was inactive on *Rhodnius neglectus*[K18765]. Fruit juice was active on *Leptinotarsa decemlineata*[J08287].

Larvicidal activity. Water extract of dried latex was active on *Culex quinquefasciatus*, LC_{100} 0.004 ml/ml. Concentration given in g of fresh plant material per ml of water needed for 100% mortality in six hours. Tested in 100 ml of water[M19731].

Molluscicidal activity. Water extract of oven-dried fruit was inactive on *Biophalaria pfeifferi*[T14178].

Ovulation inhibition effect. Ethanol (95%), water, and petroleum ether extracts administered orally to rabbits at a dose of 100.0 mg/kg were inactive[A02478].

Plant germination inhibition. Chloroform extract of dried leaves wa active vs *Amaranthus spinosus* (49.5% inhibition). Chlorform extract of dried seeds was active vs *Amaranthus spinosus*, 58% inhibition[T03367].

Radical scavenging effect. Fresh fruit juice, at a concentration of 20.0 microliters was active[M22633]. Juice of unripe, dried fruit was active. IC_{50} 25.0 mg/ml when scavenging of 1,1-diphenyl-1-2-picrylhydrazyl radicals was assayed, and IC_{50} 67.1 mg/ml when scavenging of hydroxyl radicals was assayed[K14611].

Semen coagulation. Ethanol/water (1:1) extract of aerial parts at a concentration of 2.0% was inactive on the spermatozoa of rats[W00374].

Skeletal muscle relaxant effect (central). Ethanol (100%) extract of dried leaves administered intraperitoneally to rats at a dose of 50.0 mg/kg was active[T16133].

Smooth muscle stimulant activity. Ethanol (95%) extract of dried seeds was active on the ileum of guinea pigs vs ACh, and barium-induced contractions[T07645]. Ethanol (95%), and water extracts of seeds were active on the rat intestine. The activity was not blocked by atropine or antihistamine[T06395].

Spasmolytic activity. Butanol extract of dried leaves, at a concentration of 0.2 mg/ml was active on the ileum of guinea pigs. 35.67% reduction in contraction was seen vs ACh-induced contractions; 53.37% reduction vs KCl-induced contractions. Chloroform extract was inactive vs ACh-, and KCl-induced contractions. Isopentyl alcohol extract was active, 89.34% reduction vs ACh-induced contractions, and 72.43% reduction vs KCl-induced contractions. Methanol extract was active, 20.17% reduction vs ACh-induced contractions, and inactive vs KCl-induced contractions[M27323].

Spermicidal activity. Water extract of seeds was active in rodents. The effect was 100% reversible after three months[T10128].

Spermicidal effect. Dried seeds administered by gastric intubation to male rats at a dose of 20.0 mg/animal was inactive[T02688]. Ethanol/water (1:1) extract of aerial parts at a concentration of 2.0% was inactive on the spermatozoa of rats[W00374].

Superoxide radical scavenging activity. Juice of unripe, dried fruit was active. IC_{50} 114.5 mg/ml when scavenging of superoxide was assayed[K14611].

Toxicity assessment (quantitative). Ethanol (95%) extract of dried seeds when administered intraperitoneally to rats

LD_{50} 208.0 mg/kg[T07645]. Ethanol/water (1:1) extract of aerial parts administered intraperitoneally to mice produce LD_{50} >1.0 gm/kg[W00374].

Tranquilizing effect. Ethanol (100%) extract of dried leaves administered intraperitoneally to rats at a dose of 10.0 mg/kg was active[T16133].

Tumor promotion inhibition. Methanol extract of fresh fruit in cell culture at a concentration of 200.0 mg was inactive on Epstein-Barr virus. Vs 12-0-hexadecanoyl-phorbol-13-acetate-induced Epstein-Barr virus activation[T15279].

Uterine relaxation effect. Ethanol (95%) and water extracts of seeds produced weak activity on the rat uterus[A05126]. Ethanol (95%) extract of seeds was active on the rat uterus vs oxytocin-induced contractions[T07645].

Uterine stimulant effect. Ethanol (95%) extract of seeds, at a concentration of 2.0 mg/ml administered intravenously to guinea pigs was inactive on the nonpregnant uterus[W04510]. Latex, at a concentration of 0.22 ml/liters were active on the uterus of guinea pigs[A04132].

WBC-macrophage stimulant. Water extract of freeze-dried fruit at a concentration of 2.0 mg/ml was inactive. Nitrite formation was used as an index of the macrophage stimulating activity to screen effective foods[M27208].

7 | Cassia alata

L.

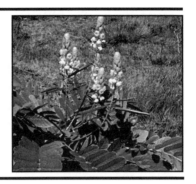

Common Names

Aaku pero	Buka Island	La'au fai lafa	Nicaragua
Akapulko	Philippines	Maliof	Papua-New Guinea
Akapulko	West Africa	Mata pasto	Brazil
Akoria	West Africa	Mhingu	Tanzania
Awunwon	West Africa	Mongrang-jangtong	India
Ayengogo	Guinea	Mula mula	India
Bai nicagi	Guinea	Mulu mulu	Papua
Bakua	Guinea	Njepaa	Sierra Leone
Balilang	Malaysia	Okpo Ndichi	Sierra Leone
Barajo	Guatemala	Palotsina	Philippines
Candelabra bush	Thailand	Pui-chi	Bangladesh
Candle tree	Malaysia	Qanabisi	Nicaragua
Christmas blossom	Nicaragua	Ringworm bush	Fiji
Chum het thet	Thailand	Ringworm bush	Guyana
Chumhet yai	Thailand	Ringworm bush	West Indies
Cortalinde	Guinea-Bissau	Ringworm cassia	Malaysia
Dadmardan	India	Ringworm shrub	Australia
Dadmurdan	Fiji	Roman candle tree	Fiji
Dadrughna	India	Sengseng	India
Galinggang hutan	Indonesia	Serocontil	Nicaragua
Gelenggang	Malaysia	Sindjo-el	Guinea-Bissau
Gelenngang	Indonesia	Sus saika	Nicaragua
Grili	Papua-New Guinea	Sus tara saika	Nicaragua
Kabaiura	Papua-New Guinea	Sus waha tara	Nicaragua
Ketapeng	Indonesia	Tarantan	West Indies
Ketepeng	Indonesia	Te'elango	West Indies
King of the forest	Jamaica	Totoncaxihuitl	Mexico
Kinkeliba	Gabon	Wasemu	Papau
Kislin	Nicaragua	Wild senna	West Indies

From: Medicinal Plants of the World *By:* Ivan A. Ross Humana Press Inc., Totowa, NJ

BOTANICAL DESCRIPTION

The shrub of the LEGUMINOSAE family may grow up to about three meters tall. leaves are pinnately compound 30- to 40-cm long, with 6–12 pairs of broad oblong leaflets, blunt at the tip, unequal at the base, the terminal pair much larger, about 15-cm long and 8-cm wide. Flowers are roundish in compact axillary racemes, golden-yellow and very showy about 20- to 30-cm long and 3–4-cm wide. the bracts are 2–3 by 1–2 cm. There are five unequal oblong 10–20 by 6–7 mm, green sepals. The petals are bright yellow ovate-orbicular to spathulate, short-clawed, 2 by 1-1.5 cm. There are 9–10 stamens; two large, four small, and three or four reduced. The anthers open via apical pores. There is only one pistil and glabrous ovary. Fruit are four-winged pods, 10–15-cm long, dark brown when ripe. There are about 50 seeds, more or less quadrangular, arranged transversely in the pod.

ORIGIN AND DISTRIBUTION

A native of tropical America, it is now widespread in warm countries. The plant grows in waste places, often along streams, banks, and in swamps.

TRADITIONAL MEDICINAL USES

Australia. Hot water extract of dried leaves is taken orally as a cathartic[W03671].

Bangladesh. Fresh leaves are squeezed and rubbed into ringworm[K10069].

Brazil. Decoction of dried leaves is taken orally as an emmenagogue and abortifacient[T16785]. Decoction of dried root is taken orally for malaria. Data were obtained by interviews with more than 8000 natives or various parts of Brazil[K07256].

Buka Island. Fresh leaves are squeezed until soft and rubbed regularly onto the affected part of the body to treat ringworm[T05034].

Fiji. Hot water extract of dried leaves and stem is used externally for ringworm and skin diseases[T10632]. The juice of the leaves and stem is squeezed out and rubbed on the affected area for ringworm and skin infections[K08933]. Infusion of dried leaves is taken orally as a blood purifier for worms and diarrhea[T10632].

Guatemala. Hot water extract of dried bark, leaves, and root is used externally for ringworm[M27151].

Guinea-Bissau. Hot water extract of root is taken orally as an emmenagogue[A00455].

Guinea. A strong decoction of hot water extract of leaves is taken orally to promote abortion, and to treat leprosy[M27151].

India. Fresh leaf juice is used for eczema. Juice from leaves is applied to affected area three times daily until cured[T10321]. Fresh leaves are crushed and used for skin diseases, especially ringworm and eczema and scabies[T07731],[T07374]. Leaf juice is used externally to treat leukoderma. A poultice of tender leaves is applied for over a month[T07731].

Ivory Coast. Decoction of dried leaves is used externally to treat infections caused by dermatophytes and orally[K13111] and externally To treat yeast infections caused by *Candida albicans* and orally to treat bacterial infections caused by *Escherichia coli*[K11576].

Jamaica. Hot water extract of dried leaves is taken orally for diabetes[T07170].

Malaysia. Decoction of root is taken orally to ease stomachache[K23166]. Hot water extract of dried leaves is taken orally as a laxative; leaves are used externally against ringworm and scabies; the sap is used externally against external ulcers[K19580].

Mexico. Hot water extract of the plant is used externally as an astringent and against inflammation of rashes; orally as a purgative, anthelmintic and to relieve fever[J01414].

Nicaragua. Fresh leaves are used externally for ringworm and athlete's foot; decoction of the fresh leaves is taken orally for stomachache. It should not be given medicinally to pregnant women; it will induce abortion[M23149].

Nigeria. Dried leaves powdered with equal amounts of *Piper Guineense*. The powder is divided into small portions and taken orally with hot "Pap" to treat indigestion. Decoction of the dried leaves is taken orally to hasten delivery during labor; a strong decoction is taken orally to cause abortion[K08933]. Decoction of dried leaves is used externally for ringworm, eczema and pustular skin infections[M30756]. Infusion of dried leaves is taken orally as a purgative[K17262]. Fresh leaf juice is used externally to treat skin infections[T05880]. Leaves mixed with fruit pulp of *Cucurbita pepo* and *Termitomyces microcarpus* (mushroom) is taken orally to treat gonorrhea[L01679]. The ground inflorescence is mixed with "Pap" and taken orally to treat constipation[K08933].

Papau-New Guinea. Dried leaves are used externally for skin eruptions such as Tinea imbricata. Crushed leaves are rubbed on the skin[T12612]. Fresh leaves are used to treat grille, a skin fungus. Crushed leaves are rubbed into the skin affected by grille[K18142,K18559]. Leaf juice is used externally for skin eruptions such as Tinea imbricata and ringworm[T09033].

Philippines. Fresh leaves are used to treat fungal infection of the skin. The leaves are crushed and rubbed vigorously on the infected area of the skin[M29360].

Sierra Leone. Decoction of dried leaves is taken orally as a laxative[T09679].

Surinam. Fresh leaves are used externally for ringworm and skin diseases[T12612].

Tanzania. Decoction of leaves is taken orally as a purgative[T16181].

Thailand. Decoction of dried leaves is taken orally for asthma[T16711]; the hot water extract is taken orally as an antipyretic[W3022A]. Hot water extract of dried entire plant is taken orally as a cathartic[W03804]. Pulverized flowers is taken orally for asthma[T16711]. Hot water extract of dried seeds is taken orally as an anthelmintic[W03804].

West Africa. Hot water extract of dried leaves is taken orally as an ecbolic and emmenagogue[T02110]. Hot water extract of fresh leaves juice is used for parasitic skin diseases[M23617]. Strong decoction of hot water extract of leaves is taken orally as an abortifacient[A00115].

West Indies. Hot water extract of flowers is used externally as an antibacterial[T00701]. Leaf teas used for intestinal worms[T00701]. Seeds are taken orally as a vermifuge[T00701].

CHEMICAL CONSTITUENTS
(ppm unless otherwise indicated)

Alatonal, St
Aloe emodin, Pl
Alquinone, Rt 10
Anthraquinone,1-5-dihydroxy-2-methyl, St
Anthraquinone,5-hydroxy-2-methyl, St
Anthraquinone glucopyranoside emodin, Pl
Beta sitosterol, Rt
Chrysarobin, lf
Chrysophanol, Pl
Chrysophanol glycoside, Lf
Dalbergin, St
Daucosterol, St
Deoxycoeluatin, Lf
Emodin, St 3.3
Fat, Sd 2.9-3.5%
Isochrysophanol, Lf
Kaempferol, Lf
Luteolin, St
Physionmonoglucoside, Lf
Phytosterol, Lf; St Bk
Protein, Sd 16.1-18.1%
Rhein, Pl
Rhein glycoside, Lf
Santal, St
Sitosterol, Lf
Tannin, Lf

PHARMACOLOGICAL ACTIVITIES AND CLINICAL TRIALS

Abortifacient effect. Ethanol/water (50%) extract of dried leaves administered by gastric intubation to rats at a dose of 125.0 mg/kg was inactive[T16785].

Analgesic activity. Ethanol (85%) extract of dried leaves administered intraperitoneally to mice at a dose of 100.0 mcg/kg was active[T15923]. Ethanol/water (1:1) extract of the aerial parts administered intraperitoneally to mice at a dose of 500.0 mg/kg was inactive vs tail pressure method[W00374].

Antibacterial activity. Chloroform extract of dried leaves at a concentration of 5.0 mcg/ml on agar plate was active on *Pseudomonas aeruginosa*, *Bacillus subtilis*, *Escherichia coli*, *Mcoccus luteus*, and *Staphylococcus aureus*[M30756]. The Chromatographic fraction undiluted on agar plate was active on several Gram positive and Gram negative organisms[T05880]. The acetic acid extract of at a concentration of 5.0 mg/ml was active on *bacillus subtilis*, *Escherichia coli*, *Mcoccus luteus*, *Pseudomonas aeruginosa*, and *Staphylococcus aureus*[M30756]. Chloroform extract of dried stem bark at a concentration of 1.0 mg/disk on agar plate was active on *Bacillus cereus*, *Bacillus subtilis*, *Pseudomonas aeruginosa*, *Salmonella paratyphi* B, *Salmonella typhi*, *Shigella dysenteriae*, *Shigella flexneri*, *Shigella sonnei*, and *Staphylococcus aureus*; inactive on *Aeromonas hydrophilia*, *Escherichia coli*, *Salmonella paratyphi* A, *Vibrio cholera*, *Vibrio mimicus* and *Vibrio parahemolyticus*. The methanol extract was active on *Bacillus cereus*, *Bacillus subtilis*, *Escherichia coli*, *Salmonella paratyphi* B, *Salmonella typhi*, *Shigella flexneri*, *Shigella sonnei*, and *Vibrio cholera*; inactive on *Aeromonas hydrophilia*, *Pseudomonas aeruginosa*, *Salmonella paratyphi* A, *Vibrio mimicus*, and *Vibrio parahemolyticus*. Active on *Shigella dysenteriae* and *Staphylococcus aureus* MIC 0.1 mg/disk. The petroleum ether extract was active on *Salmonella paratyphi* B, and *Shigella flexneri*; inactive on *Aeromonas hydrophilia*, *Bacillus cereus*, *Bacillus subtilis*, *Escherichia coli*, *Salmonella paratyphi* A, *Salmonella typhi*, *Vibrio cholera*, *Vibrio mimicus*, and *Vibrio parahemolyticus*; active on *Shigella sonnei* at a concentration of 1.4 mg/disk and *Shigella dysenteriae* and *Staphylococcus aureus* MIC 0.8 mg/disk[K11565]. Ethanol (85%) extract of dried leaves at a concentration of 10.0% on agar plate was active on *Escherichia coli*, *Proteus vulgaris*, *Pseudomonas aeruginosa*, and *Staphylococcus aureus*[M27682]. Methanol extract of the dried leaves at a concentration of 1.0 mg/disk on agar plate was active on *Bacillus subtilis*, *Escherichia coli*, *Salmonella paratyphi* B, *Shigella flexneri*, *Shigella sonnei*, and *Vibrio cholera*; inactive on *Aeromonas hydrophilia*, *Bacillus cereus*, *Pseudomonas aeruginosa*, *Salmonella paratyphi* A, *Salmonella typhi*, *Vibrio mimicus*, and *Vibrio parahemolyticus*. The methanol extract of dried leaves on agar plate showed MIC 0.2 mg/disk for *Shigella dysenteriae* and 0.4 mg/disk for *Staphylococcus aureus*. Petroleum ether extract of dried leaves at a concentration of 1.0 mg/disk on agar plate was active on *Salmonella paratyphi* B, *Shigella flexneri*, and *Shigella sonnei*; inactive on *Aeromonas hydrophilia*, *Bacillus cereus*, *Bacillus subtilis*, *Escherichia coli*, *Pseudomonas aeruginosa*, *Salmonella paratyphi* A, *Salmonella typhi*, *Staphylococcus aureus*, *Vibrio cholera*, *Vibrio mimicus*, *Vibrio parahemolyticus*, and *Shigella dysenteriae*[K11565]. Ethanol (95%) extract of dried leaves at a concentration of 100.0 mg/disk (expressed as dry weight of plant) on agar plate was active on *Bacillus subtilis* and inactive on *Escherichia coli*, *Salmonella typhosa*, *Shigella dysenteriae*, and *Staphylococcus aureus*. Water extract at a concentration of 20.0 mg/disk was inactive on *Bacillus subtilis*, *Escherichia coli*, *Salmonella typhosa*, *Shigella dysenteriae*, and *Staphylococcus aureus*[P00004]. Ethanol (95%) extract of dried leaves at a concentration of 500.0 mg/ml on agar plate was inactive on *Escherichia coli*, *Proteus mirabilis*, *Proteus vulgaris*, and *Staphylococcus epidermidis*. A concentration of 500.0 micromols/ml was inactive on *Staphylococcus aureus*[K19580]. A concentration of 5.0 mg/ml was active on *Bacillus subtilis*, *Escherichia coli*, *Mcoccus luteus*, *Pseudomonas aeruginosa*, and *Staphylococcus aureus*[M30756]. Ethanol (95%) extract of leaves on agar plate was active on *Bacillus subtilis*, *Escherichia coli*, *Klebsiella pneumonia*, *Serratia marcescens* and *Staphylococcus aureus*[T02963]. Ethanol/water (1:1) extract of the aerial parts, at a concentration of 25.0 mcg/ml on agar plate was inactive on *Bacillus subtilis*,

Escherichia coli, Salmonella typhosa, Staphylococcus aureus and *Agrobacterium tumefaciens*[W00374]. Water extract of dried leaves at variable concentrations was active on *Pseudomonas aeruginosa*, and *Staphylococcus aureus*[K07849]. The water extract of dried leaves on agar plate was active on *Escherichia coli* LC_{50} 1.0 mg/unit and MIC 1.6 mg/ml[K13111,K11576].

Anticlastogenic activity. Juice of leaves administered by gastric intubation to mice at a dose of 25.0 ml/kg was active on bone marrow cells vs mitomycin C-, dimethylnitrosamine-, and tetracycline-induced micronuclei[K17562].

Anticonvulsant activity. Ethanol/water (1:1) extract of the aerial parts administered intraperitoneally to mice at a dose of 500.0 mg/kg was inactive vs electroshock-induced convulsions[W00374].

Antifungal activity. Chloroform, acetic acid and ethanol (95%) extracts of dried leaves at concentrations of 5.0 mg/ml on agar plate showed weak activities on *Aspergillus fumigatus, Lasiodiplodia theobromae, Penicillium italicum* and *Trichophyton mentagrophytes*[M30756]. Dried leaves at a concentration of 20.0% on agar plate was inactive on *Aspergillus flavus, Aspergillus fumigatus*, Mucor species, Penicillium species, and Rhizopus species. Water extract of dried leaves at a concentrations of 80, 90, and 100.0% applied externally on human adults was active on *Malassezia furfur*. The extract was applied to the neck, hands, and trunk. Pityriasis versicolor was treated[K16191]. Methanol (85%) extract of the dried leaves at a concentration of 2.5% on agar plate was active on *Microsporum gypseum, Trichophyton mentagrophytes*, and *Trichophyton rubrum*[T15987]. Ethanol (95%) extract of dried leaves at a concentration of 500 mg/ml on agar plate was active on *Microsporum canis, Microsporum gypseum, Trichophyton mentagrophytes*, and *Trichophyton rubrum*; weakly active on *Aspergillus niger, Cladosporium werneckii, Fusarium solani*, and Penicillium species; inactive on *Candida albicans, Rhodotorula rubra*, and *Saccharomyces cerevisiae*[K19580]. Ethanol/water (1:1) extract of the aerial parts at a concentration of 25.0 mcg/ml was inactive on *Microsporum canis, Trichophyton mentagrophytes*, and *Aspergillus niger*[W00374]. Hot water extract of dried bark, leaf and root at a concentration of 1.0 ml in broth culture was inactive on *Epidermophyton floccosum, Microsporum canis, Microsporum gypseum, Trichophyton mentagrophytes* vars. Algodonosa, Granulare, and *Trichophyton rubrum*[M27151]. Juice of the dried entire plant on agar plate was inactive on *Epidermophyton floccosum, Microsporum gypseum* and *Trichophyton rubrum*[P00083]. Hot water extract of dried leaves at a concentration of 5.0% on agar plate was active on *Trichophyton mentagropytes*[T06336].

Antihistamine activity. Ethanol/water (1:1) extract of dried leaves at variable concentrations was active on guinea pig ileum[W3022A].

Antihyperglycemic activity. Petroleum ether extract of shade dried leaves administered by gastric intubation at a dose of 100.0 mg/kg to rats was active vs streptozotocin-induced hyperglycemia[T15223].

Anti-inflammatory activity. Ethanol (85%) extract of dried leaves administered intraperitoneally to mice at a dose of 100.0 mg/kg was active vs carrageenin-induced pedal edema and cotton pellet granuloma[M30962]. Ethanol/water (1:1) extract of the aerial parts administered orally to rats at a dose of 500.0 mg/kg was active vs carrageenin-induced pedal edema. Animals were dosed one hour before carrageenin injections[W00374]. Shade-dried leaves administered by gastric intubation to rats at dose of 150.0 mg/kg was active[M26843].

Antimutagenic activity. Methanol-insoluble fraction of dried flowers was active vs methylnitrosamine, methyl methane sulfonate, or tetracycline-induced genotoxicity[K17876].

Antipyretic activity. Ethanol/water (1:1) extract of dried leaves administered by gastric intubation at variable concentrations to rabbit was inactive vs yeast-induced pyrexia[W3022A].

Antispasmodic activity. Ethanol/ water (1:1) extract of dried leaves at variable concentrations was active on guinea pig ileum[W3022A]. Ethanol/water (1:1) extract of the aerial parts was inactive on guinea pig ileum vs ACh- and histamine-induced spasms[W00374].

Antitumor activity. Acid/water, ethanol (95%) and water extracts of dried leaves administered subcutaneously to mice of both sexes at doses of 0.02 gm/kg showed weak activities on Sarcoma 37[W03671].

Antiyeast activity. Chloroform, acetic acid, and ethanol (95%) extracts of dried leaves at concentrations of 5.0 mg/ml on agar plate showed weak activities on *Candida albicans*[M30756]. Dried leaves at a concentration of 20.0% on agar plate was inactive on *Candida albicans*[T15987]. Ethanol (95%) extract of dried leaves at concentrations of 20.0 and 100.0 mg/disk on agar plate were inactive on *Candida albicans*[P00004]. Ethanol/water (1:1) extract of the aerial parts at a concentration of 25.0 mcg/ml on agar plate was inactive on *Candida albicans* and *Cryptococcus neoformans*[W00374]. Juice of the dried entire plant on agar plate was inactive on *Candida albicans*, *Cryptococcus neoformans* and *Saccharomyces cerevisiae*[P00083]. Water extract of dried leaves on agar plate showed IC_{50} 28.0 mg/ml and MIC 0.39 mg/ml on *Candida albicans*[K13111,K11576].

Barbiturate potentiation. Ethanol/ water (1:1) extract of the aerial parts administered intraperitoneally to mice at a dose of 500.0 mg/kg was inactive[W00374].

Diuretic activity. Ethanol/water (1:1) extract of the aerial parts administered intraperitoneally to male rats at a dose of 250.0 mg/kg was active. Urine was collected for four hours post-treatment from saline-loaded animals[W00374].

Embryotoxic effect. Ethanol/water (50%) extract of dried leaves administered by gastric intubation to rats at a dose of 125.0 mg/kg was inactive[T16785].

Estrous cycle disruption effect. Ethanol/ water (50%) extract of dried leaves administered by gastric intubation to rats at a dose of 125.0 mg/kg was equivocal[T16785].

Hypoglycemic activity. Ethanol/ water (1:1) extract of the aerial parts administered orally to rats at a dose of 250.0 mg/kg was inactive. Less than 30% drop in blood sugar level was observed[W00374]. Hot water extract of dried leaves administered by gastric intubation to dogs at a dose of 200.0 ml/animal produced weak activity[T07170]. Petroleum ether extract of shade-dried leaves administered by gastric intubation to rats at a dose of 400.0 mg/kg was inactive[T15223].

Hypotensive activity. Ethanol/ water (1:1) extract of dried leaves administered intravenously to dogs at variable dosages was inactive[W3022A].

Hypothermic activity. Ethanol/ water (1:1) extract of the aerial parts administered intraperitoneally to mice at a dose of 500.0 mg/kg was inactive[W00374].

Laxative effect. Ethanol/water (1:1) extract of dried leaves administered orally at variable dosages to human adults was active. Patients with at least 72 hours of constipation were treated with either placebo or Cassia. Out of 24 patients treated with Cassia, 83% passed stools in 24 hours. The success rate in the placebo group was only 18%[M25326]. Hot water extract of dried leaves administered by gastric intubation at a dose of 500.0 mg/kg to rats was active. The extract had 70% of the activity of senna, *Cassia acutifolia*[M28283]. The infusion at a dose of 800.0 mg/kg was also active[K17262].

Molluscicidal activity. Ethanol (95%) and water extracts of dried trunk bark at concentrations of 10,000 ppm were inactive on *Biomphalaria glabrata* and *Biomphalaria straminea*[W02949].

Semen coagulation effect. Ethanol/water (1:1) extract of the aerial parts at a concentration of 2.0% was inactive on rat semen[W00374].

Spermicidal effect. Ethanol/water (1:1) extract of the aerial parts at a concentration of 2.0% was inactive on rat sperm[W00374].

Toxic effect (general). Ethanol (85%) extract of dried leaves administered intraperitoneally to mice at a dose of 2.0 gm/kg was inactive[T15923,M30962]. Ethanol/water (1:1) extract of dried leaves administered by gastric intubation and subcutaneously at doses of 10.0 gm/kg to mice were inactive[R00001].

Toxicity assessment (quantitative). Ethanol/water (1:1) extract of the aerial parts when administered intraperitoneally to mice showed LD_{50} 1.0 gm/kg[W00374].

Wound healing acceleration. Petrol (gasoline) extract of dried leaves applied externally to rabbits at a dose of 10.0% was active. The extract, in the form of a polyethylene glycol ointment, was applied daily to skin wound which had been inoculated with *Staphylococcus aureus* or *Pseudomonas aeruginosa*. By 21 days, area of wound was 87.6% healed over vs 56.2% on controls[T16493].

8 | Catharanthus roseus

G. Don,

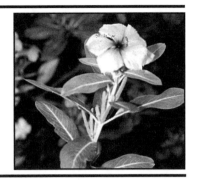

Common Names

Ainskati	India	Patti-poo	Sri Lanka
Atay-biya	Philippines	Periwinkle	Guyana
Billaganneru	India	Periwinkle	India
Boa-noite	Brazil	Periwinkle	Jamaica
Brown man's fancy	West Indies	Periwinkle	Philippines
Caca poule	Dominica	Periwinkle	USA
Chatilla	Guatemala	Periwinkle	West Indies
Chavelita	Peru	Pervenchede	French Guiana
Chichirica	Philippines	de madagascar	
Congorca	Brazil	Phaeng phoi farang	Thailand
Consumption bush	West Indies	Phang-puai-fa-rang	Thailand
Dua can	Vietnam	Pink flower	West Indies
Kantotan	Philippines	Ram goat rose	West Indies
Liluvha	Venda	Rattanjot	India
Madagascan periwinkle	Madagascar	Red rose	West Indies
Maua	Kenya	Sada bahar	India
Mini-mal	Sri Lanka	Sada-bahar	Pakistan
Nayantara	Bangladesh	Sadaphul	India
Nayantara	India	Sailor's flower	West Indies
Nichinich-so	Japan	Saponaire	Rodrigues Islands
Nichinichi-so	Japan	Tiare-tupapaku-kimo	Cook Islands
Ninfa	Mexico	Tsitsirika	Philippines
Nityakalyani	India	Ushamanjairi	India
Old maid	West Indies	White tulip	West Indies

BOTANICAL DESCRIPTION

An erect, bushy perennial herb of the APOCYNACEAE family, it grows to 75-cm high, becoming subwoody at the base and profusely branched, the stems containing some milky latex; leaves are opposite in pairs, smooth, oblong-oval, blunt, or rounded at the apex, 2.5- to 9-cm long and 1.5- to 4-cm wide, short-petioled. Flowers borne all year in upper leaf axils, are tubular, 1.5- to 4-cm long, five-lobed, flaring to a width of 5 cm; color may be white with a

From: Medicinal Plants of the World *By: Ivan A. Ross Humana Press Inc., Totowa, NJ*

yellow eye, white with a crimson eye, or lavender-pink with a crimson eye.

ORIGIN AND DISTRIBUTION

The periwinkle is believed to be native of the West Indies but was originally described from Madagascar. It is cultivated as an ornamental plant almost throughout the tropical and subtropical world. It is abundantly naturalized in many regions, particularly in arid coastal locations.

TRADITIONAL MEDICINAL USES

Australia. Hot water extract of dried leaves is taken orally for menorrhagia[W03088]. Hot water extract of leaves is taken orally by human adults for diabetes[A05524]. Hot water extract of root bark is taken orally as a febrifuge[A05524].

Brazil. Decoction of dried root is taken orally for fevers and malaria[K07977]. Hot water extract of dried leaves is taken orally for diabetes[M22746].

China. Hot water extract of the aerial parts is taken orally as a menstrual regulator[A04168,T01313]

Cook Islands. Decoction of dried leaves is taken orally to treat diabetes, hypertension and cancer. Eighteen leaves are boiled in a kettle of water, and the cool solution is drunk daily as necessary[K20471].

Dominica. Hot water extract of leaves is taken orally by pregnant women to combat primary inertia in childbirth; the tea is used to treat diabetes[W01267].

England. Hot water extract of dried entire plant is taken orally by human adults for diabetes[T09858].

Europe. Decoction of dried leaves is taken orally for diabetes mellitus[M27518].

France. Hot water extract of entire plant is taken orally as an antigalactagogue[A04168]. Hot water extract of leaves is taken orally by human adults as an antigalactagogue[T01313].

French Guiana. Hot water extract of entire plant is taken orally as a cholagogue[J10155].

India. Hot water extract of dried entire plant is taken orally by human adults for cancer[H00669]. Hot water extract of dried leaves is taken orally to Hodgkin's disease[T01745], menorrhagia and diabetes[W03088]. Hot water extract of entire plant is taken orally to treat a confirmed (by needle biopsy) case of Hodgkins disease[T00509]. Hot water extract of leaves is taken orally for menorrhagia[W00002]. Hot water extract of root and twigs is taken orally for menorrhagia[A04306]. Hot water extract of root is taken orally for menorrhagia[T01313]. Pulp of nodes mixed with cow dung is used externally for cuts and wounds[K23485].

Jamaica. Hot water extract of dried leaves is taken orally for diabetes[T07170].

Kenya. Decoction of dried root is taken orally for stomach problems[M25859].

Mexico. Infusion of whole plant is taken orally for cancer[K16948].

Mozambique. Hot water extract of leaves is taken orally for diabetes and rheumatism[01568]. Hot water extract of root is taken orally as a hypotensive and febrifuge[L01568].

North Vietnam. Hot water extract of the aerial parts is taken orally as a menstrual regulator[A04168,T01313].

Pakistan. Hot water extract of dried ovules is taken orally for diabetes[K07365].

Peru. Hot water extract of dried entire plant is taken orally by human adults for cancer, heart disease and leishmaniasis[T15323].

Philippines. Hot water extract of dried root is taken orally as an emmenagogue[T02196]. Hot water extract of leaves is taken orally for diabetes mellitus, amenorrhea, and menorrhagia[A00456]. Hot water extract of root is taken orally by pregnant women to produce abortion, as an effective emmenagogue, and for dysmenorrhea with scanty flow [T01313, A00115, A00456, A04168, A04162, A04508].

South Africa. Hot water extract of dried leaves is taken orally for menorrhagia and diabetes[W03088]. Hot water extract of leaves is taken orally for menorrhagia[T01313].

South Vietnam. Hot water extract of entire plant is taken orally by human adults as an antigalactagogue[T01313,A04168].

Taiwan. Decoction of dried entire plant is taken orally by human adults to treat diabetes mellitus[K07622] and liver disease[T14999]. Decoction of dried entire plant is taken orally to treat diabetes mellitus[K07622]. Decoction of dried root and stem is taken orally to treat diabetes mellitus[K14672].

Thailand. Hot water extract of dried entire plant is taken orally for diabetes[W01792].

USA. Hot water extract of leaves is taken orally, and dried leaves are smoked as a euphoriant[K04641].

Venda. Water extract of dried root is taken orally for venereal disease. *Catharanthus roseus* and *Ximenia caffra* are macerated and soaked in cold water for several hours to two days[T08732].

Vietnam. Hot water extract of dried aerial parts is taken orally as a drug in Vietnamese traditional medicine, listed in Vietnamese pharmacopoeia (1974 Edition)[T05058].

West Indies. Hot water extract of leafy stems is taken orally for diabetes. Hot water extract of the entire plant is taken orally for diabetes; the extract of the white variety is used for high blood pressure. Root infused in whiskey is taken orally for diabetes. Tea of white flowers and leaves is taken orally by human adults for diabetes[T00701]. Tea prepared from leaf and stem is drunk as a remedy for diabetes[L01534].

CHEMICAL CONSTITUENTS

(ppm unless otherwise indicated)

(-)Tabersonine, Pl
2-hydroxy-6-methoxy benzoic acid, Lf
3-epi ajmalicine, Call Tiss
3-hydroxy voafrine A, Pl
3-hydroxy voafrine B, Pl
3-iso ajmalicine, Pl
3'-4'-anhydro-vincaleukoblastine, Lf
4-deacetoxy vincaleukoblastine, Lf
4-deacetoxy-3'-hydroxy vincaleukoblastine, Lf
5' Phosphodiesterase, Call Tiss

7-hydroxy oindolenine ajmalicine, Call Tiss
10-geraniol hydroxylase, Pl
10-hydroxy deacetyl akuammiline, Call Tiss
11-methoxy tabersonine, Fl 0.10
16-epi vindolinine-N(B)-oxide, Pl
16-epi-19-(s) vindoline-N-oxide, Lf
16-epi-19-S-Vindolinine-N-oxide, Pl
16-epi-trans iso-sitsirikine, Lf 0.20
16-hydroxy tabersonine, Call Tiss; Rt; Cot
16-methoxy tabersonine, Cot; Hyp
17-deacetoxy leurosine, Pl
17-deactoxy vincaleukoblastine, Pl
19(s) 16-epi-vindolinine, Lf
19(s)-vindolinine, Lf
19-20-cis 16(R) iso-sitsirikine, Pl
19-20-trans 16(R) iso-sitsirikine, Pl
19-acetoxy-11-hydroxy tabersonine, Pl
19-epi ajmalicine, Pl
19-epi vindolinine, Pl
19-epi,3-iso ajmalicine, Pl
19-hydroxy-11-methoxy tabersonine, Pl
20-epi vindolinine, Pl 20.0
20-hydroxy tabersonine, Pl
21-hydroxy cyclochnerine, Pl
21'-oxo leurosine, Lf
24-methylene cholesterol, PL
Adenine phosphoribosyltransferase, Cr Gall
Adenoside diphosphate, Pl
Adenoside triphosphate, Pl
Adenosine, Lf
Ajmalicine synthetase, Pl
Ajmalicine, Call Tiss; Fl; Lf; St; Rt.
Ajmaline, Res
Akuamicine, Pl
Akuammicine, Rt 4; Lf 0.06
Akuammigine, Pl
Akuammiline, Pl
Akuammine, Pl
Alpha amyrin acetate, St
Alstonine, Rt Bk 0.01%; Rt
Ammocalline, Rt 50
Ammorosine, Rt 30
Anthranilate synthetase, Pl
Antirhine, Pl
Aparicine, Lf; Fl
Arginine, Pl
ATP sulfurylase, Pl
Bannucine, Lf 0.1
Beta sitosterol, Pl

Calmodulin, Pl
Campesterol, Pl
Cantharanthine, Pl
Carosidine, Lf; Rt
Carosine, Lf; Fl
Carotene, Lf
Cathalanceine, Pl
Catharanhine, Pl
Catharanthamine, Lf
Catharanthine, Pl; Call Tiss;
Catharanthus roseus alkaloid (Mp 300+), Lf
Catharanthus roseus alkaloid (MW 336), Pl
Catharanthus roseus alkaloid B, Pl
Catharanthus roseus alkaloid C, Pl
Catharanthus roseus alkaloid D, Pl
Catharanthus roseus iridoid glucoside
   (Mp 194-5), Pl
Catharicine, Lf; Fl
Catharine, Aer Pts
Catharosine, Aer Pts
Cathasterone, Pl
Cathenamine, Pl
Cathindine, Rt; Lf
Cathovaline, Lf
Cavincidine, Rt; Lf
Cavincine, Lf; Rt
Cholesterol, Pl
Choline, Pl
Cleavamine, Pl
Coronaridine, Pl
D-camphor, Rt 300; Bk
De-n-methyl vincaleukoblastine, Lf
Deacetoxy vincaleukoblastine, Lf
Deacetoxy vindoline, Lf; Cot; Hyp
Deacetyl aduammiline, Lf 0.3
Deacetyl akuammiline, Call Tiss
Deacetyl vincaleukoblastine, Lf
Deacetyl vindoline acetyl transferase, Lf
Deacetyl vindoline, Lf; Cot; Hyp
Deacetylvincaleukoblastine, Pl
Dehydro loganin, Lf; St
Deoxy loganin, Pl 0.30
Deoxy vincaleukoblastine, Lf
Deoxyloganin, Lf
Diacylglycerol pyrophosphate, Pl
Dihydro sitsirikine, Lf; Rt
Dihydro vindoline, Pl
Dimethyl tryptamine, Pl
Diol pseudo vincaleukoblastine, Lf
Epi-vindolinine, Lf
Extensin, Pl
Fixed oil, Sd

Fluorocarpamine, Lf
Fluorocarpamine-N-oxide, Lf
Fructose-2-6-bis-phosphate, Pl
Furfural, Lf
Geissoschizine dehydrogenase, Pl
Geissoschizine, Pl; Call Tiss
Geraniol, Pl
Glucose, Pl
Glutamine, Pl
Glycoprotein, Pl
Gomaline, Lf 0.1
Hemicellulose, Pl
Hirsutidin, Call Tiss; Fl
Horhammericine, Lf
Indole-3-acetic acid, Fl
Iso-fucosterol, Pl
Iso-leurosine, Lf
Iso-pent-2-enyl adenine riboside,
   Cr Gall 3.92 nMol/gm
Iso-pent-2-enyl adenine riboside-5'-mono-
   phosphate, Cr Gall 10.98 nMol/gm
Iso-pent-2-enyl adenine,
   Cr Gall 1.55 nMol/gm
Isositsirikine, Lf; Rt
isovallesiachotamine, Pl
Isovincoside, Pl
Isoleurodine, Pl
Isositsirikine, Pl
Kaempferol, Lf
L-(+)-bornesitol, Rt
Lanceine, Pl
Leurocolombine, Pl
Leurocristine, Pl
Leurosidine, Pl
Leurosidine-N'-B-oxide, Lf
Leurosidinine, Pl
Leurosine, Pl
Leurosine-N-oxide, Lf
Leurosinone, Lf
Leurosivine, Rt; Lf
Linoleic acid, Pl
Lirioresinol B b-D-glucoside, PL
Lochnerallol, Lf
Lochnericine, Pl 25.60
Lochneridine, Lf
Lochnerine, Pl 64.60
Lochnerinine, Pl
Lochnerivine, Rt; Lf
Lochnerol, Lf
Lochnovine, Pl
Lochrovicine, Lf
Lochrovidine, Lf

Lochrovine, Lf
Locnovidine, Pl
Loganic acid, Pl; Sd
Loganin, Lf
Maandrosine, Rt 0.05
Malic acid, Pl
Malvidin, Call Tiss; Fl
Mannoside, Pl
Minovincinine, Pl 2.0
Mitraphylline, Pl 1.0
Myricyl alcohol, Lf
N-deformyl leurocristine, Lf
N-demethyl vincaleukoblastine, Lf
Neoleurocristine, Lf
Neoleurosidine, Aer Pts
Neoleurocristine, Pl
Nor harman, Lf
Oleanolic acid, Pl
Oleic acid, Sd Oil 56.76%
Para-coumaric acid, Lf
Pericalline, Pl; Rt 0.20
Pericyclivine, Lf 0.02
Perimivine, Lf
Perividine, Lf
Perivine, Pl 9.30
Perosine, Lf; Rt 0.05
Petunidin, Fl; Call Tiss
Phosphodiesterase, Call Tiss
Phytochelatin A, Pl
Pleiocarpamine, Pl 5.0
Pleurosine, Aer Pts
Prolyl hydroxylase, Pl
Protocatechuic acid, Lf
Pseudovincaleukoblastinediol, Pl
Putrescine, Pl
Quercetin, Lf
Reserpine, Pl; Call Tiss
Resin, Rt 2.0%; Bk
Rhazimol, Lf 0.2
Ricinoleic acid, Sd Oil 3.27%
Rosamine, Lf
Roseadine, Lf
Roseoside, Lf; St
Rosicine, Lf
Rovidine, Lf
Seco loganic acid, Pl
Seco loganin, Pl
Seco loganoside, Pl
Serpentine, Pl; Call Tiss
Sitsirikine, Pl
Stigasterol, Pl
Stricosidine synthetase, Pl

Strictosideine glucosidase 1, Pl
Strictosidine glucosidase 11, Pl
Strictosidine lactam, Pl
Strictosidine synthase, Pl
Strictosidine, Pl
Sulfotransferase, Pl
Sweroside, Pl 10.0
Syringic acid, Lf
Tabersonine, Pl
Tannin, Lf
Tetrahydro alstonine, Rt 133-370; Fl;
Tetrahydroalstonine, Pl
Tetrahydroserpentine, Pl
Tryptamine, Pl
Tryptophan decarboxylase, Pl
Tryptophan synthetase, Pl
Tryptophan, Pl
Tubotaiwine, Pl
Uridine, Pl
Ursolic acid, Lf
Vallesiachotamine, Pl
Vanillic acid, Lf
Vinamidine, Lf
Vinaphamine, Lf
Vinaspine, Lf
Vinblastine, Pl
Vincadioline, Lf
Vincaleukoblastine, Pl; Lf 45-70
Vincaline 1, Rt Bk 40.0
Vincaline 11, Rt Bk 20.0
Vincamicine, Lf
Vincamine, Pl
Vincarodine, Lf 0.06
Vincathicine, Lf
Vinceine, Pl
Vincolidine, Lf
Vincoline, Lf
Vincristine, Pl
Vincubine, Pl
Vindolicine, Lf; Fl
Vindolidine, Lf
Vindoline, Pl; Call Tiss
Vindolinine, Pl
Vindolinine-N(B)oxide, Pl
Vindolinine-N-oxide, Pl
Vindorosine, Aer Pts
Vinesesine, Pl
Vinosidine, Rt, 3.0
Vinsedicine, Sd
Vinsedine, Sd
Virosine, Pl 6.1; Rt 4.0
Vivaspine, Lf

Yohimbine, Rt 0.03%
Zeatin glucosyl, Rt; Lf; Fl
Zeatin ribboside-5'-monophosphate,
   Cr Gall
Zeatin ribosyl, Rt; Fl; Lf
Zeatin, Cr Gall; Rt; Lf; Fl
Zeatin-9-riboside, Cr Gall

PHARMACOLOGICAL ACTIVITIES AND CLINICAL TRIALS

Abortifacient effect. Ethanol/water (1:1) extract of seed pods administered orally to rats at a dose of 100.0 mg/kg was inactive[W01362].

Acid phosphatase inhibition. Ethanol (95%) extract of leaves administered orally to male rats at a dose of 75.0 mg/kg daily for 24 days and autopsy on day 25 was active. The control group (10 animals) had enzyme level of 102 mg/100 mg in testes. Extract treated group was 162.5 mcg/100 mg. Control group enzyme level was 178.57 mcg/100 mg in prostate; extract treated group was 68.75 mcg/100 mg[T00768].

Acid phosphatase stimulation. Ethanol (95%) extract of leaves administered orally to male rats at a dose of 300.0 mg/kg daily for 24 days and autopsy on day 25 was active. Control group (10 animals) enzyme level was 102 mcg/100 mg in testes; extract treated group was 400 mcg/100 mg. Control group enzyme level in prostate was 178.57 mcg/100 mg; extract treated group was 447.92 mg/100 mg Ethanol (95%) extract of leaves administered orally to male rats at a dose of 75.0 mg/kg daily for 24 days and autopsy on day 25 was active. Control group (10 animals) enzyme level was 132.14 mcg/100 mg in testes; extract treated group was 427.08 mcg/100 mg. Control group enzyme level in prostate was 720.83 mcg/100 mg; extract treated group was 1183.33 mcg/100 mg[T00768].

Alkaline phosphatase stimulation. Ethanol (95%) extract of leaves administered orally to male rats at a dose of 300.0 mg/kg daily for 24 days and autopsy on day 25 was active. Control group (10 animals) enzyme

level was 1132.14 mcg/100 mg in testes; extract treated group was 954.17 mcg/100 mg. Control group enzyme level in prostate was 720.83 mcg/100 mg; extract treated group was 1716.66 mcg/100 mg[T00768].

Alkylating activity reduction. Fresh root juice and hot water extract of dried leaves produced weak activity. There was reduction of alkylating activity of ethyl methane sulfonate toward 4-para-nitrobenzylpyridine[T03555].

Animal repellent activity. Dried leaves and stem at variable concentrations was active on *Helix pomatia*[T07907].

Anithyperglycemic activity. Hot water extract of dried entire plant administered by gastric intubation to rats at a dose of 3.0 gm/kg daily for three days was inactive vs alloxan-induced hyperglycemia[T04583].

Antiascariasis activity. Alkaloid fraction of the entire plant produced weak activity on earthworm[A05806].

Antibacterial activity. Benzene extract of dried flowers, at a concentration of 5.0% on agar plate was active on *Proteus, Pseudomonas, Shigella* and *Staphylococcus* species; inactive on *Salmonella* species, and *Shigella paradysenteriae*. Benzene extract of leaves at a concentration of 5.0% on agar plate was active on *Proteus, Pseudomonas, Salmonella, Shigella* and *Staphylococcus* species[T12033]. Ethanol (70%) extract of dried leaves on agar plate was active on *Bacillus megaterium* and *Staphylococcus albus* and inactive on *Bacillus cereus* and *Staphylococcus aureus*[T06729]. Ethanol (95%) extract of fresh root on agar plate was active on *Shigella flexneri, Streptococcus faecalis,* and *Vibrio cholera* and weak activity on *Corynebacterium diptheriae, Diplococcus pneumoniae, Salmonella paratyphi* A, *Shigella dysenteriae,* and *Staphylococcus aureus*. Ethanol (95%) extract of fresh shoots on agar plate was active on *Corynebacterium diphtheriae, Diplococcus pneumoniae* and *Staphylococcus aureus*, and weak activity on *Salmonella paratyphi* B[W03491]. Total alkaloids of root, at a concentration of 500.0 mcg/ml in broth culture was inactive on *Escherichia coli*, *Salmonella typhosa*, and *Shigella dysenteriae*. Weak activity was produced on *Staphylococcus aureus* MIC 200.0 mcg/ml and *Vibrio cholera* MIC 300.0 mcg/ml[A05464]. Water extract of entire plant on agar plate at a concentration of 1:4 was inactive on *Salmonella paratyphi* A, *Salmonella typhosa*, *Shigella flexneri*; weak activity on *Escherichia coli*, *Salmonella paratyphi* B, *Staphylococcus aureus*, and *Vibrio cholera*[A05806].

Antidiuretic activity. Alkaloid fraction of the entire plant administered subcutaneously to male rats at a dose of 50.0 mg/kg was active[A05806].

Antifertility effect. Methanol/water (1:1) extract of dried leaf and stem administered orally to male rats was active[T02666].

Antifungal activity. Acetone and water extracts of dried aerial parts at a concentration of 50% on agar plate was inactive on *Neurospora crassa*; the ethanol (95%) extract was active[W04570]. Aqueous low speed supernatant of fresh leaves, at a concentration of 100.0 ml/liters in broth culture produced weak activity on *Hendersonula toroidea*[T09505]. Dried flower extract was active on *Trichophyton rubrum*[T05879]. Hot water extract of dried leaves in broth culture was active on *Trichophyton mentagrophytes*[M21411]. Hot water extract of dried stem in broth culture was active on *Trichophyton mentagrophytes* and weakly active on *Trichophyton rubrum*[T05879]. Leaves and roots on agar plate were active on *Pythium aphanidermatum*[K16304].

Antihypercholesterolemic activity. Hot water extract of dried leaves administered orally to rabbits was active[T01348].

Antihyperglycemic activity. Dried leaves in the ration of male mice at a concentration of 6.25% of the diet for 28 days was inactive vs streptozotocin-induced hyperglycemia[M27518]. Ethanol (95%) extract of dried leaves administered intragastrically to rats at a dose of 100.0 mg/kg was active. In streptozotocin-induced diabetic animals,

treatment with extract decreased serum glucose by 20.67%[T16664]. Extract at a dose of 75.0 mg/animal administered intraperitoneally was active vs streptozotocin-induced hyperglycemia[T12220]. Hot water extract of dried aerial parts administered intragastrically to dogs at a dose of 50.0 gm/kg (dry weight of plant) was inactive; a dose of 10.0 gm/kg administered intragastrically to rabbits was active vs alloxan-induced hyperglycemia[A14333]. Water extract of dried entire plant administered intravenously to rats at a dose of 10.0 mg/kg was inactive vs streptozotocin-induced hyperglycemia[K07622]. Water extract of fresh cells administered intragastrically to male rats was active vs streptozotocin-induced hyperglycemia. A 60% decrease in blood sugar was observed[K18448].

Antihypertensive activity. Total alkaloids of root administered intravenously to dogs at a dose of 4.0 mg/kg was active. There was a drop in blood of 40 to 50% for two hours in hypertension produced by slow intravenous epinephrine infusion[A05464].

Anti-inflammatory activity. Ethanol (95%) extract of dried leaves administered intraperitoneally to rats at a dose of 400.0 mg/kg was active. Edema was inhibited 65%[K11291].

Antimalarial activity. Chloroform extract of root at a dose of 400.0 mg/kg and water extract at a dose of 4.42 gm/kg administered orally to chicken produced weak activity on *Plasmodium gallinaceum*[A00785].

Antimitotic activity. Ethanol (70%) extract of leaves administered intraperitoneally to female mice was active on CA-Ehrlich ascites vs Induction of metaphase arrest in ascitic cells. Dosing was done four days after tumor cell inoculation ascitic samples removed 2, 4, 6, and 24 hours post-treatment[T00511].

Antimutagenic activity. Hot water extract of dried leaves was active on red blood cells. There was a reduction in number of micronucleated polychromatic red blood cells caused by various mutagens[T05584].

Antispasmodic activity. Total alkaloids of root, at a concentration of 1–20 was active on rabbit duodenum vs ACh-induced spasms[A05464].

Antispermatogenic effect. Hot water extract of dried leaves administered intraperitoneally to male mice at a dose of 0.2 ml/animal produced weak activity. Dosing was equivalent to 10 mg of dried material daily for 15 days followed by sacrifice. There was a slight decrease in sperm concentration from about 77 million/ml to about 52 million/ml. The levels achieved, taking all parameters together, might impair fertility, but not necessarily achieved 100% antifertility effectiveness. There was a slight decrease in motility parameters (% motility and duration of motility) and slight increase in percentage of abnormal and dead sperm[T15904]. At 10.0 mg/animal, regressive changes in seminiferous tubules and Leydig cells, increased cholesterol in testes and degeneration of all germinal elements other than were observed[T16624]. Total alkaloids administered intraperitoneally to male rats was active[A02376].

Antitumor activity. Ethanol (70%) extract of leaves administered intraperitoneally to female mice was active on CA-Ehrlich ascites[T00514]. Alkaloid fraction of dried leaves used externally was active. Ninteen patients with either flat, verruca vulgaris, plantar or genital warts were treated in this study. Six patients had all warts disappear, Seven had the majority of their warts disappear, five had 50% disappear, and one showed no response[M25836]. Alkaloid fraction of dried leaves administered intraperitoneally to mice at doses of 2.5 and 20.0 mg/kg was active on Leuk-P388, 116% and 150% ILS respectively[T03162]. Chloroform extract of leaves was active on Leuk-P388[A02006]. Ethanol (95%) extract of entire plant administered intraperitoneally to mice at a dose of 120.0 mg/kg was active on Leuk-P1534. Total alkaloids of the entire plant adminis-

tered to mice intraperitoneally at a dose of 10.0 mg/kg and orally at a 75.0 mg/kg was active on Leuk-P1534[A03910]. Leaf extract administered intravenously to human adults of both sexes at a dose of 6.0 mg/sq. m body surface was active on human cancer. Eighty percent mean reduction of leukocyte count was observed in all of the 16 patients treated. Five patients were in the terminal phase of positive chronic myelocytic leukemia, one patient had chronic myelomonocytic leukemia[N03109]. Alkaloid fraction of leaf administered intraperitoneally to mice at a dose of 35.0 mg/kg was active on CA-Ehrlich ascites, 70% ILS; a dose of 10.0 mg/kg administered intraperitoneally to rats was inactive on hepatoma, 12% TWD and a dose of 35.0 mg/kg was active on sarcoma (Yoshida ASC) 40% ILS vs resistance of heat-induced hemolysis of rat RBC[W00138].

Antiviral activity (plant pathogens) Water extract of callus tissue in cell culture was active on Tobacco Mosaic virus[T01650].

Cardiotonic activity. Ethanol (70%) extract of leaf and stem administered intravenously to guinea pigs was inactive[A05705].

CNS depressant activity. Total alkaloids of root administered intraperitoneally to rats at a dose of 120.0 mg/kg was active[A05464].

Cytotoxic activity. Alkaloid fraction of dried leaves in cell culture was active on CA-9KB, ED_{50} 0.045 mcg/ml[T03162]. Chloroform extract and culture filtrate of callus tissue in cell culture at doses of 50.0 gm (dry weight of plant) were active on Leuk-L12 10 culture. Chloroform extract of culture filtrate at a dose of 0.75 mg/ml in cell culture was active on Leuk-L1210[T09530]. Chloroform extract of leaves was active on CA-9KB[A02006]. Ethanol (95%) extract of leaves in cell culture was active on CA-9KB. ED_{50} <20.0 mcg/ml[J09860]. Ethanol (70%) extract of leaves in cell culture was active on CA-Ehrlich ascites[T00514]. Water extract of dried root in cell culture was active on CA-9KB, ED_{50} 11.0 mcg/ml[K12472]. Water extract of dried stem in cell culture was active on CA-9KB, ED_{50} <17.0 mcg/ml[K12472]. Water extract of leaves in cell culture was active on CA-9KB, ED_{50} <2.5 mcg/ml[K12472]. Ethanol (95%) extract of seed pods administered orally to rats at a dose of 100.0 mcg/kg was inactive[W01362].

Glutamate pyruvate transaminase inhibition. Ethanol/water (1:1) extract of dried entire plant at a concentration of 1.0 mg/ml in cell culture was inactive on rat liver cells vs carbon tetrachloride-induced hepatotoxicity and PGE-1-induced pedal edema[T14999].

Hyperglycemic activity. Ethanol/water (1:1) extract of dried entire plant administered orally to rabbits at a dose of 5.0 gm/kg was active. 51% increase in blood sugar. All animals died six days after dosing[W01792]. Water extract of dried entire plant administered intravenously to rats at a dose of 5.0 mg/kg was active vs streptozotocin-induced hyperglycemia[K07622].

Hypoglycemic activity. Dried leaves in the ration of male mice, at a concentration of 6.25% of the diet for 28 days, was inactive[M27518]. Ethanol (95%) extract of dried leaves administered intragastrically to rats at a dose of 100.0 mg/kg was active. Serum glucose concentration fell 26.22% in treated animals. Extract potentiated effect of exogenous insulin as well. Hot water extract administered orally to rabbits was also active[T01348]. Ethanol/water (1:1) extract of dried entire plant administered orally to rabbits at a dose of 5.0 g/kg was inactive. All the animals died within six days[W01792]. Hot water extract of dried entire plant administered by gastric intubation to rats at a dose of 3.0 gm/kg daily for three days was inactive[T04583]. Hot water extract of dried leaves (20 gm of air dried leaves) administered by gastric intubation to dogs at a dose of 200.0 ml/animal was active[T07170]. Hot water extract of the dried aerial parts administered intragastrically to dogs and rabbits at doses of 50.0 and 20.0 gm/kg (dry weight of plant) respectively was inactive[A14333].

Hypotensive activity. Total alkaloids of root administered intravenously to rabbits at a dose of 0.10 gm/kg was active[A05937]. Total alkaloids of root administered intravenously to dogs at a dose of 5.0 mg/kg was active. The was a 50 to 60% drop in blood pressure over a two hour duration[A05464]. Alkaloid fraction of the entire plant administered intravenously to dogs at a dose of 5.0 mg/kg produced weak activity[A05806].

Inotropic effect (negative). Total alkaloids of root, at a dose of 5.0 mg was active on rabbit heart[A05464].

Insect feeding deterrent. Alkaloid fraction of fresh leaves at a concentration of 0.06%, water extract at a concentration of 0.60% and methanol extract at a concentration of 0.25% of the diet were active on *Spodoptera littoralis*[T05121].

Insect sterility induction. Total alkaloids of dried leaves at a concentration of 0.5% was inactive on *Dysdercus cingulatus*. Total alkaloids of dried root at a concentration of 0.5% was active on *Dysdercus cingulatus*[T06024].

Insecticidal activity. Water extract of dried branches and leaves at variable concentrations was inactive on *Blatella germanica*. Intravenous dose of 40.0 ml/kg administered intravenously to *Periplaneta americana* was also inactive[W03405].

Insulin activity. Ethanol (95%) extract of dried leaves, at a concentration of 25.0 mg/ml was inactive. Extract did not stimulate glucose uptake or glycogen deposition, and in fact inhibited insulin's activities toward these ends[K08705].

Larvicidal activity. Petroleum ether extract of dried flower, leaf, seed, and stem, at a concentration of 100.0 ppm was active on *Anopheles stephensi* larvae; a concentration of 50.0 ppm was active on *Aedes aegypti* and a concentration of 80.0 ppm active on *Culex quinquefasciatus*[T09890].

Leukopenic activity. Alkaloid fraction of leaves administered intravenously to dogs at a dose of 2.5 mg/kg, 10 daily injections, was active[W00138]. Water extract of leaves administered intraperitoneally to rats was active[A02479].

Smooth muscle relaxant activity. Total alkaloids of root administered intravenously to dogs at a dose of 2.0 mg/kg was active[A05464].

Spasmogenic activity. Total alkaloids of root produced weak activity on rat intestine[A05937].

Toxic effect (general). Ethanol (95%) extract of leaves administered orally to male rats at a dose of 75.0 mg/kg daily for 24 days and autopsy on day 25, was active. Marked reduction in weights of testes and prostate in extract treated animals was observed[T00768]. Water extract of root administered subcutaneously to mice at a dose of 10.0 gm/kg was inactive. Total alkaloids at a dose of 0.05 gm/kg was active, 20% of the animals died[A05937].

Toxicity assessment (quantitative). Alkaloid fraction of entire plant administered intraperitoneally to mice produced a LD_{50} 4.0 ml/kg[A05940]. Total alkaloids of root administered intraperitoneally to rats produced LD_{50} 100.0 mg/kg and MLD 150.0 mg/kg[A05464].

Uterine relaxation effect. Alkaloid fraction of the entire plant was inactive on the pregnant uterus of rats[A05806].

Uterine stimulant effect. Alkaloid fraction of the entire plant was inactive on the pregnant uterus of rats. Hot water extract of root was inactive in nonpregnant uterus of cat. Total alkaloids of root were inactive in guinea pigs[A05464].

Weight loss. Ethanol (95%) extract of leaves administered orally to male rats at a doses of 75.0 and 300.0 mg/kg daily for 24 days and autopsy on day 25 was inactive[T00768]

9 | Cymbopogon citratus

(DC.) Stapf.

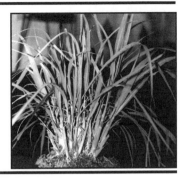

Common Names

Agin-ghas	Fiji	Lemon grass	Egypt
Agya-ghas	Fiji	Lemon grass	Guyana
Awaqa'pi l'ta	Argentina	Lemon grass	India
Bhoostrina	India	Lemon grass	Nicaragua
Black reed	USA	Lemon grass	Sierra Leone
Cana limon	Canary Islands	Lemon grass	Thailand
Capii cedron	Paraguay	Lemon grass	USA
Capim-cidrao	Brazil	Osang	Guinea
Capim-santo	Brazil	Paja de limon	Costa Rica
Chaywala ghas	Fiji	Sagadi abiruau	Nicaragua
Citronella	India	Sagadi	Nicaragua
Citronella	USA	Sakumau	Malaysia
Citronelle	Rodrigues Islands	Sitronel	Haiti
Erva cidreira capim	Brazil	Ta-khrai	Thailand
Erva-cidreira	Brazil	Tanglad	Indonesia
Fever grass	Belize	Tauj dub	USA
Fever grass	Guyana	Tauj qab	USA
Fever grass	Nicaragua	Te de limon	Guatemala
Gati-ma-nya	Ecuador	Tej-sar	Ethiopia
Ginger grass	Ecuador	Tiwahiwa	Nicaragua
Hierba de limon	Costa Rica	Vattu pulle	India
Hierba luisa	Ecuador	Yerba luisa	Easter Island
Hierba luisa	Peru	Zacate de limon	Nicaragua
Lemon grass	Argentina	Zacate limon	Belize
Lemon grass	Brazil	Zacate limon	Guatemala
Lemon grass	Ecuador	Zacate limon	Mexico

BOTANICAL DESCRIPTION

This densely tufted perennial of the GRAMINEAE family has leaf blades tapered to both ends up to 1-meter long and 5- to 10-mm wide. The flowering pannicles are rarely formed; inflorescence are 30- to 60-cm long and nodding; the partial inflorescences are paired racemes of spikelets subtended by spathes.

From: Medicinal Plants of the World *By: Ivan A. Ross Humana Press Inc., Totowa, NJ*

ORIGIN AND DISTRIBUTION

Probably originated in India, it is now wide-spread in the tropics and is frequently cultivated in gardens and along pathsides.

TRADITIONAL MEDICINAL USES

Argentina. Decoction of leaf is taken orally with "mate" tea for sore throat, empacho, and as an emetic[K23834].

Belize. Hot water extract of dried entire plant is taken orally for fever[T05011].

Canary Islands. Hot water extract of dried aerial parts is taken orally for high blood pressure and as a tranquilizer[T15880].

Colombia. Decoction of leaf is taken orally as a febrifuge[K16262].

Costa Rica. Hot water extract of leaves is taken orally as a carminative, with milk as a diaphoretic, depurative, an expectorant, and for indigestion[T01287].

Cuba. Hot water extract of dried leaves is taken orally as a hypotensive, for catarrh and rheumatism[M20030].

Egypt. Hot water extract of dried leaves and stem is taken orally as a renal antispasmodic and diuretic[N11092].

Ethiopia. Hot water extract of aerial parts is taken orally to treat stomach aches[T05018].

Fiji. Decoction of dried leaves in bath water is used for colds, coughs, fever, flu, and pneumonia[T10632].

Guatemala. Hot water extract of dried leaves is used externally for wounds, ulcers, bruises, sores, infections of the skin and mucosa, skin eruptions and erysipelas. Orally the extract is used for urinary tract infections[T15445].

Haiti. Decoction of dried leaves is taken orally for stomachache[T13846].

India. Fresh entire plant is said to repel snakes[T07374]. Two to three drops of essential oil, in hot water is taken orally for gastric troubles. For cholera, a few drops of oil with lemon juice is taken orally[T08282]. Hot water extract of dried leaves is used for bathing in cases severe headache and fever. A fomen-tation of leaves is said to give immediate relief of colds[T07374].

Indonesia. Hot water extract of the entire plant is taken orally as an emmenagogue[A00115].

Malaysia. Hot water extract of entire plant is taken orally as an emmenagogue[A06589].

Mexico. An infusion prepared from the whole plant is taken orally to treat Varix and to promote the functions of the stomach[K16948].

Paraguay. Hot water extract of dried leaves is used as an insecticide or vermifuge[K18765].

Peru. Hot water extract of dried entire plant is taken orally as an antispasmodic, stomachic and analgesic[T15323].

Thailand. Fresh entire plant is inhaled as a fragrance and eaten as a condiment[B00011]. Hot water extract of dried entire plant is taken orally as a stomachic[W03804]. Hot water extract of dried root is taken orally for diabetes[W01792].

USA. Hot water extract of entire plant is used externally by Laotian Hmong in Minnesota for healing wounds and bone fractures[T15879].

CHEMICAL CONSTITUENTS

(ppm unless otherwise indicated)

(+)-limonene, Pl
2'-0-Rhamnosyl orientin, Lf
1,4-cineole, Lf
Alpha citral, Pl
Alpha oxobisabolene, Pl
Alpha pinene, Lf 1.3%
Benzyl alcohol, Pl
Beta myrcene, EO
Beta pinene, Lf EO 1.5%
Beta sitosterol, Pl
Beta terpinene, Lf
Beta -(+)-cadinene, Pl
Borneol, Pl
Camphene, EO 0.90%
Camphor, EO 0.2%
Car-3-ene, EO 0.1%
Cellulose, Pl
Cineal, EO
Citral, Lf, Pl
Citral-A, Lf

Citral-B, Lf
Citronellal, EO
Citronellol acetate, Lf 1.3%
Citronellol, EO
Cymbopogenol, Lf
Cymbopogone, Lf
Cymbopogonol, Lf
Cymbopol, Lf
Cynaroside, Lf
D-camphor, Pl
D-citronellic acid, Lf
D-limonene, EO 5.0%
D-menthone, Pl
Dipentene, Lf
Essential oil, Pl
Eugenol, LF
Farnesol, Lf EO 2.4%
Fenchone, EO 0.3%
Furfural, Lf
Geranial, Lf EO 44.9%
Geraniol acetate, Lf EO 9.9%
Geraniol, EO
Hept-5-en-2-one,6-methyl, Lf EO 1.10%
Heptan-2-one,3-methyl, Lf EO
Hexacosyl alcohol, Lf
Humulene, EO 2.1%
Iso-orientin, Lf
L-menthol, Lf
Limonene, Lf EO
Linalool oxide, Lf EO 1.0%
Linalool, Lf, Pl
Luteolin, Lf
Luteolin-7-0-neohesperidoside, Lf
Menthol, Lf EO 0.6%
Menthone, EO 0.2%
Methyl heptenol, EO
Methyl heptenone, EO
Myrcene, Lf EO
Neral, EO 3.3-33.9%
Nerol acetate, Lf EO 7.50%
Nerol, EO
Nerolidol, Pl
Ocimene, EO 0.2%
P-Cymene, Lf
Para-coumaric acid, Lf
Perilla alcohol, EO
Phenolic substances, Lf
Phenylethyl alcohol, Pl
Terpineol, EO
Terpinolene, Pl
Triacontan 1-ol, Lf
Waxes, Lf

PHARMACOLOGICAL ACTIVITIES AND CLINICAL TRIALS

Ascaricidal activity. Fresh leaf essential oil, undiluted, was active. The oil concentration of 1:2 and 1:4 (oil/ethanol; v/v) showed high activity five days after dipping. The oil at a concentration of 1:3 (oil/ethanol; v/v) when sprayed on the ticks on cattle was active[K15932].

Analgesic activity. Ethanol (95%) extract of fresh leaves administered intragastrically to mice at a dose of 1.0 gm/kg was inactive vs tail flick response to hot water and benzoyl peroxide-induced writhing[T15876]. Fresh leaf essential oil administered intragastrically to mice was active vs acetic acid- and Iloprost-induced writhing. A dose of 20% was active vs carrageenin- and PGE-2-induced pedal edema; and inactive vs dibutyl cyclic AMP-induced hyperalgesia in paw[M27825].

Antiamebic activity. Essential oil at a concentration of 0.25 microliters/ml in broth culture was active on *Entamoeba histolytica*[K21149].

Antiascariasis activity. Ethanol (95%) extract of entire plant produced weak activity on earthworm. Paralysis was observed in 24 hours, no deaths[J08904].

Antibacterial activity. Chromatographic fraction of essential oil at a concentration of 0.05% on agar plate was active on *Bacillus subtilis*, *Escherichia coli* and *Staphylococcus aureus*. The essential oil was active on *Bacillus subtilis*, *Escherichia coli*, *Staphylococcus aureus*[M09284]; *Salmonella paratyphi* A IC_{100} 1600 ppm, *Shigella flexneri* IC_{100} 1600 ppm; strong activity on *Staphylococcus aureus* IC_{100} 400 ppm; weak activity on *Escherichia coli* IC_{90} 2400 ppm[K23904]. Essential oil on agar plate at a concentration of 0.1 ml/disc was active on *Bacillus mycoides*, *Bacillus subtilis* and *Escherichia coli*; and inactive on *Pseudomonas aeruginosa*[K17557]. Essential oil of fresh aerial parts on agar plate was active, a minimum toxic dose of 0.03% was observed for *Staphylococcus aureus*; 0.05% for *Bacillus subtilis*; 0.07% for *Escherichia coli* and 0.8%

for *Pseudomonas aeruginosa*. The effects of pH, inoculum size and strength of nutrient broth were studied[T11226]. Essential oil on agar plate was active on *Escherichia coli* and *Staphylococcus aureus*. The extract was also active when the volatile oil extract was oxidized via the active oxygen method[K11513]. Essential oil at a concentration of 20.0 mg/ml on agar plate was active on *Bacillus subtilis* and *Staphylococcus aureus*; weak activity on *Escherichia coli* and *Pseudomonas aeruginosa*[M24523]. Fresh stem, water, and hot water extracts of fresh stem at concentrations of 0.5 ml/disk on agar plate were inactive on *Bacillus subtilis* H-17(Rec+) and M-45(Rec-)[T07988]. Tincture of dried leaves (extract of 10 gm plant material in 100 ml ethanol), at a concentration of 30.0 microliters/disk on agar plate was inactive on *Escherichia coli*, *Pseudomonas aeruginosa*, and *Staphylococcus aureus*[T15445].

Anticonvulsant activity. Hot water extract of leaves (10 gm powder/150 ml water) administered by gastric intubation to mice at a dose of 20–40 ml/kg was inactive vs transcorneal electroshock and pentylenetetrazole-induced contractions[T14776].

Antifilarial activity. Fresh leaves was active on *Setaria digitata*. LC$_{100}$ 75,000 ppm[M25236].

Antifungal activity. Distillate of leaf essential oil on agar plate was active on *Curvularia lunata*, *Rhizopus* species, *Ustilaginoidea virens* and *Ustilago maydis*[M22780]. The essential oil at a concentration of 3000 ppm on agar plate was active on *Aspergilllus niger*[K16266]. Dried entire plant at a concentration of 2.0% (expressed as dry weight of plant) on agar plate was active on *Absidia spinosa*, *Alternaria alternata*, *Ceratocystis paradoxa*, *Choanephora cucurbitarum*, *Colletotrichum denatium*, *Drechslera maydis*, *Fusarium solani*, *Geotrichum candidum*, *Melanconium fuligineum*, *Myrothecium roridum*, *Phytophthora* species, *Pleurotus ostreatus*, *Pythium aphanidermatum*, *Rhizopus msporus*, *Sclerotium rolfsii*, *Sordaria fimicola*,

Thanatephorus cucumeris, *Tricholoma crassum*, *Ustilago maydis*, and *Volvariella volvacea* [P00089]. Essential oil at a concentration of 0.1 ml/disk on agar plate was inactive on *Trichophyton rubrum*[K17557]. Concentration of 0.25% was active on *Aspergillus niger*. On agar plate the essential oil was active on *Trichophyton mentagrophytes* MIC 0.08% and *Aspergillus fumigatus* MIC 0.1%[M20737]. Concentration of 20.0 mg/ml on agar plate was active on *Trichophyton mentagrophytes* and weak activity on *Aspergillus flavus*[M24523]. On agar plate, the essential oil was active on several plant pathogenic fungi[A05953].

Anti-inflammatory activity. Hot water extract of dried leaves administered intragastrically to rats at a dose of 15.0 ml/kg was active vs carrageenin-induced pedal edema[M20030].

Antimutagenic activity. Water extract of commercial sample of aerial parts at a concentration of 50.0 mg (expressed as dry weight of plant) was active on *Salmonella typhimurium* TA98 vs TRP-P-2-induced mutation. Metabolic activation was required for activity[M20801]. Ethanol (80%) extract of freeze-dried aerial parts at a concentration of 0.5 mg/plate on agar plate was active on *Salmonella typhimurium* TA100 vs 2-amino-3-methylimidazo[4,5-F]quinoline-, n-methyl-n'-nitro-n-nitroso-guanidine(MNNG)- and furylfuramide(AF-2); and on TA98 vs aflatoxin B1-, 2-amino-6-methyl-dipyrido[1,2-A:3',2'-D]imidazole- and 2-aminodipyrido-1,2-A:3'2'-D-imidazole-induced mutagenesis. A concentration of 2.5 mg/plate was active on TA100 and TA98 vs Benzo(A)Pyrene- and 3-Amino-1-Methyl-5H-Pyrido[4,3-B]Indole-induced mutagenesis, respectively. A concentration of 5.0 mg/plate was active on TA98 vs 3-Amino-1,4-Dimethyl-5H-Pyrid[4,3-B]Indole (TRP-P-1) induced-mutagenesis and a concentration of 10.0 mg/plate was active on TA100 and TA98 metabolic activation was not required of activity[K17723].

Antimycobacterial activity. Essential oil at a concentration of 20.40 mg/ml on agar plate was active on *Mycobacterium smegatis*[M24523].

Antioxidant activity. Leaf and stem taken orally by human adults was active. Biological activity reported has been patented[M30208].

Antispasmodic activity. Unsaponifiable fraction of dried leaf and stem was active on rabbit ileum[N11092].

Antispermatogenic effect. Hot water extract of oven-dried leaves administered by gastric intubation to female rats at a dose of 20–40 ml/kg was inactive. Dose contained 2 mg leaf powder/150 ml water. Dosing for 70 days[T12574].

Antistress activity. Hot water extract of leaves (2 g powder/150 ml water) administered by gastric intubation to mice at a dose of 40.0 ml/kg was inactive[T14776].

Antiyeast activity. Dried entire plant at a concentration of 2.0% (expressed as dry weight of plant) on agar plate was active on *Saccharomyces cerevisiae*[P00089]. Essential oil at a concentration of 20.0 mg/ml on agar plate was active on *Cryptococcus neoformansi* and *Saccharomyces cerevisiae*[M24523]. Essential oil on agar plate was active on *Candida albicans* and *Candida pseudotropicalis*, MIC 0.05%[M20737]. Tincture of dried leaves (extract of 10 gm plant material in 100 microliters ethanol), at a concentration of 30.0 ml/disk on agar plate was inactive on *Candida albicans*[T15445].

Anxiolytic effect. Hot water extract of oven-dried leaves taken orally by human adults at a dose of 2–10 gm/person was inactive. Eighteen volunteers were exposed to an anxiety state using the Stroop color-word test. There were no differences in the pulse rates and error rates between the placebo and treated groups[T12445].

Barbiturate potentiation. Hot water extract of leaves (10 gm powder/150 ml water) administered by gastric intubation to mice at a dose of 20.40 ml/kg was inactive. Lyo-philized extract (2 gm powder/150 ml water) administered intraperitoneally to mice was inactive[T14776].

Barbiturate sleeping time decrease. Hot water extract of leaves (10 gm powder/150 ml water) administered by gastric intubation to mice at a dose of 20.40 ml/kg was inactive; lyophilized extract (2 gm powder/150 ml water) administered intraperitoneally to mice was inactive[T14776].

Cataleptic effect. Hot water extract of leaves (2 gm powder/150 ml water) administered by gastric intubation to rats at a dose of 20.40 ml/kg was inactive[T14776].

CNS depressant activity. Hot water extract of fresh leaves (10 leaves/150 ml water) administered by gastric intubation and intraperitoneally to mice at doses of 20.0 ml/kg was inactive vs Rotarod test. Hot water extract of leaves (10 gm powder/150 ml water) administered intraperitoneally and by gastric intubation to mice at doses of 20.40 ml/kg was inactive vs Rotarod test[T14776]. Hot water extract of oven-dried leaves taken orally by human adults at a dose of 4.0 gm/day was active. Did not significantly effect sleep parameters in 50 healthy volunteers[T12445].

Conditioned avoidance response decrease. Hot water extract of leaves (2 gm powder/150 ml water) administered by gastric intubation to rats at a dose of 40.0 ml/kg was inactive[T14776].

Dermatitis producing effect. Essential oil applied externally to male human adults was active[K19502].

Diuretic activity. Hot water extract of dried leaves administered intragastrically to rats at a dose of 25.0 ml/kg produced weak activity[M20030].

Embryotoxic effect. Hot water extract of oven dried leaves administered by gastric intubation to pregnant rats at a dose of 20–40 ml/kg was inactive[T12574].

Estrous cycle disruption effect. Hot water extract of oven-dried leaves (2 mg of leaf powder/150 ml water) administered by gastric intubation to female rats at a dose of 40.0 ml/kg daily for 30 days was inactive[T12574].

Glutamate oxaloacetate transaminase stimulation. Essential oil in the ration of rats at a dose of 1500 ppm was active[K08820].

Glutamate pyruvate transaminase stimulation. Essential oil in the ration of rats at a dose of 1500 ppm was active[K08820].

Glutathione-S-transferase induction. Essential oil administered intragastrically to mice at a dose of 30.0 mg/animal was active on small intestine; inactive on liver and stomach. Dose was given every two days for a total of three doses[M30046].

Hyperglycemic activity. Hot water extract of oven-dried leaves (2 mg of leaf powder/150 ml water) administered by gastric intubation to rats at a dose of 20–40 ml/kg daily for eight weeks was inactive[T12574].

Hyperthermic activity. Hot water extract of oven-dried leaves (2 mg of leaf powder/150 ml water) administered by gastric intubation to rats at a dose of 20–40 ml/kg daily for eight weeks was inactive[T12574].

Hyperthermic effect. Hot water extract of leaves (2 gm powder/150 ml water) administered by gastric intubation to rats at a dose of 20.0 ml/kg was inactive[T14776].

Hypocholesterolemic activity. Essential oil taken orally by human adults at a dose of 140.0 mg/day was active. Twenty-two volunteers were given lemon grass oil capsules for three months. After 60 days, cholesterol level fell modestly, not significantly for a group of eight responding subjects, but it was stable for 14 resistant subjects. A posttest showed no difference between responders and resistors after the oil was withdrawn[M21093].

Hypoglycemic activity. Hot water extract of dried root administered orally to rabbits at a dose of 2.5 gm/kg was inactive[W01792]. Hot water extract of oven dried leaves (2 mg of leaf powder/150 ml water) administered by gastric intubation to rats at a dose of 20–40 ml/kg daily for eight weeks was inactive[T12574].

Hypotensive activity. Hot water extract of dried leaves administered intravenously to rats at doses of 1.0[M29843], and 3.0 ml/animal was active. Blood pressure fell by more than 30%[M20030].

Hypothermic activity. Hot water extract of fresh leaves (two leaves/150 ml water) administered intraperitoneally to rats at a dose of 40.0 ml/kg was active. Results significant at $P < 0.05$ level. Hot water extract of leaves (2 gm powder/150 ml water) administered by gastric intubation at a dose of 20.0 ml/kg was inactive; a dose of 40.0 ml/kg administered intraperitoneally to rats was active. Results significant at $P < 0.05$ level[T14776]. Hot water extract of oven-dried leaves (2 mg of leaf powder/150 ml water) administered by gastric intubation to rats at a dose of 20–40 ml/kg daily for eight weeks was inactive[T12574].

Immunomodulator activity. Essential oil in the ration of rats at a dose of 1500 ppm was inactive. Polymorphocyte, eosinophil, and monocyte counts were unaltered[K08820].

Inotropic effect positive. Hot water extract of dried leaves at a concentration of 320.0 ml was inactive on guinea pig's atrium[M29843].

Insecticidal activity. Petroleum ether extract of dried leaves at a concentration of 50.0 mcg was inactive on *Rhodnius neglectus*[K18765]. Petroleum ether extract of dried leaves at a concentration of 1.0 gm/liter was inactive on *Lutzomyia longipalpis*[M31056].

Intestinal motility inhibition. Hot water extract of fresh leaves (10 leaves/150 ml water) administered by gastric intubation to rats at a dose of 20.40 ml/kg was inactive vs charcoal meal intestinal transport assay. Hot water extract of leaves (10 gm powder/150 ml water) administered by gastric intubation to mice at a dose of 20.40 ml/kg was inactive; intraperitoneally, at a dose of 40.0 ml/kg the extract was active. Results significant at $P < 0.001$ level vs charcoal meal intestinal transport assay[T14776].

Intestinal motility stimulation. Hot water extract of fresh leaves (10 leaves/150 ml water) administered by gastric intubation to rats at a dose of 20.40 ml/kg was inactive vs charcoal meal intestinal transport assay. Hot water extract of leaves (10 gm powder/ 150 ml water) administered by gastric intubation to mice at a dose of 20.40 ml/kg was inactive vs charcoal meal intestinal transport assay[T14776].

Larvicidal activity. Fresh leaf essential oil was active. The oil was diluted with 95% ethanol and tested on larvae and engorged female cattle ticks. It showed high activity at concentrations of 1:8, 1:12, and 1:16 (oil/ ethanol; v/v)[K15932]. Water extract of dried leaves at a concentration of 0.03 gm/ml (gm of plant material per ml water) was inactive on *Culex quinquefasciatus*[M19731].

Mating inhibition. Hot water extract of oven dried leaves (2 mg of leaf powder/ 150 ml water) administered by gastric intubation to male rats at a dose of 20–40 ml/kg daily for 70 days was inactive[T12574].

Mitogenic activity. Hot water extract of oven dried leaves (2 mg of leaf powder/ 150 ml water) administered by gastric intubation to pregnant rats at a dose of 40 ml/kg daily during the entire pregnancy was inactive[T12574]. Fresh stem, water and hot water extracts of fresh stem at concentrations of 0.5 ml/disk on agar plate were inactive on *Bacillus subtilis* H-17(Rec+) and M-45(Rec-)[T07988].

Ovulation inhibition effect. Hot water extract of oven dried leaves (2 mg of leaf powder/150 ml water) administered by gastric intubation to female rats at a dose of 20–40 ml/kg daily for 51 days was inactive[T12574].

Spontaneous activity reduction. Hot water extract of leaves (10 gm powder/150 ml water) administered by gastric intubation to mice at a dose of 20.40 ml/kg was inactive[T14776].

Spontaneous activity stimulation. Hot water extract of leaves (10 gm powder/150 ml water) administered by gastric intubation to mice at a dose of 20.40 ml/kg was inactive[T14776].

Spore germination inhibitor. Essential oil at a concentration of 0.1% was active on *Aspergillus fumigatus*[M20737].

Toxic effect. Hot water extract of oven dried leaves (2 mg of leaf powder/150 ml water) administered by gastric intubation to rats at a dose of 20–40 ml/kg daily for eight weeks was inactive[T12574]. The hot water extract taken orally by human adults at a dose of 2–10 gm/day (dry weight of plant) was inactive. Serum levels of glucose, urea, creatinine, cholesterol, triglycerides, lipids, SGOT, SGPT, alkaline phosphatase, total protein, albumin, LDH, CPK, total bilirubin, and indirect bilirubin were unchanged after dosing for two weeks. A slight elevation of direct bilirubin and amylase was seen in some patients[T12574].

Weight loss. Hot water extract of oven-dried leaves (2 mg of leaf powder/150 ml water) administered by gastric intubation to rats at a dose of 20–40 ml/kg daily for eight weeks was inactive[T12574].

10 | Cyperus rotundus

L.

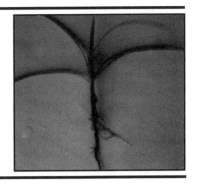

Common Names

Bhada	India	Motha sedge	India
Chido	India	Motha sedge	India
Co cu	Malaysia	Mothe	Nepal
Coquinho	Madeira	Musta	India
Cu gau	Malaysia	Mustaka	India
Cu gau	Vietnam	Mustha	India
Eldeis	Sudan	Mutha	India
Galingale	Madeira	Muthanga	India
Haeo muu	Thailand	Nut grass	Brazil
Haeo-mu	Thailand	Nut grass	Guyana
Haew muu	Thailand	Nut grass	Hawaii
Hama-suge	Japan	Nut grass	India
Herbe a oignons	New Caledonia	Nut grass	Japan
Hsiang fu	Vietnam	Nut grass	Nepal
Hsiang fu-tzu	China	Nutsedge	Hawaii
Hsiang-fu	China	Nutt grass	Iran
Hsiang-fu-tzu	China	Oniani tita	Cook Islands
Huai-mao ts'ao	China	Purple nutsedge	Hawaii
Hui-t'ou ch'ing	China	Purple nutsedge	Japan
Huong phu	Malaysia	Rhizoma cyperii	Taiwan
Hyang-boo-ja	Malaysia	S-s'ad	Morocco
Japanese nutgrass	Japan	Se'd	Qatar
Karimuthan	India	Sha-ts'ao	China
Ko-bushi	Japan	Siru	Nepal
Kobushi	Japan	Souchet rond	Vietnam
Koraikizhangu	India	T'ien-t'ou ts'ao	China
Korchijhan	India	Tamusayt	Morocco
Kraval chruk	Malaysia	Tiao ma tsung	China
Kravanh chruk	Malaysia	Tungamuste	India
Mathe	India	Tungamusti	India
Moothoo	India	Tungamuthalu	India
Moth	India	Xiang fu	China
Motha	India	Xiangfu	China

From: Medicinal Plants of the World *By: Ivan A. Ross Humana Press Inc., Totowa, NJ*

BOTANICAL DESCRIPTION

Cyperus rotundus is a plant of the GRAM-INEAE family, consisting of stems that are tuberous at the base, rising singly from a creeping, underground root-stock, about 10- to 25-cm tall. leaves are linear, broadly grooved on the upper surface, and dark green in color. Flowers are in rather small inflorescence with 2–4 bracts. The longest bracts are usually longer than the inflorescence, but some are shorter. The inflorescence consists of a few slender branches, with the longest usually not more than about 7.5-cm spikes, consisting of about 2–10 spikelets. Each spikelet is narrow and flattened; glumes rather narrow, blunt, closely overlapping with three stamens, three-branched. The nut is oblong-ovate, nearly half as long as the glume, strongly 3-angled, yellow, black when ripe.

ORIGIN AND DISTRIBUTION

Originated in India, it is now widely distributed in the tropics and subtropics. Because of its capacity to compete and adapt to diverse conditions, it has been recorded in more countries than any other weed in the world.

TRADITIONAL MEDICINAL USES

Cambodia. Hot water extract of dried tuber is taken orally for liver complaints with jaundice, and for malarial fevers[T10183].

China. Decoction of dried entire plant is taken orally for worms coming out of both the mouth and anus. *Cyperus rotundus, Berberis aristata, Embelia ribes, Piper longum,* and *Baliospermum* are used in the decoction. Mixed and honey and "Patola" (unidentified), the decoction is administered orally to bring unconscious patients to consciousness. For skin disease, decoction of *Tinospora cordifolia, Cyperus rotundus,* and *Zingiber officinale* is mixed with equal quantity of decoction of *Aconitum heterophyllum* and taken orally[T14489]. For chronic bloody diarrhea with abdominal pain, decoction of *Coleus vetiveroides, Aconitum heterophyllum, Cyperus rotundus* and *Holarrhea antidysenterica* are taken orally[T14489]. Dried tuber mixed with *Rehmannia glutinosa* (root), *Scutellaria baicalensis* (root), *Phellodendron amurense* (bark), and *Ailanthus blandulosa* (bark) administered as a vaginal suppository; is used for leukorrhea with thirst, constipation, weak pulse, abdominal pain, and backache in patients with vaginal cancer[W01791]. Hot water extract of dried rhizome is taken orally to restore menstrual regularity, to alleviate pain, and for dysmenorrhea[T03785]. Hot water extract of tuber is used for dysmenorrhea[A03411]; as a galactogogue; as an emmenagogue[A04581,K03661]; to promote difficult labor[K03661]; as an emmenagogue and for dysmenorrhea, in doses of 5–8 gm[K04768].

Cook Islands. Infusion of fresh bulb taken orally as a treatment for sore throat. Twenty to thirty bulbs, a handful of *Pandanus tectoris* bark, and a handful of *Chrysopagon acriculatus* leaves are crushed into the water of four green coconuts. Half the mixture is drunk hot and the remainder cold. The treatment lasts for three days[K20471].

Europe. Used to induce menses[A04537].

India. Hot water extract of the tuber is taken orally to relieve thirst; to decrease palpitations; to reduce weight; as an aphrodisiac; to strengthen memory; to stimulate appetite; as a stomachic; as a carminative; as an astringent; as a tonic; as a diuretic; and as an anthelmintic. The extract is used against alcoholism. One gram each of *Piper nigrum, Piper longum, Santalum album, Pterrocarpus santalinus, Nardostachys jatamansi, Symplocos racemosa, Andropogon muricatus, Elettaria cardamomum, Berris aristata, Plumbago zeylanica* and *Cyperus rotundus,* plus 5 gm *Woodfordia floribunda* are soaked in one liter of water, with sugar and raisins, and fermented 30 days, strained, and matured for 90 days, then taken orally[T16172].

Hot water extract of the tuber is taken orally as a diaphoretic; as a tonic; as a diuretic and as a demulcent. Externally as an astringent and tuber paste is applied to the breast as a galactogogue[T10183]. Decoction of dried root is taken orally for diarrhea[K17122]. Decoction of *Melia azedarach* is mixed with bulbous root of *Cyperus rotundus* and taken orally as a treatment for dermatitis[M27166]. Extract of the root is taken as an emmenagogue[A04132]. Extract of the tuber is taken orally as an emmenagogue[A04132]. Hot water extract is taken orally as an anthelmintic and as an emmenagogue[W03487]. Hot water extract of dried entire plant is taken orally for fever. This is also used as an anti-inflammatory agent in Ayurveda[T09366]. Essential oil of the root is used externally as a treatment for dermatitis[M27166]. Hot water extract of dried leaves is taken orally for blood motions. Tuber and leaves taken with bark, flowers and young fruit of *Plumbago zeylani*[M23219]. Hot water extract of dried rhizome is taken orally as a stimulant, as an anthelmintic, as a stomachic, and as a carminative. Decocted with the leaves of *Solanum nigrum*, is taken orally for recurring fever. The extract is also taken orally as an insect repellent, for dysentery and for stomach disorders[T10133]. Hot water extract of dried root is used as a diaphoretic and as an astringent[M22542]. Hot water extract of dried tuber is taken orally in Ayurvedic and Unani medicine as an emmenagogue[T05894]. Tuber is boiled in milk and given orally to improve digestion in infants[T08282]. A paste of the tuber is applied around the navel and throat to relieve pain, especially that caused by roundworms[T08282]. Hot water extract of rhizome is taken orally as an emmenagogue[A00115], and to regulate fat metabolism[A05171]. Rhizome made into a paste is applied to the breast as a galactagogue[A00115]. Tubers and rhizomes, crushed and boiled in goat's milk are taken orally for colic; to treat diarrhea; to treat vomiting in children and to relieve flatulence in children[T07731].

Indochina. Hot water extract of dried tuber is taken orally to aid childbirth, and for indigestion in infants[T10183]. Hot water extract of tuber is administered orally to women in childbirth[A05825,A06589]. Rhizome is given to women in childbirth[A00115].

Indonesia. Hot water extract is taken orally to promote menses[A00682]. Hot water extract of dried tuber is taken orally for urinary disorders[T10183].

Japan. Extract of the tuber is taken orally in Chinese medicine for women's diseases[A03690]. Hot water extract of fresh tuber is used externally to promote hair growth[T06579]. Hot water extract of the rhizome is taken orally as an emmenagogue[A04611].

Malaysia. Extract of the rhizome is taken orally an emmenagogue[A04766]. Hot water extract of tuber is taken orally an emmenagogue medicine[A06589].

Nepal. Hot water extract of the tuber is administered orally as a diuretic; as an anthelmintic, and as an emmenagogue[A00020].

New Caledonia. Hot water extract of rhizomes is taken orally as an emmenagogue[A04174].

Nigeria. Hot water extract of fresh root is used externally as an astringent; as a carminative; as an antimalarial and as a tonic[T06510].

Paraguay. Hot water extract is taken orally as a contraceptive[T15375].

Philippines. Hot water extract of dried tuber is taken orally for dysentery[T10183].

Puerto Rico. Hot water extract of dried entire plant is taken orally for kidney calculi[T14280].

South Korea. Hot water extract of rhizome is used for protection of the liver[T00325], and to induce menstruation and abortion[W00346]. Hot water extract of the dried rhizome is taken orally as an abortifacient and as an emmenagogue[T10290].

Sri Lanka. Hot water extract of dried tuber is taken orally as an astringent, as a stomachic, as a carminative, as a cholagogue, for anorexia, for diarrhea and dysentery, for liver congestion, for laryngitis, for bronchitis, pneumonia, and as an antiseptic. For scorpion stings, ulcers, and acne, a paste of tubers with lime juice is applied to the affected area[T10183].

Sudan. Hot water extract of dried entire plant is taken orally for indigestion and as an antiemetic[T10633], and as an astringent[T07856]. Hot water extract of dried root is taken orally as an antidiarrheal, and as an antiemetic[T10633].

Taiwan. Hot water extract of dried rhizome is taken orally for liver disease[T14999].

Tanzania. Fresh tuber is used in traditional medicine[T10354]. Hot water extract of dried tuber is taken orally to aid in childbirth[T03389].

Thailand. Hot water extract of dried rhizome is taken orally for blood purification and as an antipyretic[W3022A].

Vietnam. Hot water extract of dried tuber is taken orally as a diuretic, as an emmen-agogue and for uterine hemorrhage[T10183]. Hot water extract of rhizome is taken orally for difficult delivery[A04766]. Hot water extract of the tuber is taken orally as an emmenagogue[A05825].

CHEMICAL CONSTITUENTS

(ppm unless otherwise indicated)

(+)Copadiene, EO
2-Carboxy-arabinitol, Lf 34 nMol/g
4-A,5-a-oxidoeudesm-11-en-3-a-ol, Rh
1,8-Cineole, Rt
4,7-Dimethyl-tetral-1-one, Tu 7
10,12-Peroxy-calamenene, Tu
Alkaloids, Rt 0.21–0.24%
Alpha copaene, Rh, EO
Alpha cyperone, Rt 0.15–0.50%
Alpha cyperone, Tu, Rt, Rh 700
Alpha humulene, Rh,Tu
Alpha rotundol, Rh
Alpha rotunol, Rt
Alpha rotunol, Tu
Alpha selinene, Tu
Arsenic, Rh 0.29
Ascorbic acid, Rt 90
Aureusidin, Inf
Beta caryophyllene, Rh, EO
Beta cyperone, Rh
Beta elemene, Tu,Rh
Beta guaiene, Rt

Beta pinene, Rt
Beta rotundol, Rh
Beta rotunol, Rt
Beta rotunol, Tu
Beta santalene, Rt
Betaseliene, Rh
Beta selinene, Rt
Beta selinene, Tu
Calamine, Rh, EO
Calcium, Rh 0.318%
Camphene, Rt
Caryophylla-6-one, Tu
Caryophyllene, Tu
Caryophyllene-6-7-oxide, Tu
Caryophyllene-a-oxide, Tu
Caryophyllenol, Tu, EO
Chlorophyll A, Lf
Chlorophyll B, Lf
Cineol, Tu
Copaene, Rt
Copper, Rh 10
Cyperene II, Rh
Cyperene, EO, Tu, Rh
Cyperenone, Tb, Rh 115
Cyperol, EO, Tu
Cyperolone, Rh
Cyperotundone, EO
D-Copadiene, Rt
D-Epoxyguaiene, Rt
D-Fructose, Rt, Sh
D-Glucose, Rt, Sh
Delta-cadinene, Rh, EO
EO, Rt 0.5–1.0%
Epoxy-guaiene, EO
Ferulic acid, Tu
Flavonoids, Rt 1.25%
Fluoride, Rh 3.7
Gamma cymene, Rt
Humulene, Rh,Tu
Iron, Rh 430, Sh
Iso-kobusone, Rt, Rh
Isocyperol, Rh, Tu
Kobusone, Rt, Rh
Limonene, EO
Linoleic acid, Rh
Linolenic acid, Rh
Luteolin, Inf, Lf
Magnesium, Rh 0.15%
Manganese, Rh 28
Mustakone, Rt
Myristic acid, Rh
Oleanolic acid, Tu

Oleanolic acid-3-0-neohesperidoside, Tu
Oleic acid, Rh
P-cymol, Rt
P-hydroxy-benzoic acid, Tu
Para-coumaric acid, Tu
Patchoulenol acetate, Tu
Patchoulenone, Tu 30
Patchouylenone, Rh
Pectin, Rt 3.72%
Phosphorus, Sh
Pinene, Tu
Polyphenols, Rt 1.62%
Potassium, Rh 1.01%
Protocatechuic acid, Tu
Resin, Rt 4.21%
Rhamnetin-3-0-rhamnosyl(1,4)rhamnoside, Tu
Rotundene, Rt
Rotundenol, Rt
Rotundone, Rt
Selinatriene, Rt
Sitosterol, Rt
Sodium, Rh 254
Starch, Rt 9.2%
Stearic acid, Rh
Sucrose, Sh
Sugars, Rt 13.2-14.4%
Sugenol, Rh
Sugeonol acetate, Tu
Sugeonol, Rh
Sugeonyl acetate, Rh
Sugetriol triacetate, Tu
Sugetriol, Rh
Vanillic acid, Tu
Zinc, Rh 33

PHARMACOLOGICAL ACTIVITIES AND CLINICAL TRIALS

Abortifacient effect. Ethanol/water (1:1) extract at a dose of 100.0 mg/kg administered orally to pregnant rats was inactive[T02678].

Adrenergic receptor blockade (A-2). Water extract of dried rhizome was inactive. The extract did not have any inhibitory effect on angiotensin II[M20450].

Aflatoxin inactivation. Water extract of dried leaf at a concentration of 1.0 ml was active on *Asperigillus flavus*[M27387].

Aldose reductase inhibition. Hot water extract at a concentration of 0.1 mg/ml produced strong activity. The effect was tested on bovine lens aldase reductase[K11985].

Analgesic activity. Ethanol (95%) extract of the entire plant (cultivated in Saudi Arabia) administered to mouse at a dose of 500.0 mg/kg by gastric intubation was inactive vs hot plate method[M21425]. Ethanol (95%), and hot water extracts of dried rhizome, at a dose of 12.7 gm/kg administered intraperitoneally to mice were inactive vs hot plate method. Hot water extract administered orally at a dose of 12.7 gm/kg was also inactive vs acetic acid writhing inhibition test[T01727]. Alkaloid fraction, essential oil, and decoction of dried rhizome administered to mice by gastric intubation were active vs acetic acid-induced writhing[K17215].

Anthelmintic activity. Hot water extract of leaf administered to mouse was inactive on *Nippostrongylus brasiliense*, *Trichostrongylus axei* and *Syphacia obvelata*[K03517]. Hot water extract of tuber administered orally to mice was inactive on *Nippostrongylus brasiliense*, *Syphacia obvelata*, and *Trichostrongylus axei*[K03517].

Antialcoholic activity. Fermented tuber at a dose of 5.0 ml/animal in the ration of rats was active. Dose given daily for 90 days reversed alcohol-induced changes on performance of neurologic tests, EEG and EKG, fat deposition in liver and signs of hemorrhage, demyelination and spongiosis in brain. Fermented extract of the following plants, referred to as the SKV Indian herbal formula were used: *Piper nigrum*, *Piper longum*, *Santalum album*, *Pterocarpus santalinus*, *Nardostachys jatamansi*, *Symplocos racemosa*, *Andropogon muricatus*, *Elettaria cardamomum*, and *Berber aristata*. Also included: *Plumbago zeylanica*, *Cyperus rotundus*, *Woodfordia floribunda* and raisins. Rats were given the herbal formula (SKV) for three months vs rats fed alcohol for six months[T16122,T16172].

Antibacterial activity. Chloroform and methanol extracts of dried entire plant, when tested on agar plate were active and the water extract was inactive on *Bacillus subtilis, Escherichia coli, Pseudomonas aeruginosa* and *staphylococcus aureus*[T10633] Decoction of dried entire plant at MIC 125.0 mg/ml on agar plate was inactive on *E. coli, Klebsiella pneumoniae*, and *P. aeruginosa*. At MIC 15.63 mg/ml the decoction had weak activity on *Staphylococcus aureus*, and *Staphylococcus epidermidis*. At MIC 31.25 mg/ml weak activity was shown on *Bacillus cereus, Bacillus subtilis Bordetella bronchiseptica, Mcoccus flavus, Proteus vulgaris*, and *Sarcina lutea*. At MIC 62.5 mg/ml the decoction was inactive on *Salmonella typhi*[T15296]. Essential oil of dried rhizome undiluted on agar plate was active on *Staphylococcus aureus*[W03527]. Decoction of dried rhizome produced weak activity on *Streptococcus mutans* on agar plate. MIC 62.5 mg/ml[M22285]. Ethanol (95%) extract at a concentration of 100.0 mg/disk and water extract of 20.0 mg/disk, on agar plate were inactive on *Bacillus subtilis, E. coli, Salmonella typhosa, Shigella dysenteriae* and *Staphylococcus aureus*. Dose expressed as dry weight of plant[P00004]. Ethanol (95%), and petroleum ether extracts of shade dried rhizomes, on agar plate were inactive on *Enterobacter cloacae, E. coli, Klebsiella pneumoniae, Proteus vulgaris, Pseudomonas aeruginosa, Serratia marcescens, Staphylococcus aureus* and *Streptococcus faecalis*. MIC >3.0 mg/ml[K19323]. Chloroform, and methanol extracts of dried roots on agar plate were active, on *Bacillus subtilis, Escherichia coli, Pseudomonas aeruginosa* and *Staphylococcus aureus*. The water extract was inactive[T10633]. Decoction of dried stem on agar plate was active on *Pseudomonas aeruginosa, Salmonella paratyphi, Shigella sonnei, Staphylococcus aureus, Vibrio parahemolyticus*, and *Yersinia enterolitica*. The decoction was inactive on *Bacillus subtilis, Escherichia coli, Klebsiella pneumonia* and *Proteus mirabilis*[M21419]. Chloroform and methanol extracts of dried stem on agar plate were

active on *Bacillus subtilis, E. coli, Pseudomonas aeruginosa, and Staphylococcus aureus*. The water extract was inactive[T10633]. Methanol extract of dried tuber at a concentration of 1.0% on agar plate was inactive on *Escherichia coli*. The extract produced weak activity on *Staphylococcus aureus*[T03389]. Water extract of fresh tuber at a concentration of 1.0% on agar plate was inactive on *Neisseria gonorrhea*[T10354].

Anticonvulsant activity. Ethanol (70%) extract of fresh roots at variable dosage levels administered intraperitoneally to both sexes of mice was active vs metrazole-induced and strychnine-induced convulsions[T06510].

Anticrustacean activity. Chloroform extract of dried root was active on *Artemia salina* larvae. LD_{50} 86.25 mg/ml. Water and methanol extracts were inactive with LD_{50} of 1.0 mg/ml for each. Assay system is intended to predict for antitumor activity[M25594].

Antidiarrheal activity. Ethanol/water (1:1) extract of dried roots at a concentration of 300.0 mg was inactive on guinea pig and rabbit ileum vs coliinte rotoxin-induced diarrhea[K17122].

Antiemetic activity. A commercial sample of roots administered by gastric intubation to pigeon at a dose of 80.0 mg/kg was active vs reserpine-induced emesis[M18896].

Antifungal activity. Rhizome, when tested on agar plate was active on *Colletotrichum chardonianum, Phytophthora capsici* and *Sclerotinia sclerotiorum*[A02761]. Water extract of fresh shoots, undiluted on agar plate was inactive on *Helminthosporium turcicum*[W01223].

Antihepatotoxic activity. Methanol extract of rhizome at a dose of 670.0 mg/kg administered to mouse orally was active in CCl_4-treated mice[T00325]. Methanol extract of dried rhizome at a dose of 670.0 mg/kg administered by gastric intubation to mouse showed strong activity vs CCl_4-induced hepatotoxicity[T10568]. Methanol extract of dried rhizome was active in rats. Activity was measured in terms of the elongation of hexobarbital sleeping time after CCl_4 treatment. Elongation of sleeping time indicated negative results vs CCl_4-induced hepatotoxicity[T09552]. Dried tuber when administered to mice was active. The duration of hexobarbital sleeping time was used as a measurement for this activity vs CCl_4-induced hepatotoxicity[T11767]. Ether extract of dried tuber at a dose of 300.0 mg/kg administered to mice by gastric intubation was inactive vs CCl_4-induced hepatotoxicity[T08733]. Water and methanol/water(1:1) extracts of dried rhizome administered intraperitoneally to mice were active vs CCl_4-induced hepatotoxicity[T02459,T03560].

Antihistamine activity. Ethanol/ water (1:1) extract of dried rhizome at a concentration of 0.001 gm/ml was active on guinea pig ileum[W3022A].

Antihypertensive activity. Dried roots at a dose of 2.0 gm/day taken by human adults was active. Sixty four patients were given this drug for two months. There was a significant reduction in weight. Blood pressure was lowered in hypertensive patients, but not in normotensive patients. Side effects were mild with some nausea initially, and appetite suppression in 12 subjects[T11229].

Anti-implantation effect. Ethanol/water (1:1) extract of dried rhizome at a dose of 100.0 mg/kg administered orally to female rats was inactive[T02678].

Anti-inflammatory activity. Chloroform extract of dried roots at a dose of 10.0 mg/kg administered intraperitoneally to rats, and water extract at a dose of 500.0 mg/kg administered by gastric intubation were active vs carrageenin-induced pedal edema[T08524]. Water extract at a dose of 2.0% by ophthalmic administration to human adults was active. Decreased redness and reduction in pain and ocular discharge in patients with conjunctivitis[T07439]. Methanol extract at a dose of 10.0 mg/kg, and 5.0 mg/kg administered intraperitoneally to rats was

active vs carrageenin-induced edema, and formalin-induced pedal edema respectively. Petroleum ether extract at a dose of 10.0 mg/kg intraperitoneally to rats was also active[A03170]. Water extract of rhizome was inactive in albumin stabilizing assay[A02047].

Antimalarial activity. Ethanol/water (50%) extract of dried aerial parts at a concentration of 100 mcg/ml was inactive on *Plasmodium berghei*. The extract was toxic at this dose. The extract when administered by gastric intubation to mouse at a dose of 1.0 gm/kg, was active on *Plasmodium berghei*. With daily dosing for four days, inhibition was 49%[M27524]. Chloroform extract of dried tuber was active on *Plasmodium falciparum*. IC_{50} 10.0 mg/ml vs hypoxanthine uptake by plasmodia[M25016]. Both methanol and petroleum ether extracts were inactive. IC_{50} 49.0 mg/ml was obtained for both extracts vs hypoxanthine uptake by plasmodia[M25016]. Hexane extract of dried tuber was active on *Plasmodium falciparum* ED_{50} 0.66 mcg/ml[H16648].

Antioxidant activity. Methanol extract of dried rhizome at a dose of 1.6 g/kg administered by gastric intubation to mouse was inactive vs ethanol-induced lipid peroxidation in mouse liver. Dose expressed as dry weight of plant[M20450].

Antipyretic activity. Ethanol (95%) extract of the entire plant (cultivated in Saudi Arabia) administered to mouse at a dose of 500.0 mg/kg by gastric intubation was active vs yeast-induced pyrexia[M21425]. Water extract of dried rhizome at a dose of 0.5 gm/kg administered by gastric intubation to rats was active. Effect was seen 4.5 hours after treatment vs yeast-induced pyrexia[M29225]. Methanol extract of dried roots at a dose of 5.0 mg/kg administered intraperitoneally to rats was active vs pyrexia induced by yeast injection[A03170].

Antiradiation activity. Methanol extract of dried rhizome at a dose of 1000 mg/kg administered intraperitoneally to mice was inactive vs soft X-ray irradiation at lethal dose[T14342].

Antiscleroderma activity. Hot water extract of dried rhizome taken by human adults of both sexes was active. Thirty cases of generalized scleroderma were treated. The results claimed to be satisfactory in 28/30 cases. The preparation contained *Codonopsis pilosula* (Root); *Astragalusi* (Root); *Cinnamomum cassia* (Bark); *Rehmannia glutinosa* (Root); *Paeonia rubra* (Root); *Carthamus tinctorius* (Flower); *Polygonum multiflorum*; *Millettia* species; *Salvia miltiorrhiza* (Root); *Cyperus rotundus* (Rhizome) and *Glycyrrhiza uralensis* (Root)[T02279].

Antispasmodic activity. Ethanol (95%) extract of dried rhizome, at a concentration of 200.0 mcg/ml was active on guinea pig ileum vs histamine-induced contractions and barium-induced contractions. Water extract was inactive vs barium-induced contractions, and showed weak activity vs histamine-induced contractions[T08047]. Ethanol/water (1:1) extract of dried rhizome at a concentration of 0.001 gm/ml was active on guinea pig ileum[W3022A]. Methanol extract of rhizome at a concentration of 1.0 mg/ml on rat ileum was active vs ACh-induced contractions[A04754].

Antitumor activity. Water extract of the dried rhizome at a concentration of 100.0 mg/ml was active on Sarcoma 180(ASC) in mice[M19777]. Hot water extract of dried seeds administered intravaginally to human adults was active. Lacryma-Jobi uterine mycoma was treated. In 52.9% of cases the symptoms completely disappear and in 27.2% the tumors were reduced in size. A mixture was employed that contained *Angelica sinensis*, *Curcuma zedoaria*, *Prunus persica*, *Dipsacus asper*, *Cyperus rotundus*, *Prunella vulgaris*, *Achyranthes bidentata*, *Vaccaria segetalis*, *Sparganium stoloniferum*, *Laminaria japonica* and *coix*[T04479]. Ethanol (defatted with petroleum ether) extract of dried tuber at a dose of 500.0 mg/kg administered to mice intraperitoneally was active on CA-Erlich-ascites, and inactive on LEUK-SN36 and Sarcoma 180(ASC)[T04688].

Antiviral activity. Decoction of dried entire plant taken orally by human adult was active. A patient with a typical chronic infectious hepatitis was treated with good results using a decoction of *Salvia miltiorrhiza*, *Isatis tinctoria*, *Taraxacum mongolicum*, *Paeonia lactiflora*, *Atractylodes macrocephala* and *Rehmannia glutinosa*[M20727]. Hot water extract of dried rhizome at a concentration of 0.5 mg/ml in cell culture was inactive on Herpes Simplex 1 virus, Measles virus, and Poliovirus 1[K16835].

Antiyeast activity. Ethanol (95%) extract of dried rhizome at a concentration of 100.0 mg/disk, and water extract at a concentration of 20.0 mg/disk on agar plate, were inactive on *Candida albicans*. Dose expressed as dry weight of plant[P00004]. Ethanol (95%) extract of dried rhizome on agar plate, was inactive on *Candida albicans*. MIC >3.0 mg/ml. The petroleum ether extract, however, was active. MIC 1.0 mg/ml[K19323].

Barbiturate potentiation. Methanol (75%) extract of rhizome at a concentration of 500.0 mg/kg administered intraperitoneally to mice was inactive[T01199]. Methanol extract of dried rhizome at a dose of 500.0 mg/kg administered intraperitoneally to mice was inactive. The extract did not affect barbiturate sleeping time[T10453]. Methanol extract of rhizome at a dose of 670.0 mg/kg administered orally to mice decreases the barbiturate sleeping time in CCl_4-treated mice[T00325]. Methanol (75%) extract at a dose of 500.0 mg/kg intraperitoneally did not decrease the barbiturate sleeping time[T01199]. Ether extract of dried tuber at a dose of 300.0 mg/kg administered by gastric intubation to mice did not decrease the barbiturate sleeping time[T08733].

Bradycardia activity. Water extract of rhizome was active on the heart of frog. The extract was also active when administered intravenously to cats and rabbits[A03685].

Cardiac depressant activity. Water extract of rhizome administered to frog subcutaneously was active[A03685].

Coagulant activity. Hexane extract of dried leaves and stem was inactive[M24874].

Coronary vasodilator activity. Water extract of rhizome administered intravenously to cats, rabbit, and frog was active[A03685].

Cytotoxic activity. Hot water extract of dried aerial parts at a dose of 500 mcg/ml in cell culture showed weak activity on CA-JTC-26. The inhibition rate was 69%[M27219]. Chloroform, water, and methanol extracts at concentrations of 100.0 mcg/ml in cell cultures were inactive on CA-A549[K23071]. Acetone extract of dried rhizome at concentrations of 5.0% by cylinder plate method was inactive on CA-Erlich-Ascites 10 mm inhibition. The ether and water extracts at concentrations of 5.0% were both inactive. 15 mm inhibition. Methanol extract at 5.0% concentration was equivocal. 25 mm inhibition[K23071]. Water extract of dried roots at a concentration of 500.0 mcg/ml in cell culture was inactive on human embryonic cells, HE-1. The extract produced weak activity on CA-Mammary-Microalveolar. Ethanol (defatted with petroleum ether) extract of dried tuber in cell culture on HELA cells had an ED_{50} of 32.0 mcg/ml[T04688].

Diuretic activity. Ethanol (95%) extract of roots administered orally to dogs increased urine output 12–60%. Chloride and urea concentrations were unchanged[A03021]. Water extract of rhizome administration intraperitoneally to rats was active[A03680]. Ethanol/water (1:1) extract of dried rhizome at a dose of 340.0 mg/kg administered orally to male rats was active[T02678].

Estrogenic effect. Essential oil of the root administered subcutaneously to female mice at variable dosage levels was active[W03518].

Fibrinolytic activity. Hexane extract of dried leaves and stem was inactive[M24874].

Gamma-glutamyl transpeptidase inhibition. Fermented dried tuber at a dose of 5.0 ml/day in the ration of rats was active. Rats were given the SKV Indian herbal formula daily for 3–4 months vs rats fed alcohol for six months[T16172].

Glutamate pyruvate transaminase inhibition. Ethanol/water (1:1) extract at a concentration of 1.0 mg/ml in cell culture on rat liver cells was active vs PGE-1-induced pedal edema, but inactive vs CCl_4-induced hepatotoxicity[T14999].

Growth inhibitor activity. Water extract at a dose of 0.5% in the drinking water of mice was inactive. Strain SLN x C3H/HE F_1 obese mice treated with extract in drinking water between ages three and 32 weeks showed no lessening of obesity or decrease in glucose tolerance[K07953].

Hair stimulant effect. Ethanol (95%) extract of dried tuber, at a concentration of 0.4 gm/animal applied externally on male mice, was inactive. Dose expressed as dry weight of plant[T06579].

Hematopoietic activity. Powdered dried plant administered to human adult at variable dosages was active. Patients also received another preparation containing *Panax ginseng, Cervus elaphuus, Chinemys reevesii, Cervus* species, and *Schisandra chinensis* concomitantly over three months[T12054].

Hypertensive activity. Water extract of dried fat at a dose of 1.5 mg/kg administered intravenously to rats was active. A vasopressor and then vasodepressor response occur following administration of extract. Hypotensive response is blocked by administration of propanolol and atropine but not by chlorisondamine, prazosin, and cyproheptadine. Extract used was composed of roots of *Angelica koreana, Peucedanum japonicum, Angelica gigas, Lindera strychnifolia, Angelica dahurica, Glycyrrhiza glabra,* and *Asiasarum* species. Also included were rhizomes of *Cnidium officinale, Pinellia ternata, Cyperus rotundus,* and *Zingiber officinale,* with branches of *Cinnamomum cassia,* fruit of *Pachyma hoelen,* and *Citrus aurantium* plants[M26285].

Hypocholesterolemic activity. Fermented dried tuber at a dose of 5.0 ml/day in the ration of rats was active. Rats were given the SKV Indian herbal formula for 3–4 months vs rats fed alcohol for six months[T16172].

Hypoglycemic activity. Water extract at a dose of 0.5% in the drinking water of mice was inactive. Strain SLN x C3H/HE F₁ obese mice treated with extract in drinking water between ages three and 32 weeks showed no lessening of obesity or decrease in glucose tolerance[K07953]. Fermented dried tuber at a dose of 5.0 ml/day in the ration of rats was active. Rats were given the SKV Indian herbal formula for 3–4 months vs rats alcohol for six months[T16172].

Hypotensive activity. Ethanol/water (1:1) extract of dried rhizome at variable dosage levels administered intravenously to dogs produced weak activity[W3022A]. Water extract of rhizome administered intravenously to cats was active[A03685].

Hypothermic activity. Methanol extract of dried roots at a dose of 5.0 mg/kg administered to mice intraperitoneally was active vs aconitine-induced writhing[A03170].

Inotropic effect (positive). Water extract of rhizome was active on frogs heart[A03685].

Insect repellent activity. The essential oil was active on *Bruchus chinensis*, and *Sitophilus oryzae*[T03533]. At a concentration of 0.24% the essential oil was active on *Stegobium paniceum*[T03533] At 0.78%, it was active on *Rhizopertha dominica*[T03533].

Juvenile hormone activity. The essential oil was active on *Dysdercus koenigii*[T04002].

Molluscicidal activity. Ethanol (95%), and petroleum ether extracts of dried roots at a concentration of 250.0 ppm were inactive on *Biomphalaria pfeifferi* and *Bulinus truncatus*[T07986].

Molting activity (insect). The essential oil was active on *Dysdercus koenigii*[T04002].

Mutagenic activity. Water, and methanol extracts of commercial sample of rhizome at concentrations of 100.0 mg/ml on agar plate were inactive on *Bacillus subtilis*

H-17(Rec+), and *Salmonella typhimurium* TA100 and TA98. Metabolic activation had no effect on the results[A07240].

Plant germination inhibition. Protoplasts was active[A02750].

Plant growth inhibitor. Essential oil of roots at a concentration of 400.0 ppm, inhibited the germination and hypocotyl elongation of lettuce and white clover[T03535]. Water extract of tuber was active on white clover, *Digitaria sanguinalis* and *rumex*[A02820,T05602].

Plasma protein concentration. Fermented dried tuber at a dose of 5.0 ml/day in the ration of rats increased the plasma protein concentration. Rats were fed the SKV Indian herbal formula for 3–4 months vs rats fed alcohol for six months[T16172].

Platelet activating factor binding inhibition. Hot water extract at a concentration of 10.0 mg/ml was equivocal on rabbit platelets. 15% inhibition[K22944].

Platelet aggregation stimulation. Hexane extract of dried leaves and stem was inactive[M24874].

Prostaglandin inhibition. Chloroform and hot water extracts of dried rhizome produced strongly active and active inhibition respectively[P00126].

Prostaglandin synthetase inhibition. Hot water extract of commercial sample of rhizome at a concentration of 750.0 mg/ml was active on rabbit microsomes. Hot water extract of dried rhizome at a concentration of 750.0 mg/ml was active on rabbit microsomes[T08539].

Smooth muscle relaxant activity. Methanol extract of rhizome at a concentration of 1.0 mg/ml was inactive on rat ileum. The extract smooth muscle stimulant activity was also inactive on rat ileum. However, uterine relaxation effect on rat uterus was strongly active vs oxytocin-induced contractions. No uterine stimulant effect was shown on rat uterus[K04754].

Toxic effect (general). Ethanol/water (1:1) extract of dried rhizome at a dose of 10.0

g/kg administered to mice by gastric intubation and subcutaneously were inactive. Dose expressed as dry weight of plant[W3022A].

Toxicity assessment (quantitative). Ethanol (95%) extract of roots administered intraperitoneally to mice produced a LD_{50} of 90.0 gm/kg[A03021]. Ethanol (defatted with petroleum ether) extract of dried tuber administered intraperitoneally to mice produced a LD_{50} >0.5 gm/kg[T04688]. Ethanol/water (1:1) extract of dried rhizome when administered intraperitoneally to both sexes of mouse the LD_{50} was 681.0 mg/kg[T02678].

Uric acid decrease. Fermented dried tuber at a dose of 5.0 ml/day in the ration of rats was active. Rats were fed the SKV Indian herbal formula for 3–4 months vs rats fed alcohol for six months[T16172].

Weight Loss. Dried root taken by human adults orally at a dose of 2.0 g/day was active. Sixty-four obese patients were given this drug twice daily for two months. There was a significant reduction in weight. Blood pressure was lowered in hypertensive patients, but not in normotensive patients. Side effects were mild with some nausea initially, and appetite suppression in 12 subjects[T11229].

11 | Curcuma longa
L.

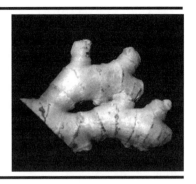

Common Names

Acafrao	Brazil	Pasupu	India
Ango	Brazil	Rajani	India
Ango hina	Brazil	Rame	Indonesia
Asabi-e-safr	Arabic Countries	Renga	Cook Islands
Avea	Arabic Countries	Rerega	Cook Islands
Besar	Nepal	Saffran vert	Mauritius
Cago	Nepal	Safran	Mauritius
Curcuma	Nepal	Safran	Rodrigues Islands
Curcuma	Iran	Tale'a	Rodrigues Islands
Dilau	India	Temoe lawak	Rodrigues Islands
Dilaw	Philippines	Temu kunyit	Malaysia
Goeratji	Indonesia	Temu-lawak	Indonesia
Haldi	Fiji	Tumeric	Japan
Haldi	India	Tumeric	Nepal
Haledo	Nepal	Tumeric	Thailand
Halodhi	India	Turmeric	Thailand
Hardi	Fiji	Turmeric	Brazil
Haridra	Malaysia	Turmeric	India
Huang chiang	Malaysia	Turmeric	Iran
Javanese turmeric	Indonesia	Turmeric	Japan
Kakoenji	Indonesia	Turmeric	Malaysia
Kalo haledo	Nepal	Turmeric	Marquesas Islands
Kerqum	Morocco	Turmeric	Mauritius
Khamin chan	Thailand	Turmeric	Nepal
Kiko eka	Marquesas Islands	Turmeric	Sri Lanka
Koening	Indonesia	Turmeric	Taiwan
Koenir	Indonesia	Turmeric	USA
Koenjet	Indonesia	Ukon	India
Kondin	Indonesia	Ukon	Japan
Kurcum	Oman	Ukon	Taiwan
Mena	Rotuma	Ul Gum	South Korea
Nghe	Vietnam	Warse	Oman
Nisha	India	Wong keong	Malaysia
Oendre	Indonesia	Wong keung	Malaysia
		Zardchoobeh	Iran

From: Medicinal Plants of the World *By: Ivan A. Ross Humana Press Inc., Totowa, NJ*

BOTANICAL DESCRIPTION

A stemless rhizomatous herb of the ZINGIBERACEAE family; with fleshy rhizome, branched, with bright orange to yellow within. Leaves are large, elongated and borne at the top of the non-woody underground stem, with overlapping petioles. Leaves are light green, 30–40 cm long and 8–12 cm wide with thin ellipse-shaped or elongate lance-shaped blades. The pale yellow cylindrical inflorescence 10–15 by 6–8 cm develops in the center of the leaves. It consists of curved bracts, each with at least two yellow flowers, except in the upper part, where the bracts are white or pink. A stamen with short filament, broad and constricted at the apex is found in the floret. The anther is versatile and usually spurred at the base. The ovaries consists of three-locules each containing two ovules. The capsules are ellipsoid. Seeds are rare.

ORIGIN AND DISTRIBUTION

Native to India but is cultivated in the tropics.

TRADITIONAL MEDICINAL USES

Arabic countries. Hot water extract of dried rhizome is taken orally and in the form of a pessary in Unani medicine as an abortifacient[T06813].

Brazil. Dried rhizome is used to protect against snakebite[K08492].

China. Hot water extract of dried tuber is taken orally in traditional medicine to improve circulation and to dissolve blood clots[T07146]. Oils of dried fruit together with oils of *Zingiber officinale*, *Saussurea lappa*, *Sansevieria roxburghiana*, and *Rubia cordifolia* are mixed with salt, buttermilk, and rice and massaged onto patient during fever. The mixture is also taken orally for cough. Essential oil of dried fruit is taken orally to bring unconscious patients to consciousness. mixed with honey and leaf of "patola"[T14489].

Cook Islands. Decoction of dried rhizome is taken orally for urinary tract ailments.

Skin of *Pandanus tectorius* fruit, combined with *Ocimum basilicum* leaves or grated rhizome of *Curcuma longa*, is boiled and then taken. Grated rhizome is used externally to treat septic puncture wounds[T09553]. Three dried roots covered by a leaf of *Syzygium malaccensis* is crushed and squeezed into the water of six green coconuts, the solution is taken orally daily for three days. Urinary infection is treated by drinking a mixture of two dried roots with 12 leaves and a piece of bark of *Syzygium malaccencse* squeezed into the juice of coconut. After three days of treatment of purge is taken with coconut or castor oil[K20471].

England. Dried rhizome, together with *Curcuma aromatica*, licorice, sulfur and ferrous sulfate is taken orally for amenorrhea[W03029].

Fiji. Poultice of dried rhizome and boiled rice is applied to boils to bring to a head, it is applied externally to aid healing of sprains, bruises and open wounds, and ophthalmic for eye diseases[T10632].

Haiti. Extract of dried rhizome is taken to treat liver complaints[K23019].

Hawaii. Water extract of the bulb is taken orally for asthma[K18991]. Hot water extract of dried entire plant is taken orally for renal or urinary calculi[T13960].

India. Fresh rhizome, ground with cow milk and castor oil is applied externally to treat paronychia[K11282]. To prevent stomach disorders, three to five ml of fresh juice is taken regularly on an empty stomach[T09230]. Hot water extract of dried rhizome is taken orally for slow lactation[A00041], to regulate fat metabolism[A05171], for diabetes[A14379], as a tonic, carminative, for diarrhea, dropsy, jaundice, and liver diseases[T09230]. Externally, the dried rhizome is used on fresh wounds, as a counter-irritant on insect stings, to facilitate the scabbing process in chickenpox and smallpox. The dried rhizome is taken orally as an anthelmintic, for urinary diseases, for liver diseases and jaundice, and as a cancer remedy[H01195]. Dried rhizome mixed with latex of *Carthamus tinctorius* is taken orally for tonsilitis[K11282]. Dried rhizome powder mixed with the juice of *Aloe vera* is used externally to treat wounds. The powder mixed with *Murraya paniculata* paste is used externally for fractured bones. Powder mixed with *Helicteres isora* and tumeric powder is used externally for cuts and wounds[M27166]. Hot water extract of powder is taken orally as a tonic[T03115]. *Curcuma longa* rhizome and *Calotropis procera* root is kept together for 20 days, ground up and a pinch is taken in the morning with milk cream for three days to obtain relief from headache[T06479]. *Curcuma longa* rhizome and leaves of *Aristolochia indica* leaves are made into a paste and applied to the forehead, two applications per day heals headache quickly[T07823]. A paste of rhizome and leaves of *Zornia diphylla* is applied to dislocated limb joints for relief. A paste of *Ocimum sanctum* leaf and *Curcuma longa* rhizome is applied externally to snakebite and other bites or stings. *Aristolochia indica* root grounded with *Curcuma longa* rhizome is applied externally to snakebite and skin diseases[T08282]. *Datura stramonium* and *Curcuma longa* rhizome are made into a paste and used externally for pimples. For sprains, *Cissampelos pareira* roots and *Curcuma longa* rhizome are made into a paste and applied on the affected location[T09390]. One handful of *Leucas linifolia* plants, 50 grams of *Brassica campestris* seed, and one average *Curcuma longa* rhizome are ground into a paste and applied to the forehead daily at sunrise for seven days for migraine[T10321]. Root ground with *Oroxylum indicum* stem bark, is made into pills. Five grams are taken twice a day for 10 days for jaundice[T13856]. Rhizome is used externally as an insect repellant[W03417]. Hot water extract of rhizome is taken orally as an emmenagogue[A00115], and externally[K25892] and orally[A04132] as an antivenin. Water extract of dried root mixed with *Alangium salvifolium* powder is used externally for wounds and vaginal discharge[M27166]. Hot water extract of dried root is taken orally as an anti-inflammatory agent in Ayurvedic medicine[T09366].

Indonesia. Hot water extract of rhizome is taken orally and by female adults to promote menses[A00682]. Tuber is taken orally as a laxative after menses, leukorrhea of postpartum recovery. Tuber is used externally for scabies. Water extract of tuber mixed with *Acorus calamus* and vinegar is taken orally for postpartum recovery. Tuber ground with water is used externally for swellings and rheumatism[T06756].

Iran. Powder of dried rhizome is taken orally as a digestant and as an antiflatulant[I00004].

Japan. Hot water extract of dried rhizome is taken orally as an aromatic stomachic, diuretic, and for jaundice and menstrual pain in Oriental medicine[N19806]. In Chinese medicine it is used to inhibit blood coagulation (Oketsu)[T09546]. Hot water extract of fresh rhizome is taken orally as a cholagogue[M20141].

Malaysia. Dried rhizome mixed with camphor in a paste form is worn externally as an abortifacient[A03602]. Hot water extract of the dried rhizome is taken orally for amenorrhea[A04361].

Marquesas Island. Root mixed with other plants is burnt and the vagina exposed to the smoke to treat prolonged menstruation[A03442]. Decoction of dried root is taken orally for hepatitis and liver troubles[T13846].

Mauritius. Hot water extract of dried root is taken orally for three days as an emmenagogue[T02146]. Hot water extract of rhizome is used as an emmenagogue[A05825].

Nepal. Hot water extract of dried rhizome is used externally for skin diseases[T01728]. Hot water extract of rhizome is taken orally as an anthelmintic[K25257]. Dried rhizome is used as for fistula. Surgical thread is dipped in solution of ash of *Achyranthes aspera*, then in latex of *Euphorbia antiquorum*, and then coated with powder of *Curcuma longa*.

Thread is pierced through the fistula and healing occurs[H05351].

Philippines. Decoction of fresh root is taken orally to treat fever in infants and to treat bleeding during pregnancy. Fresh root juice is taken orally to decrease the pain of early labor[T10116].

South Korea. Hot water extract of dried rhizome is taken orally as a contraceptive, abortifacient, emmenagogue[T10290] and to induce menstruation[W00346].

Taiwan. Hot water extract of dried rhizome is taken orally as a diuretic, an aromatic stomachic and for jaundice[H06015].

USA. Dried rhizome in a proprietary product called "pseudo hard-on pills" contains *Albus simila* (25%), *Curcuma longa* (50%) and *Purus saccharum* and *Zingiber officinale* (10%) is taken orally as an aphrodisiac[T00337].

Vietnam. Hot water extract of dried rhizome is taken orally as a drug in traditional medicine. Listed in the Vietnamese pharmacopeia (1974 edition)[T05058].

CHEMICAL CONSTITUENTS

(ppm unless otherwise indicated)

2-Hydroxy-methyly anthraquinone, Rh
4-Hydroxy bisabola-2-10-dien-9-one, Rh 5.1
4-Hydroxy cinnamoyl-(feruloyl)-methane, Rh 180
4-Hydroxy-cinnamoyl methane, Rh
4-Hydroxy-feruloxyl methane, Rh
4-Methoxy bisabola-3-10-dien-2-one, Rh 13.5
5-Hydroxy bisabola-2-10-dien-9-one, Rh 0.3
5-Hydroxy procurcumenol, Rh 0.6
5'-Methoxy curcumin, Rh 20
Alpha atlantone, Rt
Alpha curcumene, Rh
Alpha phellandrene, Rh EO; Rt Call
Alpha pinene, Tu; Rh EO 0.53%
Alpha turmerine, Rh 3.7%
Alpha turmerone, Rh
Beta bisabolene, Rh
Beta pinene, Tu; Rh EO 0.27%
Beta sesquiphellandrene, Rh
Beta sitosterol, Rh
Beta turmerone, Rh
Bis-(4-hydroxy-cinnamoyl), Rh

Bis-(para-hydroxy-cinnamoyl) methane, Rh 0.136%
Bis-demethoxy curcumin, Rh 6.6-7500; Pl; Tu; Rt 400
Bisabola-3-10-diene,2-5-dihydroxy, Rh 3.2
Bisabolene, Rt
Bisacumol, Rh 2.1
Borneol, Rh
Caffeic acid, Rh 5
Campesterol, Rh
Camphene, Tu
Camphor, Rh 60
Caryophylene, Tu, Rh
Cholesterol, Rh
Cineol, Rh 2.92%
Curcumene, Tu
Curcumenol, Rh 64.5; Rh EO 2.13%
Curcumenone, Rh 26.3
Curcumin, Rh
Curdione, Tu
Curlone, Rh 120
Curzerenone C, Rh EO 2.04%
Curzerenone, Tu
Cyclocurcumin, Rh 13.3
Dehydro curdione, Rh 4.5
Demethoxy curcumin, Rh; Rt; Pl
Di-feruloyl methane, Rh
Di-para-coumaroyl methane, Rh
Epi-procurcumenol, Rh 1.3
Eugenol, Rh EO 0.21%
Feruloyl-para-coumaroyl methane, Rh
Gamma atlantone, Rt
Germacron-(4S',5S)-epoxide, Rh 0.7
Germacron-13-al, Rh 0.6
Germacrone, Rh
Germacrone,4(S)-5(S)-epoxy, Rh
Guaiacol, Rh
Hepta-1-4-6-triene-3-one,1-7-bis-(4 benzenoid-hydroxy-phenyl), Rh 2.6
Hepta-1-6-diene-3-5-dione,1-(4-hydroxy-3-methoxy-phenyl)-7-(3-4-dihydroxy-phenyl), Rh 3.9
Iso-borneol, Rh 0.2%
Iso-procurcumenol, Rh 1.6
Limonene, Rh EO 0.23%; Tu
Linalool, Rh EO 0.16%; Tu
Mono-demethoxy curcumin, Rh
Ortho coumaric acid, Lf
Para coumaric acid, 345
Para cymene, Rh
Para-hydroxy-cinnamoyl feruloyl methane, Rh
Para-tolyl-methyl-carbinol, Rh

Penta-trans-1-trans-4-dien-3-one,1-5-bis-(4-hydroxy-3-methoxy-phenyl), Rh 26.6
Penta-trans-4-dien-3-one,1(4-hydroxy-3-methoxy-phenyl)-5-(4-hydroxy-phenyl), Rh 13.3
Procurcumenol, Rh 0.1
Protocatechuic acid, Lf
Sabinene, Rh EO; Rt
Saturated fatty acids, Rh
Stigmasterol, Rh
Syringic acid, Lf
Terpinene, Tu; Rh EO 2.72%
Terpineol, Rh EO 0.05%
Tolyl-methyl-carbinol, Rh
Turmerin, Tu
Turmerone AR, Rh
Turmerone, Rt; Rh EO 27.07%
Turmeronol A, Rh 282
Turmeronol B, Rh 192.8
Ukonan A, Rh 33-6600
Ukonan B, Rh 47
Ukonan C, Rh 52-315
Ukonan D, Rh 40.8
Unsaturated fatty acids, Rh
Vanillic acid, Lf
Zedoarondiol, Rh 35
Zingiberene, Rh EO 8.14%; Rt

PHARMACOLOGICAL ACTIVITIES AND CLINICAL TRIALS

Abortifacient effect. Hot water extract of dried root taken orally by pregnant human was inactive. A mixture of the following was given in the form of a decoction to a number of pregnant women. No toxic effects were noted. Dosing was three times daily for three days. The mixture contained *Angelica sinensis* (root), *Ligusticum wallichii* (root), *Prunus persica* (seed), *Carthamus tinctorius* (flowers), *Paeonia obvata* (root), *Achyranthes bidentata* (root), *Leonurus sibiricus* (aerial parts), *Lycopus lucidus* var. Hirta (leaf) and *Curcuma longa* (root), and *Campsis grandiflora* (flowers)[W02856].

Adrenal hypertrophy effect. Water extract of dried rhizome together with a mixture of *Levisticum officinale*, *Artemisia cappilaris* and *Chrysanthemum indicum* was active when administered to mice[K09096].

Alkaline phosphatase inhibition. Water extract of of fresh rhizome administered intragastric to ducklings at a concentration of 50.0 mg/day was active vs aflatoxin B-1 hepatotoxicity. Enzyme was measured in the serum[K15267].

Alkaline phosphatase stimulation. Methanol extract of dried rhizome administered intraperitoneally to rats at a dose of 100.0 mg/kg was active vs alpha naphthyl-isothiocyanate-induced hepatotoxicity[M27764].

Allergenic activity. Commercial sample of rhizome powder wsa active on human adults. Reaction to patch tests occurred most commonly in patients who were regularly exposed to the substance, or who already had dermatitis on the fingertips. Previously unexposed patients had few reactions (i.e., not irritant reactions)[M17058].

Antiamebic activity. Ethanol/water (1:1) extract of of rhizome at a concentration of 125.0 mcg/ml in broth culture was active on *Endameba histolytica*[A03335].

Antiasthmatic activity. Dried rhizome taken orally by human adults at a dose of 250.0 mg/person was active. Administration to 26 (11 male and 15 female) patients with bronchial asthma, once daily for three weeks. No side effects were observed. The preparation also contained *Glycyrrhiza glabra*[T03554]. A dose of 6–12 gm/person daily for 15–20 days was active. One hundred seven patients with "tamak swasa vatapradhan" (chronic bronchitis or asthma) ages 31–50 had fair to good response[T03115].

Antibacterial activity. Chloroform ethanol (95%) water and petroleum ether extracts of dried rhizome at a concentration of 250.0 mg/ml on agar plate were active on *Bacillus subtilis*, *Escherichia coli*, *Pseudomonas aeruginosa* and *Staphylococcus aureus*[K19538]. Ethanol (95%) extract at a concentration of 10.0 mg/ml was inactive on *Corynebacterium diptheriae*, *Diplococcus pneumoniae*, *Staphylococcus aureus*, *Streptococcus viridans*, and

Streptococcus pyogenes[M29966]. Water extract at a concentration of 10.0 mg/ml was inactive on *Corynebacterium diptheriae* and *Diplococcus pneumoniae*, and produced weak activity on *Staphylococcus aureus, Streptococcus viridans,* and *Streptococcus pyogenes*[M29966]. Essential oil of rhizome, on agar plate was inactive on *Bacillus cereus, Escherichia coli, Pseudomonas aeruginosa,* and *Staphylococcus aureus*[T14976]. Ethanol (95%) extract of rhizome in broth culture was active on *Lactobacillus acidophilus* and *Staphylococcus aureus*; equivocal on *Escherichia coli* and inactive on *Salmonella typhosa*[A03335]. Undiluted essential oil on agar plate was inactive on *Bacillus cereus, Escherichia coli, Pseudomonas aeruginosa,* and *Staphylococcus aureus*[T06640]. Water and hot water extracts of dried rhizome, on agar plate at a concentration of 0.5 ml/disc was inactive on *Bacillus subtilis* H-17(REC+) and H-17(REC-). Rhizome on agar plate at variable concentrations was active on *Bacillus subtilis* H-17(REC+)[T07988].

Anticoagulant activity. Chromatographic fraction of dried rhizome administered intraperitoneally to mice at a dose of 0.08 gm/kg was active. Results significant at P < 0.05 level. Ethyl acetate extract of dried rhizome administered intraperitoneally to mice at a dose of 0.1 gm/kg produced strong activity. Results significant at P < 0.01 level. The water extract at a dose of 0.1 gm/kg was equivocal[T09546].

Anticomplement activity. Polysaccharide fraction of dried rhizome administered intraperitoneally to guinea pigs at a dose of 100.0 mg/kg as active[T12554].

Anticonvulsant activity. Ethanol/water (1:1) extract of rhizome administered intraperitoneally to mice at a dose of 250.0 mg/kg was inactive vs electroshock[A03335].

Anticrustacean activity. Ethanol (95%) extract of dried rhizome was inactive on *Artemia salina.* The assay system was intended to predict for antitumor activity[K08041].

Antiedema activity. Methanol extract of dried rhizome administered to mice at a dose 2.0 mg/ear was active vs 12-0-tetradecanoylphorbol-13-acetate(TPA)-induced ear inflammation. Inhibition ratio (IR) was 71[T09546].

Antifungal activity. Chloroform, and ethanol (95%) extracts of dried rhizome, on agar plate were active and water extract produced weak activity on *Epidermophyton floccosum, Microsporum gypseum* and *Trichophyton rubrum*[P00083]. Essential oil of dried rhizome on agar plate at a concentration of 1:100 was active on *Trichoderma viride, Aspergillus flavus, Microsporum gypseum,* and *Trichophyton mentagrophytes*[T06638]. Water extract of dried rhizome at a concentration of 10.0 mg/ml on agar plate was inactive on *Microsporum canis, Microsporum gypseum, Phialophora jeanselmei,* and *Piedraia hortae* and weakly active on *Trichophyton mentagrophytes*[M29966]. Essential oil of dried rhizome on agar plate at a concentration of 1:100 was active on *Curvularia oryzae, Helminthosporum oryzae, Penicillum corymbiferum, Penicillum javanicum,* and *Penicillum lilacinum*[T06638]. Essential oil on agar plate was equivocal on *Aspergillus aegypticus*; active on *Trichoderma viride* and inactive on *Penicillium cyclopium*[T14976]. A concentration of 3000 ppm on agar plate was active on *Aspergillus niger*[K16266]. Undiluted essential oil on agar plate was inactive on *Penicillium cyclopium, Trichoderma viride* and *Aspergillus aegyptiacus*[T06640]. Fresh leaf essential oil at a concentration of 5000 ppm on agar plate produced weak activity on *Aspergillus flavus*[T16185].

Antihepatotoxic activity. Ethanol/water (1:1) extract of dried rhizome in rat-liver cell culture, and when administered intraperitoneally to mice was active vs carbon tetrachloride-induced hepatotoxicity[N19806]. Methanol extract administered intraperitoneally to mice at a dose of 100.0 mg/kg produced weak activity vs carbon tetrachloride hepatotoxicity[K18804]. Hot water extract of dried rhizome in cell culture at a concentration of 1.0 mg/plate was active on hepatocytes, measured by leakage of LDH and ASAT[K23019]. Methanol extract of dried rhizome administered intraperitoneally to rats of both sexes, at a dose of 300.0 mg/kg, produced weak activity vs alpha-naphthyl-isothiocyanate-induced hepatotoxicity. Methanol extract administered subcutaneously to rats of both sexes, at a dose of 100.0 mg/kg was inactive vs carbon tetrachloride-induced hepatotoxicity[T16952]. Methanol-insoluble fraction of dried rhizome administered intragastric to ducklings at a dose of 10.0 mg/animal was active vs aflatoxin B1-induced hepatotoxicity. Mixture of tumeric, fresh garlic, asafoetida, curcumin, ellagic acid, and butylated hydroxy toluene and butylated hydroxy anisole were used[K17144].

Antihypercholesterolemic activity. Ethanol/water (1:1) extract of dried rhizome administered intragastric to rats at a dose of 30.0 mg/gm (dry weight of plant), every six hours for 48 hours, was active vs triton-induced hypercholesterolemia[M21237]. Ether and ethanol (95%) extracts of rhizome, administered by gastric intubation to rabbit at a dose of 1.0 gm/animal were inactive vs cholesterol-loaded animals[W03093].

Antihyperglyceridemia effect. Ethanol/water (1:1) extract of dried rhizome administered intragastric to rats at a dose of 30.0 mg/gm (dry weight of plant), every six hours for 48 hours, was active vs triton-induced hypercholesterolemia[M21237].

Antihyperlipemic activity. Ethanol/water (1:1) extract of dried rhizome administered intragastric to rats at a dose of 30.0 mg/gm (dry weight of plant), every six hours for 48 hours, was active vs triton-induced hypercholesterolemia[M21237]. Ether and ethanol (95%) extracts of rhizome, administered by gastric intubation to rabbits at a dose of 1.0 gm/animal were inactive vs cholesterol-loaded animals[W03093].

Anti-implantation effect. Ethanol (95%) extract of dried rhizome administered orally to rats at a dose of 100.0 mg/kg was active. A 60.0% reduction in pregnancies (4/10) was observed. A dose of 200.0 mg/kg produced a 70.0% reduction. The petroleum ether and water extracts at a dose of 100.0 mg/kg produced 80.0% reduction and a dose 200.0 mg/kg a 100.0% reduction[J08548].

Anti-inflammatory activity. Ethanol (95%) extract of dried rhizome administered intraperitoneally to male rats at a dose of 100.0 mg/kg was active vs granuloma pouch model. Doses 200.0, 400.0, and 800.0 mg/kg were active vs carrageenin-induced pedal edema. A dose of 50.0 mg/kg was inactive vs granuloma pouch model. Water extract at doses of 5, 10, 20, 40, and 80 mg/kg were active vs carrageenin-induced rat pedal edema. A dose of 10.0 mg/kg was inactive vs granuloma pouch model, a dose of 20.0 mg/kg was active. Petroleum ether extract at a dose of 12.5 mg/kg was inactive vs granuloma pouch model, 25.0 mg/kg was active vs granuloma pouch model but inactive vs carrageenin-induced rat pedal edema. A dose of 50.0 mg/kg was active vs carrageenin-induced rat pedal edema[K01337]. Rhizome taken orally by human adults at a dose of 50.0 mg/person was active. The clinical efficacy of a herbomineral formulation containing roots of *Withania sonifera*, the stems of *Boswellia serrata*, rhizomes of *Curcuma longa* and a zinc complex (Articulin-F) was evaluated in a randomized, double-blind placebo-controlled, cross-over study in patients with osteoarthritis. After one month single blind run-in period, 42 patients with osteoarthritis were randomly allocated to receive either a drug treatment or a matching placebo for a period of three months. After a 15-day wash-out period the patients were transferred to the other treatment for a further period of three months. Clinical efficacy was evaluated every two weeks on the basis of severity of pain, morning stiffness, ritchie articular index, joint score, disability score, and grip strength. Other parameters like erythrocyte sedimentation rate and radiological examination were carried out on a monthly basis. Treatment with the herbomineral formation produced a significant drop in severity of pain and disability score. Radiological assessment, however, did not show any significant changes in both the groups. Side effects observed with this formulation did not necesitate withdrawal of treatment[M28176]. Polysaccharide fraction of dried rhizome administered intraperitoneally to rats at a dose of 100.0 mg/kg was active vs adjuvant-induced arthritis. Results significant at P < 0.01 level[T12554]. Root essential oil, administered orally to rats at a dose of 0.1 ml/kg was active vs carageenin-induced pedal edema[A05570].

Anti-ischemic effect. Rhizome administered intragastric to rats at a dose of 5.0 gm/kg was active on the heart. The dose also contained nicotinic acid. The dose was given daily for seven days during the last two of which isoproterenol was also given. Isoproterenol-induced ischemic effects on the heart were prevented[M26052].

Antimutagenic activity. Hot water extract of dried rhizome on agar plate at concentrations of 40.0 mg/plate and at the minimum toxic dose were inactive on *Salmonella typhimurium* TA100, vs aflatoxin-B1-induced mutagenesis. Metabolic activation had no effect on the results. Dried rhizome extract (type of extract not stated) on agar plate at a concentration of 50.0 mg/ml was inactive on *Salmonella typhimurium* TA1535 vs aflatoxin- and mitomycin-induced mutagenesis[M29342]. Water extract of rhizome at a concentration of 0.33 mg/ml was active on rat-liver-microsomes. The formation of labeled benzo[a]pyrene-DNA adducts was inhibited[K23394]. Infusion at a concentration of 25.0 mcg/plate on agar plate was active on *Salmonella typhimurium* TA100. 1-methyl-3-

nitro-1-nitrosoguanidine-induced mutagenesis was inhibited by 25%. There was a 38% inhibition of 4-nitro-D-phenylenediamine-induced mutagenesis of *Salmonella typhimurium* TA98. Infusion of rhizome administered intragastric to mice at a dose of 3.0 mg/animal was active. The incidence of benzo[a]pyrene-induced forestomach tumors was reduced by 53% by pretreatment with the extract. Intraperitoneal administration of the infusion was active. The formation of benzo[a]pyrene-induced bone marrow micronucleated cells was decreased 40% by pretreatment with the extract[K07408]. Powdered rhizome at a concentration of 0.033 mg/ml was active on rat-liver-microsomes. Formation of labeled benzo-[a]pyrene-DNA adducts was inhibited[K23394]. Powdered rhizome administered intragastric to rats at a dose of 0.5% of the diet was active. Animals fed the diet for one month before being given 3-methylcholanthrene intraperitoneally, produced urine with reduced mutagenicity on *Salmonella typhimurium* Strains TA100 and TA98, with or without activation with S9, as assessed by Ames test[T16608].

Antimycobacterial activity. Ethanol (95%) extract of entire plant in broth culture was active on *Mycobacterium tuberculosis* H37RVTMC 102. The extract was used in a dilution of 1:80[M27150]. Leaf juice on agar plate produced weak activity on *Mycobacterium tuberculosis* MIC <1:40[A03634].

Antinematodal activity. Water extract of rhizome at a concentration of 10.0 mg/ml produced weak activity and methanol extract at a concentration of 1.0 mg/ml was active on *Toxacara canis*[M29965].

Antioxidant activity. Hexane and methanol extracts of rhizome at concentrations of 0.1% were active[T09888]. Hexane extract of dried rhizome at a concentration of 0.06% was inactive when tested on lard. The methanol extract was active[T08288]. Hot water extract of a commercial sample of tuber, at a concentration of 100.0 ng/mcl was active vs protection of DNA against peroxidative injury[M19431]. Water extract of rhizome was active on rat brain vs Fe^{2+}/ascorbate-Fe^{2+}/TBH-induced lipid peroxidation. The biological activity was highly dose-dependent, IC_{50} 100.0 mcg/ml. The extract was also active vs Lipid peroxidation induced by TBARS, IC_{50} 50.0 mcg/ml[K21634].

Antispasmodic activity. Ethanol/water (1:1) extract of rhizome was active on the ileum of guinea pigs[A03335].

Antispermatogenic effect. Root in the ration of male mice at a concentration of 0.5% and to male rats at a concentration of 0.15% of the diet was inactive[W03048].

Antitumor activity. Ethanol (95%) extract administered intraperitoneally to mice at a dose of 100.0 mg/kg was inactive on Sarcoma 180(ASC), the water extract was active[M23643]. Hot water extract of dried root administered intraperitoneally to mice at variable dosage levels was active on CA-Ehrlich-Ascites. A mixture of *Bufo bufo*, *Solanum nigrum*, *Solanum lyratum*, *Duchesnea indica*, *Angelica sinensis*, *Curcuma longa*, and *Salvia miltiorrhiza* was used[T07449]. Methanol extract of dried rhizome administered intraperitoneally to mice at a dose of 0.03 gm/kg was inactive on LEUK-SN36. A dose of 0.1 gm/kg was active[T04205]. Polysaccharide fraction of dried rhizome administered intraperitoneally to mice at a dose of 100.0 mg/kg was active on Sarcoma 180 (solid)[T12554]. Water and methanol extracts administered intraperitoneally to mice at doses of 150.0 mg/kg on days 5, 6, and 7 were inactive on CA-Ehrlich-Ascites[H01040]. Water extract of dried rhizome administered to mice at a dose of 100.0 mg/kg was active on Sarcoma (ASC)[M19777].

Antiulcer activity. Ethanol (95%) extract of dried rhizome administered intragastric to rats at a dose of 500.0 mg/kg was active vs hydrochloric acid- sodium chloride-, sodium hydroxide-, hypothermic-resistant stress-, ethanol-, pylorus ligation-, indomethacin-, reserpine-, and cysteamine-induced ulcers[M23497]. Powdered dried rhizome taken orally by human adults of both sexes, at a dose of 250.0 mg/day produced weak activity. In a clinical study in Thailand with sixty patients, the control group received an antacid. The treatment was given before meals and at bedtime, for two weeks[K18790].

Antiviral activity. Hot water extract of dried rhizome in cell culture was active on vesicular stomatitis virus. The prescription included 10 gm each of *Curcuma longa* rhizome, *Rheum officinale* root, *Cimicifuga foetida* rhizome, *Anemarrhena asaphodeloides* rhizome, *Areca catechu* seed, *Magnolia officinalis* bark, and *Scutellaria baicalensis* root, also included are 5 gm *Amomum tsaoko* fruit, together with insects *Bombyx mori* and *Cryptotympana pustulata*[M25607]. Water extract of dried rhizome in cell culture at a concentration of 10.0% was inactive on Herpes virus Type 2, Influenza virus A2(Manheim 57), Poliovirus ll and Vaccinia virus[T09507].

Antiyeast activity. Chloroform, ethanol (95%), and water extracts of dried rhizome, on agar plate were inactive on *Candida albicans*, *Cryptococcus neoformans*, and *Saccharomyces cerevisae*[P00083]. Dried oleoresin at a concentration of 500.0 ppm on agar plate was active on *Debaryomyces hansenii* vs ascospore production. Inactive on *Candida lipolytica* vs pseudomycelium production; *Hansenula anomala* vs pseudomycelium and ascospore production; *Lodderomyces elongisporus* vs pseudomycelium production; *Rhodotorula rubra* vs pseudomycelium production; *Saccharomyces cerevisiae* vs pseudomycelium and ascospore production; *Torulopsis glabrata* vs pseudomycelium production. In broth culture the oleoresin was inactive on *Candida lipolytica*, *Debaryomyces hansenii*, *Hansenula anomala*, *Kloeckera apiculata*, *Lodderomyces elongisporus*, *Rhodotorula rubra*, *Saccharomyces cerevisiae*, and *Torulopsis glabrata* vs biomass production[T15123]. Water extract of rhizome on agar plate at a concentration of 10.0 mg/ml was inactive on *Candida albicans* and *Candida tropicalis*[M29966].

Apoptosis induction. Hexane extract of rhizome in cell culture was active on LEUK-HL60[K25671].

Arachidonate metabolism inhibition. Ether extract of dried tuber at a concentration of 100.0 mcg/ml was inactive on platelets vs AA incorporation into platelet phospholipids[T15693].

Ascaricidal activity. Root essential oil, at a concentration of 0.2% was active. Forty five minutes exposure killed all the worms. A 0.2% piperazine citrate solution required 50 minutes exposure to kill all the worms[T00549].

Carcinogenesis inhibition. Dried rhizome powder in the ration of female mice at a dose of 2.0% of the diet/day produced weak activity. Animals were 12 months of age at start of experiment vs DMBA-induced carcinogenesis. A dose of 5.0% of the diet/day was active at 8, 12, and 2 months of age to start the experiment and strongly active at six months of age to start the experiment vs DMBA-induced carcinogenesis[K24869]. Ethanol (95%) extract of dried rhizome in the ration of female mice at a dose of 5.0% of the diet vs benzo(a)pyrene-induced carcinogenesis; and on female hamster (Syrian) vs methylnitrosamine-induced carcinogenesis. A dose of 2.0% was inactive in mice vs benzo(a)pyrene-induced carcinogenesis[K18745]. Ethanol (95%) extract of rhizome at a dose of 5.0% of the diet in the ration of Syrian hamster was active vs methyl (acetoxymethyl) nitrosamine (DMN-OAC)-induced oral carcinogenesis, synergism with *Piper betel*[K21173]. Powdered root in the ration of mice at a dose of 2.0% of the diet was active vs Benzo(a)pyrene-induced tumorgenesis[M30100]. Rhizome in the ration of hamsters (Syrian) at a dose of 5.0% of the diet was active vs DMN-OAC-induced oral carcinogenesis. When a combination treatments of betel-leaf extract and tumeric; Beta carotene and tumeric; or alpha-tocopherol and tumeric were used the doses were active vs methyl nitrosamine-induced carcinogenesis[K14086]. A dose of 160.0 mg/per gm of diet was active vs 3'-methyl-4-dimethylaminoazobenzene-induced carcinogenesis[K09214]. Rhizome in the ration of rats at a concentration of 0.1% of the diet was active vs benzo[a]pyrene-induced carcinogenesis[K10660].

Cardiotonic activity. Ethanol/water (1:1) extract of rhizome administered by perfusion was inactive on the heart of the guinea pig[A03335].

Catalase stimulation. Rhizome in the ration of rats at a concentration of 1.0% of the diet produced weak activity[K16225].

Choleretic activity. Essential oil of fresh rhizome, administered intragastric to rats at a dose of 300.0 mg/kg was active[M20141].

Chromosome aberrations induced. Hot water extract of dried rhizome administered intraperitoneally to mice was inactive on bone marrow vs cyclophosphamide-induced damage[M30769]. Water extract of fresh tuber, at a concentration of 4.0% was active. Assayed was done on root of *Allium cepa.*, chromosome breakage was observed[K14943].

Clastogenic activity. Hot water extract of dried rhizome administered intraperitoneally to mice was inactive on bone marrow vs cyclophosphamide-induced damage[M30769]. Methanol extract of root administered intraperitoneally to mice at a dose of 500 mg/kg was active[T14094].

CNS depressant activity. Ethanol/water (1:1) extract of rhizome administered intraperitoneally to mouse at a dose of 250.0 mg/kg was active[A03335].

Cytochrome B-5 increase. Powdered rhizome administered intragastric to mice at a dose of 4.0 gm/kg was active. Assay was done in pups presuming translactational exposure[K25126].

Cytochrome B-5 inhibition. Powdered root in the ration of mice at a dose of 5.0% of the diet was active[M30100].

Cytochrome P-450 induction. Powdered rhizome administered intragastric to mice at a dose of 4.0 gm/kg was active. Assay was done in pups presuming translactational exposure[K25126].

Cytochrome P-450 inhibition. Powdered root in the ration of mice at a dose of 5.0% of the diet was active[M30100]. Water extract of rhizome at a concentration of 3.0 mg/ml was active on rat liver microsomes[K23394].

Cytotoxic activity. Ethanol/water (1:1) extract of rhizome in cell culture at a concentration of 1.0 mg/ml was active on human lymphocytes, human leukemic lymphocytes and Dalton's lymphoma[H01195]. Ethanol/water (1:1) extract of rhizome in cell culture was inactive on CA-9KB, $ED_{50} >$ 20.0 mcg/ml[A03335]. Ether and petroleum ether extract of rhizome in cell culture were active on LEUK-L1210, ED_{50} 10.0 and 5.0 mcg/ml respectively[T13791]. Ether extract of dried rhizome in cell culture was active on hepatoma HTC[T02632]. Water extract at a concentration of 500.0 mcg/ml produced weak activity on CA-Mammary-Microalveolar[M26592]. Petroleum ether extract of dried rhizome in cell culture was active on LEUK-L1210. ED_{50} 1.8 mcg/ml[M22787]. Water extract of dried rhizome in cell culture at a concentration of 0.1 mg/ml was inactive on HELA cells. Methanol extract produced strong activity[H01040].

Desaturase-Delta-5 inhibition. Ethanol (95%) extract of fresh rhizome at a concentration of 0.1% was active. The effect was assayed by looking at the ratio of Dihomo-gamma-linolenic acid to arachidonic acid in cell-free preparations of *Mortierella alpina* IS-4[K07766].

Diuretic activity. Rhizome in the ration of rats that were fed a low thiamine diet showed no change in urinary or fecal excretion[W04316].

Embryotoxic effect. Ethanol (95%) extract of rhizome administered orally to rats at a doses of 100.0 and 200.0 mg/kg produced 70% and 80% inhibition of pregnancy respectively. Water extract produced 80% and 100% inhibition respectively, and petroleum ether extract produced 80% and 100% inhibition respectively[N00186]. Ethanol (95%), water and petroleum ether extracts of rhizome administered orally to rats at doses of 100.0 mg/kg was active[W00335].

Food consumption reduction. Powdered rhizome administered intragastric to rats at a dose of 10.0% of the diet was inactive[T16608].

Gastric secretory inhibition. Water extract at a dose of 132.0 mg/kg and methanol extract at a dose of 155.0 mg/kg of entire plant, administered intragastric to rabbit were active. Gastric juice was collected by catheter[M20895].

Gastrointestinal disorders. Powdered dried rhizome taken orally by human adults at a dose of 500.0 mg/person was active. A randomized double-blind study was conducted to examine the efficacy of treating dyspepsia with given extract. Patients were given the dose four times per day after meals and before bed for seven days. Eighty patients were assigned to control or treatment groups. A statistically significant 87% of the treatment and 53% of the group showed improvement, though patient satisfaction ran only 50 and 47%[T16521].

Genotoxicity activity. Rhizome administered by gastric intubation to mice at doses of 2.5, 5.0 and 7.5 gm/kg were inactive[T07727].

Glutamate oxaloacetate transaminase inhibition. Hot water extract of dried rhizome administered subcutaneously to mice at a dose of 20.0 gm/kg was active vs carbon tetrachloride-induced hepatotoxicity. The dose represents the amount of crude drug equivalent. Results significant at P <0.01 level[T08190].

Glutamate oxaloacetate transaminase stimulation. Methanol extract of dried rhizome administered intraperitoneally to rats at a dose of 100.0 mg/kg was active vs

Alpha-naphthylisothiocyanate-induced hepatotoxicity[M27764].

Glutamate pyruvate transaminase inhibition. Hot water extract of dried rhizome administered subcutaneously to mice at a dose of 20.0 gm/kg (the amount of crude drug equivalent) was active vs carbon tetrachloride-induced hepatotoxicity. Results significant at P < 0.01 level[T08190]. Water extract of fresh rhizome in the ration of ducklings at a concentration of 50.0 mg/day was active vs aflatoxin B-1 hepatotoxicity. Enzyme was measured in the serum[K15267].

Glutamate pyruvate transaminase stimulation. Methanol extract of dried rhizome administered intraperitoneally to rats at a dose of 100.0 mg/kg was active vs Alpha-naphthylisothiocyanate-induced hepatotoxicity[M27764]. Water extract of fresh rhizome in the ration of ducklings at a concentration of 50.0 mg/day was active vs aflatoxin B-1 hepatotoxicity. Enzyme was measured in the serum[K15267].

Glutathione formation induction. Powdered root in the ration of mice at a dose of 5.0% of the diet was active[M30100].

Glutathione peroxidase stimulation. Rhizome in the ration of rats at a concentration of 1.0% of the diet produced weak activity[K16225].

Glutathione-S-Transferase induction. Powdered rhizome administered intragastric to mice at a dose of 4.0 gm/kg was active. Assay was done in pups presuming translactational exposure[K25126]. Powdered root in the ration of mice at a dose of 5.0% of the diet was active[M30100]. Rhizome administered intragastric to mice at a concentration of 4.0 gm/kg was active. Progeny's liver looked at after translactational exposure other significant enzyme include soluble sulfhydryl cytochrome B5 cytochrome P450[K25332].

GRAS status. Rhizome and root obtained GRAS status by United States of America Food and Drug Administration in 1976 (Sect. 582.10) and the essential oil (Sect. 582.20) as flavoring agents[K00040].

Hyaluronidase inhibition. Root essential oil, administered orally to male mice at a dose of 0.1 ml/kg was active[A05570].

Hypoglycemic activity. Water extract of rhizome administered orally to rabbits at a dose of 10.0 mg/kg was inactive[A14379]. Drop in blood sugar of 15 mg relative to inert-treated control indicated positive results[A14379].

Hypothermic activity. Ethanol/water (1:1) extract of rhizome, administered intraperitoneally to mice at a dose of 250.0 mg/kg was inactive[A03335].

Immunostimulant activity. Polysaccharide fraction of dried rhizome administered intraperitoneally to mice at a dose of 100.0 mg/kg for five days was inactive vs SRBC challenge. A dose of 200.0 mg/kg was active, results significant at P < 0.01 level[T12554].

Immunosuppressant activity. Water extract of rhizome administered by gastric intubation to rats at a dose of 100.0 mg/kg was active. Daily dosing for 10 days to typhoid bacillus-sheep RBC stimulated animals showed the antibody titre to be significantly inhibited[T06208]. Hot water extract of rhizome administered intraperitoneally to rats was active[T04890].

Insect repellent activity. Petroleum ether extract of dried rhizome at variable concentrations was active on *Rhyzopertha dominica*, *Sitophilus granarius* and *Tribolium castaneum*[T07420]. Petroleum ether extract of root at a concentration of 680.0 mcg/sq. cm was active on *Tribolium castaneum*[T05122]. Root essential oil was active on *Aedes aegypti*[W00135].

Insecticide activity. Methanol extract of dried rhizome was active on *Spodoptera litura* larvae[T09361]. Powdered rhizome applied externally to human adults was active. *Azadirachta indica* leaves and *Curcuma longa* root were ground to form a paste 4:1 by weight. This was spread over the entire body daily. Nintey seven percent of 814 cases of scabies were cured within 15 days of treatment[K07698]. Water extract of dried root, at variable concentrations was inactive on *Blatella germanica* and *Oncopelatus fasciatus*. Intravenous dose of 40.0 ml/kg produce weak activity on *Periplaneta americana*[W03405].

Interferon induction stimulation. Hot water extract of dried rhizome administered intragastric to mice at a dose of 0.4 ml/animal for seven days was active. The prescription also included 10 gm each of *Curcuma longa* rhizome, *Rheum officinale* root, *Cimicifuga foetida* rhizome, *Anemarrhena asaphodeloides* rhizome, *Areca catechu* seed, *Magnolia officinalis* bark and *Scutellaria baicalensis* root, also included are 5 gm *Amomum tsaoko* fruit, together with insects *Bombyx mori* and *Cryptotympana pustulata*. A dose of 0.6 ml/animal administered intraperitoneally was also active[M25607].

Intestinal absorption inhibition. Water extract of dried rhizome at a concentration of 1.0%, administered by perfusion produced weak activity in rats vs absorption of sulfaguanidine. Methanol and water extracts at a concentration of 0.1% were inactive[T15727].

Lactate dehydrogenase stimulation. Methanol extract of dried rhizome administered intraperitoneally to rats at a dose of 100.0 mg/kg was active vs Alphanaphthylisothiocyanate-induced hepatotoxicity[M27764].

Leukopenic activity. Water extract of rhizome administered intragastric to mouse at a dose of 100.0 mg/kg was active[M31104].

Lipid peroxide formation inhibition. Hot water extract of a commercial sample of tuber was active. IC_{50} 200.0 ng/mcl[M19431]. Hot water extract of dried rhizome in cell culture at a concentration of 1.0 mg/plate was inactive on hepatocytes monitored by production of malonaldehyde[K23019].

Liver regeneration stimulation. Commercial sample of oleoresin at a concentration of 0.6% of the diet in the ration of male rats was inactive. Partially hepatectomized animals were dosed daily for seven days[T05564].

Mutagenic activity. Bulb on agar plate at a concentration of 50.0 mcg/plate was active on *Salmonella typhimurium* TA1535 and inactive on *Salmonella typhimurium* TA1537 and TA1538[T16468]. Infusion on agar plate at a concentration of 200.0 mcg/plate was inactive on *Salmonella typhimurium* TA100 and TA98. Metabolic activation had no effect on the results[K07408]. Chloroform/methanol (2:1) extract of rhizome on agar plate at a concentration of 10.0 mg/plate produced complete growth inhibition of the Pig-Kidney LLC-PK1 and Trophoblastic-Placenta cells, thus it was impossible to interpret the results. Effect was the same with or without metabolic activation. Water extract of rhizome on agar plate at a concentration of 100.0 mg/plate was inactive on Pig-Kidney-LLC-PK-1 and Trophoblastic-Placenta cells. The effect was the same with or without metabolic activation[T04521]. Ethanol (95%) extract of dried rhizome on agar plate at a concentration of 10.0 mg/plate was active on *Salmonella typhimurium* TA102, and inactive on *Salmonella typhimurium* TA98[K08041]. Ethanol (95%) extract of dried rhizome on agar plate at a concentration of 250.0 mcg/plate was inactive on *Salmonella typhimurium* TA98, TA100, and TA1535. Metabolic activation had no effect on the results[K14566]. Ethanol (95%) extract of fresh rhizome, on agar plate at a concentration of 360.0 mcg/plate was inactive on *Salmonella typhimurium* TA100, TA98, TA1535, and TA1538. Metabolic activation had no effect on the results[K14566]. Ethanol (95%) extract of root, on agar plate at a concentration of 15.0 mg/plate was active on *Salmonella typhimurium* TA98. Streptomycin dependent strains of TA98 were tested. Metabolic activation had no effect on the results[T12546]. Hot water and methanol extracts of rhizome on agar plate at concentrations of 50.0 mg/disc (expressed as dry weight of plant) were inactive on *Salmonella typhimurium* TA98 and TA100. Effect was the same with or without metabolic activation. Histidine was removed from the extract prior to testing[T06535]. Resin on agar plate at a concentration of 160.0 mcg/plate was inactive on *Salmonella typhimurium* TA100, TA98 and TA1535[T08621]. Water extract of dried rhizome at a concentration of 50.0 mg/ml on agar plate was inactive on *Salmonella typhimurium* TA1535. Mutagenicity was assayed by SOS UMU test. Metabolic activation had no effect on the results[M29342]. Water, and hot water extracts of dried rhizome, on agar plate at a concentration of 0.5 ml/disc, and rhizome at variable concentrations were inactive on *Bacillus subtilis* M-45(REC-) and H-17(REC+)[T07988].

Myocardial uptake of 86-RB enhanced. Hot water extract of dried tuber administered intraperitoneally to mice at variable dosage levels was inactive, as evidenced by uptake of 86-RB by the myocardium[T07146].

Necrotic effect. Ethanol (95%) extract of rhizome on agar plate at a concentration of 250.0 mcg/plate was inactive on *Salmonella typhimurium* TA1538. Metabolic activation had no effect on the results[K14566].

Nematocidal activity. Hexane extract of dried rhizome was active on *Toxacara canis*[H12627].

Nitrosation inhibition. Rhizome at variable concentrations was active on *Salmonella typhimurium* TA100 and TA1535 vs nitrosation of methylurea[T15244].

Ovulation inhibition effect. Ethanol (95%), water and petroleum ether extracts of rhizome administered orally to rabbits at doses of 100.0 and 200.0 mg/kg were inactive[J08548]. Water and petroleum ether extracts of rhizome administered orally to rabbits at doses of 100.0 mg/kg were inactive[W00335].

Phagocytosis capacity increased. Polysaccharide fraction of dried rhizome administered intraperitoneally to mice at a dose of 100.0 mg/kg was active. vs clearance of colloidal carbon. Results significant at P < 0.01 level[T12554].

Plant extract on agar plate at a concentration of 0.5% was inactive and stimulated acid production on *Escherichia coli*, *Streptococcus faecalis*, *Streptococcus lactis* and active on *Lactobacillus acidophilus* and *Lactobacillus plantarum*.[N00137].

Plasma bilirubin decrease. Methanol extract of dried rhizome administered intraperitoneally to rats at a dose of 100.0 mg/kg was inactive vs Alpha-naphthylisothiocyanate-induced hepatotoxicity[M27764].

Platelet aggregation inhibition. Ether extract of dried tuber at a concentration of 100.0 mcg/ml was inactive. vs collagen-, and ADP-induced aggregation and A23187 used as ionophore, vs calcium ionophore-induced aggregation. A concentration of 50.0 mcg/ml was active vs arachidonic acid-induced aggregation[T15693]. Water extract of dried rhizome was active on the platelets of human adults and rabbits. The dose consist of a mixture of *Levisticum officinale*, *Artemisia cappilaris*, *Curcuma longa*, and *Chrysanthemum indicum*[K09096].

Protease(HIV) inhibition. Water extract of rhizome at a concentration of 200.0 mcg/ml was equivocal[K21241].

Radical scavenging effect. Hot water extract of dried rhizome at a concentration of 250.0 mg/liter was inactive when measured by decolorization of diphenylpicryl hydroxyl radical solution. There was six percent decoloration[K23019].

RBC synthesis antagonist. Water extract of rhizome administered intragastric to mice at a dose of 100.0 mg/kg was active[M31104].

Spasmogenic activity. Methanol extract of dried rhizome at a concentration of 5.0 mg/ml was inactive on the ileum of rats[T16652].

Spasmolytic activity. Methanol extract of dried rhizome at a concentration of 5.0 mg/ml was inactive on the ileum of rats vs ACh-induced contractions[T16652].

Sulfhydryl-containing compounds increased. Powdered rhizome administered intragastric to mice at a dose of 4.0 gm/kg was active. Assay was done on pups, presuming translactational exposure[K25126]. Water extract of rhizome at a concentration of 50.0 mcg/ml was active on rat brain. There was a decrease in the depletion of sulhydryl containing compounds induced by promoters of lipid peroxidation[K21634].

Superoxide dismutase stimulation. Rhizome in the ration of rats at a concentration of 1.0% of the diet produced weak activity[K16225].

Taenicide activity. Root essential oil at a concentration of 0.2% was active on *Taenia saginata*. Forty two minutes of exposure was required to kill all the worms. A 0.2% piperazine citrate solution required 60 minutes exposure to kill all the worms[T00549].

Teratogenic activity. Ethanol (95%), water and petroleum ether extracts of rhizome administered orally to female rabbits at doses of 200.0 mg/kg were inactive[J08548]. Root in the ration of female mice and rats, at a concentration of 0.5% of the diet for seven days, was inactive[T03084].

Thromboxane B-2 synthesis inhibition. Ether extract of dried tuber at a concentration of 100.0 mcg/ml was active on platelets vs calcium ionophore A23187 stimulation of platelets. A concentration of 62.5 mcg/ml was active, 12-HETE synthesis was stimulated[T15693].

Toxic effect (general). Ethanol (95%) extract of rhizome administered intragastric to mice at a dose of 100.0 mg/kg was inactive[M31104]. Ethanol (95%) extract of rhizome in the ration of male guinea pigs, and female monkeys at variable dosage levels for three weeks was inactive. No toxic effects or abnormal morphological or histological results was observed. Doses of 300.0 mg/kg and 2.5 gm/kg in the ration of Rhesus monkeys and rats of both sexes was inactive. Dosing was only on the first day, followed by control diet for three weeks[T02456].

Toxic effect. Commercial sample of oleoresin, at variable dosage levels, in the ration of pigs was active. Animals were fed dietary levels of the oleoresin equal to 60, 296, and 1551 mg/kg/day for 102–109 days. All dose levels showed a significant dose-dependent increase in liver and thyroid weight. A reduction on weight gain and feed conversion efficiency was observed in the high dose group. The two higher dose groups showed evidence of thyroidal hyperplasia, epithelial changes in the urinary bladder and kidney, and pericholangitis[T12438].

Toxicity assessment (quantitative). Ethanol (95%) extract of rhizome administered intraperitoneally to mice produced LD_{50} 3.98 gm/kg; water extract LD_{50} 430.0 mg/kg and petroleum ether extract LD_{50} 525.0 mg/kg[K01337]. Ethanol/water (1:1) extract of rhizome administered intraperitoneally to mice produced LD_{50} 500.0 mg/kg[A03335].

Tyrosinase inhibition. Methanol extract of dried rhizome at a concentration of 167.0 mcg/ml was active[K20239]. An extract of skin-lightening cosmetics contain extracts of *Syzygium aromaticum*, *Curcuma longa*, *Areca catechu*, and/or *Sauesurea lappa* (comprising melanin inhibitors) in addition to base materials showed tyrosinase-inhibiting activity[K25491].

Uterine stimulant effect. Methanol extract of dried rhizome at a concentration of 5.0 mg/ml was inactive on the uterus of rats[T16652]. Methanol/water (1:1) extract of leaves, at a dose of 10.0 mcg/ml was active on the uterus (unspecified condition) of hamsters[A03566].

WBC-macrophage stimulant. Water extract of freeze-dried rhizome at a concentration of 2.0 mg/ml was inactive. Nitrite formation was used as an index of the macrophage stimulating activity to screen effective foods[M27208].

Weight gain inhibition. Powdered rhizome administered intragastric to rats at a dose of 10.0% of the diet was inactive[T16608].

12 | Hibiscus rosa-sinensis

L.

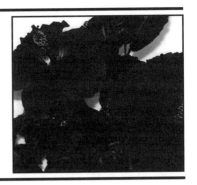

Common Names

Ampolo	Nicaragua	Gwo fle baye	Trinidad
Antolanagan	Philippines	Gwo waz baya	Trinidad
Ardhol	Fiji	Hibiscus	Easter Island
Aroganan	China	Hibiscus	Guyana
Avispa	Nicaragua	Hibiscus	Vietnam
Banban	Papua-New Guinea	Hindu-ma-pangi	Bangladesh
Bunga raya	Malaysia	Hong can	Vietnam
Chemparathy	India	Jaba	India
China rosa	Kuwait	Jabaphool	India
China rose	India	Japa	India
China rose plant	India	Japa puspi	Nepal
Chinese hibiscus	Nepal	Japakusum	India
Choon kin phee	Malaysia	Jasum	Fiji
Chou blak	Haiti	Jasum	India
Chuan chin pi	Malaysia	Jasunt	India
Chuan chin pi	Vietnam	Jaswand	India
Chuen kan pi	Malaysia	Jia pushpa	India
Cucarda	Peru	Joba	India
Dam but	Vietnam	Kaute	India
Dasani	India	Kaute'enua	Cook Islands
Dok mai	Vietnam	Kaute'enua	Rarotonga
Double hibiscus	Trinidad	Kauti	Rarotonga
Fencing flower	Trinidad	Kayaga	China
Fla baya	Trinidad	Kembang sepatu	Indonesia
Fleur barriere	Trinidad	Koute	Indonesia
Flores rosa	Guam	Lagitua	New Britain
Foulsepatte	Rodrigues Islands	Lelegurua	New Britain
Fu-yong-pi	China	Loloru	New Britain
Ghanti phul	Nepal	Mandaar	India
Gros rose	French Guiana	Mandara	India
Gudhal	India	Rose de chine	Vietnam
Gumamila	Philippines	Rose of China	China
Gurhal	India	Rose-cayenne	Guadeloupe
Gwo fla bays	Trinidad	Roz kaiyen	Guadeloupe

From: Medicinal Plants of the World *By: Ivan A. Ross Humana Press Inc., Totowa, NJ*

Sadaphool	India	Shoe flower plant	Kuwait
Sambathoochedi	India	Takuragan	China
Senicikobia	India	Tapulaga	China
Senitoa yaloyalo	India	Tiare kalova kalova	Papua-New Guinea
Shoe black	Nicaragua	Tulipan	Mexico
Shoe flower	Indonesia	Wavu wavu	Indonesia
Shoe flower	Nepal	Woz baya	Trinidad

BOTANICAL DESCRIPTION

A shrub of the MALVACEAE family with long slender branches up to about six meters tall. They are arranged spirally on the stem, ovate, have long stalks and measure up to 15 cm long and 10 cm wide. Flowers are borne singly in the axils of the upper leaves, usually on rather long stalks. They have an epicalyx of 5–7 bracteoles about 1 cm long and cupular calyx about 2.5 cm long. The corolla is short-lived of five very showy contorted-overlapping petals. Many varieties exist differing in size and color corolla, in single or double forms. The fruit (very rarely formed) is a capsule about 3 cm long.

ORIGIN AND DISTRIBUTION

A native of south-eastern Asia. Very commonly cultivated and relict by old habitations and cultivations in a wide range of situations. Now commonly found throughout the tropics, and as a houseplant throughout the world. Most ornamental varieties are hybrids, many of them resulting from crosses with the African *H. schizopetalus*.

TRADITIONAL MEDICINAL USES

Bangladesh. A decoction of the flower with green betel nut is given to regulate the menstrual cycle[K10069].

China. Hot water extract of flowers is taken orally as an emmenagogue and a tonic[W02290]. Hot water extract of the bark is taken orally as an emmenagogue[A06589]. Water extract of trunk bark is taken orally as an emmenagogue[A02296].

Cook Islands. Hot water extract of dried flowers and leaves is used for ailing infants.

Flowers, or sometimes leaves with or without *Gardenia taitensis* leaves, are boiled or fried in coconut cream. It is then taken internally or used as a massage. Hot water extract of dried leaves and flowers is taken orally for gonorrhea. Infusion is taken orally as an abortifacient[T09553].

East Indies. Hot water extract of flowers is taken orally to regulate menstruation and for abortion[A06589]. Leaf juice is administered orally by midwives to stimulate expulsion of afterbirth. Given with *Vernonia cinerea*[A06589].

Fiji. Fresh leaf juice is taken orally for easier delivery in childbirth and for diarrhea[T10632]. Hot water extract of flowers and leaves is taken orally to ease childbirth[M00729]. Infusion of dried flowers is taken orally to aid digestion[T10632].

French Guiana. Hot water extract of flowers is taken orally for the grippe[J10155].

Ghana. Peeled twig is used as a chewstick[T03316].

Guadeloupe. Hot water extract of flowers is taken orally as a sodorific and antitussive. Syrup is made by boiling unopened flowers, and drunk with sugar[T07660].

Guam. Leaves are applied to affected parts for draining abscesses[A01962].

Haiti. Decoction of dried flowers is taken orally for flu and cough[T13846]. Decoction of dried leaves is taken orally for flu, coughs and stomach pain; for eye problems macerated leaves is used in a bath for the head[T13846].

Hawaii. Flowers are eaten to produce lactation[W00534].

India. Decoction of dried flowers is taken orally for abortion[K16006]. Hot water extract is taken orally as an antifertility agent[T02635].

The hot water extract is used as a contraceptive in Ayurvedic medicine. For this the flowers with their sexual parts (pistil and stamens) are taken orally by the female concerned. Four to five flowers make one dose and 2–3 doses are taken per day at intervals of 5–6 hours[T06787]. Dried buds are eaten as a treatment for diabetes. One unopened flower (mature bud) is chewed and eaten per day early in the morning before taking meals, for up to ten days or until the level of blood sugar is reduced to the tolerance limit. This treatment is said to be good in managing the disease but is not a permanent cure[M24146]. Fresh buds are taken orally by women to produce complete sterilization. Three flower buds are collected just before blooming and mixed with the water left after washing rice. One such bud makes one dose. The female is given one dose orally daily on the 4th, 5th, and 6th days of the menses. The application is repeated for 3–4 months for permanent sterilization[T06787]. Flowers and leaves are taken orally for constipation and painful bowel motion. The leaves and flowers are churned into a mucilaginous juice with water and filtered. About half a cup of the filtrate is taken by mouth every day before going to bed[K23365]. Hot water extract of dried stems is taken orally as a diuretic[T03906]. Hot water extract of flowers is taken orally for menorrhagia, bronchitis[A00041], as an emmenagogue[A00468], for treatment of menarche, flower decoction along with "Jaggary" is drunk[K11282], and as a contraceptive in Ayurvedic medicine[L02359]. Hot water extract of the aerial parts is taken orally as an aphrodisiac and emmenagogue[W01378]. Hot water of leaves is taken orally as an aperient, laxative, anodyne and to expel the placenta after childbirth; externally, in combination with juice of *Veronia cineria*, it is used as an emmolient[L02359]. Root juice is taken orally as an abortifacient. Five mililiters each of root juice of *Plumbago rosea* and *Hibiscus rosa-sinensis* is given on an empty stomach along with red-colored brain of a species of fresh water fish locally known as "Magur"[T09302]. Hot water extract of root is taken orally as a demulcent and for coughs[L02359].

Indonesia. Flowers are taken orally to regulate menstruation, to cause abortion[A00115] and as an emmenagogue[A04162]. Juice of leaves is taken orally by women in labor[A00115].

Japan. Decoction of fresh leaves is taken orally as an antidiarrheal[H12480].

Kuwait. Flowers are taken orally by females as an emmenagogue and by males as an aphrodisiac[L02255].

Malaysia. Hot water extract of roots is taken orally for fevers and venereal diseases[A06589]. Infusion of hot water extract of flowers is taken orally as an expectorant[A06589]. Water extract of the bark is taken orally as an emmenagogue[A04361].

Mexico. Infusion of bark, leaves and flowers are taken orally to treat dysentery[K16948].

Nepal. Hot water extract of roots is taken orally for coughs[A00020]. Powdered dried flowers administered intravaginally to accelerate parturition. Two to four teaspoonfuls are given during labor pains[K23191].

New Britain (East). Hot water extract of flowers is taken orally to regulate menstruation[M00729].

New Caledonia. Decoction of hot water extract of flowers is taken orally as an emmenagogue and as an abortifacient[A04174].

New Ireland. Water extract of fresh flowers and leaves is taken orally to induce labor. Flowers and young leaves are soaked in coconut water and the solution in taken to induce labor in the Northern Province[T02699].

Papau-New Guinea. Flowers are taken orally to relieve labor pains[A00614]. Hot water extract of flowers and leaves is taken orally to induce labor. Leaves and flowers are soaked in coconut juice for several hours then taken[M00729].

Peru. Hot water extract of dried flowers is taken orally by males as a contraceptive and by females as an emmenagogue[T15323]. Hot water extract of dried stems is taken orally as a contraceptive and emmenagogue[T15323].

Philippines. Fresh flowers are bruised and applied to tumors and inflammations; water extract is taken orally in bronchial catarrh for a sodorific effect[A02296]. Hot water extract of bark is used externally as an emmolient[A04508]. Hot water extract of flowers is used externally as an emmolient[A04508]; paste of flowerbud is applied topically to cancerous swellings[A05825]. Hot water extract of roots is used externally as an emollient[A04508]. Juice of leaves, together with leaves of *Vernonia cinerea*, is used to stimulate expulsion of the afterbirth[A00115]. The hot water extract is used externally as an emmolient[A04508].

Rarotonga. Decoction of fresh leaves is taken orally to treat women for irregular menstrual periods[A08575]. Infusion of fresh flowers is taken orally as an abortifacient[K08575].

Samoa. Hot water extract of flowers and leaves id taken orally to ease childbirth[M00729]. Water extract of fresh flowers and leaves is taken orally to induce labor[T02699].

South Africa. Leaves are cooked and eaten as spinach in Matabeleland and Nyasaland[A05825].

Trinidad. Decoction[K03665] and infusion[T00701] of hot water extract of flowers is taken orally for amenorrhea.

Vanuata. Decoction made from the petals is taken orally for amenorrhea and to induce abortion[K18109]. Decoction of leaves is taken orally to treat uterine hemorrhage. Squeeze eight leaves with water, then boil a few minutes. Drink the preparation repeatedly as necessary. To induce sterility. Squeeze a large handful of leaves into 250 ml of water. Drink all at once during menstruation. Repeat during the following period[K18109]. Decoction of stem bark is taken orally for menorrhagia. Grate a handful of bark, prepare a decoction, cool it and drink of a maximum of two or three doses. Infusion of leaves is taken orally for menorrhagia. Six leaves crushed in water, and brought to a boil is taken orally[K18109].

Vietnam. Flowers are taken orally for dysmenorrhea[A00115] and as an abortive[A04766]. Hot water extract of dried leaves is a drug in traditional medicine[T05058]. Water extract of bark is taken orally as an emmenagogue[A04766,A00115].

CHEMICAL CONSTITUENTS

(ppm unless otherwise indicated)

Apigenidin, Fl
Arachidic acid, Lf
Behenic acid, Lf
Campesterol, Pl
Catalase, Pt,Lf
Cholesterol, Pl
Citric acid, Fl
Cyanidin, Fl
Cyanidin diglucoside, Fl
Cyanin, Fl
Dec-9-yn-1-oic acid, St Bk
Dec-9-yn-1-oic acid methyl ester, St Bk
Dec-9-ynoic acid, St Bk 1.2
Dec-9-ynoic acid methyl ester, St Bk 4.6; Rt Bk 0.8
Decanoic acid, Lf
Docosan-1-ol, Lf
N-Docosane, Lf
N-Dotriacontane, Lf
N-Eicosane, Lf
Ergosterol, Pl
Fructose, Fl
Gentisic acid, Lf
Glucose, Fl
Heneicosan-1-ol, Lf
N-Heneicosane, Lf
Heneicosanoic acid, Lf
N-Hentriacontane, Fl 0.102%; Lf
Heptacosan-1-ol, Lf
N-Heptacosane, Lf
Heptacosanoic acid, Lf
N-Heptadecane, Lf
Heptadecanoic acid methyl ester, St Bk
Hexacosan-1-ol, Lf
N-Hexacosane, Lf
N-Hexadecane, Lf
Hexacosanoic acid, Lf
Hibiscus mucilage Rl, Lf 1166
Lauric acid, Lf
Lignoceric acid, Lf
Malvalic acid, Lf
Malvalic acid methyl ester, Rt Bk

Margaric acid, Lf
Montanyl alcohol, Lf
Myristic acid, Lf
Non-8-yn-1-oic acid, St Bk
Non-8-yn-1-oic acid methyl ester, St Bk
Non-8-ynoic acid, St Bk
Non-8-ynoic acid methyl ester, St Bk; Rt Bk
N-Nonacosane, Lf
N-Nonadecane, Lf
Nonadecanoic acid, Lf
Nonanoic acid, Lf
Octacosan-1-ol, Lf
Iso-octacosan-1-ol, Lf
N-Octacosane, Lf
Octacosanoic acid, Lf
Octadecandienoic acid, Lf
N-Octadecane, Lf
Octanoic acid, Lf
Oxalic acid, Fl
Palmitic acid, Lf
Pelargonidin, Fl
Pentacosan-1-ol, Lf
N-Pentacosane, Lf
Pentacosanoic acid, Lf
Pentadencanoic acid, Lf
Quercetin, Fl 300
Quercetin-3-7-di-o-beta-D-glucoside, Pt
Quercetin-3-di-o-beta-D-glucoside, Pt
Quercetin-3-0-beta-D-sophorotriosid, Pt
Beta sitosterol, Lf, St, St Bk 40.8, Pl
Stearic acid, Lf
Sterculic acid Lf
Sterculic acid methyl esther, Rt Bk 36.1
Stigmasterol, Pl
Sucrose, Fl
Taraxeryl acetate, Lf, St
Tartaric acid, Fl
Tetracosan-1-ol, Lf
N-Triacontan-1-ol, Lf
Iso-triancontan-1-ol, Lf
N-Triacontane, Lf
Tricosan-1-ol, Lf
N-Tricosane, Lf
Tricosanoic acid, Lf
Tridecanoic acid, Lf
Undecanoic acid, Lf

PHARMACOLOGICAL ACTIVITIES AND CLINICAL TRIALS

Abortifacient effect. Ethanol (95%), water and petroleum ether, extracts of leaves, flowers and roots administered orally, dried roots by gastric intubation, and dried leaves subcutaneously to rats at doses of 200.0, 200.0, and 150.0 mg/kg respectively were inactive. Ethanol (95%), water and petroleum ether extracts of stem administered orally, and of dried stem administered by gastric intubation to rats at doses of 200.0 mg/kg were inactive[W01362]. Ethanol/water (1:1) extract of the dried entire plant, administered by gastric intubation to rats at a dose of 200.0 mg/kg was inactive[T10126]. Water insoluble and ether-soluble fractions of a total benzene extract of dried flowers, administered by gastric intubation to rats at a dose of 186.0 mg/kg was active[T04410]; ether-soluble and water-insoluble fractions of a total benzene extract, at a doses of 73.0 mg/kg were active[T10130]. Ethanol (90%), water and petroleum ether extracts of dried flowers, administered by gastric intubation at doses of 200.0, 200.0, and 150.0 mg/kg respectively were inactive[T08135].

Acid phosphatase stimulation. The effect of the 50 % ethanolic and benzene extracts of *H. rosa-sinensis* flowers, on the estrogen dependent enzyme (acid and alkaline phosphatase) activity of rat uterus, was studied. A significant increase in the acid phosphatase and decrease in alkaline phosphatase was reported with both the extracts, the effect being dose-related for both the enzymes. The antiestrogenic property of the ethanolic and benzene extracts was further confirmed in rats by a significant reduction in the fresh uterine content of protein, non-protein, nitrogen and total solid matter. Benzene and ethanol/water (1:1) extracts of flowers, administered orally to female rats daily for 12–18 days at doses of 75.0 mg/kg were equivocal. At doses of 150.0 mg/kg and 300.0 mg/kg both extracts were active[T01570].

Alkaline phosphatase inhibition. Benzene and ethanol/water (1:1) extracts of flowers, administered orally to rats daily for 12–18 days were active at doses of 75.0 mg/kg, 150.0 mg/kg, and 300.0 mg/kg[T01570].

Analgesic activity. Ethanol (70%) extract of dried leaves administered orally to mice at a dose of 125.0 mg/kg was active vs inhibition of aconitine-induced writhing[T01802].

Androgenic effect. Benzene extract of dried flowers administered by gastric intubation and ethanol (95%) extract administered orally to normal male[T04212] and castrated[T01782] rats at doses of 250.0 mg/kg were inactive[A02434].

Anti-FSH activity. Ethanol (95%) extract of flowers, administered orally to rats at a dose of 150.0 mg/animal was active[A02434].

Antiestrogenic effect. Benzene extract of dried flowers, administered by gastric intubation to rats at as dose of 200.0 mg/kg was equivocal and active at a dose of 250.0 mg/kg. The extract was also active when administered orally to mice at a dose of 1 gm/kg, and subcutaneously at a dose of 250.0 mg/kg. The ethanol/water (1:1) extract was equivocal in rats when administered by gastric intubation at a dose of 200.0 mg/kg, and active when administered orally at a dose of 150.0 mg/kg[T02650]. Studies with the total benzene extract of *H. rosa-sinensis* flowers revealed antiestrogenic activity in bilaterally ovariectomized immature albino rats. It disrupts the estrous cycle in rats, depending on the dose and duration of treatment. The extract led to a reduction in the weights of the ovary, uterus and pituitary. Ovaries showed follicular atresia and uterine atrophic changes. These effects could be reversed 30 days after withdrawal of the plant extract. In guinea pigs the benzene and ethanolic extract of the flowers led to an increase in the ovarian weight as well as in the weight and diameter if the corpora lutea, indicating an antiestrogenic activity. Benzene extract of the flowers, administered orally to ovariectomized rats at doses of 50.0, 100.0, 150.0, 200.0, and 250.0 mg/kg were active. Ethanol (95%) extract of the flowers, administered orally to ovariectomized rats was inactive at a dose of 100.0 mg/kg and

active at doses of 150.0, 200.0, and 250.0 mg/kg[T00888]. Ethanol/water (1:1) extract was active at a dose of 75.0 mg/kg, reduction of glycogen content in uterus of treated animals is claimed indicative of antiestrogenic activity[T00850].

Antifertility effect. Ethanol (95%) extract of dried flowers, taken orally by human females at doses of 750.0 mg/person was active. The dose was divided and taken three times daily from the 7th to the 22nd day of the menstrual cycle. A total of 21 women, 15–35 years of age were in the test group. Seven of the women discontinued the treatment for one reason or another. Three of the seven women discontinued treatment due to nonassociated illness. No pregnancies have developed in the 14 women after up to 20 months[T03949]. In another trial, women between the ages of 18 and 45 were given Vidangadi yoga, and herbal medicine consisting of *Embelia ribes* seeds, *Hibiscus rosa-sinensis* flowers and *Ferula foetida* oleoresin mixed in equal amounts. Eight hundred-miligram tablets were given three times per day with water or milk during menstruation for six days. Of the 1083 patients enrolled in the study, 83.1% did not become pregnant. Five hundred continued treatment for 36 cycles or more. No toxic effect was observed[T11017].

Antifungal activity. Ethanol/water (50%) extract of dried leaves was active on *Rhizoctonia solani*. Mycelial inhibition was 34.50%[T16358].

Antigonadotropin effect. Benzene extract of dried flowers, administered by gastric intubation to male and female rats at doses of 250.0 mg/kg were active[T04012].

Antihypertensive activity. In an uncontrolled clinical study on 20 patients of mild to moderate hypertension, powdered flowers (6–9 g per day in divided doses) were reported to produce significant reduction in the blood pressure, the effect on the diastolic pressure being more marked than on systolic.

Anti-implantation effect. Benzene extract of dried flowers, administered by gastric intubation to mice at a dose of 1.0 gm/kg was active. Dosing was done on days 1–4 of gestation, in the morning[T09869]. The extract was inactive at a dose of 250.0 mg/kg with dosing on days 1–3[T04012], and at 750.0 mg/kg administered orally to mice[T13682]. Benzene extract of leaves and stem bark, administered by gastric intubation to rats at a doses of 250.0 mg/kg showed 12.5% activity [L01413]. Benzene extract of petals, administered orally to rats at a dose of 100.0 mg/kg was active[A02176]. Ethanol/water (1:1) extract of the aerial parts, administered orally to mice at a dose of 100.0 mg/kg was inactive[A04819]. Hibiscus has been investigated extensively for its antifertility effect. Different parts of the plant have been screened for their effect on the reproductive system. The benzene extract of H. rosa-sinensis flowers (100 mg/kg) revealed post-coital antifertility effect in female albino rats, leading to 80% reduction in the implantation site on the 10th day of pregnancy. The fetal loss in the rats was within the normal range, indicating the absence of any abortifacient effect in the benzene extract. The petroleum ether extract was devoid of antifertility effect whereas the ether and ethanolic extracts of the flower petals however, a change in the sex ratio of the pups born was observed, the incidence of male:female pups born being higher in the extract-treated rats. Benzene extract of flowers, administered orally to rats at doses of 50.0 and 250.0 mg/kg were active[K01147,K02033,M01121]. Ethanol (95%) extract of flowers, administered orally to rats at a dose of 250.0 mg/kg showed weak activity. Water and petroleum ether extracts of flowers, administered orally to rats at doses of 250.0 mg/kg were inactive[K02033].

Anti-inflammatory activity. Ethanol (70%) extract of dried leaves, administered intraperitoneally to rats at a dose of 100.0 mg/kg was active vs carrageenin-induced pedal edema[T01802].

Antipyretic activity. Ethanol (70%) extract of dried leaves, administered intraperitoneally to rats at a dose of 100.0 mg/kg was active vs brewer's yeast-induced pyrexia[T01802]. Ethanol/water (1:1) extract of the aerial parts, administered intraperitoneally to mice at a dose of 500.0 mg/kg was active[A04819].

Antispasmodic activity. Ethanol/water (1:1) extract of the aerial parts was active on guinea pig's ileum vs ACh and histamine-induced spasms[A04819].

Antispermatogenic effect. Benzene extract of dried flowers, administered by gastric intubation to rats at a dose of 250.0 mg/kg was active. The animals were dosed daily for 30 days. Spermatogenesis was arrested at the early spermatid stage. The tubules showed disquamation of genital elements in the lumen. The tubules consisted of spermatogonia, sertoli cells, spermatocytes and degenerated spermatids. Leydig cells were atrophic. After 45 days of treatment a general derangement in the tubules was observed. The spermatocytes were darkly stained and between them empty spaces were seen suggesting disappearance of tubular elements. After 60 days treatment, marked degenerative changes were noticed in the seminferous tubules. Hypoplasia of all germinal elements excluding spermatogonia was observed. Reduction in weight of testes, epididymis, seminal vesicles, prostate, and pituitary was noted after treatment[T04012]. Ethanol (95%) extract of the dried flowers, administered by gastric intubation to rats at doses of 50.0 mg/animal and 150.0 mg/animal with daily dosing for 30 days were inactive. With daily dosing for 15 days of 250.0 mg/animal, cells in seminiferous tubules showed degranulation and vacuolization, absence of sperm and decrease in tubular diameter, interstitial cells were not affected. Daily dosing for 30 days caused a complete disorganization of the testicular architecture and shrinkage of the seminiferous tubules and complete destruction of spermatogonial cells. Germinal epithelium was affected and the leydig cells were absent. Cells of sertoli were the least affected[W02604]. Ethanol (95%) extract of flowers, administered orally to rams and rats at doses of 250.0 mg/animal and 150.0 mg/animal respectively were active[A02434].

Antiviral activity. Ethanol (80%) extract of freeze-dried plant, in cell culture at variable concentrations was equivocal on Coxsakie B2 virus, measles virus and polio virus I. and inactive on adenovirus, Herpes virus type I and Semlicki-forest virus vs plaque-inhibition[T06435].

Barbiturate potentiation. Ethanol/water (1:1) extract of the aerial parts, administered intraperitoneally to mice at a dose of 500.0 mg/kg was active[A04819].

Beta-glucuronidase inhibition. Benzene and Ethanol/water (1:1) extracts of dried flowers, administered by gastric intubation to normal and ovariectomized female rats at doses of 200.0 mg/kg, with dosing on days 1–5, were active[T12126].

Beta-glucuronidase stimulation. Benzene and ethanol/water (1:1) extract of dried flowers, administered by gastric intubation to ovariectomized rats at doses of 200.0 mg/kg with dosing on days 1–5, produced weak activity[T12126].

CNS depressant activity. Ethanol/water (1:1) extract of the aerial parts, administered intraperitoneally to mice at a dose of 500.0 mg/kg was active[A04819].

Embryotoxic effect. Benzene extract of dried flowers, administered by gastric intubation to pregnant rats at doses of 100.0, 150.0, and 186.0 mg/kg with dosing on days 1–10, were active. The ether-soluble and water insoluble fractions of the total benzene extracts were also active[T04410]. Water extract at doses of 200.0 and 270.0 mg/kg[T08135] and ethanol (95%) extract at 200.0 mg/kg[K16006], administered by gastric intubation to pregnant rats were inactive. Petro-

leum ether extract of dried flowers, administered by gastric intubation to pregnant rats at a dose of 150.0 mg/kg was inactive[T08135]. Benzene extract of flowers, administered by gastric intubation to rats at a dose of 250.0 mg/kg was active; ethanol (95%) water and petroleum ether extracts at doses of 200.0, 200.0, and 150.0 mg/kg administered orally to rats respectively were inactive[W01362]. Ethanol (95%), water and petroleum ether extracts of leaves and roots administered orally, dried roots and dried leaves by gastric intubation to rats at doses of 200.0, 200.0, and 150.0 mg/kg respectively, were inactive. Ethanol (90%), water and petroleum ether extracts of stem, administered orally and dried stem by gastric intubation to rats were inactive[W01362].

Estrogenic effect. Benzene extract of dried flowers, administered subcutaneously to infant mice[T01782] and by gastric intubation to female rats[T04012] at doses of 250.0 mg/kg were inactive.

Estrous cycle disruption effect. Benzene extract of flowers, administered orally to rats at a dose of 50.0 mg/kg was active[K04766].

Gonadotropin synthesis inhibition. Benzene extract of flowers, administered orally to rats at a dose of 250.0 mg/kg was active[L00242].

Hypotensive activity. Ethanol/ water (1:1) extract of the aerial parts, administered intravenously to dogs at a dose of 50.0 mg/kg was active[A04819].

Hypothermic activity. Ethanol/water (1:1) extract of the aerial parts, administered intraperitoneally to mice at a dose of 500.0 mg/kg was active[A04819].

Inotropic effect positive. Hot water extract of dried leaves, at a concentration of 320.0 microliters was inactive on guinea pig atrium[M29843].

Juvenile hormone activity. Acetone extract of dried stem produced weak activity on *Dysdercus cingulatus*[T01351].

Lactate-dehydrogenase-X inhibition. Benzene extract of dried flowers, administered subcutaneously to male *Rhinopoma kinneari* at a dose of 7.5 mg/animal was equivocal[T04005] and the hot water extract was active[T03946]. Enzyme levels measured in testes daily after a single injection of the extract.

Luteotropic effect. Benzene extract of dried flowers, administered by gastric intubation to guinea pigs at doses of 150.0 and 300.0 mg/kg were active. Results significant at P < 0.005 level. At a dose of dose of 75.0 mg/kg the extract was inactive. The ethanol/water (1:1) extract at doses of 150.0 and 300.0 mg/kg were inactive[T06358].

Menstruation induction effect. Water extract of leaves, was active on the non-pregnant uterus of rabbits and inactive on the non-pregnant uterus of rats[A03522].

Ovulation inhibition effect. Ethanol/water (1:1) extract of the aerial parts, administered orally to rabbits at a dose of 50.0 mg/kg was inactive vs copper acetate-induced ovulation[W01378].

Plant germination inhibition. Methanol extract of fresh stem bark was active on lettuce seeds[H01446].

Radical scavenging effect. Ethanol/water (1:1) extract of dried entire plant at a concentration of 5.0 mcg/ml was inactive vs superoxide anion, estimated by the neotetrazolium method[K21650].

Teratogenic activity. Ethanol (95%) extract of dried flowers, administered by gastric intubation to pregnant rats at a dose of 270.0 mg/kg was inactive[K16006]. Benzene extract of petals, administered orally to rats at a dose of 100.0 mg/kg was inactive[A02176].

Toxicity assessment (quantitative). Ethanol (70%) extract of dried leaves when administered intraperitoneally to mice LD_{50} 1.533 gm/kg[T01802]. Ethanol/water (1:1) extract of the aerial parts, administered intraperitoneally to both sexes of mice produced a LD_{50} 1.0 gm/kg[A04819].

13 | Hibiscus sabdariffa

Gaertn.

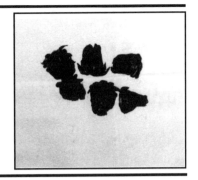

Common Names

Abuya	Congo-Brazzaville	Lal ambari	India
Baquitche	Guinea-Bissau	Mesta	Bangladesh
Basap	Senegal	Nsa	Congo-Brazzaville
Bisap	Senegal	Otesse	Guinea-Bissau
Bondio	Senegal	Patwa	India
Cutcha	Guinea-Bissau	Red roselle	India
Dakouma	Senegal	Red sorrel	Egypt
Fasab	Senegal	Red sorrel	Germany
Folere	Guinea-Bissau	Red sorrel	India
Gogu	India	Red sorrel	Senegal
Hamaiga	Nicaragua	Rosa de Jamaica	Guatemala
Ibuya	Congo-Brazzaville	Rosella	Egypt
Indian sorrel	Senegal	Roselle	Egypt
Indian sorrel	Senegal	Roselle hemp	Senegal
Inkulu	Congo-Brazzaville	Roselle	India
Jericho rose	Germany	Roselle	Iraq
Karkade	Egypt	Roselle	Japan
Karkade	Germany	Roselle	Mexico
Karkade	Italy	Roselle	Senegal
Karkade	Somaliland	Roxella-red sorrel	Thailand
Karkadeh	Sudan	Satui	Sierra Leone
Karkadesh	Egypt	Sawa sawa	Sierra Leone
Krachiap daeng	Thailand	Senegal bisap	Senegal
Kuges	Senegal	Sudan tea	East Africa
		Susur	Indonesia

BOTANICAL DESCRIPTION

The plant is an erect annual herb of the MALVACEAE family with a reddish cylindrical stem, nearly glabrous. Leaves are simple, having petiole, blade 3–5 lobed or parted, the lobes serrated or obtusely toothed. Flowers are solitary, axially, nearly sessile, 5- to 7-cm in diameter; consisting of epicalyx–segments 8–12, distinct, lanceolate to linear, adnate at base of the calyx; calyx is thick, red, and fleshy, cup-like, deeply parted, prominently 10-nerved; pet-

From: Medicinal Plants of the World *By:* Ivan A. Ross Humana Press Inc., Totowa, NJ

als 5, yellow, twice as long as calyx. Stamens are numerous; the filaments united into a staminal column; style single, five-branched near summit, stiga capitate. The fruit is capsule, ovoid, pointed, 1- to 2-cm long, shorter than the calyx, having densely sharp and stiff hairs.

ORIGIN AND DISTRIBUTION

A native to the tropics, it is extensively cultivated for its succulent fleshy edible calyx, and the stems yields a fairly strong fiber.

TRADITIONAL MEDICINAL USES

Africa. Hot water extract of seeds is taken as a diuretic and tonic[J09596]. Seed oil is used externally to heal sores on camels[09596].

Brazil. Hot water extract of root is taken orally as a stomachic and externally as an emollient[J09596].

Cameroon. Hot water extract of dried leaves is taken orally as an anthelmintic[T14170].

Congo. Hot water extract of leaves is taken orally to expedite delivery[A04171].

East Africa. Hot water extract of leaves is taken orally to relieve coughs[T09596]. Unripe fruit juice is taken orally with salt, pepper, asafetida, and molasses as a remedy for biliousness. Hot water extract of leaves is used as a flavoring agent, a diuretic, choleretic, febrifuge, hypotensive, to decrease viscosity of blood and to stimulate intestinal peristalsis. Externally the extract is used for sores and wounds [J09596].

Egypt. Decoction of hot water extract of the calyx is taken with sugar three times daily for high blood pressure[T00687]. Hot water extract of the entire plant is taken orally for heart and nerve diseases, as a laxative, to reduce weight, as a diuretic, to activate and neutralize hepatic secretion, to activate gastric secretion, as a digestive, for arteriosclerosis, as a diaphoretic, to give a euphoric impression, and as an intestinal antiseptic[A03932]. Leaf essential oil is taken orally to treat cancer[J02774].

Guatemala. Hot water extract of dried calyx is taken orally as a diuretic and for renal inflammation[T15295].

Guinea–Bissau. Seeds are taken orally by males as an aphrodisiac[J09596].

India. Hot water extract of leaves is taken orally as a diuretic, choleretic, febrifuge, hypotensive, to decrease blood viscosity, and to stimulate intestinal peristalsis[J09596]. Water extract of seed is taken orally to relieve dysuria and strangury, for mild cases of dyspepsia, and to relieve debility[T09596].

Mexico. Hot water extract of leaves is taken orally as a diuretic, choleretic, febrifuge, for hypotension, to decrease viscosity of the blood and to stimulate intestinal peristalsis[T09596].

Senegal. Hot water extract of leaves is used externally on wounds[TA06024], and orally to lower blood pressure[J09596]. Hot water extract of flowers is taken orally to combat fatigue, for indigestion, as a diaphoretic, cholagogue, and diuretic[A06024].

Sierra Leone. Decoction of dried leaves is taken orally to treat postpartum hemorrhage, to initiate contractions; as a diuretic during pregnancy (mixed with leaves of *Dialium guineensis*[T08806]).

Sudan. Hot water extract of flowers is taken orally as a blood purifier[A04407]. Hot water extract of the dried flowers is taken orally for coughs[T05013].

Thailand. Decoction of dried calyx is taken orally for dried calyx[T16711].

CHEMICAL CONSTITUENTS
(ppm unless otherwise indicated)

3-Methyl-1-butanol, Lf, Fr, Sd
Acetic acid, Fr, Sd
Alpha terpinyl acetate, Fr, Lf, Sd
Aluminum, Fl 125
Anisaldehyde, Fr, Lf, Sd
Anthocyanins, Cx 1.5%
Ascorbic acid, Fl 0.01–0.11%
Ascorbic acid, Fr 0.054–0.375%
Ash, Fl 0.6–7.7%; Lf 1.00–1.11%
Aspartic acid,
Behenic acid, Sd

Benzaldehyde, Fr
Benzyl alcohol, Fr, Lf
Beta carotene, Lf 41-555; Fl 0–21
Beta sitosteol–beta-D-galactopyranoside, Pl
Beta sitosterol, Sd (61.3% Sterols)
Beta sitosterol-beta-D-galactoside, Lf
Beta sitosteryl benzoate, Lf
Butyric acid, Fr
Calcium oxalate, Fr
Calcium, Fl 0.11-1.74%; Lf 0.213–1.479%; Sd 0.32-0.60%
Campesterol, Sd (16.5% Sterols)
Caprylic acid, Fr, Sd
Carbohydrates, Fl 9.20–76.50%; Sd 55.7%
Cellulose, Sd 16.8%
Cholesterol Sd (5.1% Sterols)
Chromium, Fl 54
Chrysanthemin, Fl
Cis–12,13-epoxy-cis-9-octadecenoic acid, Sd (4.5% Lipids)
Citric acid, Fr 3.74–17.00%
Cobalt, Fl 38
Cyanidin-3-sambubioside, Cx
Cyanin, Fl
Delphinidin, Cx
Delphinidin-3-glucoside, Cx
Delphinidin–3–sambubioside, Cx
Delphinin, Fl
Ergosterol, Sd (3.2% Sterols)
Ethanol, Lf, Fr, Sd
Eugenol, EO
Fat, Fl, 0.1-11%; Lf 0.3–3.3%; Sd 16.8-22.3%
Fiber, Fl 1.0–14.8%; Lf 1.3–11.4%; Sd 12.0%
Formic acid, Fr, Sd
Furfural, EO
Glycolic acid Fl
Gossipetin, Fl
Gossypetin-3-glucoside, Fl
Gossypol, Sd 25.2%
Hexadecanoic acid, Sd
Hibiscetin, Fl
Hibiscic acid, Fl 1.5-2.3%
Hibiscin chloride
Hibiscin, Fl
Hibiscitrin, Pe
Hibiscretin, Fl
Iron, Fl 1-536; Lf 15-333
Isoamyl alcohol, Lf, Fr, Sd
Isopropyl alcohol, Lf, Fr, Sd
Lauric acid, Sd
Levulinic acid methyl ester, EO
Linoleic acid, Sd (14.4% Lipids)

Linolenic acid, Sd
Magnesium, Fl 0.224%
Malic acid, Lf 1.25%; St 0.6%; Fl 6.5%
Malvalic acid, Sd (1.3% Lipids)
Malvin, Fl
Manganese, Fl 0.151%
Methanol, Lf, Fr, Sd
Mucilage, Cx
Myristic acid, Sd (2.1% Lipids)
Myrtillin, Fl
Niacin, Fl -71; Lf 12-132
Nitrogen, Sd 3.29%
Oleic acid, Sd (34.0% Lipids)
Oxalic acid, Fl
Palmitic acid, Sd (35.2% Lipids)
Palmitoleic acid, Sd (2.0% Lipids)
Pectin, Fr 1.02%; Cx 3.19%
Pelargonic acid, Fr, Sd
Pentosans, Sd 15.8%
Phosphorus, Fl 180-4,348; Sd 6,000; Lf 480–6,458
Potassium, Fl 0.94%
Propionic acid, Fr, Sd
Protein, Fl 7.0-11.0%
Protocatechuic acid, Fl
Quercetin, Fr
Resin, Cx
Riboflavin, Fl 0-4; Lf 1–31
Sabdaretin, Fl
Sabdaritrin, Fl
Saponin, Rt
Selenium, Fl 143
Silicon, Fl 91
Sodium, Fl 382
Starch, Sd 11.1%
Stearic acid, Sd (3.4% Lipids)
Sterculic acid, Sd (2.9% Lipids)
Stigasterol, Sd
Sucrose, Cx 0.24%
Sulfur, Sd 0.4%
Tannic acid, Fr
Tartaric acid, Rt
Thiamin, Fl 0–3; Lf 0–12
Tin, Fl 10
Utalonic acid, Fl
Water, Lf 85.6%; Sd 7.6–12.9%; Fl 84.5-88.2%
Zinc, Tr, Fl

PHARMACOLOGICAL ACTIVITIES AND CLINICAL TRIALS

Acid phosphatase inhibition. Dried calyx, at a concentration of 10.0% of the diet in the ration of rats showed weak activity. Rats were fed cholic acid vs cholesterol-loaded animals[K08332].

Acidifying activity. Decoction of dried fruit juice administered orally to male human adults at a dose of 24.0 gm/day was inactive[K19490].

Alkaline phosphatase inhibition. Dried calyx, at a concentration of 10.0% of diet in the ration of rats, showed weak activity. Rats were fed cholic acid vs cholesterol-loaded animals[K08332].

Anthelmintic activity. Ethanol (95%) extract of dried leaves at a concentration of 50.0 mg/ml was inactive on *Lumbricus terrestris*[T14170].

Antibacterial activity. Seed oil, on agar plate was active on *Bacillus anthracis*, *Staphylococcus albus*, and inactive on *Proteus vulgaris* and *Pseudomonas aeruginosa*[T02040].

Antiedema activity. Methanol extract of flowers applied externally to mice at a dose of 2.0 mg/ear was active. Inhibition ratio (IR) was 17 vs 12-0-tetradecanoyl-phorbol-13-acetate (TPA)-induced ear inflammation[K11173].

Antifungal activity. Ethanol/water (1:1) extract of dried leaves at a concentration of 250.0 mg/ml on agar plate was active on *Aspergillus fumigatus*, *Aspergillus niger*, *Botrytis cinerea*, *Penicillium digitatum*, *Rhizopus nigricans*, *Trichophyton mentagrophytes*, and inactive on *Aspergillus niger*. Dose expressed as dry weight of plant[T16238]. Flowers, at a dose of 10.0 g/liter in broth culture was inactive on *Aspergillus flavus*. Aflatoxin formation decreased[T08142]. Water extract of dried flowers at a concentration of 500 mg/ml on agar plate, was active on *Aspergillus fumigatus*, *Botrytis cinerea*, *Fusarium oxysporum*, *Penicillium digitatum*, *Rhizopus nigricans, and Trichophyton mentagrophytes,* and inactive on *Aspergillus niger*. Dose expressed as dry weight of plant[T12725].

Antihypercholesterolemic activity. Dried calyx at a concentration of 5.0% of the diet in the ration of rats was active. Rats were fed cholic acid vs cholesterol-loaded animals[K08332].

Antihyperlipemic activity. Dried calyx at a concentration of 5.0% of the diet in the ration of rats was active. Rats were fed cholic acid vs cholesterol-loaded animals[K08332].

Antihypertriglyceridemia effect. Dried calyx at a concentration of 5.0% of the diet in the ration of rats was active. Rats were fed cholic acid vs cholesterol-loaded animals[K08332].

Anti-inflammatory activity. Decoction of dried fruit administered orally to human adults at a dose of 3.0 gm/person was active. In this clinical trial, 50 patients with kidney stones were treated with extract three times a day for seven days to one year. The extract showed anti-inflammatory action after operation. Dose expressed as dry weight of plant[P00098].

Antischistosomal activity. Water extract of dried seeds at a concentration of 10,000 ppm was inactive on *Schistosoma mansoni*[M26095]. Water extract of dried sepals at a concentration of 100.0 ppm was active on *Schistosoma mansoni*[M26095].

Antitoxic activity. Flowers, at a dose of 1.0 gm/liter in broth culture was active on *Aspergillus flavus*. The production of aflatoxin was inhibited[T08142].

Antiviral activity. Water extract of dried flowers at a concentration of 10% in cell culture was active on herpes virus type 2 and Vaccina virus and inactive on Influenza virus and Polio virus II[T09507].

Antiyeast activity. Ethanol/water (1:1) extract of dried leaves at a concentration of 250.0 mg/ml on agar plate was inactive on *Candida albicans* and active on *Saccharomyces pastorianus*. Dose expressed as dry weight of plant[T16238]. Water extract of dried flowers at a concentration of 500 mg/ml on agar plate was inactive on *Candida albicans* and active on *Saccharomyces pastorianus*. Dose expressed as dry weight of plant[T12725].

Choleretic activity. Water extract of flowers taken orally by human adults was active[A03087].

Creatinine level decrease. Decoction of dried fruit juice administered orally to male adults at a dose of 24.0 gm/day was active[K19490].

Cytotoxic activity. Ethanol (70%) extract of flowers, in cell culture was active on CA–Erlich–Ascites. Greatest effect only after 24 hours exposure[T00514]. Water extract of dried flowers at a concentration of 10.0% on cell culture produced weak activity on HELA cells[T09507].

Diuretic activity. Decoction of dried calyx administered by gastric intubation to rats at a dose of 1.0 gm/kg produced strong activity[T15295]. Water extract of flowers taken orally by human adults was active[A03087].

Estrogenic effect. Water extract of dried calyx administered intraperitoneally to female at a dose of 500.0 mg/kg was active. Results significant at $P < 0.001$ level[T15927].

Feeding deterrent (insect). Acetone extract of dried shoots, undiluted, was active on *Diacrisia obliqua*[T10822].

Genitourinary effect. Decoction of dried fruit juice administered orally to male adults at a dose of 24.0 gm/day was active. Decrease urinary levels of sodium, potassium, phosphate, uric acid, and calcium was demonstrated[K19490].

Glutamate-oxaloacetate-transaminase inhibition. Dried calyx, at concentration of 10.0% of the diet in the ration of rats was active. Rats were fed cholic acid vs cholesterol-loaded animals[K08332].

Glutamate-pyruvate-transaminase inhibition. Dried calyx, at a concentration of 10.0% of the diet in the ration of rats showed weak activity. Rats were fed cholic acid vs cholesterol-loaded animals[K08332].

Hypotensive activity. Ethanol (95%) extract of dried calyx administered intravenously to dogs at a dose of 200.0 mg/kg produced weak activity[T03823]. Water extract of dried calyx administered intravenously to cats at a dose of 25.0 mg/animal was active. Animals were anesthetized with alpha-chloralose. Effect blocked by atropine[M26310].

Water extract of flowers taken orally by human adults was active[A03087]. Water extract of flowers administered intravenously to dogs produced weak activity[A03597].

Intestinal motility inhibition. Water extract of dried calyx administered to dogs at a dose of 5.0% was active. Oral transit time assayed by first detection of phthalylsulphasalazine in blood. This dose was also active in rats. Assayed by transit of graphite-agar suspension[M30497].

Laxative effect. Water extract of flowers taken orally by human adults was active[A03087].

Mutagenic activity. Dried fruit on agar plate at a concentration of 50.0 mcg/plate was activity on *Salmonella typhimrium* TA100 and TA98. Metabolic activation required to obtain positive results[M09083]. Seed oil was active on *Salmonella typhimurium* TA100 and TA98. Metabolic activation was not required for activity[Ti3966].

Smooth muscle relaxant activity. Hot water extract of dried petals was active on the aorta of rats. IC_{50} 0.53 mg/ml vs ACh-induced contractions and IC_{50} 2.53 mg/ml when de-endotheliazed muscle strips were used[K16061]. Water extract of dried calyx, at a concentration of 2.0% was active on the ileum of rabbits. Effect not influenced by phentolamine, propanolol, haloperidol, and guanethidine[M30497].

Spasmogenic activity. Water extract of dried calyx at a concentration of 0.4 mg/ml was active on the frog rectus abdominus muscle. The effect was slightly antagonized by tubocurarine. A concentration of 1.0 mg/ml was active on rabbit's uterus. The effect was blocked by indomethacin and hydrocortisone, but not by atropine or cyperoheptadine[M26310]. The extract, at a concentration of 0.16% was active on the ileum of rabbits. Effect blocked by atropine[M30497].

Spasmolytic activity. Water extract of dried calyx at a concentration of 0.4 mg/ml was active on the rectus abdominus muscle of frogs. Effect antagonized by tubocurarine vs ACh-induced contractions. The extract was also active on the uterus of rats vs rhythmic contractions. Effect not antagonized by rantidine or propanolol. At a concentration of 5.0 mg/ml the extract was active on the tracheal chain of guinea pig vs ACh-, histamine-, and serotonin-induced contractions; active on the aorta of rabbits. Effect not antagonized by atropine, propanolol, or ranitidine vs norepinephrine-induced contractions[M26310]. At 10.0 mg/ml, the extract was active in one the diaphragms of rats. Physostigine and suxamethonium enhanced the effect vs electrically induced contractions[M26310]. Water extract of dried petals at a concentration of 0.6 mg/ml was active on the aorta of rats vs norepinephrine-induced contractions, and inactive vs K+-induced contractions[K23418].

Toxicity assessment. Hot water extract of dried calyx administered by gastric intubation to rabbits produced LD_{50} 129.1 gm/kg[T03823].

Uricosuric activity. Decoction of dried calyx administered to rats at a dose of 1.0 gm/kg was active[T15295].

Uterine relaxation effect. Water extract of flowers was active on the uterus of rats[A03597].

14 | Jatropha curcas

Miers.

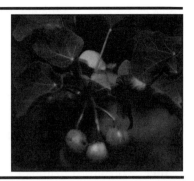

Common Names

American purging nut	South Africa	Physic nut	Nigeria
Ba dau me	Vietnam	Physic nut	South Africa
Bagbherenda	Fiji	Physic nut	Thailand
Barbados purging nut	South Africa	Physic nut	Virgin Islands
Bi ni da zugu	Nigeria	Physicnut bush	Fiji
Big purge nut	South Africa	Piao branco	Brazil
Black vomit nut	South Africa	Pignon d'inde	Rodrigues Islands
Botuje	Nigeria	Pindi	India
Cantal–muluung	Somalia	Pinnao de purga	Brazil
Cuta	Mexico	Pinon botija	Cape Verde Islands
Datiwan	Nepal	Pinon	Guatemala
Dinon	Puerto Rico	Pinon	Mexico
Eso botuje	Nigeria	Pinon	Peru
Etamanane	Senegal	Pinoncillo	Mexico
Fiki	Tonga	Punnetang	India
Habb el meluk	Sudan	Purge nut bush	West Indies
Habb–el–meluk	Mexico	Purge nut bush	West Indies
Jarak pagar	Indonesia	Purging nut	South Africa
Kananeranda	India	Purging nut	Thailand
Kasla	Philippines	Purging physic	Nicaragua
Lapalapa	Nigeria	Purgueira	Guinea–Bissau
Lohong	Vietnam	Ram jyoti	Nepal
Ma feng shu	Indonesia	Ramjeevan	Nepal
Medisiyen blen	West Indies	Ratanjyot	India
Mupfure–donga	Venda	Sabuu dam	Thailand
Nepalamu	India	Saimal	Nepal
Owulo idu	Nigeria	Sajiba	Nepal
Pe–fo–tze	Vietnam	Sajiwa	Nepal
Perchnut	West Indies	Sajiwan	Nepal
Physic nut bush	Fiji	Sajiyon	Nepal
Physic nut	Ghana	Satiman–G	Nepal
Physic nut	Guam	Sdatiwan	Nepal
Physic nut	Guyana	Seemanepaalam	India
Physic nut	Nepal	Tartago	Puerto Rico

From: Medicinal Plants of the World *By: Ivan A. Ross Humana Press Inc., Totowa, NJ*

Tong–chou	Vietnam	Ungume	Guinea–Bissau
Tubaang–bakod	Cape Verde Islands	Wedsiyen	Haiti
Tubang–bakod	Philippines	White physic nut	West Indies
Tubatuba	Guam	Wiriwiri	Fiji
Udukaju	Thailand		

BOTANICAL DESCRIPTION

A glabrous erect branched shrub of the EUPHORBIACEAE family, 2- to 5-meters high and has stout cylindrical green branches with viscid milky or reddish sap. Leaves are orbicular-ovate, angular or somewhat three- or five-lobed, 10- to 15-cm long, acuminate, base cordate with long petioles. Cymes are axillary, peduncled, the flowers greenish or greenish–white, 6- to 8-mm in diameter. The male and female borne at different times in the same inflorescence; petals 6- to 7-mm long. The petals are reflexed, stamens 10, the filaments of the inner five, connate. Capsules at first fleshy, becoming dry, of two or three cocci, subspherical, 2.5- to 4-cm diameter with seeds blackish, about 2-cm long.

The two species commonly found in the tropics, J. curcass, Linn., (physic nut) and J. Gossypifolia L. (bellyache bush), are the most widely used species in traditional medicine. No chemotaxonomic delimitation has been reported, and the species appear to have similar uses in folk medicine, same chemical constituents, and similar pharmacological activity. This profile mainly concerns J. curcass, but references are made on J. gossypifolia.

ORIGIN AND DISTRIBUTION

Native of tropical America it is now widespread. Rather common, particularly near habitations.

TRADITIONAL MEDICINAL USES

Brazil. Dried entire plant is taken orally, for sinusitis. Luffa operculata fruit and Jatropha curcas latex are mixed, practitioners advise caution in use because the latex is caustic[T08730].

Hot water extract of root is taken orally, as an Anthelmintic[W00408]. Infusion of dried leaf, seed or stem orally, is used for toothache, fever, and headache[K16654].

Cambodia. Seed extract taken orally as an abortifacient[A00115].

Cape Verde Islands. Hot water extract of the leaf is used to induce the secretion of milk especially in women recently given birth[W02885].

Colombia. Leaf decoction is used orally as a febrifuge[K16262].

Egypt. Hot water extract of seed is taken orally, for jaundice[L00484].

Fiji. Fresh leaf juice is taken orally for diarrhea, fever, and as a hemostatic. Fresh stem juice is used externally for sores and sprains. Stem juice is put in bath water[T10632].

Guam. Seeds when taken orally has been reported to be toxic. As few as three fruits may be fatal. In other cases, one to four seeds is purgative. Symptoms include irritation of throat, and intense abdominal pain. Also included are vomiting, dizziness, restlessness, muscular spasms, may become drowsy, then collapse (skin clammy, slow pulse), smoke victims show mydriasis[A05675].

Guatemala. Hot water extract of the leaf is taken orally as a treatment for dysentery[W01280].

Guinea-Bissau. Hot water extract of the leaf is administered orally to accelerate secretion of milk in postpartum women[A00455].

Haiti. Dried leaf decoction is taken orally, for edema, flu, and for cough. Fresh latex is rubbed on the tongue for buccal thrush. It is also used for burns, and cutaneous infections. In the treatment of bruises, the leaves are applied in sequence until one of them sticks onto the skin. This is allowed to dry, and then is replaced with another leaf until the bruise is healed[T13846].

India. Dried branches are applied externally, for joint pains. Young branches are warmed in the fire then placed on the affected joint[T10133]. Dried entire plant is taken orally as a purgative[K11284]. Fresh latex is used for toothache. Teeth are cleaned with the stem or leaf juice is applied to the painful tooth[T10321]. Fresh leaf juice is taken orally for epilepsy. Leaf juice is mixed with garlic powder and camphor and taken twice a day for four days[M23219]. Fresh leaves are used for guinea worms. Leaves are warmed and tied locally over the swelling to promote suppuration[M28491]. Hot water extract of seeds is taken orally as an abortifacient. The extract is also used for intestinal parasites. One seed is ground and soaked in water and small amounts of the extracts are drunk[M27166].

Indonesia. Hot water extract of stem is taken orally, to treat matrix cancer and stomach cancer. Mixed with *Ageratum conyzoides*, *Eclipta alba*, and *Spilanthes acmella*, taken after meals in morning and evening[A05827].

Ivory Coast. Fresh leaves are used as a hemostatic[T15327].

Mexico. Fresh sap is taken orally for mouth sores. Sap is rubbed on sore. The sap is also taken orally for whooping cough[T08016]. Latex is used to treat mouth infections[K16948].

Nepal. Hot water extract of leaf is taken orally as a lactagogue[A00020].

Nigeria. Decoction of root is taken orally to treat venereal disease. Dried leaf juice is used externally, to treat ringworm. Juice from the leaves are applied to affected part with cotton. Fresh latex is used to treat coated tongues. The latex is applied to the affected part of the tongue. Hot water extract of dried leaf is taken orally to treat diarrhea. Ten to fifteen leaves crushed with potash and added to 1–2 glasses of water. The liquid can be stored and taken when

required. Decoction made from young leaves is taken orally, as treatment for fever. Decoction prepared from the leaves are administered as a rectal injection to treat jaundice[K08933]. Hot water extract of dried seed is taken orally to treat arthritis[T05549]. Hot water extract of fresh root is taken orally for jaundice, as an antirheumatic and for dysentery. Infusion of fresh leaf and root is used externally as a treatment for ringworm. The infusion is used orally as an antipyretic and as an anticonvulsant[T06510].

Peru. Hot water extract of dried seed is taken orally, as a purgative[T15323].

Philippines. Fresh leaves are used to treat fever. Leaves are pasted on the temples or on the forehead. The fresh bark is used to treat fractures and sprains. Strips of bark are either blanched over steam or rolled over a low flame, then secured with bandage over the affected area[M29360].

Senegal. Fresh leaf juice is applied as an eye wash for eye diseases. The juice is also used externally for wounds and sores[M24038]. Hot water extract of dried entire plant is taken orally as a treatment for leprosy. Hot water extract of dried exudate is used for open sores. Hot water extract of dried leaves is taken orally as a treatment for odontalgia, syphilis, and for lung diseases. The extract is used externally for sores and for abscesses. Hot water extract of dried seed is administered orally as a treatment for enteralgia[M21947]. The seed is taken orally for stomachache[M24038].

Somalia. Infusion of dried seed is administered orally to treat constipation. Three seeds are roasted, peel is removed and the kernel crushed and added to a cup of tea. Tea is drunk and followed by 1–2 liters of milk. Purgation follows in 1–3 hours[A05675].

South Africa Decoction of dried seed is taken orally as a purgative[M27166].

Sudan. Seeds are used as an oral contraceptive[A04839] and as an Anthelmintic[T00368].

Thailand. Seed oil is administered orally as a laxative. Seed oil is taken and mixed with a little chili[T11371]. The entire plant is taken orally as a purgative[T12027].

Tonga. Infusion of dried leaves is taken orally to treat vaginal bleeding[T08685].

Venda. Decoction of dried root is administered orally as a treatment for toothache. The decoction is used to rinse the oral cavity. The decoction is also taken orally for sore throat[T08732].

Vietnam. Seed oil is taken orally as an abortive[A04766] and as an emmenaogue[A04942].

Virgin Islands. Hot water extract of the entire plant is administered orally as a treatment for the common cold, either alone or in combinations with other plants[W00903].

West Africa. Hot water extract of dried leaves are used externally for guinea worm. Hot water extract of seed oil is used externally for parasitic skin diseases as a rubefacient[M23617].

West Indies. Hot water extract of the leaf is taken orally for heart troubles[T00701].

Zaire. Infusion of dried leaf is taken orally for diarrhea, chest pains, coughs, anemia, urinary tract infections, diabetes, dental caries, and infected wounds. Externally, the infusion is used for infected wounds, and for skin diseases[K18012].

CHEMICAL CONSTITUENTS

(ppm unless otherwise indicated)

7-Keto-beta sitosterol, Sd
Alpha amyrin, Lf 67
Apigenin, Lf
Arabinose, Sd
Arachidic acid, Sd 0.180–0.288%
Ash, Sd 4.5%
Beta amyrin, Bk
Beta sitosterol, Sd
Beta sitosterol-beta-D-glucoside, Lf
Campesterol, Lf
Carbohydrates, Sd 33.5%
Curcain, Lx
Curcin, Sd
Curculathyrane A, Pl
Curculathyrane B, Pl

Curcusone A, Rt 0.0132%
Curcusone B, Rt 0.0127%
Curcusone C, Rt 0.001%
Curcusone D, Rt 0.004%
Daucosterol, Lf 0.014%
Dulcitol, Sd
Fat, Sd 30-48%
Fiber, Sd 15.5%
Friedelin, St 8
Friedelinol, St 0.001%
Fructose, Sd
Galactose, Sd
Glucose, Sd
Ikshusterol, Lf 27
Isovitexin, Lf
J. curcas flavonoid II, Lf 0.04%
J. curcas triterpene, Lf 0.05%
Jatropha curcas flavonoid I, Lf 0.065%
Jatropha factor C-1, Sd 65
Jatropha factor C-2, Sd 65
Jatrophin, Rt
Jatrophol, Rt
Jatropholone A, Rt
Jatropholone B, Rt
Jatropholone, Rt
Lignoceric acid, Sd Ol
Linoleic acid, Sd 8.796–16.224%
Linolenic acid, Sd 0.330–0.528%
Myristic acid, Sd 0.540–0.864%
N–1–triacontanol, Lf
Oleic acid, Sd 10.944–19.968%
Palmitic acid, Sd 3.9900–6.5325%
Palmitoleic acid, Sd 0.420–0.672%
Phorbol,12-deoxy–16–hydroxy, Sd Ol
Protein, Sd 16.2-18.6%
Raffinose, Sd
Rhamnose, Sd
Scoparone, St 10
Stachyose, Sd
Starch, Sd
Stearic acid, Sd 2.640–8.736%
Stigast-5-ene-3-beta, 7-alpha-diol, Lf
Stigast-5-ene-3-beta, 7-beta-diol, Lf 8
Stigasterol, Lf 0.025%
Sucrose, Sd
Tannin, Re 11.6-18.7%
Taraxasterol, Bk, Rt
Tomentin, Rt
Triacontan-1-ol, Lf 36
Vitexin, Lf
Water, Sd 6.6%
Xylose, Sd

PHARMACOLOGICAL ACTIVITIES AND CLINICAL TRIALS

Analgesic activity. Ethanol/water (1:1) extract of the aerial parts administered to mice intraperitoneally at a dose of 0.25 mg/kg was inactive vs tail pressure method[W00374].

Antibacterial activity. Ethanol/water (1:1) extract of the aerial parts at a concentration of 25 mcg/ml on agar plate was inactive against *Bacillus subtilis, E. coli, Salmonella typhosa*, and *Agrobacterium tumefaciens*[W00374]. Ethyl acetate extract of dried aerial parts at a concentration of 1.0 mg/disk on agar plate was inactive against *E. coli* and *Staphylococcus aureus*. Water extract of the dried aerial parts at a concentration of 1.0 mg/disk on agar plate was inactive against *E. coli* and *Staphylococcus aureus*[T16253]. Methanol extract of dried leaves at a concentration of 10 mg/ml on agar plate was inactive against *Escherichia coli, Klebsiella pneumoniae, Salmonella typhimurium, Pseudomonas aeruginosa*, and *Streptococcus mutans*. The extract was active against *Staphylococcus aureus*, MIC 125.0 mcg/ml[K18012]. A 95% ethanol extract of sun-dried leaves at a concentration of 50.0 mg/ml on agar plate was active against *Staphylococcus aureus* and inactive on *Bacillus subtilis*. Extract of 10 ml/g plant material. 0.1 ml extract placed in well on plate[T14752]. Ethanol (95%) extract of dried root and stem at a concentration of 10.0 mg/ml on agar plate was inactive on *Corynebacterium diptheriae* and *Diplococcus pneumoniae*, weakly active on *Staphylococcus aureus, Streptococcus pyogenes*, and *Streptococcus viridans*. Water extract of dried root and stem at a concentration of 10.0 mg/ml on agar plate was inactive on *Corynebacterium diptheriae* and *Diplococcus pneumoniae*, and weakly active on *Staphylococcus aureus, Streptococcus pyogenes* and *Streptococcus viridans*[M29966]. Methanol extract of dried seeds at a concentration of 2.0 mg/ml on agar plate was active on *Corynebacterium diptheriae* and *Pseudomonas aeruginosa* and inactive on *Neisseria* species, *Salmonella* species, *Staphylococcus aureus, Streptobacillus* species, and *Streptococcus* species[M27767].

Anticonvulsant activity. Ethanol/water extract (1:1) of the aerial parts at a concentration of 0.25 mg/kg administered intraperitoneally to mice was inactive vs electroshock-induced convulsions[W00374]. Ethanol (70%) extract of fresh root given to mice, both sexes, intraperitoneally was active vs metrazole-induced convulsions and weakly active vs strychnine-induced convulsions[T06510].

Antifungal activity. Ethanol/water (1:1) extract of the aerial parts at a concentration of 25 mcg/ml on agar plate was inactive against *Microsporum canis, Trichophyton mentagrophytes* and *Aspergillus niger*[W00374]. Ethyl acetate extract of the dried aerial parts at a concentration of 0.13 mg/ml on agar plate was active against *Msporum canis* but inactive against *Microsporum fulvum, M. gypseum*, and *Trichophyton gallinae*. Water extract of the dried aerial parts on agar plate was inactive against *M. canis, M. fulvum, M. Gypseum* and *Trichophyton gallinae*[T16353]. Acetone/water (50:50) extract of fresh latex on agar plate was inactive against *Microsporum gypseum* and *Trichophyton mentagrophytes*[M21482]. Methanol extract of dried leaves at a concentration of 10.0 mg/ml on agar plate was inactive against *Aspergillus niger* and *Microsporum gypseum*[K18012]. Ethanol (95%) extract of sun-dried leaves at a concentration of 50 mg/ml on agar plate was inactive on *Aspergillus niger*. Extract of 10 ml/gm plant material. 0.1 ml extract placed in well on plate[T14752].

Anticrustacean activity. Ethanol extract of dried seeds (defatted with petroleum ether) was inactive on *Artemia salina*. LD$_{50}$ > 1.0 mg/ml[T04904].

Antifertility effects. Fruit, when fed to female rats in the ration at a dose of 3.3% of the diet, exhibited 100% effect. Seeds, when fed to female rats in the ration at a dose of 3.3% of the diet exhibited 100% effect[A04839].

Anti-inflammatory activity. Ethanol/water (1:1) extract of the aerial parts at a dose of 0.25 mg/kg administered to male rats orally was inactive vs carrageenin-induced pedal edema. The animals were dosed one hour before carrageenin injections[W00374].

Antischistosomal activity. Ethanol (95%) extract of the plant at a concentration of 2000 mg/ml was inactive against Schistosoma, *Hematobium cercariae*, *H. Miracida*, and *H. ova*[T08931].

Antispasmodic activity. Ethanol/water (1:1) extract of the aerial parts administered to guinea pigs was inactive vs ACh. and histamine-induced spasms[W00374].

Antitumor activity. Chloroform extract of leaves and twigs at a dose of 12.5 mg/kg administered intraperitoneally to mice was active, 40% ILS. At a dose of 25.0 mg/kg 32% ILS, at 50.0 mg/kg 57% ILS on LEUK-P388. Ethanol (95%) extract of leaves and twigs at a dose of 100.0 mg/kg intraperitoneally in mice was active, 35% ILS, at a dose 25.0 mg/kg 41% ILS, and at 50.0 mg/kg 33% ILS on LEUK-P388. Petroleum ether extract of leaves and twigs administered intraperitoneally to mice was inactive on LEUK-P388[M00721]. Ethanol (defatted with petroleum ether) extract of dried seeds administered intraperitoneally to mice was inactive on LEUK–P388[T05868].

Antiviral activity. Ethyl acetate extract of the dried aerial parts in cell culture was active against Cytomegalovirus with LC_{50} 7.0 mcg/ml. Virus exposed to extract before infecting host cells[M29360]. LC_{50} > 100 mcg/ml (inactive) when infected host cells exposed to extract[T16253]. Ethyl acetate extract of the dried aerial parts in cell culture was active against Sindbis virus LC_{50} 88.0 mcg/ml. Infected host cells exposed to extract[M29360]. LC_{50} < 1.0 mcg/ml was active when virus exposed to extract before infecting host cells. Water extract of the dried aerial parts in cell culture was active against Cytomegalovirus, LC_{50} 22.0 mcg/ml when virus exposed to extract before infecting host cells. When infected host cells exposed to extract, a LC_{50} > 100 mcg/ml is obtained (inactive). Water extract of the dried aerial parts in cells culture against Sindbis virus was active, LC_{50} 32.0 mcg/ml when infected host cells exposed to extract. The extract is also active LC_{50} < 1.0 mcg/ml when virus exposed to extract before infecting host cells[T16253]. Methanol extract of dried leaves at a concentration of 100 mcg/ml in cell culture was weakly active against HIV virus[K21223]. Water extract of fresh leaves in cell culture was active against Tobacco Mosaic virus. The viral inhibitory activity was 40%[K09718].

Antiyeast activity. Ethanol/water (1:1) extract at a concentration of 25 mcg/ml on agar plate was inactive against *Candida albicans* and *Crytoccccus neoformans*[W00374]. Ethyl acetate extract of the dried aerial parts at a concentration of 1.0 mg/disk on agar plate was inactive against *Candida albicans* and *Saccharomyces cerevisiae*. The water extract at the same conditions was also inactive[T16253].

Barbiturate potentiation. Ethanol/water (1:1) extract of the aerial parts at a dose of 0.25 mg/kg administered to mice intraperitoneally was positive[W00374].

Cardiac effect. Methanol extract of dried seeds exhibited a negative chronotropic effect and a negative inotropic effect on the guinea pig atrium[T08446].

Crown gall inhibition. Ethyl acetate extract of the dried aerial parts in cell culture had a LC_{50} 1.4 mcg/ml (active). Assay system is intended to predict for antitumor activity. Water extract was also active with LC_{50} > 3.0 mcg/ml[T16253]. Ethanol (defatted with petroleum ether) extract of dried seeds at a concentration of 2.0 mg/ml on potato disk was inactive on *Agrobacterium tumefaciens*. Hexane extract was also inactive. Assay system was intended to predict for antitumor activity[T05868].

Cytotoxic activity. Ethanol/water (1:1) extract of leaves in cell culture was active against CA–9KB. $ED_{50} < 20.0$ mcg/ml[T08931]. Methanol extract of dried leaves at a concentration of 100.0 mcg/ml in cell culture was inactive against several human tumors[K21223]. Chloroform extract of leaves and twigs in cell culture was active on LEUK–P388, ED_{50} 1.1 mcg/ml and inactive on CA–9KB with $ED_{50} > 20.0$ mcg/ml[M00721]. Ethanol (95%) extract of leaves and twigs in cell culture was active on LEUK-P388, ED_{50} 2.4 mcg/ml, but inactive on CA-9KB, $ED_{50} > 20.0$ mcg/ml. Petroleum ether extract of leaves and twigs in cell culture was inactive on CA-9KB, $ED_{50} > 20.0$ mcg/ml, and also inactive on LEUK-P388, $ED_{50} > 20.0$ mcg/ml[M00721]. Ethanol (defatted with petroleum ether) extract of dried seeds in cell culture was active on LEUK-P388. ED_{50} 9.0 mcg/ml[T10632,M23219]. The extract was inactive on CA–9KB $ED_{50} > 30.0$ mcg/ml[T04904,T05868].

Diuretic activity. Ethanol/water (1:1) extract of the aerial parts at a dose of 0.125 mg/kg administered intraperitoneally to male rats was positive. Saline-loaded animals were used and urine was collected for four hours after dosing[W00374].

Glutamate dehydrogenase Stimulation. Dried seeds in the ration of chicken at a concentration of 0.5% of the diet was active. Sorbitol-dehydrogenase was also stimulated[K10612].

Hemolytic activity. Seed oil showed an ED_{100} 0.1 mg/ml on rabbit RBC in cell culture[K20893].

Hemostatic activity. Fifty percent concentrate of fresh leaf extract was active on human whole blood[T15327].

Hypoglycemic activity. Ethanol/water (1:1) extract of the aerial parts at a dose of 250 mg/kg administered orally to rats was inactive. There was less than 30% drop in blood sugar level[W00374].

Hypothermic activity. Ethanol/water (1:1) extract of the aerial parts at a dose of 0.25 mg/kg administered intraperitoneally to mice was inactive[W00374].

Irritant activity. Acetone extract of a commercial sample of seeds at a dose of 1.8 mcg/ear in mice was active. ID_{50} (24 hours). Seed oil at a dose of 25.0 mcg/ear exhibited weak activity. ID_{50} (24 hours)[N19357].

Larvicidal activity. Ethanol (95%) extract of dried fruits and leaves at a concentration of 100 ppm was weakly active against *Aedes fluviatilis*[K11645]. Methanol extract of dried leaves at a concentration of 10.0 mcg/ml on agar plate was inactive against *Candida albicans*[K18012].

Molluscicidal activity. Aqueous slurry (homogenate) of fresh entire plant was inactive against *Lymnaea columella*, $LD_{100} > 1$ M ppm. Aqueous slurry of the fruits, roots and leaves when tested was inactive against *Lymnaea cubensis*, $LD_{100} > 1$ M ppm[T04621]. Methanol extract of dried leaves at a concentration of 100 ppm was inactive against *Bulinus globosus*[T03107]. Ethanol (95%) extract of dried fruits and leaves at a concentration of 100 ppm was inactive against *Biomphalaria glabrata*. Hexane extract of the dried fruits and leaves at a concentration of 100 ppm was inactive against *Biomphalaria glabrata*[M17600]. Benzene extract of fresh fruit pulp was active against *Oncomelania hupensis*. LD_{50} 40 ppm. Butanol extract of fresh fruit pulp was active against *Oncomelania hupensis*. LD_{50} 45 ppm. Methyl chloride extract of fresh fruit pulp was active against *Oncomelania hupensis quadrasi*. LD_{50} 65 ppm. Water extract of fresh fruit pulp was active against *Oncomelania hupensis*. LD_{50} 50 ppm. Water extract of fresh fruit pulp was active against *Oncomelania hupensis quadrasi*. LD_{50} 18–25 ppm. LD_{90} 27–48 ppm. Methanol extract of fresh fruit pulp was active against *Oncomelania hupensis quadrasi*. LD_{50} 6.7 ppm[T04260]. Ethanol (95%) extract of dried root at a concentration of 100.0 ppm was active on *Bulinus truncatus*, 65% mortality. The water extract at a concentration of 160 ppm was weakly active, with 50% mortality[T04646]. Methanol extract of dried seed pods at a concentration of 100.0 ppm was inactive on *Bulinus globosus*[T03107]. Methanol extract of dried stembark at a concentra-tion of 100.0 ppm was inactive on *Bulinus globosus*[T03107].

Semen coagulation. Ethanol/water (1:1) extract of the aerial parts at a concentration of 2% was inactive in rats[W00374].

Spasmolytic activity. Butanol extract of dried leaves at a concentration of 0.2 mg/ml was active on guinea pig ileum. A 90.45% reduction in contraction was seen, vs ACh-induced contractions. A 28.49% reduction was seen vs KCl-induced contractions. Methanol extract of dried leaves at a concentration of 0.2 mg/ml was inactive on guinea pig ileum, vs ACh- and KCl-induced contractions[M27323].

Spermicidal effect. Ethanol/water (1:1) extract of the aerial parts was inactive in rats[W00374].

Toxicity assessment (quantitative). Ethanol/water (1:1) extract of the aerial parts administered intraperitoneally to mice demonstrated LD_{50} at 0.5 gm/kg[W00374]. Seed oil administered intragastrically to rats caused severe diarrhea and gastrointestinal inflammation. LD_{50} 6.0 ml/kg[K20893]. Fresh fruit pulp administered by gastric intubation at a dose of 10 gm/kg per day for three consecutive days gave a 100% mortality. 10 gm/kg given as a single dose was inactive[T04260].

Water extract of seed administered subcutaneously to mouse had a MLD_{50} 300.0 mcg/animal[W00298]. Seed oil administered subcutaneously to mice was active. LD_{100} 1.0 ml/animal. The toxic element is destroyed by heat[W04255]. Ethanol (95%) extract, methanol (70%) extract, and water extract of dried seeds, at doses of 500.0 mg/kg administered intraperitoneally to mice showed weak activity and caused some depression. Seed oil in the ration of rats at a dose of 15.0% of the diet was inactive. Roasted seeds, in the ration of rats at a dose of 48.0% of the diet, was active[T08446]. Seeds taken by children mistaken for edible nuts exhibited marked nausea, abdominal pain, and vomiting and some patients had diarrhea. Recovery was rapid[T15609]. Dried seeds fed to chicken in the ration at a concentration of 0.5% of the diet caused death. Toxic signs included poor growth, locomotor disturbances, and dullness. Also animals had hepatic, intestinal and renal lesions and significant increases in serum GOT, SHD, GDH, and total protein levels. Other signs included congested heart and its blood vessels, intestine and renal cortex, hepatocyte necrosis, erosion of intestinal mucous membranes, degeneration of renal tubular cells, and an increase in hepatic and cardiac lipid levels[K10612,K10618]. Water extract of fresh seeds at a dose of 5.0 mg/kg administered intraperitoneally to mice caused death within three days. Fresh seeds in the ration of mice at a dose of 25% of the diet caused death within 11 days[M17379].

15 | Lantana camara L.

Gaertn.

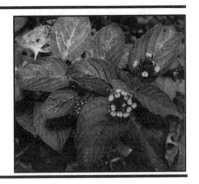

Common Names

Ach man	Guatemala	Mvuti	Tanzania
Aruppu	India	Orozus	Mexico
Big sage	West Indies	Orozuz	Mexico
Bonboye	West Indies	Panj phuli	India
Bunchberry	India	Pasarin	Panama
Bunga taya ayam	Guatemala	Pasarrion	Panama
Camara	Brazil	Pha-ka-krong	Guatemala
Camara	Canary Islands	Phakaa drong	Thailand
Cambara de espinto	Guatemala	Phakas krong	Thailand
Cariaquita	Colombia	Pink-edge red lantana	Australia
Cariaquito	West Indies	Prickly lantana	Guatemala
Carraquillo	Colombia	Ramtana	Guatemala
Cidreirarana	Brazil	Sanguinaria	Colombia
Common lantana	China	Siete negritos	Guatemala
Common lantana	China	Skastajat stuki	Mexico
Cuasquito	Guatemala	Sweet sage	Guyana
Cuencas de oro	Puerto Rico	Talatala	Guatemala
Frutilla	Mexico	Tembelekan	Guatemala
Gandheriya	India	Ti–plomb	West Indies
Gurupacha	Colombia	Tshidzimbambule	Venda
Hedge flower	Thailand	Venturosa	Canary Islands
Kayakit	West Indies	Venturosa	Colombia
Kiwepe	Tanzania	Verveine	West Indies
Lantana	Australia	Vielle fille	Rodrigues Islands
Lantana	India	White sage	Guatemala
Large leaf lantana	Guatemala	White sage	West Indies
Latora moa	Guatemala	Wild sage	India
Maviyakuku	Rwanda	Yellow sage	Guatemala
Mille fleurs	West Indies	Wild sage	West Indies
Mkinda	Tanzania		

From: Medicinal Plants of the World *By: Ivan A. Ross Humana Press Inc., Totowa, NJ*

BOTANICAL DESCRIPTION

An erect, branching shrub of the VERBENACEAE family, 0.5- to 2-meters high. Stems are four-angled, armed with hooked prickles. Leaves opposite, blade ovate, 4- to 10-cm long, with coarse surfaces and toothed margins. Flowers are dense, long-stalked, flat-topped, head-like, axillary spikes about 2.5-cm across. Corolla sympetalous, with a curved tube and a spreading limb about 8-mm wide, and it is yellow, orange, red, or pink in color. Fruit is a shiny, dark purple or black, globose drupe are 5- to 6-mm wide.

ORIGIN AND DISTRIBUTION

A native of tropical America, it is now a weed throughout the tropics, especially in coconut plantations, pastures, and waste places. The natural distribution now extends northwards to Texas and South Carolina. It has also become naturalized in many places, and forms impenetrable thickets in Ceylon and Indonesia.

TRADITIONAL MEDICINAL USES

Australia. Fresh fruit is eaten as a food. Mashed fresh leaves are applied to the skin to treat neurodermatitis, eczema, rashes, psoriasis, tinea, chicken pox, boils, bites, and to stop bleeding in traumatic injuries. Infusion is taken orally to treat whooping cough, catarrh, pulmonary problems, epidemic parotiditis, and to reduce fever. Decoction is used to treat aphids. Boil 500 gm of leaves in one liter of water, strain, and spray[K19791].

Brazil. Decoction of dried aerial parts is used externally as a treatment for mange[T15975]. Decoction of dried leaves is taken orally for malaria, for fevers, colds, headache, and as a tonic and febrifuge[T15975,K07977,K16654]. Dried plant is given orally to cows to treat mange[K18765].

Canary Islands. Infusion of the dried aerial parts is taken orally by pregnant women as an abortifacient[T10928].

Colombia. Decoction of hot water extract of the entire plant is taken orally to facili-

tate childbirth. Infusion of the hot water extract is taken orally as an emmenagogue[A00709]. Hot water extract of dried entire plant is taken orally as an emmenagogue[T15375].

East Africa. Ash from dried leaves is mixed with salt and taken orally for sore throat, cough, and toothache. Leaves are chewed for toothache. Vapor of boiling leaves is inhaled for headache and colds. Hot water extract of dried leaves is taken orally as a diaphoretic, stimulant, for jaundice, chest diseases, and for rheumatism. Fresh fruit is said to be toxic to children, although there is disagreement. Hot water extract of dried root is taken orally as a febrifuge; and for malaria, including quinine-resistant cases. Toxicity has been reported in sheep and cattle[T10828].

Guatemala. Decoction of dried leaves is taken orally to treat rheumatism. Decoction of *Lantana camara* and *Slaix chilensis* is used. The decoction is also taken orally to treat constipation and eczema. Infusion of dried leaves is taken orally as a tonic and stimulant[K19791]. Hot water extract is used externally for wounds, ulcers, bruises, sores, and infections of the skin and mucosa[T15445].

India. Ash of the entire plant is used externally for chronic ulcers[T08191]. Fresh leaves when ingested are reported to cause photodermatitis in domestic animals; it may also cause death[M25120]. Water extract of fresh leaves is applied to the eye to for eye injuries[M27166].

Indonesia. Decoction of fresh root is taken orally to treat gonorrhea and leukorrhea. Pounded fresh leaves are applied to the skin to treat boils. Leaves are taken orally to treat intestinal spasm, and as an emetic. Infusion is taken orally to treat rheumatism and as a diaphoretic. Tincture of fresh bark is taken orally as a tonic. Water extract of fresh flowers is given orally to children to treat cough[K19791]. Crushed leaves are applied on wounds[T10133]. Hot water extract of leaves are taken orally as a diaphoretic, carminative, and antiseptic[T15475].

Kenya. Dried stem is used as toothbrush[M25859].

Mexico. Dried leaves boiled with barley is given orally to women in childbirth. The decoction is taken orally to relieve indigestion, to treat rheumatism, as a stomach tonic, and to treat snakebite (poultice of crushed leaves are applied to the wound)[K19791]. The whole plant is rubbed with cold water to treat chills[K16948]. Water extract of fresh root is taken orally for dysentery; gastrointestinal pain, toothache, uterine hemorrhage, and excess menstrual discharge. Water extract of fresh shoots is taken orally for rashes. Used medicinally for "magical" illnesses comprising a variety of physiological illnesses and symptoms[T09735]. Infusion of dried fruits and leaves is taken orally for coughs[T08016]. Decoction of the leaf is taken orally as an appetizer and as a vomitive[K16948].

Nigeria. Infusion of fresh leaves and root is taken orally as an antiasthmatic, tonic, and as an anticonvulsant. Hot water extract of the fresh leaves and root is taken orally as an anticonvulsant[T06510].

Panama. Decoction of dried leaves are taken orally to treat colds and stomach afflictions[K19791]. Extract of the entire plant is taken orally for digestive disorders. For skin diseases, decoction of the whole plant in warm water is applied to affected skin areas[T01287].

Rwanda. Decoction of dried leaves is taken orally for malaria[M31549].

Southeast Asia. Pounded dried leaves are applied to the skin as a treatment for cuts; to treat swelling. Lotion is prepared from pounded leaves to treat rheumatism. Infusion of the dried leaves is taken orally to treat bilious fevers (usually have emetic effect)[K19791].

Surinam. Infusion of dried entire plant is used as a herbal bath[K19791].

Tanzania. Decoction of dried root is taken orally for stomachache and against vomit-ing. A grain of another plant species is added. Water extract is used externally for itching and rashes[T10828]. Fresh leaves are used in traditional medicine[T10354].

Thailand. Decoction of dried entire plant is taken orally for asthma. Crushed roasted leaves are used as a poultice for anti-inflammatory affections[T16711].

Tonga. Fresh leaf juice is applied cuts to prevent infection[K19791].

USA. Extract of the plant is taken orally as a carminative[K19791].

Venda. Fresh leaves macerated in cold water for several hours to two days is used as a eye drop for eye injury[T08732].

Venezuela. Hot water extract of dried stem is taken orally as an emmenagogue[T15375].

Vietnam. Leaf tea is taken orally as an emmenagogue[A04942].

West Africa. Infusion of dried leaves is taken orally to treat coughs, colds; as a diaphoretic; stimulant; to treat jaundice and chest pains. Used in bath for rheumatism[K19791].

West Indies. Hot water extract of leaves taken orally is a common remedy for dysmenorrhea[A03403,T00701] and fever[T00701]. Decoction of dried leaves is taken orally for cough, flu, and indigestion[T13846].

CHEMICAL CONSTITUENTS

(ppm unless otherwise indicated)

1-Triacontanol, Lf
3-Ketoursolic acid, Lf
8-Epi-loganin, Rt 70
Ajugose, Rt 0.19%
Aldehydes, Lf 12-14
Alpha amyrin, Lf, St
Alpha cellulose, St 30.6%
Alpha pinene, Lf
Amylase, Lf
Arachidic acid, Aer
Ash, Fr 3.7%; Sh 10.29%; St 3.5%
Beta sitosterol, Sd
Cadinene, Lf
Cadinol, Lf
Calcium, Fr 0.11%; Sh 0.61%
Camaric acid, Aer 0.119%
Camarinic acid, Aer 11.6

Camaroside, Lf 0.0181%
Camerene, Lf
Caryophyllene, Lf 0.04-0.16%
Catalase, Lf
Cedrene, Pl
Cineole, Lf
Cis-nerolidol, Pl
Citral, Lf
Diodantunezone, Rt
Dipentene, Lf
Essential oils, Fl 0.07%; Lf 0.05-0.32%
Eugenol, Lf
Farnesol, Pl
Fat, Sd 9.0–48.0%
Furfural, Lf
Furfuroids, St 21.6%
Gamma terpinene, Lf
Geniposide, Rt
Geraniol, Lf
Glucose, Aer
Glucosidasae, Lf
Glycine, Lf
Icterogenin, Lf
Invertase, Lf
Iso–diodantunezone, Rt
Isocamarene, Lf
Lamiridoside, Rt
Lancamacrone, Pl
Lantabetulic acid, Pl
Lantadene–A, Lf 0.3–0.7%
Lantadene–B, Lf 0.2%
Lantadenes, Lf 0.2–1.7%
Lantaiursolic acid, Rt 24
Lantanic acid, Lf
Lantanilic acid, Pl
Lantanolic acid, Lf
Lantanose A, Rt 310
Lantanose B, Rt 94
Lantic acid, Lf
Lantoic acid, Lf
Leucine, Lf
Lignin, St 14.0%
Linalool, Lf
Linoleic acid, Aer
Lipase, Lf
Magnesium, Fr 0.146%
Maltose, Aer
Manganese, Sh 308–412
Methyl-3-oxo–ursolate, Lf
Myristic acid, Aer
Nitrogen, Sh 0.88%
Oleanolic acid, Aer 57

Oleanonic acid, Lf 0.0241%
Oleic acid, Aer
Oxidase, Lf
P-cymene, Lf
Palmitic acid, Aer
Phellandral, Lf
Phellandrene, Lf 50–240
Phellandrone, Lf
Phosphorous, Sh 0.15%
Pomolic acid, Aer 9.5
Potassium, Sh 0.9%
Protein, Fr 5.1%; Sd 35.1%
Rhamnose, Aer
Sodium, Lf 0.82%
Stachyose, Rt 0.0695
Sugar, Fr 18%
Tannase, Lf
Tannin, Lf
Terpineol, Lf
Theveside, Rt 14–900, Lf 800,
Theviridoside, Rt 320–500
Trans–nerolidol, Pl
Triacontan–1–ol, Aer
Tyrosine, Lf
Valine, Lf
Verbascose, Rt 0.081%
Verbascoside, Pl
Verbascotetracose, Rt 0.043%
Water, Fr 76%

PHARMACOLOGICAL ACTIVITIES AND CLINICAL TRIALS

Acid phosphatase stimulation. Dried leaves administered to guinea pigs by gastric intubation were active[M05080].

Analgesic activity. Ethanol (95%) extract of leaves administered intraperitoneally to rats was only active with high doses[T00435].

Aniline hydroxylase induction. Dried leaves administered to guinea pigs by gastric intubation at a dose of 2.0 gm/kg was inactive[T08119].

Antibacterial activity. Decoction of dried leaves, in broth culture, was inactive on *Bacillus subtilis*, *Klebsiella pneumonia*, *Proteus vulgaris*, *Pseudomonas aeruginosa*, *Salmonella typhi*, *Sarcina lutea*, *Staphylococcus albus*, *Staphylococcus aureus*, and *Streptococcus mutans*[M18378]. Essential oil on agar plate was inactive on *Bacillus cereus*, *Escherichia coli*, *Pseudomonas aeruginosa*, and *Staphylococcus* *aureus*[T14976]. Ethanol (70%) extract of root, at a concentration of 100.0 mg/ml in broth culture, was inactive on *Bacillus subtilis* and *Escherichia coli*[T00693]. Fresh essential oil at undiluted concentration on agar plate was active on *Pseudomonas aeruginosa* and *Staphylococcus aureus*. The oil was inactive on *Bacillus cereus*, and *Escherichia coli*[T06640]. Leaf essential oil, at undiluted concentration on agar plate, was active on *Bacillus subtilis*, zone of inhibition 13.0 mm; *Escherichia coli*, zone of inhibition 9.5 mm; *Sarcina lutea*, zone of inhibition 12.0 mm; and weak activity on *Staphylococcus aureus*, zone of inhibition 2.5 mm[T01545]. Petroleum ether extract of dried leaves, in broth culture was active on *Salmonella typhi*, MIC 0.63 mg/ml; *Bacillus subtilis*, MIC 1.25 mg/ml, and *Sarcina lutea*, MIC 1.25 mg/ml. The extract was inactive on *Klebsiella pneumoniae*, *Proteus vulgaris*, *Pseudomonas aeruginosa*, *Staphylococcus albus*, *Staphylococcus aureus*, and *Streptococcus mutans*[M18378]. Saline extract of leaves, at a concentration of 1:10, on agar plate was active on *Staphylococcus aureus*[W01047]. Tincture of dried leaves (10 g of leaves in 100 ml ethanol), at a concentration of 0.1 ml/disk, on agar plate was active on *Bacillus subtilis*. The tincture was inactive on *Proteus vulgaris*, *Pseudomonas aeruginosa*, *Salmonella typhi*, *Shigella flexneri*, *Staphylococcus aureus*, and *Streptococcus pyogenes*. At 30 ml/disk, the tincture was active on *Pseudomonas aeruginosa* and inactive on *Escherichia coli*[T15445]. Water extract of fresh leaves at a concentration of 1.0% on agar plate was inactive on *Neisseria gonorrhea*[T10354].

Anticonvulsant activity. Ethanol (70%) extract of fresh leaves administered intraperitoneally to mice of both sexes at variable dosage levels was active vs metrazole and strychnine-induced convulsions[T06510].

Antifungal activity (plant pathogen). Ethanol (70%) extract of root, at a concentration of 100.0 mcg/ml, in broth culture was inactive on *Penicillium crustosum*[T00693].

Water extract of fresh leaves at a concentration of 1.0% was active on *Aspergillus niger* vs rot of tomato fruits caused by *A. niger* and aggravated by *Drosophila bucksii*[T15148]. Water extract of fresh shoots at undiluted concentration on agar plate was inactive on *Helminthosporium turcicum*[W01223].

Antifungal activity. Dried leaves undiluted on agar plate was active on *Aspergillus fumigatus* and *Aspergillus niger*[T11794]. Essential oil at undiluted concentration on agar plate was active on Alternaria species, *Aspergillus candidus*, *A. flavus*, *A. nidulans*, *A. niger*, *Cladosporium herbarum*, *Cunninghamella echinulata*, *Helminthosporium saccharii*, *Microsporum gypseum*, *Mucor mucedo*, *Penicillum digitatum*, *Rhizopus nigricans*, *Trichophyton rubrum*, and *Trichothecium roseum*. No activity was observed for *Fusarium oxysporum* and *Aspergillus fumigatus*[K08673]. Essential oil on agar plate was inactive on *Trichoderma viride*, *Aspergillus aegyptiacus* and *Penicillium cylopium*[T14976]. Ethanol/water (1:1) extract of dried seeds at a concentration of 10%/disk, on agar plate was inactive on *Aspergillus niger*[T08445]. Fresh essential oil at undiluted concentration on agar plate was inactive on *Penicillium cyclopium*, *Trichoderma viride*, and *Aspergillus aegyptiacus*[T06640]. Methanol extract of dried leaves at a concentration of 0.03% on agar plate was inactive on *Trichophyton mentagrophytes*[T06031]. Water extract of fresh leaves at a concentration of 1:1 on agar plate was active on *Fusarium oxysporum* F. Sp. Lentis. Extract represented 1 g dried leaf in 1.0 ml water[K18143].

Antihemorrhagic activity. Dried leaves applied externally on wounds as a paste was effective on 80% of the cases. Leaves taken orally by human adults checked bleeding in 94% of the cases of rectal and 100% of nasal bleeding[T12460].

Antimalarial activity. Chloroform extract of dried root bark showed weak activity on *Plasmodium falciparum*; IC_{50} 49.0 mcg/ml. The methanol extract was inactive; IC_{50}

499.0 mcg/ml, and the petroleum ether extract was active; IC_{50} 10.0 mcg/ml vs hypoxanthine uptake by Plasmodia[M25016].

Antimutagenic activity. Methanol extract of dried leaves, at a concentration of 50.0 microliters/disk on agar plate was inactive on *Escherichia coli B/R–WP2–TRP*[T08867].

Antimycoplasmal activity. Petroleum ether extract and decoction of dried leaves in broth culture were inactive on *Mycoplasma hominis* and *Mycoplasma pneumoniae*[M18378].

Antitrichomonal activity. Methanol extract of dried leaves at a concentration of 1.0 mg/ml was inactive on *Trichomonas vaginalis*[M31549]. Dried leaves, undiluted on agar plate was active on *Candida vaginalis*[T11794]. Ethanol (70%) extract of root at a concentration of 100.0 mcg/ml in broth culture was inactive on *saccharomyces cerevisiae*[T00693]. Methanol extract of dried leaves at a concentration of 0.03% on agar plate was inactive on *Candida albicans*[T06031]. Petroleum ether extract and decoction of dried leaves in broth culture were inactive on *Candida albicans*, *Candida tropicalis*, and *Saccharomyces cerevisae*[M18378].

ATPase(mg++) stimulation. Dried leaves administered by gastric intubation to guinea pigs at a dose of 2.0 gm/kg was equivocal. Results significant at $P < 0.001$ level[T08119]. At daily dosing for three days, the activity was positive[T05377].

ATPase(Na+/Ca++) stimulation. Dried leaves administered to guinea pigs by gastric intubation at a dose of 2.0 g/kg, was active. Results significant at $P < 0.001$ level[T08119].

Bile lithogenic suppression. Leaves administered orally to ewe at a dose of 100.0 gm/animal was active[K03660].

Bronchodilator activity. Hot water extract of dried leaves administered intravenously to guinea, at a dose of 1.5 ml/animal, was inactive[M29843].

Cathepsin B induction. Dried leaves administered by gastric intubation to guinea pigs was active[M05080].

CNS depressant activity. Ethanol (70%) extract of fresh leaves administered to mice of both sexes intraperitoneally, at variable dosage levels was active[T06510]. Ethanol (95%) extract of leaves administered intraperitoneally to mice was active[T00435].

Cytochrome C reductase inhibition. Dried leaves at a dose of 2.0 gm/kg administered to guinea pigs by gastric intubation was equivocal[T08119].

Cytochrome oxidase induction. Dried leaves, at a dose of 2.0 gm/kg administered to guinea pigs by gastric intubation, was active when dosed daily for three days[T05377].

Cytochrome P-450 induction. Dried leaves at a dose of 2.0 gm/kg administered by gastric intubation to guinea pigs was inactive[T08119].

Dermatitis producing effect. Dried leaves applied externally on a 50-year-old patient with recurrent contact dermatitis was active. The patient was patch tested to determine sensitivity[M25250]. Ethanol (95%) extract of fresh leaves, at a dose of 2.0 mg/kg administered by gastric intubation to rats was active. Rats developed photodermatitis within three minutes of being exposed to sunlight[M25120]. Fresh leaves, used externally on human adults was active vs patch test. 1.82% of 207 patients were sensitive[T14330].

Enzyme activity. Dried entire plant given to guinea pigs was active on acid phosphatase stimulation, results significant at $P < 0.01$ level. The plant was inactive on alkaline phosphatase stimulation and inhibition; active on BUN raising effect; glutamate dehydrogenase stimulation, results significant at $P < 0.01$ level; glutamate oxaloacetate transaminase stimulation, results significant at $P < 0.01$ level; glutamate pyruvate transaminase inhibition result significant at $P < 0.05$ level; lactate dehydrogenase stimulation, results significant at $P < 0.01$ level; sorbitol dehydrogenase stimulation, results significant at $P < 0.01$ level[T10651]. Dried leaves, at a dose of

2.0 gm/kg administered to guinea pigs by gastric intubation, was equivocal. NADH–ferricyanide reductase inhibition. Results significant at P < 0.001 level[T08119]. An increase in the activity of glucokinase, and aldolase in the hepatic postmitochondrial fraction[M05080]. At daily dosing for three days, glutamate dehydrogenase stimulation was active[T05377]. The dose was active on glutathione-S-transferase induction[T08119].

Gall bladder paralysis. Entire plant administered to ewe at a dose of 600.0 gm/animal orally was active[L01365].

Glucose-6-Phosphatase inhibition. Dried leaves, at a dose of 2.0 gm/kg administered to guinea pigs by gastric intubation, was active[M05080].

Glutamate oxaloacetate transaminase stimulation. Dried leaves, at a dose of 6.0 gm/kg administered to cows by gastric intubation, was active[W04173].

Hair inhibition effect. Dried shoots administered to guinea pigs orally, at a dose of 20.0 gm/kg was active. the animals developed alopecia[T03008].

Hematopoietic activity. Dried entire plant increased the number of erythrocytes, and leukocytes. Results significant at P < 0.01 level[T10651].

Hemotoxic activity. Dried leaves administered to ewe by gastric intubation was active. It decreased blood's ability to coagulate[T08527].

Hepatotoxic activity. Dried aerial parts administered to buffalo, cow, ewe, and guinea pigs, orally caused obstructive jaundice, photosensitization, and rise in serum glutamic oxaloacetic transaminase activity, and histopathological changes in different organs of ewe; histopathological changes in liver and kidneys in cows; histopathological changes in various organs in guinea pigs[T05878]. Dried entire plant in the ration of cow was active[M25859]. Dried flowers administered to guinea pigs orally at a dose of 20.0 gm/kg was inactive[T03008]. Dried leaves in the ration of cows was active. The chief signs were photosensitization and jaundice. Dried leaves, at a dose of 6.0 gm/kg administered by gastric intubation to cows was active. Serum bilirubin increase, and autopsy showed liver damage[W04173]. At 2.0 gm/kg administered by gastric intubation to guinea pigs, there was a decrease in protein content of hepatic microsomes and in the ratios of phospholipid:protein and cholesterol:protein[T08119]. Dosing guinea pigs daily for three days, decreased in dry weight, DNA, RNA, and protein content of liver at necropsy[T03591]. When administered orally to guinea pigs at a dose of 6.0 gm/kg, serum bilirubin increased markedly. Dried shoots administered orally to guinea pigs at a dose of 20.0 gm/kg was inactive[T03008]. Leaves administered to ewe orally at a dose of 200.0 g/animal was active[M00352].

Hypertensive activity. Ethanol (95%) extract of leaves administered intravenously to dogs was active[T00435].

Hypotensive activity. Alkaloid fraction of dried leaves when administered to dogs intravenously, showed acceleration of respiration and "shivering"[W03885]. Ethanol (95%) extract of leaves administered intraperitoneally to mice was active[T00435].

Immunosuppressant activity. Powdered dried leaves at a dose of 200.0 mg/kg administered orally to sheep, was active. Sheep showed suppression of both cellular and humoral immunity[M28758].

Insect repellent activity. Water extract of fresh leaves at a concentration of 1.0% was active vs rot of tomato fruits caused by *Aspergillus niger* and aggravated by *Drosophila bucksii*[T15148].

Insecticidal activity. Petroleum ether extract of dried leaves at a concentration of 1.0 gm/liter was inactive on *Lutzomyia longipalpis*[M31056]. Ethanol (95%), and petroleum ether extracts of dried plant at concentrations of 50.0 mcg were inactive on *Rhodnius neglectus*[K18765]. Petroleum ether extract of the entire plant at a concentration of 100.0 ppm was active on *Culex quinquefasciatus*. 42% mortality[T08384].

Juvenile hormone activity. Dried leaves was active on *Dysdercus koenigii*[T04002].

Lactate dehydrogenase stimulation. Dried leaves administered by gastric intubation to guinea pigs was active[M05080].

Lipid peroxide formation inhibition. Dried leaves fed to guinea pigs in the ration was active[T06540].

Liver effects. Ethanol (95%) extract of fresh leaves, at a dose of 1.0 gm/kg administered by gastric intubation to rats was active. Bromosulphalein was injected into rats and excretion by the liver into bile was measured. Excretion was impaired indicating impaired liver function[M25120].

Molluscicidal activity. Aqueous homogenate of the fresh entire plant was inactive on *Lymnaea columella* and *L. cubensis*. Fruits, leaves and roots were tested[T04621]. Ethanol (80%) extract, at a concentration of 200.0 mg/liter was inactive on *Biomphalaria pfeifferi* and *Bulinus truncatus*[M26126]. Ethanol (95%), and water extracts of dried stem bark at concentrations of 1000 ppm, showed weak activities on *Biomphalaria glabrata* and *Biomphalaria straminea*[W02949]. Powdered dried leaves, at a concentration of 10,000 ppm, produced weak activity[T13890].

Molting activity (insect). Dried leaves was active on *Dysdercus koenigii*[T04002].

NADH reductase stimulation. Dried leaves, at a dose of 2.0 gm/kg administered to guinea pigs by gastric intubation, was active when dosed daily for three days[T05377].

NADPH-cytochrome C reductase stimulation. Dried leaves at a dose of 2.0 g/kg administered to guinea pigs by gastric intubation was equivocal[T08119].

Nephrotoxic activity. Dried leaves at a dose of 2.0 gm/kg administered to guinea pigs by gastric intubation at daily dosing for three days decreased in dry weight DNA, RNA and protein of kidneys at necropsy[T03591].

Nucleotidase inhibition. Dried leaves, at a dose of 2.0 gm/kg administered to guinea pigs by gastric intubation was equivocal[T08119].

Pharmacokinetics. Dried aerial parts administered to ewe intraruminal at a dose of 4.0 gm/kg showed most of the toxin was retained in the rumen; it was readily absorbed in the small intestine, as well as the stomach and large intestine[M05465].

Pheromone (insect sex attractant). Ether extract of leaves and twigs was active on male Mediterranean fruit fly; equivocal on *Aspiculurus tetraptera*, male and female *Dacus dorsalis*, and male and female melon fly[T10330].

Pheromone (insect sex attractant and signaling) Ether extract of the aerial parts was active on *Dacus dorsalis* (male) and equivocal on *Aspiculurus tetraptera*, *Dacus dorsalis* (female), Mediterranean fruit fly (male), and melon fly[T10330].

Pheromone (signaling). Ether extract of leaves and twigs was active on male Mediterranean fruit fly; equivocal on *Aspiculurus tetraptera*, *Dacus dorsalis* (females and males), and melon fly (males and females)[T10330].

Photosensitizer activity. Aerial parts in the ration of livestock was active[K13618]. Dried leaves in the ration of cows was active[W04174].

Plant germination inhibition. Chloroform extract of dried leaves was equivocal vs *Amaranthus spinosus* (13% inhibition)[T03367]. The water extract at a concentration of 50.0% was active. The effect was tested in spores of *Cyclosporum dentatus*. Methanol and water extracts of dried root at concentrations of 50.0 ppm were active on beans[T09735], and the spores of *Cyclosporum dentatus*[T15561], respectively. Water extract of dried inflorescence at a concentration of 50.0% was active on spores of *Cyclosporum dentatus*. Water extract of dried stem, at concentration of 50.0% was active. The effect was tested in spores of *Cyclosporum dentatus*[T15561].

Plasma bilirubin increase. The dried entire plant fed to guinea pigs was active[T10651].

Protein synthesis inhibition. Dried leaves, at a dose of 6.0 gm/kg administered orally to guinea pigs, was active[T03008].

Respiratory depressant. Ethanol (95%) extract of leaves administered intravenously to dogs was active[T00435].

Smooth muscle relaxant activity. Ethanol (95%) extract of leaves was active on rat duodenum. Tissue become refractory with high concentrations[T00435].

Smooth muscle stimulant activity. Alkaloid fraction of dried leaves was active on rat intestine[W03885]. Ethanol (95%) and water extracts of bark and leaves at concentrations of 0.1 mg/ml were active on guinea pig ileum[M22196].

Succinate dehydrogenase stimulation. Dried leaves at a dose of 2.0 g/kg administered to guinea pigs by gastric intubation was active with daily dosing for three days[T05377].

Toxic effect. Chromatographic fraction of dried leaves, at a dose of 125.0 mg/kg administered to guinea pigs by gastric intubation was active. Treated animals became icterus, sedated, and photosensitive. Bilirubin levels were generally elevated[M17781]. The ethanol (95%) extract administered to rats was also active[W04097]. The dried leaves when administered to cows at a dose of 6.0 gm/kg by gastric intubation was active. Autopsy showed liver damage and gastroenteritis[W04173]. At a dose of 2.0 gm/kg dried leaves administered by gastric intubation to guinea pigs was active. The dose caused a decrease in hepatic mitochondrial protein content. The phospholipid to protein ratio did not change, but there was a marked increase in the cholesterol to protein ratio and the cholesterol to phospholipid ratio. Mitochondrial swelling, in the absence of or presence of ascorbic acid, decreased in hepatic mitochondria from Lantana-intoxicated guinea pigs. Daily dosing for three days produced toxicity, including yellowness of conjunctiva and ears and photosensitization within five days[T05377]. At a dose of 6.0% g/kg, dried leaves administered to rabbits by gastric intubation was active. Toxicity included ictericity, anorexia, and decreased fecal output. Hepatotoxicity was observed histo-pathologically[M20781]. Dried entire plant at a dose of 4.0 gm/animal administered to buffalo by gastric intubation was active[T01545]. Fresh entire plant administered to steer by gastric intubation at variable dosage levels, produce toxicities that included weakness, anorexia, icterus, constipation, dehydration, photosensitization, depression, and hepatotoxicities. When administered orally, icterus, hydrothorax, and dehydration were evident. Numerous hepatotoxicities and renal toxicities were seen[M24764]. Fresh leaves in the ration of dogs was active. Kidney and liver damage on a German Shepherd was reported. Other cases are reported on sheep, guinea pigs, horses, cattle, and others. The leaves in the ration of cattle, a dose of 350.0 mg/animal caused photosensitization, dermatitis, liver and kidney damage, intestinal hemorrhage, paralysis of the gall bladder and death in 1–4 days[K20147]. Water extract of fruit administered to rats intraperitoneally was active, 2/2 deaths. The extract of unripe fruits caused 4/5 deaths[K00334].

Toxicity assessment (quantitative). Ethanol/water (1:1) extract of the entire plant administered to mice intraperitoneally produced $LD_{50} > 1.0$ gm/kg[A04819].

UDP-glucuronyl transferase inhibition. Dried leaves administered to guinea pigs by gastric intubation to guinea pigs was active. Results significant at $P < 0.001$ level[T08119].

Uterine relaxation effect. Alkaloid fraction of dried leaves was active on rat uterus. There was inhibition of motility[W03885].

Uterine stimulant effect. Water extract of root was inactive on rat uterus[A03531].

Xanthine oxidase stimulation. Dried fruit, at a dose of 20.0 gm/kg, when administered to guinea pigs orally was inactive. Enzymes were measured in liver and kidney. Dried leaves at a dose of 6.0 gm/kg administered to guinea pigs orally was active. Enzyme was measured in liver and kidney[T03008]. Dried shoots administered to guinea pigs at a dose of 20.0 gm/kg was inactive. Enzyme measured in liver and kidney[T03008].

16 | Macuna pruriens

(L) DC.

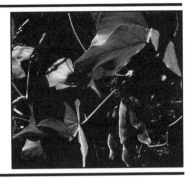

Common Names

Alkushi	Pakistan	Kavanch	India
Alkusi	India	Kawach	India
Atmagupta	India	Kawanch	India
Baidhok	India	Kawanch	Pakistan
Belki	India	Kawanh	India
Cigu	Thailand	Kerainch	India
Cowage	India	Kewanch	India
Cowhage	Nepal	Konch	India
Cowitch	Trinidad	Konchkari	Pakistan
Cowitch	Guyana	Kowez	India
Cowitch vine	Virgin Islands	Metaftum	Guinea–Bissau
Cussu	India	Mijeh	Thailand
Demar pirkok	Panama	Nipay	Philippines
Dulagondi	India	Pois a gratter	Trinidad
Ganhoma	Guinea–Bissau	Poua grate	Guadeloupe
Goncha	Pakistan	Pwa grate	Haiti
Horseeye bean	Thailand	Pwa gwate	Trinidad
Kaocho	Nepal	Sijeh	Thailand
Kapikachchhu	India	Taingilotra	Madagascar
Kapikachchu	India	Tainkilotra	Madagascar
Kauso	Nepal	Talcodja	Guinea–Bissau
Kausva	Nepal	Vetvet bean	Japan
Kavach	India	Wanduru–me	Sri Lanka

BOTANICAL DESCRIPTION

A vine of the PAPILIONACEAE family. The seeds of *Macuna pruriens* are black in color with pale brown specks, uniform in shape, 9- to 12-mm long with funicular hilum and cellular pit growth around the hilum. The seed coat is hard, thick, and glossy. The embryo completely fills the seed and is made up of two large fleshy cotyledons. Transverse section of seed shows an outer testa with a palisade epidermis made up of a rod-shaped macrosclereids with thickened anticlinal walls.

ORIGIN AND DISTRIBUTION

Originated in India, it is now commonly found throughout the tropics.

From: Medicinal Plants of the World *By:* Ivan A. Ross *Humana Press Inc., Totowa, NJ*

TRADITIONAL MEDICINAL USES

Brazil. Alcohol extract of dried seeds is taken orally as a nerve tonic. Alcohol and water extracts are taken orally as aphrodisiac[K20642].

Guadeloupe. Seeds crushed and mixed with syrup is given orally to infants as a vermifuge[T07660].

India. Hot water extract of dried fruit is administered orally to children in cases of stomach worms. Overdoses are fatal[T07201]. Water extract of leaves is taken orally as a nerve tonic, in dysentery, as an aphrodisiac, and for scorpion stings[M27166]. Powdered pod trichomes is taken orally as an anthelmintic. About four to five pod hairs are taken along with milk or buttermilk[K23365]. Hot water extract of root is taken orally as an emmenagogue[A04132]. Dried root is used for rheumatism and gout. Roots of *Macuna pruriens* and *Hymenodictyon excelsum* heated in mustard oil, which is then rubbed on the affected area[M23826]. Hot water extract of dried root is taken orally for delirium in Ayurvedic and Unani medicine[T05894]. Dried powdered root is taken orally with honey as a blood purifier, diuretic, and to dissolve kidney stones[T07731]. Fresh root is taken orally to relieve dysmenorrhea, paving the way for effective conception in future menstrual cycles. Paste made from *Macuna pruriens*, *Pygaeopremna herbacea*, *Tephrosia purpurea*, and *Gardenia turgida* roots, plus a few cloves of *Allium sativum* is given. Twenty grams of the paste is given on day three of menstruation[T09302]. Seeds are taken orally by male human adults to cure night dreams and impotency, to promote fertility, and as an aphrodisiac to increase seminal fluid and manly vigor[A04300]. Hot water extract of boiled seeds is taken by male human adults as an aphrodisiac[A06590]. Powdered seeds, taken with milk (five gm three times a day with sufficient quantity of milk), is used for diarrhea[K23294]. As an aphrodisiac, two seeds are powdered and taken with a cup of cow's milk[K23365]. Decoction of seed is taken orally for scorpion stings and snakebite[M27166]. Hot water extract of seeds is taken orally as a Nervine[T05894]. Seeds taken orally, is used as an aphrodisiac in Ayurveda and Unani medicine[T05894]. Decoction of dried seeds is taken orally for abortion[K16006], as an aphrodisiac[T03102] and sexual debility[T03252]. For persistent coughs, seeds are placed over a red hot plate or burning charcoal, and the fumes inhaled through the mouth[T07823]. Decoction of dried seeds together with *Terminalia arjuna* and *Sida retusa* is taken orally for pulmonary tuberculosis[T16239]. Fresh seeds cooked in goat's milk are taken orally as an aphrodisiac and for seminal weakness and impotence[T07731]. Hot water extract of dried seed pods is taken orally as an Anthelmintic in Ayurvedic and Unani medicine[T05894].

Guinea–Bissau. Plant juice is taken orally as an emmenagogue. Seed is taken orally as an aphrodisiac[A00455].

Haiti. Decoction of dried fruit is taken orally for intestinal parasites[T13846].

Ivory Coast. Hot water extract of the entire plant is taken orally as an emmenagogue[A01966].

Madagascar. Decoction of water extract of seeds is taken orally as an aphrodisiac (120 gm/seeds in one liter milk)[A04923].

Mozambique. Hot water extract of seeds is taken orally as an aphrodisiac[L01568].

Nepal. Hot water extract of seeds is taken orally as an aphrodisiac[A00020].

Nigeria. Dried leaf extract is used to treat snakebite[K20898].

Pakistan. Hot water extract of seeds is taken orally as an aphrodisiac[A01908].

Philippines. Fresh stem sap is used to treat sore/wind burns. A fresh stem is cut off on both ends, and the sap is blown from one end to the other over the mouth of the child[M29360].

Thailand. Dried leaves and stem are used for burns and cuts. *Oroxylum indicum* bark and *Macuna pruriens* leaves are pounded together and applied to burns and cuts[T11371].

Trinidad. Crushed seeds are taken orally with molasses for intestinal worms[A00701].

Virgin Islands. Hot water extract of the entire plant is taken orally for worms[W00903].

CHEMICAL CONSTITUENTS

(ppm unless otherwise indicated)

1-Methyl-3–carboxy-6,7-dihydroxy-1,2,3,4–Tetrahydroisoquinolone, Sd
5-Hydroxytryptamine, Sd, Pod trich, Fr, Lf, St
5-Methoxy tryptamine,N-N-dimethyl, Lf 25; St, Fr
5-Methoxy-N,N-dimethyltryptamine-N-oxide, Sd
5-Oxyindole-3-alkylamine, Sd
6–Methoxyharman, Lf
Alanine, Sd 0.54–1.16%
Arachidic acid, Sd 65–1,385
Arginine, Sd 1.24–2.6%
Ash, Sd 3.0-4.4%
Aspartic acid, Sd 1.99–4.21%
Behenic acid, Sd 140–2,265
Beta carboline, Sd
Beta sitosterol, Sd
Bufotenine, Lf, St, Fr
Calcium, Sd 1,320–1,600
Carbohydrates, Sd 52.9–66.7%
Choline, Lf, Sd, Sh, St, Rt
Cis-12,13-epoxyoctadec–trans-9-cis-acid, Sd
Cis–12,13–epoxyoctadec–trans-9-enoic-acid, Sd
Cis-12-1-octadec-trans-9-enoic acid, Sd 01.0%
Cystine, Sd 1,400–2,965
DOPA, Sd 0.24–4.80%
Fat, Sd 0.7–6.3%
Fiber, Sd 4.6–9.5%
Gallic acid, Sd
Glutamic acid, 1.91–4.04%
Glutathione, Sd
Glycine, Sd 0.72–1.53%
Histidine, Sd 0.33–0.69%
Iron, Sd 200
Isoleucine, Sd 0.75–1.59%
Kilocalories, Sd 0.34–0.40%
Lecithin, Sd 10%
Leucine, Sd 1.18–2.52%
Linoleic acid, Sd 715–30,680
Linolenic acid, Sd 265–5,800
Lysine, Sd 0.97–2.10%
Macuna pruriens alkaloid P, Sd 27
Macuna pruriens alkaloid Q, Sd
Macuna pruriens alkaloid R, Sd 66
Macuna pruriens alkaloid S, Sd 33
Macuna pruriens alkaloid X, Sd
Methionine, Sd 1,875–3,975
Mucunadine, Sd
Mucunain, Sd
Mucunine, Sd
Myristic acid, Sd 15–125
N,N-Dimethyltryptamine, Sd, St, Fr, Lf 60
N,N-Dimethyltryptamine-N-oxide, Sd
Niacin, Sd 17–34
Nicotine, Sd
Oleic acid, Sd 735–11,400
Palmitic acid, Sd 0.14–3.38%
Palmitoleic acid, Sd 35–630
Phenylalanine, Sd 0.75–1.59%
Phosphorus, Sd 0.32–0.47%
Proline, Sd 0.92–1.96%
Protein, Sd 15.5–33.1%
Prurienidine, Sd 110
Prurieninine, Sd 11
Riboflavin, Sd 1.1–2.7
Saponins, Sd 2.1%
Serine, Sd 0.77–1.62%
Serotonin, Sd
Stearic acid, Sd 390–12,475
Thiamin, Sd 1.4–5.7
Threo-12-octadec–trans–9-enoic acid, Sd Ol
Threo–12-1,octadec–cis–9-enoic acid, Sd Ol
Threonine, Sd 0.63–1.33%
Tryptamine, Sd
Tyrosine, Sd 0.798–1.691%
Valine, Sd 0.86–1.82%
Vernolic acid, Sd Ol 4.0%
Water, Sd 9.1–11.4%

(Amino acids calculated by multiplying by protein/6.25 mg/gm N.)

PHARMACOLOGICAL ACTIVITIES AND CLINICAL TRIALS

Anabolic activity. Plant administered orally to castrated adult and young male mice at a dose of 7.70 mg/animal was active. Animals were pretreated with testosterone over a period of four days. The plant was mixed with *Lactuca scariola*, *Hygrophila spinosa*, *Parmelia parlata*, *Argyreia speciosa*, *Tribulus terrestris*, and *Leptadenia reticulata*. When administered to infant mice at a dose of 22.0 mg/animal, the mixture was active. There was increased maltase activity of dorsoventral prostate and increase in fructose content of seminal vesicles[W00486].

Analgesic activity. Ethanol (95%) extract of dried fruit trichomes administered intragastrically to rats at a dose of 2.0 gm/kg was active vs acetic acid-induced writhing. 1.0 gm/kg was active vs hot plate method[K12860]. Ethanol (95%) extract of dried leaves administered intragastrically to rats at a dose of 1.0 gm/kg was active vs hot plate method and acetic acid-induced writhing[K12860].

Anticoagulant activity. Water extract of dried leaves at a concentration of 1.0 mg/ml was active on human whole blood[K20898].

Antigalactagogue effect. Seeds taken by human adults orally at a dose of 15.0 gm/animal was inactive. The subjects had hyperprolactinemia and galactorrhea. Both subjects had a history of secondary amenorrhea and primary sterility. Daily dosing (divided doses) for 24 weeks in one subject and 10 weeks in a second subject[T02368].

Antihypercholesterolemic activity. Decoction of dried leaves administered intragastrically to rats at a dose of 5.0 gm/kg was active vs diet- and triton-induced hypercholesterolemia[M22106].

Antihyperlipemic activity. Decoction of dried leaves administered intragastrically to rats at a dose of 5.0 gm/kg was active vs diet- and triton-induced hypercholesterolemia[M22106].

Anti-inflammatory activity. Ethanol (95%) extract of dried fruit trichomes administered intragastrically to rats at a dose of 3.0 gm/kg was active vs carrageen induced pedal edema. Ethanol (95%) extract of dried leaves administered intragastrically to rats at a dose of 1.0 gm/kg was active vs carrageenin-induced pedal edema[K12860].

Antiparkinson activity. Methanol extract of dried seeds administered intraperitoneally to rats at a dose of 200.0 mg/kg was active. An alcohol-insoluble methanol extract, free from L-DOPA was tested. Seeds administered by gastric intubation to rats at a dose of 400.0 mg/kg was active[T06167].

Seeds taken orally by human adults at a dose of 15–40 gm/person was active. L–DOPA content was about 4.5–5.5%. The study involved 33 patients with Parkinson's disease[T03294].

Antipyretic activity. Ethanol (95%) extract of dried fruit trichomes administered intragastrically to rats at a dose of 1.0 gm/kg was active vs yeast-induced pyrexia. Ethanol (95%) extract of dried leaves administered intragastrically to rats at a dose of 1.0 gm/kg was active vs yeast-induced pyrexia[K12860].

Antiradiation effect. Methanol extract of dried prothallus administered intraperitoneally to mice at a dose of 100 mg/kg was inactive vs soft X-ray irradiation at lethal dose[T14342].

Antispasmodic activity. Ethanol/water (1:1) extract of fruit was active on guinea pig ileum vs ACh- and histamine-induced spasms. Ethanol/water (1:1) extract of root was active on guinea pig ileum vs ACh- and histamine-induced spasms[A03335].

Aphrodisiac activity. Plant administered orally to male human adults was active. A clinical trial involving 133 subjects ranging in age from 18–46 years presented cases of improper erection, night emissions, premature ejaculations, spermatorrhoea, functional impotence ,and/or oligospermia. Of all patients, 71.4% claimed to be aided by the drug with no side effects[T01692]. Seeds taken by male human adults at variable dosage levels was active. The product contained a mixture of *Orchis mascula*, *Hygrophila spinosa*, *Lactuca scariola*, *Macuna pruriens*, *Parmelia parlata*, *Argyreia speciosa*, *Tribulus terrestris*, and *Leptadenia reticulata* (known as speman). The study involving 21 infertile oligospermic patients in the age group of 25–35 years. Dosing with speman was two tablets three times daily for four weeks. Semen and blood samples were collected for analysis. Fifty percent of the subjects showed improvement of prostatic function as assessed by the activity of maltase and by the citric acid content, with increase in the activity of amylase and maltase and a decrease in post-treatment levels of glycogen in seminal fluid. No marked change in seminal vesicular function was noted[T04226]. Ether and ethanol (95%) extracts of seeds administered intraperitoneally to rats were inactive. No effect on social behavior, including homosexual mounting, sniffing, lying over one another, and so forth, was observed[T03102].

Bronchodilator activity. Hot water extract of dried seeds administered intravenously to guinea pig at a dose of 1.5 ml/animal was inactive[M29843].

Cholinesterase inhibition. Methanol extract of seeds administered intraperitoneally to rats at a dose of 200.0 mg/kg was inactive. An alcohol-insoluble methanol extract, free from L-DOPA, was tested[T06167].

Cytotoxic activity. Ethanol/water (1:1) extract of fruit in cell culture was inactive on CA–9KB. $ED_{50} > 20.0$ mcg/ml. Ethanol/water (1:1) extract of root in cell culture was inactive on CA-9KB. $ED_{50} > 20.0$ mcg/ml[A03335].

Embryotoxic effect. Water extract of seeds administered intragastrically to pregnant rats at a dose of 175.0 mg/kg was inactive[K16006].

Fertility promotion effect. Dried entire plant extract taken orally by male human adults at a dose of 96.0 mg/day was active. Thirty-five patients with oligospermia were given two tablets three times per day for three months. Total sperm count and sperm motility improved[T12794].

FSH release inhibition. Seeds taken orally by male human adults at variable dosage levels was equivocal. The product contained a mixture of *Orchis mascula*, *Hygrophila spinosa*, *Lactuca scariola*, *Macuna pruriens*, *Parmelia parlata*, *Argyreia speciosa*, *Tribulus terrestris*, and *Leptadenia reticulata* (known as speman). Dosing was two tables three times daily for four days[T04226].

FSH synthesis stimulation. Seeds taken by male human adults orally at variable dosage levels was equivocal. The product contained a mixture of *Orchis mascula*, *Hygrophila spinosa*, *Lactuca scariola*, *Macuna pruriens*,

Parmelia parlata, *Argyreia speciosa*, *Tribulus terrestris*, and *Leptadenia reticulata* (known as speman). Dosing was two tablets three times daily for four days[T04226].

Genitourinary effect. Water extract of the entire plant administered orally to mice at a dose of 5.0 mg/day was active. The mice received a single dose of cadmium chloride (1 mg) plus test preparation of placebo for up to 60 days. The test group showed fewer toxic effects than the control group on the seminiferous tubules, epididymis, and spermatids. The test preparation contained *Orchis mascula*, *Lactuca serriola*, *Asteracantha longifolia*, *Macuna pruriens*, *Parmelia perlata*, *Argyreia speciosa*, *Tribulus terrestris*, and *Leptadenia reticulata*, and gold[T15943].

Gonadotropin release stimulation. Seeds taken by male human adults orally at variable dosage levels was equivocal. The product contained a mixture of *Orchis mascula*, *Hygrophila spinosa*, *Lactuca scariola*, *Macuna pruriens*, *Parmelia parlata*, *Argyreia speciosa*, *Tribulus terrestris*, and *Leptadenia reticulata* (known as speman). Dosing was two tablets three times daily for four days[T04226].

Gonadotropin synthesis stimulation. Seeds taken by male human adults orally at variable dosage levels was equivocal. The product contained a mixture of *Orchis mascula*, *Hygrophila spinosa*, *Lactuca scariola*, *Macuna pruriens*, *Parmelia parlata*, *Argyreia speciosa*, *Tribulus terrestris*, and *Leptadenia reticulata* (known as speman). Dosing was two tablets three times daily for four days[T04226].

Hypocholesterolemic activity. Seeds in the ration of rats was active[A14339].

Hypoglycemic activity. Ethanol/water (1:1) extract of fruit administered orally to rats at a dose of 250.0 mg/kg was active. More than 30% drop in blood sugar level was observed. Ethanol/water (1:1) extract of root administered orally to rats at a dose of 250.0 mg/kg was active. More than 30% drop in blood sugar level was observed[A03335]. Ethanol/water (1:1) extract of seeds administered orally to rats at a dose of 250.0 mg/kg was inactive. Less than 30% drop in blood sugar level was observed[W00374]. Seeds in the ration of rats was active[A14339].

LH-release inhibition. Seeds taken by male human adults orally at variable dosage levels was equivocal. The product contained a mixture of *Orchis mascula, Hygrophila spinosa, Lactuca scariola, Macuna pruriens, Parmelia parlata, Argyreia speciosa, Tribulus terrestris* and *Leptadenia reticulata* (known as speman). Dosing was two tablets three times daily for four days[T04226].

LH-release stimulation. Seeds taken by male human adults orally at variable dosage levels was equivocal. The product contained a mixture of *Orchis mascula, Hygrophila spinosa, Lactuca scariola, Macuna pruriens, Parmelia parlata, Argyreia speciosa, Tribulus terrestris* and *Leptadenia reticulata* (known as speman). Dosing was two tablets three times daily for four days[T04226].

LH-synthesis stimulation. Seeds taken by male human adults orally at variable dosage levels was equivocal. The product used contained a mixture of *Orchis mascula, Hygrophila spinosa, Lactuca scariola, Macuna pruriens, Parmelia parlata, Argyreia speciosa, Tribulus terrestris,* and *Leptadenia reticulata* (known as speman). Dosing was two tablets three times daily for four days[T04226].

Nematocidal activity. Decoction of a commercial sample of seeds at a concentration of 10.0 mg/ml was inactive on *Toxacara canis*[M26175]. Water extract of dried seeds at a concentration of 10.0 mg/ml was inactive on *Toxacara canis*; the methanol extract at a concentration of 1.0 mg/ml showed weak activity[M28316].

Penis erectile stimulant. Extract of dried seeds taken orally by human adults was active. Improvement in erection, duration of coitus, and postcoital satisfaction has been observed in 56 cases treated for four weeks[T14366].

Plant growth inhibitor. Dried seeds exhibited allelopathic effect in field tests[K10998]. The acid fraction of ethanol (80%) extract inhibited the growth of *Lactuca sativa* seedlings[M27351].

Prolactin inhibition. Seeds taken orally by female human adults at a dose of 15.0 gm/person was inactive. Subjects had hyperprolactinemia and galactorrhea. Both subjects had a history of secondary amenorrhea and primary sterility. Daily dosing (divided doses) for 24 weeks in one subject and 10 weeks in a second subject. Inhibition of prolactin response to chlorpromazine injection in five subjects was positive[T02367].

Prostate treatment. Hot water extract of the entire plant administered orally to human adults was active. Forty-five patients with prostatitis were given the test preparation, and 10 more patients served as untreated controls. Of 38 patients with benign hypertrophy in the test group, 28 improved and did not need surgery. All of the controls needed surgery. The test preparation contained *Orchis mascula, Lactuca serriola, Asteracantha longifolia, Macuna pruriens, Parmelia perlata, Argyreia speciosa, Tribulus terrestris, Leptadenia reticulata ,* and gold[T15944].

Spermatogenic effect. Seeds taken orally by human adults at variable dosage levels was equivocal. A group of 30 oligospermic infertilities in the age group of 24–46 years were studied over four months. Dosing was three times daily. Increases in magnesium content and in sperm count was reported. The product used contained a mixture of *Orchis mascula, Hygrophila spinosa, Lactuca scariola, Macuna pruriens, Parmelia parlata, Argyreia speciosa, Tribulus terrestris,* and *Leptadenia reticulata* (known as speman)[T04225]. Speman, used in a study involving 40 subjects to improve fertility, was active. Most of the patients claimed marked improvement relative to showing better semen profiles[T03252].

Taenicide activity. Ethanol (95%) and water extracts were active on *Taenia solium*[T08066].

Teratogenic activity. Water extract of seeds administered intragastrically to pregnant rats at a dose of 175.0 mg/kg was active[K16006].

Toxic effect. Water extract of seeds in the ration of rats at variable dosage levels was active. Feeding caused weight loss unless supplemented with L-methionine and L-tryptophan. The protein fraction of the seeds was incorporated into the experimental ration[T06797].

Toxicity assessment. Ethanol/water (1:1) extract of fruit administered intraperitoneally to mice tolerated a maximum dose of 1.0 gm/kg[A03335]. Ethanol/water (1:1) extract of root when administered intraperitoneally to mice the maximum tolerated dose was 250.0 mg/kg[A03335].

M. pruriens is an ingredient of several commercial preparations claimed to have beneficial effects in the management of various sexual disorders. One such preparation is Tenex forte, which has other constituents like musk, saffron, yohimbine hydrochloride, nuxvomica pulvis, *makardhwaj shilajeet, Orchis mascula, Withania somnifera, Sida cordifolia, Bombax malabaricum, Argyreia speciosa,* and *Swarnamakshik bhasma,* as well as Mustong, which contains M. *pruriens, Glycyrrhiza glabra, Withania somnifera, Tribulus terrestris, Myristica fragrans,* and *Tinospora.* Some uncontrolled clinical studies have claimed to have found these compound preparations effective in improving libido and performance in man.

17 | Mangifera indica

L.

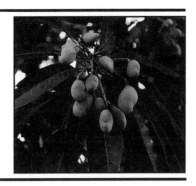

Common Names

Aam	Fiji	Mango	Guam
Aam	India	Mango	Guatemala
Aamp	Nepal	Mango	Guyana
Aanp	Nepal	Mango	Haiti
Alfonso mango	India	Mango	India
Am	India	Mango	Ivory Coast
Am	Pakistan	Mango	Mexico
Amba	Oman	Mango	Nepal
Amm	India	Mango	Nicaragua
Amp	Nepal	Mango	Pakistan
Amra	India	Mango	Peru
Amva	India	Mango	Puerto Rico
Andok–ntang	Guinea	Mango	Sudan
Asm	India	Mango	Tanzania
Bo–amb	India	Mango	Tonga
Bowen mango	USA	Mango	Venezuela
Bumango	Senegal	Mango dusa	Nicaragua
Chamorro	Guam	Mango tree	India
Embe	Tanzania	Mangofruit	India
Maamidi	India	Mangu	Nicaragua
Mam–maram	India	Mangue	Rodrigues Islands
Manga	Brazil	Mangueira	Brazil
Mangga	Guam	Mankro	Nicaragua
Mangguo	China	Mave	India
Mango	China	Mwembe	Tanzania
Mango	Brazil	Oegkoti–tong	India
Mango	Canary Islands	Ondwa	Guinea
Mango	Curacao	Pauh	Indonesia
Mango	Egypt	Skin mango	Brazil
Mango	Fiji	Vi papaa	Rarotonga

From: Medicinal Plants of the World *By:* Ivan A. Ross Humana Press Inc., Totowa, NJ

BOTANICAL DESCRIPTION

Trees of the ANACARDIACEAE family vary in sizes, according to variety and can be from 3- to 30-meters tall, typically heavy-branched from a stout trunk. Leaves spirally arranged on the branches, lanceolate-elliptical, pointed at both ends, the blades mostly up to about 25-cm long and 8-cm wide, sometimes much larger, reddish, and thinly flaccid when first formed (new flush). Inflorescences are large terminal pannicles of small polygamous, fragrant, yellow to pinkish flowers. Fruit is a drupe, variously shaped, according to the variety, from ellipsoid to obliquely reniform, 5- to 15-cm long.

ORIGIN AND DISTRIBUTION

Records indicate that mango has been in cultivation on the Indian subcontinent for well over 4,000 years. It is a native of tropical Asia and introduced wherever the climate is sufficiently warm and damp. It is now completely naturalized in many parts of the tropics and subtropics and here and there a component of mature secondary vegetation.

TRADITIONAL MEDICINAL USES

Brazil. Decoction of dried bark is used to treat scabies[K18765].

Canary Islands. Dried oleoresin is used for food. Hot water extract of dried bark is taken orally for diarrhea. Hot water extract of fresh fruit is taken orally as an anthelmintic[T15880].

Curacao. Decoction of hot water extract[A05332] or tea[A05449] of leaves is drunk for high blood pressure; three cups a day, three days in succession. Some take the decoction every day.

Fiji. Fresh kernel is eaten for dysentery and asthma; juice is used as a nose drop for sinus trouble. Fresh leaf juice in coconut oil is used externally for heat rash and burns. Hot water extract of dried bark is taken orally for syphilis. Unripe fresh fruit pulp, mixed with curd is used for indigestion and stomachache[T10632].

Guam. The fruit has been reported to cause rash called mango dermatitis on human adults[A05675].

Haiti. Water extract of dried bark is taken orally for liver trouble[T13846].

India. Decoction of dried bark is used for diabetes. Ten grams of dried leaves of *Zanthoxylum armatum* boiled in eight liters of water along with 125 gm of mixture having equal parts of bark of *Acacia nilotica*, *Mangifera indica*, and *Syzygium cumini* until the quantity of water is reduced to two liters. Fifty milliliters of decoction is taken twice a day after meals[M24146]. Hot water extract of the dried bark is taken orally for leukorrhea, bleeding hemorrhoids, and lung hemorrhage[T09230]. Decoction of stem bark is used to treat menarche. Decoction is taken orally with cow's milk[K11282]. Decoction is taken orally of the vapor is inhaled to treat jaundice[K23156]. It is taken to prevention conception. As a contraceptive, the stem bark of the young mango plant which has not flowered even once constitutes the contraceptive. Fifty grams of fine stem bark powder is said to be administered with alcoholic wine for preventing conception. It is said to be effective enough to cause abortion safely up to six months after conception[T14570,T01694]. Dried seed powder is applied to the head to remove dandruff. The kernel starch is eaten as a famine food[T08282]. Extract of flowers is used in diarrhea and dysentery[J02755]. Fresh leaf juice is used for treating inflammation of the eye; it is applied on eyes (protecting eyelids) twice daily[K23171]. For styes, petiole juice is applied to the stye during the time it is painful or irritated. For permanent cure, apply when pus has started oozing[T10321]. Fruit is used as a laxative, diuretic, diaphoretic, astringent, and refrigerant[J02755]. Hot water extract of dried leaves is taken orally for diabetes[A14379,T09230], diarrhea and hiccups[T09230]. Dried leaves is used to prevent tooth decay. Powder or decoction is applied to teeth with finger or brush[M20879]. Hot water extract of kernel is taken orally as an Anthelmintic, aphrodisiac, laxative and tonic[W00384]. Hot water extract of the bark is used as an astringent, tonic[J02755], and for menorrhagia[W03487]. Water extract of leaves is taken orally for coughs, asthma, dysentery, and diarrhea[J02755].

Malaysia. Hot water extract of seed is taken orally for menorrhagia[A06590].

Nepal. Hot water extract of fruit is administered intravaginally to human in hemorrhages from the uterus. Hot water extract of seeds is taken orally for asthma[A00020].

Nicaragua. Phenol/water extract of inner bark is used externally for wounds[M23149].

Panama. Fruit is eaten as a laxative. Hot water extract of leaves is used to treat rheumatism. Decoction of 15–20 leaves in one liter of water is prepared. Leaves are chewed for toothache and gum disorders[T01287].

Peru. Hot water extract of dried fruit is taken orally medicinally[T15323].

Rarotonga. Fresh fruit rind is eaten as a refreshing tonic[K08575].

Senegal. Hot water extract of dried bark is used orally for mouth sores, odontalgia, and as a mouthwash for toothache. The extract is taken orally for dysentery and diarrhea; it is used externally for cutaneous affections. Hot water extract of dried leaves is taken orally for bronchitis, toothache, angina, and blennorrhagia. Hot water extract of oleoresin is taken orally for syphilis[M21947].

Sri Lanka. Bruised bark and leaves of *Ervatania dichotoma*, bark of *Mangifera indica* and *Ficus glomerata* are boiled in coconut oil and applied to abraded skin of ulcers and fistulae as an astringent and antiseptic[T08443].

Tanzania. Decoction of dried stem bark is used orally for toothache. Decoction of root is taken orally for malaria[T16181].

Tonga. Infusion of dried leaves is used for syndrome locally called Kita Fa' ele, consisting of fever, chills, dizziness, and lower abdominal pain presumed to result from insufficient rest during puerperium. *Mangifera indica, Diospyros lateriflora, Bischofia javanica,*

Pittosporum arborescens, and *Colubrina asiatica* are used in the preparation[T08685].

Zaire. Infusion of dried stem bark is taken orally for diarrhea, chest pains, coughs, anemia, urinary tract infections, and diabetes. Externally, the infusion is used for infected wounds and skin diseases and as an oral application for dental caries[K18012].

Particular care should be taken in using the shoots and flowers, since they may be contaminated with fungal toxins. Mycotoxins are among the most important chemical hazards in the rural countryside.

CHEMICAL CONSTITUENTS
(ppm unless otherwise indicated)

1-3-5-6-7-Pentamethoxy xanthone, Sh
1-3-6-7-Tetramethoxy xanthone, Sh
2-Ethyl hexanol, Pan
2-Octene, Fl
4-Phenyl-n-butyl gallate, Fl
5-912-Cis-heptadecenyl), Fr Pe
5-Dehydro-avenasterol, Ker
5-Heptadec-cis-2-enyl resorcinol, Lx
5-Methyl furfur-2-al, Fr Pu
5-Pentadecyl resorcinol, Fr Pe
6-Phenyl-N-hexyl gallate, Fl
7-Dehydro-avenosterol, Ker
Acetaldehyde, Fr
Acetic acid ethyl ester, Fr
Acetic acid methyl ester, Fr
Acetic acid N-butyl ester, Fr
Acetophenone, Fr Pu
Acetyl furan, Fr Pu
Alanine, Fr 0.051-0.565%
Allo-aromadendrene, Lf EO
Alpha amyrenone, Sd Ol
Alpha amyrin, Rt Bk 33.3
Alpha amyrin, St Bk 43.7-100
Alpha cubebene, Lf EO
Alpha farnesene, Lf EO
Alpha guaiene, Lf EO
Alpha humulene, Fr Pu
Alpha phellandrene, Fl
Alpha phellandrene, Fr Pu
Alpha pinene, Fl
Alpha pinene, Lf EO; Fr Pu
Alpha terpinolene, Lf EO
Alpha thujene, Lf EO
Alpha tocopherol, Fr

Ambolic acid, Pl
Ambonic acid, Pl
Amentoflavone, Bk
Arachidic acid, Ker
Arachidonic acid, Sd Ol
Arginine, Fr 0.019–0.340%
Ascorbic acid, Fr 0.003–0.176%;
    Lf 0.053–0.243%
Ash, Lf 1.9–13.3%; Fr 0.470–2.914%;
    Sd 3.66%
Aspartic acid, Fr 0.042–0.410%
Benzaldehyde, Fr Pu
Beta amyrenone, Sd Ol
Beta amyrin, Rt Bk 50; St Bk 43.7–100
Beta bulnesene, Lf EO
Beta caryophyllene, Lf EO
Beta elemene, Lf EO
Beta myrcene, EO
Beta ocimene, Lf EO
Beta phellandrene, Fr Pu
Beta pinene, Lf EO
Beta selinene, Fr Pu
Beta sitosterol, Rt Bk; Fr Pe; St Bk; Lf; Sd; Pn
Beta carotene, Fr 11–96; Lf 6–44
Beta pinene, Fl
Bis-2-ethyl hexanyl-phthalate, Pan
Boron, Fr 0.5–17.5
Calcium, Fr 0.0092–0.1400%; Lf 0.029–
    2.93%
Campesterol, Ker
Camphene, Lf EO
Car-3-ene, Fr Pu; Lf EO
Carbohydrates, Fr 17.000–92.939%; Lf
    16.5–54.0%
Carbonate, Sd 900
Carotenoids, Fr 10–165
Caryophyllene, Fr Pu
Catalase, Fr
Catechin oxidase, Fr
Chlorine, Fr 205
Cholesterol, Ker
Cis–ocimene, EO
Cis–zeatin riboside, Sd
Cis–zeatin, Sd
Citric acid, Fr
Citrostadienol, Ker
Copper, Fr 1.1–16.6
Cycloartenol, St Bk 0.07%
Cycloartenone, Sd OL
Cyclobranol, Ker
Cyclosadol, Ker
Cystine, Fr 70–350

D–arabinose, Fl
Dammaradienol, Ker
Dammarendiol II, St Bk 20
Daucosterol, St Bk 3.7
Delta cadinene, Lf EO
Delta elemene, Lf EO
Dimethyl sulfide, Fr Pu
Dipentene, Fl
Eicos–9–en-1-oic acid, Ker
Elaidic acid, Ker
Elemicin, Lf EO
Ellagic acid, Pn
EO, Fl 400
Estragole, Lf EO
Eugenol methyl ester, Lf EO
Euxanthone, Lf
Fat, Fr 0.100–1.689%; Lf 0.40–3.8%;
    Sd 10.7%
Fatty acids, Sd Ol
Fiber, Fr 0.8–4.9%; Lf 1.6–21.1%
Friedelan-3-beta-ol, Rt Bk
Friedelin, Rt Bk
Friedelinol, Ker
Fructose, Fr 2.57–4.83%
Fructose,1-6-phosphatase, Fr
Furfural, Fr Pu
Furfurol, Re 1.8%
GABA, Fr
Galactose, Fl; Pn
Gallic acid, Fl 9.0%; Fr Pu; Pn; Lf
Gallicin, Pn
Gallotannic acid, Fl 15.0%
Gamma terpinene, Lf EO; Fr Pu
Gentisic acid, Lf
Geraniol, Fl
Germanicol, Ker
Glochidonol, Sh
Glucose, Fr 1.00–4.32%
Glutamic acid, Fr 0.06–0.68%
Glycine, Fr 0.021–0.190%
Gramisterol, Ker
Heptadecan-1-oic acid, Ker
Hexadec-7-en-oic acid, Ker
Hexadec-9-en-1-oic acid, Ker
Histidine, Fr 0.012-0.120%
Homo-mangiferin, Lf
Hopane-1-beta-3-beta-22-triol, St Bk
Humulene, Lf EO
Indicene, Lf EO
Indicoside A, St Bk
Indicoside B, St Bk
Iodine, Fr 0.016

Iron, Fr 1-243; Lf 62
Iso-mangiferin, Lf
Iso-quercitrin methyl ether, Sh
Isoleucine, Fr 0.018–0.200%
Isomangiferolic acid, Pl
Kaempferol methyl ether, Sh
Kaempferol, Lf
Kilocalories, Fr 0.0590–0.3554%
Laccase, Fr
Lauric acid, Ker
Lauric acid, Fr 10-55
Leucine, Fr 0.031–0.295%
Limonene, Fr Pu; Fl
Linalool, Lf EO
Linoleic acid, Fr 140-765; Sd Ol
Linolenic acid, Fr 370-2023; Sd Ol; Fr Pe
Lophenol, Ker
Lupenone, Sh; Sd Ol
Lupeol, Sh; Lf; Ker
Lysine, Fr 0.041–0.320%
Magnesium, Fr 84–875
Malic acid, Fr 0.67–3.66%
Manganese, Fr 0.2-12.2
Mangiferic acid, Fr
Mangiferin, Bk; Fr Pe; Lf; Rt Bk
Mangiferine, Fr
Mangiferol, Bk
Mangiferolic acid, Rt Bk; St Bk
Mangiferonic acid methyl ester, St Bk 20
Mangiferonic acid, Pl
Meso inositol, Fr Pe
Methionine, Fr 50–550
Methyl cyclohexane, Fr Pu
Myrcene, Lf EO
Myricetin methyl ester, Sh
Myristic acid, 90–492
N-hentriacontane, Galls
N-heptacosane, Galls
N-nonacosane, Galls
N-octadecane, Pn
N-octane, Pr Pu
N-octyl gallate, Fl
N-pentacosane, Galls
N-pentyl gallate, Fl
N-propyl gallate, Fl
N-texatriacontane, Galls
Neo-beta carotene-B, Fr 19.2
Neo-beta carotene-U, Fr 7.3
Neoxanthophyll, Fr
Nerol, Fl
Neryl acetate, Fl
Niacin, Fr 6.5-63; Lf 22-100

Nonadecan-1-oic acid, Ker
Obtusifoliol, Ker
Ocimene, Lf EO
Ocotillol, St Bk 12.5
Octacosan-1-ol, Pn
Octadeca-6-9-dien-1-oic acid, Ker
Octadeca-cis-9-cis-15-dienoic acid, Fr
Octdeca-3-6-9-trien-1-oic acid, Ker
Octillol II, St Bk 50
Oleic acid, Sd Ol; Fr Pe
Oleic acid, Fr 540–2,950
Oxalic acid, Fr 300
P–coumaric acid, Pl
Palmitic acid, Fr 0.0520–0.2843%
Palmitoleic acid, Fr 0.0480–0.2625%
Pantothenic acid, Fr 1.6–8.8
Para cymene, Fr Pu
Pentadecan–1–oic acid, Ker
Peonidin-3-galactoside, Fr Pe
Peroxidase, Fr
Phenylacetaldehyde, Fr Pu
Phenylalanine, Fr 0.017-0.370%
Phosphorous, Fr 0.0103-0.1050%; Lf 0.072-
   0.380%
Phytin, Fr
Potassium, Fr 0.1080-0.9475%
Proline, Fr 0.018-0.200%
Propionaldehyde, Fr
Protein, Fr 0.5-6.0%; Lf 3.0-7.8%; Sd 9.5%
Protocatechuic acid, Lf
Quercetin methyl ether, Sh
Quercetin, Pl
Quercitrin methyl ether, Sh
Riboflavin, Fr 0.5-3.3; Lf 0.6-2.7
Rutin, Lf 5.2%
Sabinene, Lf EO
Serine, Fr 0.022-0.315%
Silica, Sd 0.41%
Sodium, Fr 13-143
Starch, Sd 72.8%
Stearic acid, Fr 30-164; Sd Ol; Ker
Stigast-7-en-3-beta-ol, Ker
Stigasterol, Ker
Succinic acid, Fr
Sucrose, Fr 6.67-12.58%
Sugars, Fr 11.2-20.5%; Sd 1.07%
Sulfur, Fr 70-615; Sd 2,300
Tannin, Fl 15.0%; Sd 0.11%
Taraxerol, Lf
Taraxerone, Lf
Terpinene, Lf EO
Thiamin, Fr 0.4-3.4; Lf 0.4-1.8

Threonine, Fr 0.019-0.225%
Toluene, Fr Pu
Trans-zeatin ribose, Sd
Trans-zeatin, Sd
Trichloro ethylene, Fr Pu
Tridecan-1-oic acid, Ker
Tryptophan, Fr 80-700
Tyrosine, Fr 0.01-0.16%
Ursolic acid, Sh
Valencene, Fr Pu
Valine, Fr 0.026-0.27%
Vitamin-B6, Fr 1.3-7.3
Water, Fr 75.43-90.00%; Lf 78.2%
Xanthophyll, Fr 42
Zinc, Fr 0.4-11.4

PHARMACOLOGICAL ACTIVITIES AND CLINICAL TRIALS

Allergenic activity. Fresh fruit eaten by human adult was active. A male presented with periorbital edema, facial erythema, widespread urticaria, and dyspnea 20 minutes after eating a mango fruit. Pulse was 100 beats/min, blood pressure 104/72. Anaphylaxis was diagnosed. He was treated with intravenous hydrocortisone and chlorpheniramine maleate and recovered. Prick testing with mango juice produced a wheal within five minutes. The patient has a history of asthma, eczema, hay fever, and drug allergy[M29141]. Powder commercial sample of fruits was active on human adults. Reactions to patch tests occurred most commonly in patients who were regularly exposed to the substance, or who already had dermatitis on the fingertips. Previously unexposed patients had reactions (i.e., not irritant reactions)[M17058].
Anthelmintic activity. Hot water extract of kernel, at a concentration of 1:50, was active on *Haemonchus contortus*[W00384].
Antibacterial activity. Ethanol (95%) extract of dried leaves on agar plate was active on *Escherichia coli* and *Staphylococcus aureus*[W03693]. Water extract was active on *Actinomycete* species and plaque bacteria. Commercial dentifrices were tested alone and in combination with plant extracts against plaque bacteria in the paper disk

assay. The addition of plant extracts significantly increased the zone of inhibition relative to that of the dentifrices[M20879]. The extract was active on *Bacteroides gingivalis* vs two clinical isolates, *Pseudomonas saccharophila* (clinical isolate), *Streptococcus salivarius* vs five clinical isolates, *Streptococcus viridans* vs 40 clinical isolates. Water extract taken orally by human adults was active. Fifty patients with chronic suppurative peridontitis were given leaf extracts of *Mangifera indica*, *Camellia sinensis*, *Murray koenigii*, *Ocimum basilicum* or *Azadirachta*. Bacterial populations declined by 50%, and 40 patients showed improvement[M20879]. Hot water extract, undiluted on agar plate was inactive on *Escherichia coli* and *Staphylococcus aureus*[W03693]. Ethanol (95%) extract of fresh kernel on agar plate was active on *Agrobacterium tumefaciens* MIC 1.5 mg/ml; *Sarcina lutea* MIC 2.0 mg/ml; *Staphylococcus aureus* MIC 2.0 mg/ml; *Bacillus firmis* MIC 3.0 mg/ml; *Escherichia coli* MIC 3.0 mg/ml; *Proteus vulgaris* MIC 3.0 mg/ml and *Pseudomonas aeruginosa* MIC 4.0 mg/ml[M20550]. Hot water extract of dried leaves on agar plate was active on *Sarcina lutea* and *Staphylococcus aureus*[W01818]. Methanol extract of dried stem bark at a concentration of 10.0 mg/ml on agar plate was inactive on *Escherichia coli*, *Pseudomonas aeruginosa*, *Salmonella typhimurium* and *Streptococcus mutans*. The extract was active on *Klebsiella pneumonia* and *Staphylococcus aureus* MIC 125.0 mcg/ml. The tannin fraction of dried stem bark, on agar plate was active on *Citrobacter diversus* at a dose of 110.0 mcg/ml; *Salmonella enteritidis* at a dose of 120.0 mg/ml; *Staphylococcus aureus* at a concentration of 145.0 mcg/ml; *Escherichia piracoli*, *Klebsiella pneumonia*, and *Shigella flexneri* at a concentration of 200.0 mcg/ml; weak activity was shown on *Escherichia coli*, at a concentration of 225.0 mcg/ml[K21572].
Antifungal activity. Ethanol (95%) extract of fresh kernel, at a concentration of 5.0 mg/

ml on agar plate was active on *Trichophyton mentagrophytes*[M20550]. Hot water extract of dried leaves on agar plate was inactive on *Aspergillus niger*[W01818]. Methanol extract of dried stem bark, at a concentration of 10.0 mg/ml was inactive on *Aspergillus niger* and *Microsporum gypseum*[K18012].

Anti-inflammatory activity. Ethanol (95%) extract of fresh kernel, at a dose of 50.0 mg/kg administered by gastric intubation to rats was active vs carrageenin-induced pedal edema, 5-HT-induced pedal edema, bradykinin-induced pedal edema, turpentine-induced pleurisy, granuloma pouch, cotton pellet granuloma, and adjuvant-induced arthritis. The extract was inactive vs dextran-induced pedal edema, prostaglandin-induced pedal edema, and weakly active vs formaldehyde-induced arthritis[M20550].

Antimalarial activity. Water extract of bark at a dose of 7.82 gm/kg administered orally to chicken was inactive on *Plasmodium gallinaceum*[A00785].

Antimycobacterial activity. Hot water extract of dried leaves on agar plate was inactive on *Mycobacterium phlei*[W01818].

Antinematodal activity. Water extract of dried leaves at variable concentrations was active on *Meloidogyne incognita*[T07251].

Antitumor activity. Ethanol/water (1:1) extract of dried aerial parts administered intraperitoneally to mice at a dose of 250.0 mg/kg was inactive on Leuk-P388[T10126].

Antiviral activity. Ethanol (80%) extract of freeze-dried leaves in cell culture, at variable dosages was equivocal on Coxsackie B2 virus, measles virus, and Polio virus; inactive on adenovirus, herpes virus type 1, and Semilicki-forest virus vs plaque-inhibition[T06435]. Methanol extract of dried stem bark, at a concentration of 100.0 mcg/ml in cell culture, showed weak activity on HIV virus[K21223]. Undiluted leaf juice was inactive on bean mosaic virus. Reduction of infectiousness was measured[T09049].

Antiyeast activity. Ethanol (60%) extract of dried leaves on agar plate was inactive on *Candida albicans*[M31296]. Ethanol (95%) extract of fresh kernel at a concentration of 5.0 mg/kg on agar plate, was active on *Candida lunata* and inactive on *Candida albicans*[M20550]. Hot water extract of dried leaves on agar plate was inactive on *Saccharomyces cerevisiae*[W01818]. Methanol extract of dried stem bark, at a concentration of 10.0 mg/ml, on agar plate was inactive on *Candida albicans*[K18012].

Ascaricidal activity. Ethanol (95%) extract of dried seeds was active on *Ascaris lumbricoides*[T08066].

Cytotoxic activity. Ethanol/water (1:1) of dried aerial parts at a concentration of 25.0 mg/ml was inactive on CA-9KB[T10126]. Methanol extract of dried stem bark, at a concentration of 100.0 mcg/ml, was equivocal on CA-HS-578-T, CA-mammary-MF-7, CA-mammary-MF-7/ADR, human breast cancer cell lines BT-549, MDA-MB-231, MDA-MB-435, MDA-N, T47-D, leukemia cell line CCRF-CEM; inactive on RPMI-8226 cells and weakly active on CA-colon-KM12, CA-HCT-15, CA-human-colon COLO-205, CA-human-colon-HCT116, CA-human-nonsmall-cell-lung HOP-62, CA-human-ovarian OVCAR-3, CA-human-ovarian OVCAR-4, CA-human-ovarian OVCAR-5, CA-human-ovarian-SKOV-3, cancer cell line-human CNS-SNB75, human CNS cancer cell line SF-268, human CNS cancer cell line SF-295, human CNS cancer cell line SF-539, human CNS cancer cell line SNB-19, human CNS cancer cell line U251, human colon cancer cell line HCC-2998, human colon cancer cell line HT29, human colon cancer cell line SW620, human leukemia cell line HL-60-TB, human leukemia cell line MOLT-4, human melanoma cell line MALME-3M, human melanoma cell line SK-MEL-2, human melanoma cell line SK-MEL-5, human nonsmall cell lung cancer cell line

A549(ATCC), human nonsmall cell lung cancer cell line EKVX, human nonsmall cell lung cancer cell line HOP-92, human nonsmall cell lung cancer cell line NCI-H226, human nonsmall cell lung cancer cell line NCI-H23, human nonsmall cell lung cancer cell line NCI-H322M, human nonsmall cell lung cancer cell line NCI-H460, human nonsmall cell lung cancer cell line NCI-H522, human ovarian adenocarcinoma IGROV-1, human ovarian cancer cell line OVCAR-8, human renal cancer cell line 786-0, human renal cancer cell line A498, human renal cancer cell line CAKI-1, human renal cancer cell line SN-12C, human renal cancer cell line TK-10, human renal cancer cell line UO-31, Leuk-K562, Leuk-SR, Melanoma-LOX IMVI, Melanoma-M14, Melanoma-SK-MEL-28, Melanoma-UACC-257, Melanoma-UACC-62, and Mycobacterium fortuitum[M21223]. Water extract of freeze-dried fruit was active on Leuk-P815. Tumor-toxic activity was evaluated by culturing Mastocytoma P815 cells with macrophage cells and measuring the incorporation of 3H-Thimidine radioactivity[M27208].

Dermatitis producing effect. Fresh fruit applied externally to male human children was active. Cross-sensitivity as a result of the presence of phenols with 15-C side chains[K19400].

Estrogenic effect. Methanol extract of leaves administered subcutaneously to mice was active[A05970].

Hypoglycemic activity. Fibers of fresh fruit at a concentration of 9.0% was active. Fibrous waste from processing fruit slowed the rate of activity of amylase in potato starch and slowed the diffusion of glucose in a dialysis experiment[K08691]. Water extract of dried leaves administered orally to rabbits at a dose of 10.0 mg/kg was active. Drop in blood sugar of 15 mg relative to inert-treated control indicated positive results[A14379].

Insecticidal activity. Petroleum ether extract of dried bark, at a concentration of 50.0 mcg was active on Rhodnius neglectus[K18765].

Interleukin induction. Water extract of freeze-dried fruits produced weak activity. IL-1 activity was measured by the IL-1 dependent growth of a T-helper cell line[M27208].

Juvenile hormone activity. Acetone extract of stem was active[J08616].

Larvicidal activity. Water extract of dried cotyledons, at a concentration of 0.03 gm/ml, was inactive on Culex quinquefasciatus. Concentrations given in grams of fresh plant material per ml water[M19731].

Molluscicidal activity. Aqueous slurry (Homogenate) of fresh entire plant was inactive on Lymnaea columella and L. cubensis. LD_{100} for both > 1 M ppm[T04621]. Water extract of oven-dried leaves produced weak activity on Biophalaria pfeifferi[T14178]. Water saturated with fresh leaf essential oil, at a concentration of 1:10 was inactive on Biomphalaria glabrata[T07475].

Mutagenic activity. Seed oil was inactive on Salmonella typhimurium TA100 and TA98. Metabolic activation has no effect on the results[T13699].

Nutritional value. Seed oil in the ration of rats, at a dose of 10.0% of the diet was active. Animals showed good growth performance and feed efficiency. It is rich in stearic and oleic acids and low in linoleic acid. The experiment was carried out over three generations of rats[M05253].

Plant germination effect. Water extracts of dried bark, dried leaves and dried stem, at concentrations of 500 gm/liter produced weak activity on the seeds of Cuscuta reflexa after six days of exposure to the extract[M31053].

Plant growth inhibitor. Water extracts of dried leaves, dried stem, and dried bark, at concentrations of 500.0 gm/liter produced weak activity. Cuscuta reflexa seedling length, weight and dry weight measured after six days exposure to the extract[M31053].

Spasmolytic activity. Butanol extract of dried trunk bark, at a concentration of 0.2 mg/ml was active on guinea pig ileum. 45.12% reduction in contractions was seen vs ACh-induced contractions; 37.43% reduction in contractions seen vs KCl-induced contractions. Isopentyl alcohol extract of trunk bark, at a concentration of 0.2 mg/ml, showed 87.34% reduction in contractions vs ACh-induced contractions and 76.54% reduction in contractions vs KCl-induced contractions. Methanol extract of dried trunk bark, at a concentration of 0.2 mg/ml, showed 34.00% reduction in contractions vs ACh-induced contractions and 20.17% reduction in contractions vs KCl-induced contractions[M27323].

Teratogenic activity. Seed oil in the ration of rats, at a dose of 10.0% of the diet was inactive. The experiment was carried out over three generations. There was no difference in litter size, birth weight, or weanling weight over controls fed cocoa-butter fat[M05253].

Toxic effect (general). Seed oil in the ration of rats, at a dose of 10.0% of the diet was inactive. There was no effect on organ weights, cholesterol, triglyceride, and lipid content of serum and liver, mating behavior, litter size, birth weight, or mortality over controls fed cocoa-butter fat. Experiments were carried out over three generations[M05253].

Toxicity assessment (quantitative). Ethanol/water (1:1) extract of dried aerial parts administered intraperitoneally to mice produced a $LD_{50} > 1000$ mg/kg[T10126].

Tumor promotion inhibition. Methanol extract of fresh fruit, at a concentration of 200.0 mcg in cell culture was inactive on Epstein-Barr virus vs 12-0-hexadecanoyl-phorbol-13-acetate-induced Epstein-Barr virus activation[T15279].

Uterine stimulant effect. Ethanol/water (1:1) extract of dried aerial parts was active on rat uterus[T10126]. Water extract of kernel was inactive on nonpregnant uterus of guinea pigs[A04219].

WBC-Macrophage stimulant. Water extract of freeze-dried fruits, at a concentration of 2.0 mg/ml produced weak activity on macrophages. Nitrile formation was used as an index of the macrophage stimulating activity to screen effective foods[M27208].

Weight increase. Seed oil in the ration of rats at a dose of 10.0% of the diet produced weak activity. The experiment was carried out over three generations. The first generation showed a slight weight increase over controls fed cocoa butter fat[M05253].

18 | Manihot esculenta
Crantz.

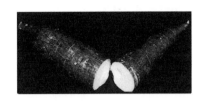

Common Names

Aikavitu	Nicaragua	Manioka	Samoa
Anaha	Nicaragua	Maniota	Venezuela
Belaselika	Nicaragua	Mannyok	Venezuela
Cassava	Brazil	Merelesita	Venezuela
Cassava	Nicaragua	Muhoko	Tanzania
Cassava	Guyana	Nao harnaka	Papua-New Guinea
Cassava	Nigeria	Noumea	Papua-New Guinea
Cassava	Tanzania	Sakarkanda	Papua-New Guinea
Cassava	Thailand	Sakarkanda	Fiji
Cassava	Venezuela	Sokobale	Fiji
Cassava	Zaire	Tapioka	Samoa
Coci	Zaire	Tapioka	Venezuela
Itk	Nicaragua	Tavioka	Venezuela
Kasaleka	Nicaragua	Vula'tolu	Venezuela
Kasera	Nicaragua	Yabia	Venezuela
Kasera	Fiji	Yabia damu	Venezuela
Katafaga	Fiji	Yauhra	Nicaragua
Manioc	Central Africa	Yuca	Guatemala
Manioc	Rodrigues Islands	Yuca	Nicaragua
Manioc	Sri Lanka	Yuca	Puerto Rico

BOTANICAL DESCRIPTION

A perennial shrub of the EUPHOR-BIACEAE family, it has slender little-branched erect nodose glaborous stems, arising from a stock bearing thick tuberous roots; usually growing to about three meters high. Leaves are spirally arranged, long-stalk to a blade deeply divided into three to seven linear to elleptic-lanceolate lobes, exuding a milky sap when broken. Flowers are not often formed because plants are harvested in loose panicles before flowering takes place. Fruit is a small capsule; seeds are mottled and about 12-mm long.

ORIGIN AND DISTRIBUTION

Native probably of Brazil, it is now widespread in the tropics and subtropics. It is also cultivated and sometimes relict.

TRADITIONAL MEDICINAL USES

Central Africa. Leaf juice is taken orally as an abortifacient[A04153].

From: Medicinal Plants of the World *By: Ivan A. Ross Humana Press Inc., Totowa, NJ*

Colombia. Dried leaves crushed together with leaves of *Tabernaemontana undulata* are boiled to produce a tea that is considered an excellent vermifuge[J10345].

Fiji. Juice of grated tubers is taken orally for constipation and indigestion. Boiled tubers are eaten for diarrhea[T10632].

Haiti. Macerated dried leaves are put in a bath, or applied to the forehead for headache; for cutaneous infections leaves are used in a bath[T13846].

Ivory Coast. Hot water extract of leaves is taken orally as an emmemagogue[A01966].

Samoa. Stem inserted into the uterus and rotated as a means of inducing abortion[A00368]. Boiled tuber is taken orally for diarrhea[T13846].

Venezuela. Fresh pulverized tuber is eaten for diarrhea[K08575].

CHEMICAL CONSTITUENTS

(ppm unless otherwise indicated)

Alanine, Rt 0.87–.0.28%
Aluminum, Rt 10–77
Amentoflavone, Lf
Arginine, Rt 0.314–0.997%
Ascorbic acid, Lf 0.08–1.00%; Rt 0.01–0.15%
Ash, Lf 2.7–13.5%; Rt 0.50–3.43%
Aspartic acid, Rt 0.181–0.575%
Beta carotene, Rt 14–150
Boron, Rt 0.6–7.5
Caffeic acid, Rt
Calcium, Rt 0.019–0.289%; Lf 0.145–1.000%
Calcium oxalate, Rt 170–505
Carbohydrates, Rt 26.92–85.49%
Citrates, Rt 0.26–1.148%
Copper, Rt 0.0001–0.00038
Cystine, Rt 650–2065
Dehydroascorbic acid, Rt 52–154
Ent-kaurene, Rt
Ent-primara-8(14)-15-diene, Rt
Fat, Lf 0.2–2.0%; Rt 0.10–1.24%
Fiber, Rt 2.10–8.86%
Glutamic acid, Rt 0.47–1.49%
Glycine, Rt 640–2030
HCN, Lf 0.018–0.180%; St; Flour; Tuber; Rt Bk 1351
Histidine, Rt 0.045–0.143%
Hydrogen sulfide, Lf 42–8573

Iron, Lf 28–1500; Rt 2–114
Iso-linamarin, Tb 0.79%
Isoleucine, Rt 610–1935%
Kilocalories, Lf 498–3957; Rt 1200–3810
Lauric acid, Rt 10–32
Leucine, Rt 900–2860
Linamarin, Seedling, Tb 0.042–0.393%
Linoleic acid, Rt 440–1400
Linolenic acid, Rt 230–730
Linustatin, Seedling
Lotaustralin, Seedling, Rt
Lysine, Rt 1000–3175
Magnesium, Rt 290–2100
Malates, Rt 2060–6095
Manganese, Rt 0.5–2.5
Methionine, Rt 0.104–0.330%
Methyl linamarin, Tb 80–113
Neo linustatin, Seedling
Niacin, Lf 15–75; Rt 6–44
Oleic acid, Rt 0.104–0.330%
Oxalate, Rt 0.015–0.142%
Oxalic acid, Rt 171, Lf 0.635%
Palmitic acid, Rt 950–3015
Phenylalanine, Rt 0.06–0.19%
Phosphorous, Lf 560–2800; Rt 310–2225
Podocarpusflavone A, Lf
Potassium, Rt 0.238–2.426%
Proline, Rt 0.0760–0.2415%
Protein, Lf 5.1–30.3%; Rt 0.4–9.8%
Quercetin, Rt
Quercetin-3-0-a-L-rhamnosyl-glucoside, Lf
Riboflavin, Lf 3–15; Rt 2–3.2
Scopoletin, Rt
Serine, Rt 760–2425
Sodium, Rt 62–2655
Stachene(+), Rt
Starch, Rt 28.00–82.84%
Stearic acid, Rt 70–220
Succinates, Rt 0.34–1.05%
Sugars, Rt 0.34–3.37%
Sulfur, Rt 54–250
Thiamin, Lf 2–10; Rt 0.3–7.1
Threonine, Rt 650–2065
Tryptophan, Rt 430–1365
Tyrosine, Rt 400–1270
Valine, Rt 0.079–0.251%
Water, Lf 74.8–81.0%; Rt 60.7–69.4%
Yucalexin A–16, Rt 0.1
Yucalexin A–19, Rt 2.8
Yucalexin B'–11, Rt 3
Yucalexin B–14, Rt 1.1
Yucalexin B–18, Rt 1.9

Yucalexin B–20, Rt 1
Yucalexin B–22, Rt 1.4
Yucalexin B–5, Rt 0.6
Yucalexin B–6, Rt 2.5
Yucalexin B–7, Rt1.3
Yucalexin B–9, Rt 18.3
Yucalexin P–10, Rt 2.1
Yucalexin P–12, Rt 2.1
Yucalexin P–13, Rt 0.3
Yucalexin P–15, Rt 1.4
Yucalexin P–17, Rt 0.3
Yucalexin P–21, Rt 0.5
Yucalexin P–4, Rt 0.4
Yucalexin P–8, Rt 6.9
Zinc, Rt 4–19

PHARMACOLOGICAL ACTIVITIES AND CLINICAL TRIALS

Antibacterial activity. Ethyl acetate extract of dried aerial parts at a concentration of 1.0 mg/ml on agar plate was active on *Staphylococcus aureus*. Water and acetic acid extracts of the dried aerial parts at concentrations of 1.0 mg/disk were inactive on *Escherichia coli* and the water extract was inactive on *Staphylococcus aureus*[T16253].

Anticrustacean activity. Ethyl acetate extract of dried aerial parts produced weak activity on *Artemia salina* LC_{50} 2390 mcg/ml. The water extract was inactive, LC_{50} 4430 mcg/ml[T16253].

Antifertility effect. Fresh root in the ration of female rats at a concentration of 100.0% of the diet was active. Significant reduction in frequency of pregnancy was observed. The average number of the litter and birth weights was significantly reduced[T01280].

Antifungal activity. Acetic extract of dried aerial parts at a concentration of < 0.13 mg/ml on agar plate was active on *Microsporum canis*, *Microsporum fulvum*, *Microsporum gypseum*, and *Trichophytum gallinae*; the water extract was active on *Microsporum canis* and inactive on *Microsporum fulvum*, *Microsporum gypseum*, and *Trichophytum gallinae*[T16253]. Water extract of fresh leaves on agar plate was inactive on *Ustilago nuda* and strong activity was reported on *Ustilago maydis*[T08889].

Antihypercholesterolemic activity. Dried root in the ration of rats at a dose of 68.0 gm/animal was active. The animals were fed the ration daily for three months. There was an overall decrease in serum levels; however, high density lipid cholesterol was increased, as compared to rats fed rice. Results significant at P < 0.01 level[M05256].

Antihyperlipemic activity. Dried root in the ration of rats at a dose of 68.0 gm/animal was active. Animals were fed the ration daily for three months. There were significant decreases in lipid and cholesterol levels over animals fed rice[M05256].

Antithyroid activity. Dried root ingested by human adults was active[T04575].

Antitumor activity. Ethanol (95%) extract of dried root administered intraperitoneally to mice at a dose of 100.0 mcg/kg was inactive on Sarcoma 180 (ASC); the water extract was active at the same dose[M23643].

Antiviral activity. Ethyl acetate extract of dried aerial parts in cell culture was active on Cytomegalovirus, LC_{50} 0.14 mcg/ml when the virus is exposed to the extract before infecting hosts cells; Sindbis virus, LC_{50} 5.2 mg/ml when virus is exposed to extract before infecting host cells and LC_{50} 6.1 mg/ml when the infected host cells were exposed to the extract. The extract was inactive on Cytomegalovirus when hosts cells were exposed to the extract LC_{50} > 100 mcg/ml. Water extract of dried aerial parts in cell culture was active on Cytomegalovirus LC_{50} 0.18 mcg/ml and Sindbis virus LC_{50} 26.0 mcg/ml when virus were exposed to the extract before infecting hosts cells; Sindbis virus LC_{50} 3.2 mcg/ml when infected host cells were exposed to the extract; inactive on Cytomegalovirus LC_{50} > 100 when infected hosts cells were exposed the extract[T16253].

Antiyeast activity. Ethyl acetate and water extracts of dried aerial parts at concentrations of 1.0 mg/disk were inactive on *Candida albicans* and *Saccharomyces cerevisiae*[T16253].

Crown gall tumor inhibition. Water and acetic acid extracts of dried aerial parts in cell culture were active. LC_{50} 0.03 mcg/ml and 0.32 mcg/ml respectively were observed. Assay system is intended to predict for antitumor activity[T16253].

Diabetogenic activity. Dried tuber in the ration of dogs was active. Animals were fed diet in which cassava (rice, in controls) provided the carbohydrate. After 14 weeks, the plasma amino acid index of gluconeogenesis was 5.077 times greater in the cassava-fed compared to control animals. This value was 1.912 times greater than controls in a third group fed rice and HCN. Plasma lipase activity was significantly elevated in cassava-fed vs controls. Plasma thiocyanate levels were elevated in both cassava- and HCN-fed animals, but significantly more so in the latter. Pancreas showed hemorrhage, necrosis, fibrosis, and atrophy of acinar tissue and fibrosis of islets. Hemorrhage was less prominent and fibrosis more so in HCN-fed animals[M29790].

Embryotoxic effect. Dried root flour in the ration of pregnant rats at a dose of 80.0% of the diet was inactive. Dosing was on day 1–15 of gestation. Resorption occurred in 19%, and fetal malformation in 28%. Cassava starch from roots in the ration of rabbits at concentrations of 15.0, 30, and 45% of the diet was inactive[T01696].

Fish poison. Water extract of fresh root bark was active. LD_{50} 0.25%[T14676].

Glucose-6-Phosphatase dehydrogenase stimulation. Dried root in the ration of rats at a dose of 68.0 gm/animal was active. Animals were fed the ration daily for three months. Liver enzyme levels were lower than animals fed on rice[M05256].

Goitrogenic activity. Dried tuber in the ration of dogs was inactive. Animals were fed diet in which cassava (rice, in controls) provided the carbohydrate. After 14 weeks T3 level had risen by roughly 40% in each group, whereas it had fallen by 36% in a third group fed rice and HCN. Thyroid weight after 14 weeks was not significantly different between control and cassava-fed groups, although it was significantly elevated above control in HCN treated group. Thiocyanate levels were elevated in cassava and HCN-fed groups though only the latter demonstrated thyroid histopathology[M29782]. Fresh root administered to mice by gastric intubation was inactive[T10907].

Hyperglycemic activity. Fresh root ingested by human adult at variable dosage levels was inactive. A study of 110 non-insulin dependent diabetics failed to find evidence that consumption of cassava flour induces diabetes[M22228]. Tuber ingested by male human adult at a dose of 50.0 gm/person was active[M23163].

Juvenile hormone activity. Acetone extract of stem was active[J08616].

Lipid metabolism effects. Dried roots in the ration of rats at a dose of 68.0 g/animal was active. Animals were fed the ration daily for three months. Total serum cholesterol and triglyceride were lowered over rats fed rice. Glucose-6-phosphate dehydrogenase level in the liver was increased. Triglyceride lipase and lipoprotein lipase were decreased. Results were significant at $P < 0.01$ level[M05256].

Molluscicidal activity. Aqueous slurry (homogenate) of fresh entire plant was inactive on *Lymnaea columella* and *Lymnaea cubensis*. $LD_{100} > 1$ ppm[T04621]. Water extract of oven–dried leaves was inactive on *Biomphalaria pfeifferi*[T14178]. Water extract of oven-dried stem showed weak activity on *Biomphalaria pfeifferi*[T14178].

Mutagenic activity. Fresh leaves and acetone and methanol extracts of fresh leaves at concentrations of 50 mg/plate, on agar plate were active on *Salmonella typhimurium* TA98. Mutagenicity was assayed after acid or enzymatic hydrolysis after leaves were boiled. Hexane extract of fresh leaves at a concentration of 500.0 mg/plate on agar

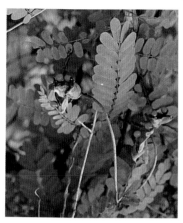

Plate 1. *Abrus precatorius* (*see* full discussion in Chapter 2).

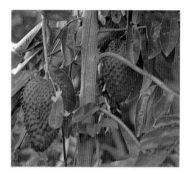

Plate 4. *Annona muricata* (*see* full discussion in Chapter 5).

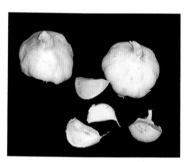

Plate 2. *Allium sativum* (*see* full discussion in Chapter 3).

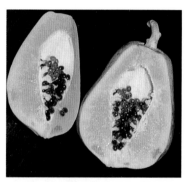

Plate 5. *Carica papaya* (*see* full discussion in Chapter 6).

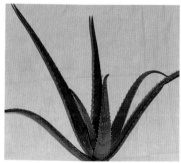

Plate 3. *Aloe vera* (*see* full discussion in Chapter 4).

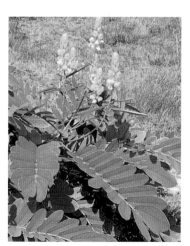

Plate 6. *Cassia alata* (*see* full discussion in Chapter 7).

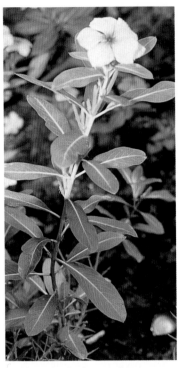

Plate 7. *Catharanthus roseus*
(*see* full discussion
in Chapter 8).

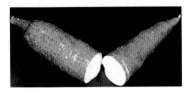

Plate 8. *Cymbopogon citratus*
(*see* full discussion
in Chapter 9).

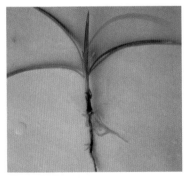

Plate 9. *Cyperus rotundus* (*see*
full discussion in Chapter 10).

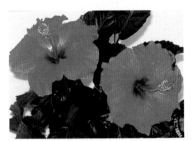

Plate 10. *Hibiscus rosa-sinensis*
(*see* full discussion
in Chapter 12).

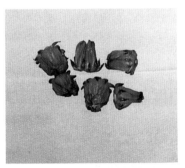

Plate 11. *Hibiscus sabdariffa*
(*see* full discussion in Chapter 13).

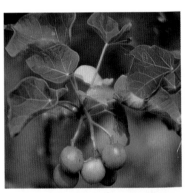

Plate 12. *Jatropha curcas* (*see*
full discussion in Chapter 14).

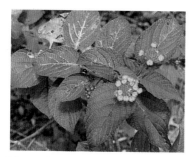

Plate 13. *Lantana camara* (*see* full discussion in Chapter 15).

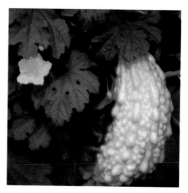

Plate 16. *Momordica charantia* (*see* full discussion in Chapter 19).

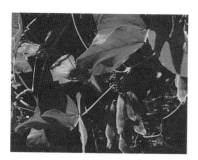

Plate 14. *Macuna pruriens* (*see* full discussion in Chapter 16).

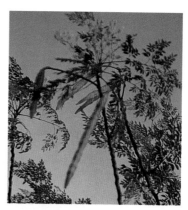

Plate 17. *Moringa pterygosperma* (*see* full discussion in Chapter 20).

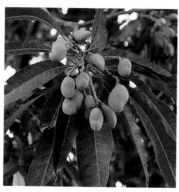

Plate 15. *Mangifera indica* (*see* full discussion in Chapter 17).

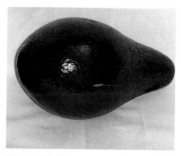

Plate 18. *Persea americana* (*see* full discussion in Chapter 21).

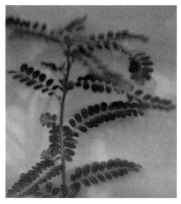

Plate 19. *Phyllanthus niruri* (*see* full discussion in Chapter 22).

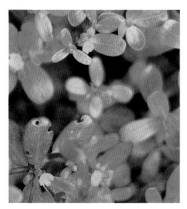

Plate 20. *Portulaca oleracea* (*see* full discussion in Chapter 23).

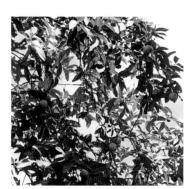

Plate 21. *Psidium guajava* (*see* full discussion in Chapter 24).

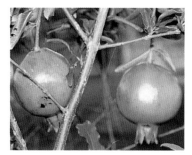

Plate 22. *Punica granatum* (*see* full discussion in Chapter 25).

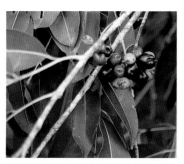

Plate 23. *Syzygium cumini* (*see* full discussion in Chapter 26).

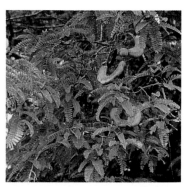

Plate 24. *Tamarindus indica* (*see* full discussion in Chapter 27).

plate was inactive on *Salmonella typhimurium* TA98. Chloroform extract of fresh leaves at a concentration of 0.1 ml/plate on agar plate was inactive on *Salmonella typhimurium* TA100, TA97, and TA98. The mutagenic effect was measured after boiling the leaves and metabolic activation had no effect on the results[M22823]. Chloroform extract of boiled root at a concentration of 0.1 ml/plate on agar plate was active on *Salmonella typhimurium* TA98, and inactive on TA97 and TA100. Metabolic activation had no effect on the results[M22823]. Chloroform extract of dried roots at a concentration of 0.1 ml/plate on agar plate was active on *Salmonella typhimuriumi* TA97 and TA98, and inactive on TA100. Mutagenic effect measured after boiling and metabolic activation had no effect on the results[M22823].

Ovulation inhibition effect. Cassava starch from root in the ration of rabbits at concentrations of 15%, 30%, and 45% of the diet was inactive[T01696].

Protein synthesis inhibition. Fresh leaves in buffer was active. IC_{50} 0.75 mg of protein per ml[M24428].

Respiration (cellular) inhibition. Dried tuber in the ration of rats at a dose of 35.0% of the diet was active. Effects were measured in the liver[M13661].

Teratogenic activity. Dried root flour in the ration of pregnant rats at a dose of 80.0% of the diet was active. Dosing was on days 1–15 of gestation. Resorption occurred in 19%, and fetal malformation in occurred in 28%. Of the abnormal fetuses, all showed growth retardation, 19% has limb defects, and 5.5% had microcephaly with open eye[T10567]. Fresh root in the ration of female rats at a concentration of 50.0% of the diet was inactive[T01280].

Thyroid Stimulating Hormone activity. Sun-dried root ingested by human adult was active[T16366].

Toxic effect (general). Hot water extract of fresh leaves taken orally by human adults at variable dosage levels was inactive. The leaves, which usually contain large quantities of cyanogenic glucosides, were processed into a traditional vegetable sauce "Mpondu" by simple methods that included blanching (10 minutes), mashing, and then boiling for 20–80 minutes. These methods enhanced the detoxification of the leaves, with blanching alone resulting in the loss of 57% of the bound (glycosidic) cyanide. It was presumed that losses of cyanide during these processes would be accounted for in volatile HCN, its derivatives, and boiling water[N15216]. Entire plant taken orally by human adult was active[T15330,T15956]. Fresh root in the ration of female rats at a concentration of 100.0% of the diet was active. There was an increased incidence of neonatal deaths among offspring, which had poor development, reduced brain weights, and increased tendency toward biting litter mates[T01280].

19 | Momordica charantia
L.

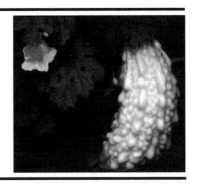

Common Names

African cucumber	USA	Cerasee	Jamaica
Amargoso	Philippines	Cerasee	Trinidad
Ampalaya	Philippines	Cerasee	West Indies
Ampalaya	USA-FL	Concombre	West Indies
Art pumpkin	West Indies	Condiamor	Belize
Asorosi	Haiti	Condiamor	Guatemala
Assorossi	Haiti	Coraillie	West Indies
Balsam apple	West Indies	Cun de amor	Puerto Rico
Balsam pear	Australia	Cundeamor	Brazil
Balsam pear	Bahamas	Cundeamor	Cuba
Balsam pear	Thailand	Cundeamor	Mexico
Balsam pear	USA	Cundeamor	Puerto Rico
Balsambirne	Bahamas	Cundeamor	USA
Balsamina	India	Embusabusu	Congo-Brazzaville
Balsamina	Peru	Eyezom	Guinea
Balsamino	Panama	Futoreishi	Japan
Ban kareli	India	Kakara	India
Baramasiya	India	Kakayi	Nigeria
Barbof	Senegal	Kakiral	India
Bitter cucumber	Thailand	Kakle	East Africa
Bitter gourd	Fiji	Kakral	India
Bitter gourd	India	Karala	India
Bitter gourd	Thailand	Karawila	Sri Lanka
Bitter gourd	USA	Karela	Fiji
Bitter melon	USA	Karela	India
Bitter pear melon	Taiwan	Karela	Nepal
Bobobo	Ivory Coast	Karela	USA
Broomweed	Nicaragua	Karela	West Indies
Caprika	West Indies	Kuguazi	West Indies
Carailla	Guyana	Lenzaa	Congo-Brazzaville
Carilla	USA	Lumba-lumba	East Africa
Carilla	West Indies	Lumbuzi	Thailand
Cerasee	Bahamas	Ma ra	Thailand
Cerasee	Bimini	Machete	Puerto Rico

From: Medicinal Plants of the World *By: Ivan A. Ross Humana Press Inc., Totowa, NJ*

Maiden apple	USA
Maiden apple	Virgin Islands
Maiden's blush	USA
Makalalaska	Nicaragua
Manamat	East Africa
Mange kuli	West Indies
Mara khee nok	Thailand
Mara	Thailand
Margoze	Rodrigues Islands
Mbosa	Congo-Brazzaville
Mbunbulu	Congo-Brazzaville
Melao-de-sao caetano	Brazil
Meleni	Brazil
Mexicaine	West Indies
Miniklalasni	Nicaragua
Momotica	Curacao
Nagareishi	Japan
Nania nania	Ivory Coast
Nara cheen	Thailand
Nguene	Ivory Coast
Nyanyra	Togo
Nyinya	East Africa
Okookoo	Nigeria
Panaminik	Nicaragua

Papayilla	Peru
Paprika	West Indies
Paroka	Guadeloupe
Pavakkachedi	India
Pepino montero	Nicaragua
Periya laut	Malaysia
Pom kouli	Guadeloupe
Pomme nerveille	West Indies
Pomme z'indiens	West Indies
Pomme-coolie	Guadeloupe
Qisaul-barri	India
Quisaul-barri	Saudi Arabia
Saga	Saudi Arabia
Serimentok	India
Seripupa	India
Sorosi	Nicaragua
Sorrow see	Belize
Sushavi	India
Tasplira	Nicaragua
Uchhe	India
Ulhimar	India
Wild balsam pear	Bahamas
Yesquin	Haiti
Zague zrou	Ivory Coast

BOTANICAL DESCRIPTION

Slender-stemmed tendril climber of the CUCURBITACEAE family, the older stem is often flattened and fluted to six meters or longer. Leaves alternate, cut into 5–7 narrow-based lobes. The lobes are mostly blunt, but have small marginal points, up to about 12-cm long, very thin-textured, and characteristically pungent-aromatic. Flowers are yellow on short (female) or long (male) peduncles that are short-lived. Fruit narrowed to both ends, ribbed with prominent tubercles on the ribs, 8- to 15-cm long, orange when ripe and then becoming softly fleshy and opening to reveal pendulous seeds covered with red pulp.

ORIGIN AND DISTRIBUTION

Originally found only in the tropics of the old world, it has been spread by man throughout all the tropical regions of the world and is commonly found on fences and shrubs and in hedgerows.

TRADITIONAL MEDICINAL USES

Africa. Hot water extract of root is taken orally as an aphrodisiac[A04179].

Asia. Fresh fruit is consumed in large amounts for the treatment of diabetes[M23109].

Australia. Fresh fruit is cooked as a vegetable, after steeping in salt water; it is used as an anthelmintic and emetic. Hot water extract of root is taken orally as an abortifacient[A05524].

Bahamas. Hot water extract of dried vine is taken orally as an emmenagogue and for early abortion[T05032].

Belize. Hot water extract of dried leaves taken frequently as a tea is used to treat diabetes[T05011].

Bimini. Fruit is eaten as a vegetable. Hot water extract of the vine is taken orally for diabetes, fevers, and as an abortifacient[T00359].

Brazil. Decoction of dried entire plant is taken orally as a vermifuge and febrifuge[T15975]. Decoction of dried stem is taken orally for fevers and malaria[K07977]. Diluted decoction (14.2%) of fresh leaves is taken orally to treat rheumatism. Cataplasm prepared from fresh leaves is applied externally to treat leprosy, especially to reduce the pain[A00499]. Dried fruit is used as insecticide. Unripe fruit is eaten to treat colds, as a purgative, and abortifacient[K19563]. Ethanol (95%) extract of the entire plant is taken orally for colic and fevers. Hot water extract of fruit is used externally to treat wounds. Fruit juice mixed with Ricinus oil in equal parts is taken orally as an anthelminitic. Hot water extract of root is taken orally as a purgative and to induce abortion and in large doses as an emetic, and the tincture is claimed to have an aphrodisiac effect[A00499]. Seeds are taken orally as an anthelmintic[W00408].

Congo. Extract of entire plant is taken orally for menstrual irregularities[A04171].

Costa Rica. Leaf extract is taken orally as an emmenagogue[T01287].

Cuba. Extract of the entire plant is taken by females to treat sterility[A00115]. Hot water extract of fruit and leaves is taken orally as an emmenagogue[W02588].

Curacao. Hot water extract of vine, decoct with sugar, is taken orally for high blood pressure[A05449].

East Africa. Hot water extract of root is taken orally as an abortifacient[W00113].

England. Hot water extract of dried fruit is taken orally for diabetes[M22031].

Fiji. Fresh fruits toasted or fried in oil is eaten for stomach worms, fever, phlegm, and diabetes. Fresh leaf juice is taken orally for hypertension, dysentery, and diabetes[T10632].

Ghana. Hot water extract of root is taken orally for malarial fever[T16158].

Guadeloupe. Water extract of fruit is taken orally for hyperglycemia[T07660].

Guam. Extract of the entire plant is used externally for malignant ulcers[W00113].

Guatemala. Hot water extract of fresh leaves is used externally for ringworm and skin fungal diseases[M27151].

Haiti. Decoction of dried aerial parts is taken orally for fever. Hot water extract of dried entire plant is taken orally for fever, to stimulate the appetite, for liver troubles, anemia, and rage; ophthalmic, the decoction is used for eye infections and externally for cutaneous infections[T13846].

India. Butanol extract of dried leaves is taken orally as a galactagogue; the hot water extract is taken orally as an emmenagogue in dysmenorrhea, for leprosy, piles, and jaundice. The leaf juice is taken orally as an anthelmintic. Fresh fruit is used as a common vegetable. Extract of the fruit is taken orally for jaundice, piles, leprosy, as an emmenagogue in dysmenorrhea, as a tonic for rheumatism and gout, and as a laxative[T05236]. Hot water extract of dried root is taken orally to induce abortion up to the fifth month of pregnancy[T04748,T14891,W04510]. Hot water extract of dried seeds is taken orally for diabetes, hepatic disorders, pain relief in gout, pain relief in rheumatism, and as an anthelmintic[M25712]. The extremely bitter effusion from boiled seeds when taken orally is said to produce instantaneous vomiting[T02487]. Hot water extract of flowers and leaves is taken orally each month to avoid childbirth through early abortion[T04902]. Hot water extract of fresh seeds is taken orally for diabetes[A14461]. Tender shoots along with young leaves of *Leucas indica*, pepper, garlic, and salt are pounded in equal quantities, made into pills and taken once a day for nine consecutive days to treat pneumonia. Shoots, ground with pepper, camphor, young leaves of *Fluggea lencopyros* and young shoots and bark of mango is taken orally for nine consecutive days to treat leukorrhagia[K11282]. Hot water extract of fruit is taken orally as an anthelmintic, antileprotic,[W00113] and as a remedy for diabetes mellitus[J03769]. Fruit eaten in large doses is considered an abortifacient[A00115]. Hot water extract of dried fruit is taken orally for diabetes[A14379]. Fresh fruit is used as an ingredient in curries[M22031]. For hydro-phobia, *Notonia grandiflora* juice is mixed with bitter gourd (*Momordica charantia* L.) powder and is taken internally[M27166]. Hot water extract of root is taken orally as an abortifacient[A04179,A00115,A05825,W00384]. Hot water extract of seeds is taken orally to produce instantaneous vomiting[T00794]. Seeds are taken orally as an anthelmintic[W00384]. Hot water extract of vine is taken orally as an emmena-gogue[A04179]. Juice of the entire plant is taken orally as an abortifacient and an emmena-gogue[A04132]. Leaves are eaten by children as a purgative[K11282] and anthelmintic[W00384]. Saponifiable fraction of unripe fruit is used as a vegetable. The juice is taken orally for diabetes mellitus[W00678]. Unripe, fresh fruit juice is taken orally for malarial fevers[M23219].

Iraq. Water extract of fruit is taken orally as an anthelmintic and for leprosy[W00113].

Ivory Coast. Leaves are crushed and the juice is drunk with palm wine as an aphrodisiac[A04941].

Jamaica. Hot water extract of dried entire plant is used as a bush tea[W04546]. Hot water extract of dried fruit is taken orally for diabetes[T07170,K20280].

Malaysia. Hot water extract of the entire plant is taken orally as an abortifacient[A03602].

Mexico. Decoction of the entire plant is taken orally to treat diabetes and dysentery[K16948]. Extract of the root is used as an aphrodisiac[A00136]. Hot water extract of leaves is taken orally as an aphrodisiac[A04179].

Nepal. Leaf juice is taken orally as a pur-gative, and emetic[A00020].

Nigeria. Fifteen to twenty dried leaves are crushed into 2–3 glasses of water, the filtrate is taken orally with salt to taste as a treat-ment for diarrhea. Decoction of dried fruit and leaves is taken orally as a laxative and as an anthelmintic[K08933]. Fresh fruit and leaf juices is taken orally as an anthelmintic. Fresh entire plant is used externally for malignant ulcers[T07722]. Fresh fruit is eaten a pot herb. Fresh leaves is eaten as a pot

herb[T06510]. Leaf extract is used to treat breast cancer[T07722].

Panama. Hot water extract of leaves is taken orally as an antipyretic, choleretic, and antidiabetic. Infuse 10–12 leaves in 1 liter of water, and take 3–4 times daily[T01287].

Peru. Hot water extract of dried fruit is taken orally as a purgative and for respira-tory conditions; externally on contusions and wounds. Hot water extract of dried seeds is taken orally as a vermifuge and for colic; externally, it is used for suppurations[T15323].

Philippines. Decoction of dried entire plant is used as a bath for newborns. It is believed that it removes disease-causing elements from the skin. The petroleum ben-zene extract is taken orally for coughs in infants[T10116]. Hot water extract of root is taken orally to produce abortions. Hot water extract of vine is taken orally as a powerful emmenagogue[A04179].

Puerto Rico. Hot water extract of dried entire plant is taken orally for diabetes[A14280]. Hot water extract of the entire plant is taken orally as a treatment for diabetes mellitus[A01947]. Hot water extract of vine is taken orally for diabetes[A00637,A04179] and is rubbed on the skin to relieve itching[A06027].

Saudi Arabia. Hot water extract of dried fruit is taken orally for rheumatism, gout, liver disorders, spleen disorders, pyrexia, colic, flatulence, menstrual suppression, and diabetes[M22673,T10348].

Senegal. Hot water extract of dried entire plant is taken orally for intestinal pain and externally as a cicatrisant[T12145].

Sri Lanka. Extract of the fruit is taken orally as an anthelmintic[W00113]. Fresh fruit juice[K17959]. and hot water extract[M17655] are taken orally for diabetes mellitus. Hot water extract of dried fruit is taken orally as a hypoglycemic agent[T08396].

Thailand. Decoction of dried fruit is taken orally as an anti-inflammatory,[T16711] and hot water extract is taken orally for dia-betes[W01792]. Hot water extract of dried entire plant is taken orally as an antipyretic[W3022A]. Hot water extract of dried leaves is taken orally as an antipyretic[W03804].

Togo. Decoction of dried leaves is taken orally for malaria[M23556].

Trinidad. Decoction of dried fruit, leaf, and stem is taken orally for diabetes (noninsulin-dependent)[M23565].

Turkey. Dried fruit juice is taken orally as a treatment for peptic ulcers[K11898]. Fresh fruit is eaten as a treatment for ulcers[K18219].

USA. Hot water extract of fruit is administered rectally as a remedy for hemorrhoids. Externally, the fruit is used for snakebite, leprosy, itching, skin, burns, and wounds. Unripe fruit is taken orally for bacillary dysentery; taken every two days, it relieves chronic colitis and in large doses it is an abortifacient. Unripe fruit juice is used externally to treat burns. Hot water extract is taken orally for thrush, as a substitute for quinine in intermittent fever, as a remedy for liver and spleen ailments, for gout and rheumatism, as a vermifuge, purgative, and for menstrual difficulties[A04179].

Venezuela. Hot water extract of root is taken orally as an antimalarial[A04179].

Virgin Islands. Fruit is taken orally for a bad heart and diabetes[W00903].

West Africa. Extract of the root together with the fruit of seeds is taken orally as an abortifacient[A00115]. Fruit is taken orally as an abortifacient[W00113] and antidiabetic remedy[T02106].

West Indies. Decoction (sweetened) of the hot water extract of leaves is taken orally as a powerful emmenagogue, for diabetes, hypertension, to treat worms, and to treat malarial fever. Fresh plant juice is taken orally for fever and to stimulate the appetite. The juice is applied ophthalmic for eye infection[T13846]. Fruit juice is taken orally for diabetes. Hot water extract of fresh or dried vine with salt is taken orally by women before and after childbirth. Seeds are taken orally as an anthelmintic. Hot water extract

of the entire plant is taken orally as a laxative and abortifacient; infusion alone or with *Bidens reptans* is drunk for menstrual troubles[T00701]. Hot water extract of vine is taken orally regularly each month by women to avoid childbirth by early abortion[A04179]. Infusion of dried leaves is used a tea which is ascribed anti-diabetic properties[M23109].

CHEMICAL CONSTITUENTS
(ppm unless otherwise indicated)

(-)-Menthol, Sd EO
5-a stigasta-7,22,25-trien-3-b-ol, Pl
5-a stigasta-7,25-dien-3-b-ol, Pl
5-Hydroxytryptamine, Fr
24-Methylene cycloartenol, Sd oil
Alanine, Sd 0.0158%
Alkaloids, Fr 380
Alpha carotene 5-6-epoxy, PC
Alpha carotene epoxide, PC
Alpha glucose, Sd
Alpha momorcharin, Sd
Alpha spinasterol, Fr
Alpha–alpha trehalose, Sd
Alpha–elaeostearic acid, 0.467–23.163%
Arginine, Sd 0.0323%
Ascorbic acid, Fr 0.057–3.645%;
    Lf 0.17–1.24%
Ascorbigen, Fr
Ash, Fr 0.4–14.2%; Lf 2.1–14.9%
Asparagine, Sd
Aspartic acid, Sd 0.009%
Beta alanine, Fr
Beta amyrin, Sd oil
Beta carotene 5-6-epoxy, PC
Beta carotene, Fr; Lf 51–330
Beta glucose, Sd
Beta momorcharin, Sd 0.08%
Beta sitosterol, Fr
Beta sitosterol-D-glucoside, Fr
Calceolarioside E, Aer
Calcium, Fr 130–4,333; Lf 0.264–1.87%
Capric acid, Sd oil
Carbohydrates, Fr 4.7–76.3%; Lf 7–61.8%
Charantin, Fr 0.035–0.15%; Sd
Charine, Fr
Cholesterol, Fr
Citrulline, Fr
Copper, Fr 30
Cryptoxanthin, Fr; PC
Cucurbita-5-24-dien-3-beta-ol,10-alpha, Sd oil

Cucurbita-5-24-diene,3-beta-7-beta-23-
   trihydroxy-7-O-beta-D-glucoside, Lf
Cucurbitacin B, Sd
Cucurbitacin K, Sd
Cycloartenol, Sd oil
Galacturonic acid, Fr
Delta carotene, PC
Diosgenin, Fr; Tc
Elasterol, Pl
Ethylene, Fr
Fat, Fr 0.2–6.0%; Lf 0.4–3.9%;
   Sd 1.0-49.6%
Fiber, Fr 1.0–25.78%; Lf 0.5–10.4%
Flavochrome, Fr
Fluoride, Fr 0.2–0.5
Fluorine, Fr 4.8
Galactouronic acid, Fr
Gamma aminobutyric acid, Fr
Gamma carotene, PC
Gentisic acid, Lf
Glutamic acid, Fr; Sd 0.0212%
Glycine, Sd 38.2
Hexadecan-1-ol, Sd EO
Histidine, Sd
Inhibitor BG-1-A, Sd
Inulin, Cal Tiss; Fr
Iodine, Fr 0.41
Iron, Fr 2–560; Lf 50–357
Iso leucine, Sd
Kilocalories, Fr 190–3,290; Lf 440–3,020
Lanosterol, Fr
Lauric acid, Fr; Sd oil
Lead, Fr 5
Lectin inhibitor A, Sd
Lectin, Sd
Leucine, Sd
Linoleic acid, Sd oil 0.07–3.8%; Fr; Cot
Linolenic acid, Sd oil, Fr, Cot
Lutein, PC
Lycopene, Sd; Fr; PC
Lysine, Sd
Magnesium, Fr 0.0195–0.38%
Manganese, Fr 10
MAP-30, Sd
Momorcharaside A, Sd
Momorcharaside B, Sd
Momorcharin 1, Sd
Momorcharin 11, Sd
Momordica agglutinin, Sd
Momordica anti-HIV protein MAP-30, Sd
Momordica chanantia cytostatic factor or
   40,000 daltons, Fr

Momordica charantia cytostatic factor or
   11,000 daltons, Fr
Momordica charantia cytostatic factor, Fr
Momordica charantia inhibitor protein, Sd
Momordica charantia lectin, Sd
Momordica charantia steroid glycoside, Fr
Momordica charantia triterpene glycoside, Cot
Momordica cucurbitane 3, Lf
Momordica cucurbitane 6, Lf
Momordica elastase inhibitor MEI-1, Sd
Momordica protein MAP-30, Fr; Sd
Momordica trypsin inhibitor MTI-1
Momordica trypsin inhibitor MTI-11
Momordicin 8, Lf
Momordicin 11, Lf
Momordicin, Fr
Momordicine 1, Lf + St 0.07%
Momordicine 111, Lf + St 0.12%
Momordicine, Lf
Momordicoside A, Sd 0.1287%
Momordicoside B, Sd 0.0090%
Momordicoside C, Sd 0.0114%
Momordicoside D, Sd 0.00228%
Momordicoside E', Fr 0.00104%
Momordicoside E, Fr 0.0037%
Momordicoside E–1, Fr 0.0756%
Momordicoside EX, Fr 0.00126%
Momordicoside F', 0.0006%
Momordicoside F, Fr 0.0072%
Momordicoside F–1, Fr 0.0434%
Momordicoside F–2, Fr 0.004%
Momordicoside G, Fr 0.01236%
Momordicoside H, Fr 0.0074%
Momordicoside I, Fr 0.0082%
Momordicoside J, Fr 0.0008%
Momordicoside K, Fr
Momordicoside L, Fr 0.0036%
Momordin 2, Sd
Momordin A, Sd
Momordin B, Sd
Momordin, Sd
Multiflorenol, Sd oil
Mutatochrome, PC
Mycose, Sd
Myristic acid, Sd oil
Nerolidol Sd EO
Niacin, Fr 3–50; Lf 15–103
Nickel, Fr 10
Nitrogen, Fr 3.38%
Oleic acid, Fr; Cot 15.58%
Ornithine, Sd 0.0063%
Oxalate, Fr 185–1,444

Oxalic acid, Fr 5
P-insulin, Sd; Fr
Palmitic acid, Fr; Sd oil; Cot 2.71–51.95%
Palmitoleic acid, Fr
Para cymene, Sd EO
Pectin, Fr
Pentadecan–1–ol, Sd EO
Peroxidase, Fr
Petroselinic acid, Sd
Phenylalanine, Fr
Phosphorus, Fr 0.032–0.83%
Phosphorus, Lf 0.054–3.3467%
Phytofluene, PC; Tr; Sd
Pipecolic acid, Fr
Polypeptide–P, Fr
Potassium, Fr 0.27–4.50%; Lf 0.51–3.30%
Proline, Fr
Protein, Fr 0.9–18.1%; Lf 5.1–37.1%
Riboflavin, Fr 0.4–9; Lf 4.6–31
Ribosome-inactivating protein 1, Sd
Ribosome-inactivating protein 2, Sd
Ribosome-inactivating protein 3, Sd
Ribosome-inactivating protein 4, Sd
Rosmarinic acid, Aer
Rubixanthin acid, Aer
Serine, Sd 0.0040%
Sodium, Fr 20–333; Lf 190–1,234
Squalene, Sd EO
Stearic acid, Sd oil 2.98–14.78%; Fr; Cot
Stigast-5-ene-3-beta-25 diol, Fr
Stigasta-5,25-dien-3-beta-ol, Pl
Stigasta-5-25(27)-dien-3-beta-ol,3-0-(6'-0-
    palmitoyl-beta-D-glucosyl), Fr
Stigasta–5–25(27)–dien–3–beta–ol,3–0–(6'–
    0–stearoyl–beta–D–glucosyl), Fr
Stigasta–5–25–dien–3–beta–ol, Fr
Stigasta–5–25–diene–3–beta–D–glucoside, Fr
Stigasta–7–22–25–trien–3–beta–ol, Fr
Stigasta–7–22–diene–3–beta–ol, Fr
Stigasterol, Fr
Sugars, Fr 3.5–4.5%
Taraxerol, Sd oil
Thiamin, Fr 0.2–12; Lf 1.3–8
Threonine, Sd 0.0017%
Titanium, Fr 100
Trehalose, Sd 0.3960%
Trypsin inhibitor MI–3, Sd
Tyrosine, Sd 0.0517%
Urease, Sd
V–insulin, Fr
Verbascoside, Aer
Vicine, Sd 0.0500–0.4000%

Water, Fr 79.5–93.4%; Lf 80.1–84.6%
Zeatin riboside, Sd
Zeatin, Sd
Zeaxanthin, PC
Zeinoxanthin, PC

PHARMACOLOGICAL ACTIVITIES AND CLINICAL TRIALS

Abortifacient effect. Ethanol/water (1:1) extract of dried aerial parts administered orally to pregnant rats at a dose of 100.0 mg/kg was inactive. Ethanol/water (1:1) extract of dried fruit administered orally to rats at a dose of 100.0 mg/kg was inactive[T02678]. Water extract of dried seed administered intraperitoneally to pregnant rats at a dose of 8.0 mg/kg was active. A fraction designated as AP–11 was tested[T00398]. Acetone extract of dried seed administered intraperitoneally to pregnant mice at a dose of 4.0 mc/gm on day 12 of pregnancy was active[T10072]. Water extract administered intraperitoneally to pregnant mice at a dose of 0.04 mg/ml was active[K21690]. Water extract of leaves administered orally to female rats at a dose of 200.0 mg/kg was inactive[W01362].

Adenyl cyclase inhibition. Dried fruit in cell culture was inactive[T08662].

Analgesic activity. Ethanol/water (1:1) extract of dried entire plant administered intragastrically to mice was inactive vs hot plate method and tail clip method. Ethanol/water (1:1) extract of dried fruit administered intragastrically to mice was inactive[K09153]. Methanol extract of dried seed administered subcutaneously, 30 minutes before challenge, was active in mice and equivocal in rats. Naloxone does not inhibit effect vs acetic acid-induced writhing[25712].

Anthelmintic activity. Ethanol (95%) extract of fruit at a concentration of 100.0 mg/ml was active on *Ascaridia galli*. Ethanol (95%) extract of fruit juice at a concentration of 0.1 ml was active on *Ascaridia galli*[K03520]. Hot water extract of seed at a concentration of 1:50 was active on *Haemonchus contortus*[W00384].

Antibacterial activity. Chloroform and ethanol (95%) extracts of dried fruit at concentrations of 250.0 mg/ml on agar plate were active on *Bacillus subtilis*, *Escherichia coli*, *Pseudomonas aeruginosa*, and *Staphylococcus aureus*. Ethanol/water (1:1) extract at a concentration of 1.0 mg/ml in broth culture was inactive on *Pseudomonas aeruginosa*. Water extract at a concentration of 250.0 mg/ml on agar plate was active on *Bacillus subtilis*, *Escherichia coli*, and *Pseudomonas aeruginosa* and inactive on *Staphylococcus aureus*. Petroleum ether extract at a concentration of 250.0 mg/ml on agar plate was active on *Bacillus subtilis* and *Pseudomonas aeruginosa* and inactive on *Staphylococcus aureus* and *Escherichia coli*[K19538]. Dried fruit on agar plate was active on *Sarcina lutea*. chloroform, ether, water, and methanol extracts of dried fruit on agar plate were active on *Escherichia coli*, *Pseudomonas aeruginosa*, *Salmonella typhosa*, *Sarcina lutea*, *Shigella dysenteriae*, and strong activity on *Staphylococcus aureus* MIC < 50.0 mg/disk. Water and methanol extracts also produced strong activity on *Bacillus subtilis*, MIC < 50.0 mg/disk. Petroleum ether extract was inactive on *Escherichia coli*, *Pseudomonas aeruginosa*, *Salmonella typhosa*, *Sarcina lutea*, *Shigella dysenteriae*, and *Staphylococcus aureus*[P00093]. Ethanol (95%) and hot water extracts of dried bark on agar plate were active on *Escherichia coli* and *Staphylococcus aureus*[W03693]. Ethanol (95%) and water extracts of dried seeds at a concentration of 10.0 mg/ml on agar plate were inactive on *Corynebacterium diphtheriae*, *Diplococcus pneumoniae*, *Staphylococcus aureus*, *Streptococcus pyogenes*, and *Streptococcus viridans*[M29966]. Ethanol (95%) extract of dried leaves undiluted on agar plate was inactive on *Staphylococcus aureus* and *Escherichia coli*; hot water extract was active[W03693]. Methanol extract of dried leaves on agar plate at a concentration of 2.0 mg/ml was active on *Corynebacterium diptheriae*, Neis-

seria species, *Pseudomonas aeruginosa*, *Salmonella* species, *Streptobacillus* species, *Streptococcus* species, and inactive on *Staphylococcus aureus*[M27767]. Ethanol/water (1:1) extract of entire plant at a concentration of 1.0 mg/ml in broth culture was inactive on *Pseudomonas aeruginosa*[K09153]. Methanol extract of dried entire plant at a concentration of 15.0 mg/ml on agar plate was active on *Sarcina lutea*[T09739]. Methanol/water (1:1) extract of leaves in broth culture was active on *Staphylococcus aureus* and inactive on *Bacillus subtilis*, *Escherichia coli*, Proteus species, *Pseudomonas aeruginosa*, and *Staphylococcus albus*[J00209]. Unsaponifiable fraction of seed oil on agar plate was active on several Gram negative organism[T07075].

Anticlastogenic activity. Fruit and leaf juice administered intraperitoneally to mice at a dose of 50.0 ml/kg was active on marrow cells vs mitomycin C-, tetracycline-, and dimethylnitrosamine-induced micronuclei[K17561].

Anticonvulsant activity. Ethanol (70%) extract of fresh fruit administered intraperitoneally to mice of both sexes at variable dosages was inactive vs metrazole- and strychnine-induced convulsions. Ethanol (70%) extract of fresh leaves administered intraperitoneally to mice of both sexes at variable dosage levels was inactive vs metrazole- and strychnine-induced convulsions[T06510]. Ethanol/water (1:1) extract of dried entire plant administered intraperitoneal to mice was inactive vs supramaximal electroshock-induced convulsions. Ethanol/water (1:1) extract of dried fruit administered intraperitoneally to mice was inactive vs hot plate and tail clip method[K09153].

Antifertility effect. Fresh leaf juice administered orally to female mice was active[W02108]. Unripe fruit juice administered by gastric intubation to male rats at a dose of 5.0 ml/kg daily for 49 days, followed by mating, was active[T05027].

Antifungal activity. Ethanol (95%) extract of dried seeds at a concentration of 10.0 mg/ml on agar plate was inactive on *Microsporum canis, Microsporum gypseum, Phialophora jeanselmei, Piedraia hortae,* and *Trichophyton mentagrophytes*[M29966]. Ethanol/water (1:1) extract of dried entire plant at a concentration of 1.0 mg/ml in broth culture was inactive on *Aspergillus fumigatus* and *Trichophyton mentagrophytes*. Ethanol/water (1:1) extract of dried fruit at a concentration of 1.0 mg/ml in broth culture was inactive on *Aspergillus fumigatus* and *Trichophyton mentagrophytes*[K09153]. Hot water extract of fresh leaves in broth culture at a concentration of 1.0 ml was inactive on *Epidermophyton floccosum, Microsporum canis, Trichophyton mentagrophytes* var. algodonosa, and granulare[M27151].

Antihepatotoxic activity. Hot water extract of dried aerial parts at a concentration of 1.0 mg/plate in cell culture was inactive on hepatocytes, measured by leakage of LDH and ASAT[K23019].

Antihistamine activity. Ethanol/water (1:1) extract of dried entire plant at a concentration of 0.01 gm/ml produced weak activity on guinea pig ileum[W3022A].

Antihypercholesterolemic activity. Acetone extract of dried fruit in the ration of rats at a dose of 250.0 mg/kg was active vs alloxan-induce hyperglycemia[M22671]. Fruit taken orally by male human adults at a dose of 2.0 gm/person was active. Ten mild diabetic patients (23–28 years of age) were used in the study. Fruit powder was given once daily for 11 days[M27532].

Antihyperglycemic activity. Acetone extract of dried fruit in the ration of rats at a dose of 250.0 mg/kg was active. Fall in blood sugar of 49% in 30 days. Blood sugar was maintained within normal limits for two weeks after treatment ceased vs alloxan-induced hyperglycemia[M22671]. Benzene extract of dried fruit administered intragastrically to rabbit at a dose of 1.0 g/kg was active. Alloxan-recovered rabbits were tested for glucose tolerance following

sample treatment vs glucose-induced hyperglycemia[M22131]. Chloroform extract of dried fruit administered intragastrically to female rats at a dose of 250.0 mg/kg was inactive vs streptozotocin-induced hyperglycemia[K19538]. Decoction of dried fruit taken orally by human adults at a dose of 500.0 mg/person was active[A14458]. Ethanol (95%) extract of dried fruit administered intragastrically to female rats at a dose of 250.0 mg/kg was active vs streptozotocin-induced hyperglycemia; 75.0 mg/kg administered intraperitoneally to rats was inactive[T12220]. Dried powdered fruit, taken orally once daily for 11 days by ten male patients with mild diabetes (23–28 years of age), at a dose of 2.0 gm/person was active[M27532]. Water extract of dried fruit administered intragastrically to female rats at a dose of 250.0 mg/kg was active vs streptozotocin-induced hyperglycemia. The effect was potentiated when used with *C. longa* and *E. officinalis*[K19538]. The water extract when administered orally to rats at a dose of 4.0 gm/day for two months was active vs alloxan-induced hyperglycemia. Onset of retinopathy was also retarded[T14959]. Acetone extract of dried fruit at a dose of 250.0 mg/kg in the ration of rats was inactive vs alloxan-induced hyperglycemia[M22671]. Decoction of dried fruit, leaves and stem administered intraperitoneally to male mice at a dose of 0.5 ml/animal was active vs streptozotocin-induced hyperglycemia. 1.0 ml of extract is equivalent to 10 gm of dried plant material. Single dose of the extract reduced plasma concentration by about 50% after five hours [M23565]. Decoction of fresh seeds taken orally by human adults at variable dosage levels was inactive. Three patients were studied; half of a seed was boiled in five cups of water until the volume was two cups. One cupful was given in the morning and one in the evening[A14461]. Methanol extract of shade dried seeds administered orally to rats at a dose of 10.0 mg/kg was active vs adrenaline-induced hyperglycemia[T14966]. Dried fruit administered intragastrically to rabbits at a dose of 1.0 gm/kg was active vs alloxan-induced hyperglycemia[M22028]. Decoction of 25% aqueous extract of dried fruit administered intragastrically to mice at a dose of 0.5 ml/animal was inactive vs alloxan-induced hyperglycemia, maximal change in blood sugar was 4.33%[M22673]. Hot water extract (25%) of dried fruit administered by gastric intubation to mice at a dose of 0.5 ml was inactive vs alloxan-induced hyperglycemia[T10348]. Dried fruit extract together with a mixture of *Litchi chinensis* saponins, oleanolic acid administered intraperitoneally to mice at a dose of 0.1 gm/kg was active. Biological activity reported has been patented[M29299]. Dried fruit taken orally by human adults was active. A diabetic woman recovered from glycosuria after taking a kind of curry. Karela was an active ingredient[M22031]. Ethanol (95%) extract of dried aerial parts and fruits administered intragastrically to rats at a dose of 250.0 mg/kg was inactive vs rats fasted for 18 hours, over fed rats, glucose-induced hyperglycemia and streptozotocin-induced hyperglycemia. With dosing for 21 days, the extract was also inactive vs glucose-induced hyperglycemia[M22670]. Ethanol (95%) extract of dried entire plant administered intragastrically to rats at a dose of 250.0 mg/kg was active vs rats fasted for 18 hours, overfed rats, glucose-induced hyperglycemia, streptozotocin-induced hyperglycemia and when dosed for 21 days vs glucose-induced hyperglycemia[M22670]. Ethanol (95%) extract of fresh fruit administered intragastrically to rats at a dose of 200.0 mg/kg was active vs streptozotocin-induced hyperglycemia. Blood sugar levels decreased 22%[K11849]. Fresh fruit administered intragastrically to rats at a dose of 15.0 g/animal, 5 g each time, three times a day for three weeks was active vs alloxan-induced hyperglycemia. Water extract of fresh fruit

administered intragastrically to rats at a dose of 1.0 g/animal for a period of three weeks was active vs alloxan-induced hyperglycemia The reduction of the initial blood sugar level decreased from 220 mg% to 105 mg%. Water extract of fresh fruit administered orally to male human adults at a dose of 1.0 g/animal was active vs alloxan-induced hyperglycemia. The subjects included (433 mg%) severe to mild (260%) diabetics, aged 42 to 70 years. Blood sugar was estimated after two, three, four, and seven weeks of treatment. The fall in blood sugar was highly significant at the termination of treatment. The overall fall in blood sugar was 54%[K12995]. Hot water extract of fresh fruit administered intragastrically to rats of both sexes at a dose of 4.0 g/animal was active vs alloxan-induced hyperglycemia[M23178]. Fresh fruit juice administered intragastrically to rabbit at a dose of 6.0 ml/kg was active vs alloxan- and glucose-induced hyperglycemia[A14328]. Ethanol (95%) extract of fruit and fruit juice administered orally to rabbits at doses of 3.0 ml/kg were active vs alloxan-induced hyperglycemia[A07281]. Fresh fruit juice taken orally by human adults at a dose of 50.0 ml/day for 8 to 11 weeks was active. Improved glucose tolerance in diabetic patients was observed. Results significant at P < 0.01 level[T12686]. When administered intragastrically to male rats at a dose of 5.0 ml/kg, the juice was active. A glucose tolerance test was used[A14525]. Fresh fruit juice administered intragastrically to rats at a dose of 10.0 ml/kg daily for 30 days was inactive vs streptozotocin-induced hyperglycemia[T16092]. Fresh fruit juice taken by human adults at a dose of 100.0 ml 30 minutes before oral glucose load in the glucose tolerance test was active. The results indicated improved glucose tolerance in 73% of patients with maturity onset diabetes. Eighteen patients participated[T12706]. Fried fruit taken orally by human adults at a dose of 0.23 kg/day for

8 to 11 weeks was active. Improved glucose tolerance in diabetic patients was observed. Results significant at P < 0.05 level[T12686]. Fruit pulp juice administered intragastrically to rats at a dose of 2.5 gm/kg was inactive vs streptozotocin-induced hyperglycemia. Methanol extract was inactive[K13947]. Hot water extract of dried fruit administered to diabetic rabbits at a dose of 10.20 mg/kg was active[P00050]. Lyophilized extract of dried fruit administered to rabbit at doses of 1.2 gm and 400 mg/kg were inactive vs alloxan-induced hyperglycemia[P00096]. Hot water extract of fresh fruit juice taken orally by human adults was active on maturity onset diabetics vs glucose-induced hyperglycemia. 73% improved glucose tolerance was observed[M17655]. Hot water extract of fruit juice administered orally to rats at a dose of 5.0 ml/kg was equivocal vs anterior pituitary extract-induced hyperglycemia[A07232]. Methanol extract of seed administered intragastrically to rats at a dose of 2.5 gm/kg was inactive vs streptozotocin-induced hyperglycemia[K13947]. Protein fraction (FM-1) of dried fruit was active on mice[M22015]. Seeds administered by gastric intubation to rabbits was active in streptozotocin-treated animals[T05236]. Water extract of fresh fruit administered intragastrically to male mice at a dose of 0.5 gm/kg was active. There was a significant decrease in nonfasting blood-glucose levels of hyperglycemia induced mice. Results significant at P < 0.01 level[K18219]. Water extract of fresh fruit administered intragastrically to mice at a dose of 16.0 gm/kg was active vs streptozotocin-induced hyperglycemia[M25031]. Water extract of seed administered orally to rabbits at a dose of 3.0 ml/kg was inactive vs alloxan-induced hyperglycemia[A07281].

Anti-implantation effect. Ethanol/water (1:1) extract of dried aerial parts administered orally to rats at a dose of 100.0 mg/kg was inactive. Ethanol/water (1:1) extract of dried fruit administered to rats

at a dose of 100.0 mg/kg was inactive[T02678]. Hot water extract of leaves administered orally to rats at a dose of 500.0 mg/kg was inactive[A04902].

Antilipolytic activity. Acetone extract of dried seed at a concentration of 500.0 mcg/plate was active on rat adipocytes vs ACTA and epinephrine bitartrate induced lipolysis. Acetone extract of unripe fresh fruit at a concentration of 500.0 mcg/plate was active on rat adipocytes vs ACTA-induced lipolysis, epinephrine bitartrate-induced lipolysis, and glucagon-induced lipolysis[T11178]. Chromatographic fraction of decorticated seed at a concentration of 300.0 mcg/ml was active on hamster adipocytes. A concentration of 250.0 mg/ml was active on rat adipocytes. Results significant at P < 0.005 level[M11890].

Antimalarial activity. Chloroform extract of aerial parts administered subcutaneously to chicken at a dose of 42.0 mg/kg was inactive on *Plasmodium gallinaceum*. A dose of 496.0 mg/kg administered subcutaneously to duckling was inactive on *Plasmodium cathemerium*. Water extract at a dose of 3.44 gm/kg administered orally to chicken was inactive on *Plasmodium gallinaceum*; a dose of 2.37 gm/kg administered orally to ducklings was inactive on *Plasmodium cathemerium* and *Plasmodium lophurae*[A00785]. Ethanol (95%) extract of dried leaves produced weak activity on *Plasmodium falciparum*. IC_{50} 68.4 mg/ml[M23556]. Water extract of dried flowers administered intragastrically to mice at a dose of 1.0 gm/kg was inactive on *Plasmodium berghei*[K07998].

Antimutagenic activity. Carbon tetrachloride and petroleum ether extracts of green fruit administered intragastrically to mice at doses of 5.0 mg/gm, given twice, were active. Methanol extract was inactive[M24272]. Methanol-insoluble fraction of dried leaves was active vs methylnitrosamine, methyl methane sulfonate, or tetracycline-induced genotoxicity[K17876].

Antimycobacterial activity. Chloroform, water, and methanol extracts of dried fruit on agar plate were active on *Mycobacterium smegatis*. The ether extract produced strong activity, MIC 2.0 mg/disk. Petroleum ether extract was inactive[P00093].

Antiprotozoan activity. Ethanol/water (1:1) extract of dried entire plant at a concentration of 125.0 mg/ml in broth culture was active on *Entamoeba histolytica*[K09153]. Ethanol/water (1:1) extract of dried fruit in culture broth was active on *Entamoeba histolytica*. IC_{100} was 25.0 mcg/ml[K09153].

Antipyretic activity. Ethanol/water (1:1) extract of dried entire plant administered by gastric intubation to rabbit at variable dosage was inactive vs yeast-induced pyrexia[W3022A].

Antispermatogenic effect. Ethanol (95%) extract of fruit administered orally to male dogs at a dose of 1.75 gm/animal was active. Animals were dosed daily for 20 days, sacrificed, and then organs examined. Seminiferous tubules lacked primary spermatocytes. 38.7% tubule contained normal spermatids. Spermatid abnormalities consisted of clear and vacuoled nuclei and formation of giant multinucleated cells. Interstitial cells did not show morphological evidence of lesions. After daily dosing for 40 days, tubule diameter decreased to 167 m (220 for controls). Testes exhibited variable degrees of spermatogenic arrest, mainly at spermatid stage disorganization, sloughing of immature cells, and giant cell formation common in damaged tubules. Daily dosing for 60 days produced seminiferous tubules completely devoid of spermatozoa. Seventy-five percent completely lacked step 1–8 spermatid. Many tubules devoid of cells except for sertoli cells and basal spermatogonia. Tubular diameters minimal and lumen of epididymis and vas deferens devoid of spermatozoa. The extract administered orally and subcutaneously to male gerbils at doses 200.0 mg/kg daily for two weeks were active. Reduction in tes-ticular weight and disruption of spermatogenesis without affecting seminal vesicles or prostate was observed[M01152].

Antitumor activity. Hot water extract of entire plant administered intraperitoneally to rats at a dose of 0.4 mg/animal produced weak activity on Sarcoma 180 (ASC). Slight increase in life span was observed. When administered orally to human adult at a dose of 15.0 ml/person three times daily for 62 days was active on cancer (human). The extract, when was administered to one lymphatic leukemia patient caused marked increase in hemoglobin content and decrease in WBC[A00706]. Water extract of fresh fruit administered intraperitoneally to mice at a dose of 100.0 mg/ml was inactive on CBA/D1 cells. Drug was preincubated with tumor cells and then injected concomitantly. The extract was also active on LEUK–L1210, drug was preincubated with tumor cell line in vitro. Weak activity was produced on LEUK–P388, drug was also preincubated with tumor cell line in vitro[T09137].

Antiulcer activity. Chloroform, ethanol (95%), and hexane extracts, and essential oil administered intragastrically to rats at doses of 500.0 mg/kg were inactive[K11898].

Antiviral activity. Ethanol/water (1:1) extract of dried fruit in cell culture at a concentration of 0.05 mg/ml was inactive on Ranikhet and Vaccinia virus[K09153].

Antiyeast activity. Chloroform, ether, and methanol extracts of dried fruit on agar plate were active on *Candida albicans*. Water extract produced strong activity, MIC 25 mg/disk. Petroleum ether extract was inactive[P00093]. Ethanol (95%) and water extracts of seeds, at a concentration of 10.0 mg/ml on agar plate, were inactive on *Candida albicans* and *Candida tropicalis*[M29966]. Ethanol/water (1:1) extract of dried entire plant at a concentration of 1.0 mg/ml in broth culture was inactive on *Candida albicans*, *Cryptococcus neoformans*, and *Sporotrichum schenckii*.

Ethanol/water (1:1) extract of dried fruit at a concentration of 1.0 mg/ml in broth culture was inactive on *Candida albicans*, *Cryptococcus neoformans*, and *Sporotrichum schenckii*[K09153].

CNS depressant activity. Ethanol (70%) extract of fresh fruit administered intraperitoneally to mice of both sexes at variable dosages was active. Ethanol (70%) extract of fresh leaves administered intraperitoneally to mice of both sexes at variable dosage levels was active[T06510].

Cytotoxic activity. Dried fruit extract in cell culture was active on CA–755 and Leuk–CML (Human)[T08662]. Fresh fruit juice in cell culture at a concentration of 0.14 mg/ml was active on Melanoma-B cell-M9. Viable cells decreased from 100% to 5% between 18 and 26 hours. The juice was also active on human lymphocytes and leukemic lymphocytes. ED_{50} 0.35 and 0.16 mg/plate, respectively[T04893]. Hot water extract of entire plant at a concentration of 4.0 mg/ml was active on HEP 2 Cells[A00706]. Water extract of dried fruit in cell culture was inactive on human lymphocytes[T08985]. Water extract of fresh fruit in cell culture was active on CBA/D1 cells. CD_{10} 50.0 mcg/ml. The activity was highly dose-dependent[T09137]. Water extract of fresh fruit in cell culture was active on human lymphoblast and lymphocytes[T01575]. Water extract of seeds in cell culture was inactive on *Sarcoma* (Yoshida ASC). $ED_{50} > 1.0$ mg/ml[A04780].

Diuretic activity. Ethanol/water (1:1) extract of dried entire plant administered intragastrically to rats at a dose of 510.7 mg/kg was inactive. Ethanol/water (1:1) extract of dried fruit administered intragastrically to rats at a dose of 510.7 mg/kg was inactive vs supramaximal electroshock-induced convulsions[K09153].

DNA Synthesis inhibition. Hot water extract of entire plant at a concentration of 0.1 mg/ml was active on sea urchin ova (antimitotic effect)[A00706]. Chromatographic fraction of dried fruit in cell culture was active on BKH-21 cells and vesicular stomatitis virus[T08985]. Ethanol (100%) extract of seed in cell culture was active on Sarcoma 180 (solid)[M27078].

Embryotoxic effect. Water[W01362] and hot water[A04902] extracts of leaves administered orally to rats at 200.0 and 500.0 mg/kg respectively were inactive.

Estrogenic effect. Hot water extract of leaves administered subcutaneously to rats at a dose of 20.0 mg/animal was inactive[A04902].

Feeding deterrent (insect). Glycoside mixture of dried cotyledons at a concentration of 2.0 mg/insect was active on *Raphidopalpa foveicollis*[T08932]. Seed oil at a concentration of 0.5% was active on *Athalia promina*[T02572].

Fructose diphosphatase inhibition. Ethanol (95%) extract of fresh fruit administered intragastrically to rats at a dose of 200.0 mg/kg was active, activity decreased 20%[K11849].

Gamma-glutamyltransferase induction. Unripe fruit juice administered intragastrically to male rats at a dose of 10.0 ml/kg was active. Results significant at $P < 0.001$ level[M17655].

Gluconeogenesis inhibition. Hot water extract of fresh fruit juice was inactive on kidneys[M17655].

Glucose absorption inhibition. Acetone extract of oven-dried fruit at a concentration of 125.0 mg/ml was active on rats small intestine. Ethanol (95%) extract was inactive on adipocytes. Aqueous high speed supernatant of fresh fruit at a concentration of 50.0 microliters was active on the small intestine and inactive on adipocytes of rats[T12135]. Water extract of fresh fruit administered intragastrically to mice at a dose of 16.0 gm/animal was inactive vs streptozotocin-induced hyperglycemia[M25031].

Glucose oxidase inhibition. Aqueous high speed supernatant of fresh fruit at a concentration of 50.0 microliters was active on rat adipocytes and liver homogenates[T12135]. Ethanol (95%) extract of oven-dried fruit at a concentration of 125.0 mg/ml was active on rat adipocytes and liver homogenates[T12135].

Glucose uptake induction. Fresh fruit juice administered by gastric intubation to rats at a dose of 10.0 mg/kg was active. Results significant at $P < 0.001$ level[T12703]. Hot water extract of fresh fruit juice was active[M17655].

Glucose-6-phosphatase dehydrogenase stimulation. Ethanol (95%) extract of fresh fruit administered intragastrically to rats at a dose of 200.0 mg/kg was active vs streptozotocin-induced hyperglycemia[K11849].

Glucose–6–phosphatase inhibition. Ethanol (95%) extract of fresh fruit administered intragastrically to rats at a dose of 200.0 mg/kg was active vs streptozotocin-induced hyperglycemia, activity decreased 23%[K11849].

Growth inhibitor activity. Hot water extract administered to rats at a dose of 2.0 mg/animal was active on fetal development[A00706].

Guanylate cyclase inhibition. Water extract of fresh fruit in cell culture was active on human lymphoblasts. ED_{50} 0.3 mg/ml[T01575]. Dried fruit extract in cell culture was active[T08662]. Ethanol (defatted with petroleum ether) extract of fresh fruit was active. ED_{50} 170.0 mcg/ml[T12861]. Water extract of fruit produced strong activity on rat colon, heart, kidney, liver, lung, and stomach. Water extracts of seed and unripe fruit were inactive on rat liver[M00425]. Water extract of leaves produced strong activity on rat liver[M00425].

Hematinic activity. Hot water extract of entire plant taken orally by human adults at a dose of 15.0 ml/person three times daily for 62 days was active. The extract was administered to one lymphatic leukemia patient caused marked increase in hemoglobin content of blood and decrease in WBC[A00706].

Hepatotoxic activity. Infusion of dried entire plant taken orally by human children at variable dosage levels was equivocal. May be associated with the development of veno-occlusive disease of the liver in Jamaican children[W04546].

Hexokinase inhibition. Aqueous high speed supernatant of fresh fruit at a concentration of 50 ml was active on rat liver homogenates. Ethanol (95%) extract of oven-dried fruit at a concentration of 125.0 mg/ml was active on rat liver homogenates[T12135].

Hyperglycemic activity. Methanol extract of a commercial sample of entire plant administered intragastrically to rat at a dose of 2.5 gm/kg was active. The result was significant at 60 minutes[K13947]. Methanol extract of seed administered intragastrically to rats at a dose of 2.5 gm/kg produced weak activity[K13947]. Protein fraction (FM-11) of dried fruit was active on mice[M22015].

Hyperlipidemic activity. Hot water extract of fresh fruit juice was active on adipose tissue vs triglyceride content of adipose tissue[TM17655].

Hypoglycemic activity. Alkaloid fraction of vine administered orally to rabbits was inactive; hot water extract was active[A00637]. Decoction of dried fruit administered intragastrically to rabbits at a dose of 200.0 mg/kg was active[A14458]. Ethanol (95%) extract of dried fruit administered intragastrically to female rats at a dose of 250.0 mg/kg was active[K09153]. Water extract of dried fruit administered orally to female rats at a dose of 250.0 mg/kg was active. The effect is potentiated if used with *C. longa* and *E. officinalis*[K19538]. At a dose of 10.0 mg/kg administered orally to rabbits, there was a drop in blood sugar of 15 mg relative to inert-treated control[A14379]. Decoction of dried fruit, leaves, and stem in the drinking water of male mice at a concentration of 0.2% was inactive. 1.0 ml of the extract is equivalent to 10 g of dried plant material. Daily dosing of the extract for 13 days followed by intraperitoneally glucose tolerance. Plasma glucose and plasma insulin were measured. There was no significant alteration of body weight, food intake, fluid intake, or plasma concentrations of glucose or insulin. Glucose tolerance, measured on day 13, was improved by treatment. Intraperitoneal administration of the decoction at a dose of 0.3 ml/animal was active, based on a glucose tolerance test. A single dose of extract was given and glucose and insulin levels were measured at 2, 4, 8, 8.5, and 9 hours. Following a single dose of the extract, basal plasma glucose concentrations were reduced after four and eight hours. Glucose tolerance was also improved eight hours after dosing. Plasma insulin levels were unaffected by the extract[M23565]. Dried fruit administered intragastrically to rabbits at a dose of 0.5 gm/kg was active[M22028]. Dried plant juice administered by gastric intubation and intravenously to rabbits were active[T08662]. Dried unripe fruit juice administered intragastrically to rabbits at a dose of 500.0 mg/animal was inactive[A14310]. Ethanol/water (1:1) and saline extracts of shade dried seeds administered orally to rats at doses of 20.0 mg/kg and methanol extract at dose of 10.0 mg/kg were active[T14966]. Ethanol/water (1:1) and water extracts of fresh fruit administered intragastrically to mice at doses of 0.5 g/kg were inactive[K18219]. Ethanol/water (1:1) extract of dried entire plant administered intragastrically to rats at a dose of 250.0 mg/kg was inactive[K09153]. Fresh fruit pulp juice administered by gastric intubation to rats at a dose of 10.0 ml/kg was active[T08396]. Fresh fruit taken by human adults at a dose of 15.0 g/day for 21 days was equivocal. The fall in blood sugar was 25% of the initial level; however statistically is insignificant[K12995]. Fresh fruit juice administered intragastrically to rabbits at a dose of 6.0 ml/kg was active[A14328]. Fruit juice administered intragastrically to rabbits at doses of 200 and 500.0 mg/animal were inactive[W00276]. Glycoside mixture of dried fruit at a dose of 10.0 mg/kg administered to rabbits was active. Lyophilized extract at doses of 1.2 gm and 400.0 mg/kg administered to rabbits were

inactive[P00096]. Hot water extract at doses of 5, 10, and 20 mg/kg were inactive[P00050]. Hot water extract of 20 g of air-dried fruit administered by gastric intubation to dogs at a dose of 200.0 ml/animal produced weak activity[T07170]. Fruit pulp juice administered intragastrically to rats at a dose of 2.5 gm/kg was active. The results significant at 60–120 minutes.[K13947]. Ethanol/water (1:1) extract of dried entire plant administered intravenous to dogs at variable dosage was inactive[W3022A].

Hypothermic activity. Ethanol/water (1:1) extract of dried entire plant administered intragastrically to rats was inactive. Ethanol/water (1:1) extract of dried fruit administered intragastrically to rats was inactive[K09153].

Insecticide activity. Ethanol (95%) extract of dried meristem at a concentration of 50.0 mcg was inactive on *Rhodnius neglectus*[K18765]. Methanol and acetic acid extract of dried fruit were inactive on *Spodoptera litura* larvae. Petroleum ether extract at a concentration of 1.0 ppm was active[P00001]. Water extract of dried leaves was inactive on *Oncopelatus fasciatus*; strong activity on *Blatella germanica*; intravenous administration at a dose of 40.0 ml/kg produced strong activity on *Periplaneta americana*[W03405].

Insulin induction. Water extract of fresh unripe fruit in cell culture at a concentration of 1.0 mg/ml was active on pancreatic islets[M21802].

Leukopenic activity. Hot water extract of entire plant taken orally by human adult at a dose of 15.0 ml/person three times daily for 62 days was active. The extract when administered to one lymphatic leukemia patient caused marked increase in hemoglobin content of blood and decrease in WBC[A00706].

Lipid metabolism effect. Acid/ethanol extract of unripe dried fruit and seeds at variable concentrations was active on adipocytes[T13897].

Lipid peroxide formation inhibition. Hot water extract of dried aerial parts at a concentration of 1.0 mg/plate in cell culture was inactive on hepatocytes and monitored by production of malonaldehyde[K23019].

Lipid synthesis stimulation. Chromatographic fraction of decorticated seed at a concentration of 500.0 mcg/ml was active on rat adipocytes. Results significant at P < 0.005 level[M11890].

Lipolytic effect. Seeds administered by gastric intubation to rabbits at a dose of 3.0 gm/animal was active in streptozotocin-treated animals[M29966].

Liver glycogen increase. Fresh fruit juice administered by gastric intubation to rats at a dose of 10.0 ml/kg was active. Results significant at P < 0.01 level[T12703]. Hot water extract of fresh fruit juice was active. Muscular glycogen level was also increased[M17655].

Metastasis inhibition. Chromatographic fraction of dried fruit in cell culture was active on vesicular stomatitis virus[T08985].

Molluscicidal activity. Aqueous slurry (homogenate) of fresh root was inactive on *Lymnaea columella* and *Lymnaea cubensis.* LD_{100} > 1000 ppm[T04621]. Ethanol (95%) and water extracts of dried fruit at concentrations of 1000 ppm produced weak activity on *Biomphalaria glabrata*, and *Biomphalaria straminea*[W02949].

Oxygen radical inhibition. Fresh fruit juice at a concentration of 0.1 ml/units was active. A heat, acid and alkali-stable component of the extract acted as scavenger of both superoxide and hydroxyl radicals. At the given concentration 90.16% scavenging of superoxide was seen. At a concentration of 0.33 ml/units 87.70% scavenging of hydroxyl radical was seen[T16453].

Parasympatholytic activity. Ethanol/water (1:1) of dried entire plant at a concentration of 0.01 gm/ml produced weak activity on guinea pig ileum[W3022A].

Plant germination inhibition. Hot water extract of entire plant at a concentration of 20.0 ppm was active vs corn, cotton, and broad beans[A00706].

Protein synthesis inhibition. Chromatographic fraction of dried fruit in cell culture was active on BHK-21 cells and vesicular stomatitis virus[T08985]. Water extract of seed was active on rabbit reticulocyte lysate[T01769]. Water extract of dried seed at a concentration of 10.0 mg/ml produced strong activity (99% inhibition) on rabbit reticulocyte lysate[K21690].

Radical scavenging effect. Hot water extract of dried aerial parts at a concentration of 250.0 mg/literwas inactive. Activity measured by discoloration of diphenylpicryl hydroxyl radical solution. Six percent decoloration was observed[K23019].

Respiration inhibition (cellular). Fresh fruit juice administered by gastric intubation to rats at a dose of 10.0 ml/kg was inactive[T12703].

Respiration stimulant (cellular). Fresh fruit juice administered by gastric intubation to rats at a dose of 10.0 ml/kg was inactive[T12703].

RNA synthesis inhibition. Ethanol (100%) extract of seed in cell culture was active on Sarcoma 180 (solid)[M27078].

Spasmolytic activity. Ethanol/water (1:1) extract of dried entire plant was inactive on rat uterus[K09153]. Ethanol/water (1:1) extract of dried fruit was inactive on the uterus of rats[K09153].

Spermicidal effect. Unripe fruit juice was active on the sperm of rats[T05027].

Toxic effect (general). Ethanol (95%) extract of fruit administered orally to male gerbils at a dose of 1.10 g/kg daily for 30 days was inactive. At dose of 150.0 mg/kg weak activity was produced. Twenty to thirty percent of the animals died within 30 days[M01152]. Ethanol/water (1:1) extract of dried entire plant administered by gastric intubation and subcutaneously to mice at doses of 10.0 g/kg (dry weight of plant) were inactive[R00001]. Alkaloid fraction of vine administered intraperitoneally to rats at a dose of 14.0 mg/kg, and to rabbits orally at a dose of 56.0 mg/animal, was inactive[A00637]. Decoction of dried fruit taken orally by human adults at a dose of 500.0

mg/person was inactive[A14458]. Fresh fruit juice administered intragastrically to rabbits at a dose of 6.0 ml/kg was active. Death occurred with 23 days when dosing continued. Two pregnant animals suffered from uterine hemorrhage and then died. When administered intraperitoneally to rats at a dose of 15.0 ml/kg death occurred within 18 hours [A14328].

Toxicity assessment (quantitative). Ethanol/water (1:1) extract of dried aerial parts administered intraperitoneally to mice of both sexes produced a LD_{50} 681.0 mg/kg[T02678]. Ethanol/water (1:1) extract of dried entire plant administered intraperitoneally to mice produced a LD_{50} of 681.0 mg/kg[K09153]. Water extract of fresh fruit administered intraperitoneally and subcutaneously to mice produced LD_{50} 16.0 and 27.0 mg/ml respectively[T09137]. Water extract of seed administered intraperitoneally to rat produced LD_{50} 25.0 mg/kg[T01769]. Ethanol/water (1:1) extract of dried fruit, when administered intraperitoneally to mice produced a LD_{50} of 681.0 mg/kg[K09153].

Trypsin inhibition. Chromatographic fraction of seed was active[H04816].

Tumor promotion inhibition. Methanol extract of fresh fruit in cell culture at a concentration of 200.0 mcg was inactive on Epstein–Barr virus vs 12-0-hexadecanoyl-phorbol-13-acetate-induced Epstein–Barr virus activation[T15279].

Uterine relaxation effect. Ethanol/water (1:1) extract of dried fruit administered to nonpregnant rats was inactive[T02678].

Uterine stimulant effect. Ethanol (95%) extract of dried root administered intravenously to guinea pigs at a dose of 10.0 mg/ml was active on the nonpregnant uterus[W04510]. Ethanol/water (1:1) extract of dried fruit administered to nonpregnant rats was inactive[T02678].

20 | Moringa pterygosperma
Gaertn.

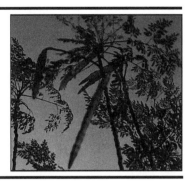

Common Names

Ba da dai	Indonesia	Malungai	Guam
Ben aile	New Claedonia	Malungal	Philippines
Ben aile	Senegal	Malunggay	Philippines
Ben nut tree	Mauritius	Mangai	India
Ben nut tree	West Indies	Maranga	Mauritius
Brede mourounge	Rodrigues Islands	Marum	Malaysia
Chum ngay	Indonesia	Marum	Thailand
Da-tha-lwon	India	Mbum	Senegal
Daintha	India	Meetho sirgavo	India
Dandalonbin	India	Meethosaragavo	India
Danthalons	India	Merunggai	Malaysia
Dhak I houm	Indonesia	Moringa	India
Diaboy	Senegal	Moringa	West Indies
Drum stick	Nepal	Moringa tree	West Indies
Drum stick tree	India	Moringue	Angola
Drumstick	India	Munaga	India
Drumstick	Sri Lanka	Munga	India
Drum stick tree	Fiji	Mungay	India
Getha	Saudi Arabia	Munigha	India
Horseradish tree	Mauritius	Muringa	India
Horse radish tree	India	Murunga	Sri Lanka
Horse radish tree	Malaysia	Murungai	India
Horse radish tree	Nepal	Musing	India
Horse-radish	India	Nebeday	Senegal
Horseradish tree	Fiji	Neboday	Senegal
Horseradish tree	Guam	Nebreday	Senegal
Horseradish tree	Nigeria	Neveday	Senegal
Horseradish tree	USA	Nevorday	Senegal
Horseradish tree	West Indies	Nevredie	Senegal
Horseradish tree	Indonesia	Noboday	Senegal
Kelor	Indonesia	Nobody	Senegal
Kelor	Malaysia	Radish tree	India
Kelor pea	Malaysia	Ramunggai	Malaysia
Ma-rum	Thailand	Ravinta	India

From: Medicinal Plants of the World *By: Ivan A. Ross Humana Press Inc., Totowa, NJ*

Sahajan	India	Shajiwan	Nepal
Sahajana	India	Shajmah	India
Sahanjana	India	Shajna	India
Sahjan	India	Shejan	India
Sahjna	India	Shigru	India
Sahjna	Pakistan	Shobanjan	Nepal
Saijan	Fiji	Shobhanjana	India
Saijan	Guyana	Sigru	India
Sainjan	India	Soanjna	Fiji
Sainjna	India	Sobhanja	India
Sajana	India	Sobhanjan	India
Sajina	India	Sobhanjana	India
Sajna	Bangladesh	Sobhanjanavriksha	India
Sajna	Fiji	Sohawjana	Nepal
Sajna	India	Sojna	India
Salijan	India	Sonth	India
Sanjna	India	Sunja	India
Sapsap	Senegal	Sunara	India
Saragavo	India	Sundan	India
Segat	India	West Indian ben	India
Segra	India	Wolof	Senegal
Sehjan	India	Yovoviti	Togo
Shahjnah	India	Zoliv	Haiti

BOTANICAL DESCRIPTION

A tree of the MORINGACEAE family that grows to 10 to 15 meters high. It is a rapidly growing tree that resembles a legume, has tripinnate leaves, a gummy bark and fragrant flowers with white petals. The brown, three-angled fruits are up to 45 cm long and have winged seeds. The flowers are 1.5 to 2 cm long. Fertile filaments are villous at the base; ovary hairy; pods 15 to 30 cm long and pendulous.

ORIGIN AND DISTRIBUTION

A native of India now found in East and Southeast Asia, Polynesia and the West Indies.

TRADITIONAL MEDICINAL USES

Andaman Islands. Fruits and leaves are taken as a vegetable[K23301].

Colombia. Hot water extract of the plant is taken orally as an abortive[T15375].

East Africa. Hot water extract of the root bark is taken orally as an abortifacient[T05825].

East Indies. Hot water extract of the root bark is taken orally as a menstrual promoter, a diuretic and as a stimulant[W02290].

Fiji. Dried leaves, grounded with garlic, salt, black pepper and turmeric is used as a treatment for dog bites. Dried leaves, grounded with black pepper is applied externally for headache[T10632]. Fresh leaf juice, mixed with honey is used as ointment for sore eyes. The fresh leaf juice is taken orally to induce vomiting (useful in poisoning)[T10632].

Guam. Hot water extract of seeds is taken orally to treat fevers, and as a tonic[A01962].

Haiti. Decoction of dried leaves is taken orally for nervous shock[T13846].

India. Fifteen grams of root bark mixed with 20 corns of black pepper is taken orally to produce abortion[W00002]. Decoction of dried leaves is taken orally for abortion[K16006]. Externally for rheumatism[M23219] and for wound healing[T05532]. Leaves made into a paste with salt is used to treat edema[T08282]. Dried fruit is taken orally for 20 days to produce sterility. A mixture of the fruits of *Clerodendrum indicum*, *Sesamum orientale*, *Moringa pterygosperma* and *Piper nigrum* is mixed with sugar[T01925]. The mixture is also taken as a tonic[T06351]. Hot water extract of the dried fruit is taken orally for headache and for giddiness[T10064]. Dried gum is applied externally for headache[M22542]. Dried seeds, after frying, are eaten[T05532]. Dried stem bark is taken orally for backache. *Moringa pterygosperma, Cuminum cyminum, Trigonellla foenumgraecum* and *Murraya koenigii* are taken[M23219]. Flowers are taken orally as a stimulant and aphrodisiac. Hot water extract is taken orally as a tonic and cholagogue[W00015]. Fresh flowers are used as a vegetable[T05532]. Fresh seed pods are used as a vegetable[T05532]. Gum is administered intravaginally to produce abortion[W00002]. Hot water extract of dried flowers is taken orally in Ayurvedic and Unani medicine as an aphrodisiac and stimulant[T05894]. Hot water extract of dried fruit and leaves is taken orally for dysentery and diarrhea[T10064]. Hot water extract of dried root and stem bark is taken orally as an abortifacient and emmenagogue[T14891]. Hot water extract of dried root bark is taken orally for fertility control[T04748]. Hot water extract of stem bark is taken orally in Ayurvedic medicine as an abortive, antipyretic, and as a tonic[A01897]. Hot water extract of the dried bark is used in Ayurvedic and Unani Medicine as an abortifacient, taken orally by pregnant women[T5894]. Hot water extract of the dried root is taken orally in Ayurvedic and Unani medicine as an abortifacient[T05894]. Juice of fresh bark is taken orally to relieve acute stomachaches. Juices of *Erythrina variegata* and *Moringa oleifera* barks are mixed. Also, for stomachache, juice of bark is mixed with *Ferula asafoetida* and salt, and given orally. Externally the juice is used as a treatment for mange in horses[W03073]. Leaf juice, mixed with honey is used as an eye ointment for conjunctivitis[K23294]. Leaves are taken orally as an aphrodiasic[A04891], and to treat wounds. Leaves are pounded with turmeric and buttermilk and applied to wounds[K11282]. Powdered dried root and stem is used externally for rheumatism pains. For asthma, and cough, 50 mg of the powder in water is taken orally. Stem bark is taken orally to produce permanent sterility. Five gram of stem bark from an old tree is ground into a paste by adding two seeds of *Piper nigrum*, one gram of *Cuminum cyminum* seeds and a few pieces of *Allium sativum*. This paste is swallowed after the third day of delivery. A bland diet is followed. This is repeated three times. After two to three months, the woman should not participate in coitus[T16478]. Fresh stem bark is used to produce abortion. The gum from the stem bark is rubbed with milk and made into a paste and applied to the vagina and up into the cervix. The gum is very tough, swells rapidly when moistened, and produces abortion by dilating the cervix[T16478].

Indonesia. Hot water extract of the plant is taken orally to provoke the menses, and as an abortive[A00682,A04766].

Malaysia. Hot water extract of the bark is taken orally to stimulate the menses[A06590]. Hot water extract of the root is taken orally for amenorrhea[A04587], and may cause abortion[A06590].

Mauritius. Hot water extract of the bark is taken orally as a purgative, vermifuge, and as an antispasmodic[W01270].

Nepal. Hot water extract of flowers is taken orally as an aphrodisiac[A00020]. Hot water extract of the dried bark is taken orally by pregnant women as an abortifacient[A00020]. Hot water extract of the root is taken orally as a stimulant; for intermittent fever; epilepsy, and as an abortifacient[A00020].

New Caledonia. Gum is taken orally as an abortifacient[A04174]. Leaves are rubbed over the breast to reduce milk flow[W04017].

Nigeria. Hot water extract of fresh root is taken orally as an analgesic, a hypotensive and as a sedative[T06510]. Hot water extract of the dried root and stem is taken orally to treat arthritis[T05549].

Philippines. Decoction of dried leaves is taken orally as a galactogogue. A decoction of *Solanum nigrum*, *Moringa pterygosperma*, and beach pebbles is used[T10116]. Extract of leaves is used as a galactagogue[A00115].

Saudi Arabia. Hot water extract of the dried fruit is taken orally for diabetes, ascites, edema, spleen enlargement, inflammatory swellings, abdominal tumors, colic, dyspepsia, fever, ulcers, paralysis, lumbago, and skin diseases[M22673,T10348].

Senegal. An entire dried plant is used for sprains in adult; headache and neuralgia in children and adults; rheumatism and arthritis by adults, rickets in children and adults; bronchitis in children and adults and as an antipyretic in children and adults. Dried exudate is used as an astringent for various medicinal purposes. Fresh inflorescence is placed in the eyes for eye problems[W04017].

Thailand. Hot water extract of dried root is taken orally as a cardiotonic, a stimulant for fainting[R00001], and as an antipyretic[W3022A].

Togo. Decoction of dried leaves and twigs is taken orally for malaria[M23556].

USA. Fresh leaves are taken orally as a diuretic[A05408].

West Indies. Flowers are boiled and the decoction taken orally as a cough remedy[L01534]. Hot water extract of root bark is used as a diuretic, stimulant, as menstrual promoter, and as an abortive[W02290]. Seeds are taken orally as a purgative[T00701]. Warmed leaves are used as a dressing for syphilitic ulcers[T00701].

CHEMICAL CONSTITUENTS

(ppm unless otherwise indicated)

3-Methoxy quercetin, Lf
4- Hydroxy phenylacetonitrile, Sd
4-Hydroxy phenylacetamide, Sd
4-Hydroxy phenylacetic acid, Sd
Alanine, Sd
Amylase, Lf
Arachidic acid, Sd Oil
Arginine, Sd
Ascorbic acid oxidase, Fr
Ascorbic acid, Fr Ju, Lf
Athomin, Rt Bk
Baurenol, Bk
Behenic acid, Sd Oil

Benzenoids, Lf
Benzyl glucosinolate, Sd
Beta sitosterol, St Bk
Beta carotene, Fr
Calcium, Fl; Fr 0.4%
Choline, Lf 0.42%; Fr 0.42%
Essential Oil, Bk 50
Gossypitin, Lf
Gum, Fl
Histidine, Sd
Hydroxy proline, Sd
Iso-butyl thiocynate, Pl
Iso-thiocynate, Pl
Kaempferol, Fl
Lauric acid, Sd Oil
Leucine, Sd
Lignoceric acid, Sd Oil
Linoleic acid, Sd Oil
Moringine, Bk; Rt Bk
Moringinine, Bk; Rt Bk
Moringyne, Sd
Myristic acid, Sd Oil
Niazicin B, Lf 1.06
Niazimicin, Lf 18.2-2.5
Niaziminin A, Lf 2.8-10.3
Niaziminin B, Lf 0.7
Niazinin A, Lf 2.3-13.7
Niazinin B, Lf 2.6-14.5
Niazirin, Lf 4.5
Niazirinin, Lf 2.7
Nicotinic acid, Fr 2; Lf 8
Oleic acid, Sd Oil 67.48%
Oxalic acid, Fr 0.042-0.101%, Lf 0.101%
Palmitic acid, Sd Oil 3.4-9.3%
Pentadecanoic acid, Sd Oil,
Phenylalanine, Sd
Phosphorus, Fr 0.45%
Potassium, Fl
Proline, Sd
Protein, Fr 2.5-19.5%; Sd 46.5%; Lf 6.7-29%
Pterygospermin, Rt; St Bk; Sd; Bk
Quercetagetin, Lf
Quercetin, Fl
Quercetin-3-glycoside, Fl
Rhamnetin, Fl
Rhamnetin-3-glycoside, Fl
Rutin, Lf 2.6%
Serine, Sd
Spirochin, Rt
Spirochine, Rt
Starch, Lf

Stearic acid, Sd Oil 7.4-10.5%
Sulfur, Rt
Threonine, Sd
Valine, Sd
Vitamin A, Lf 113 I. U./gm; Fr 1.8 I. U/gm
Vitamin B-1, Lf 0.6; Fr 0.5
Vitamin B-2, Lf 0.5; Fr 0.7
Zeatin Ribose, Fr
Zeatin, Fr

PHARMACOLOGICAL ACTIVITIES AND CLINICAL TRIALS

Abortifacient activity. Ethanol/water (1:1) extract of root, at a dose of 200.0 mg/kg, administered orally to rats was inactive[W01362]. Ethanol/water (50%) extract of leaves and twigs, at a dose of 100.0 mg/kg, administered by gastric intubation to pregnant rats was inactive[T16726]. Ethanol/water (1:1) extract of dried aerial parts when administered orally to pregnant rats was inactive[T02678]. Ethanol/water (50%) extract of the entire plant at a dose of 100.0 mg/kg, administered by gastric intubation to pregnant rats was inactive[T16726].

Adrenolytic activity. Ethanol (95%), and water extracts of leaves, when administered to dogs intravenously to dogs were inactive[A03456].

Analgesic activity. Ethanol/water (1:1) extract of dried leaves and dried stem, at a dose of 500.0 mg/kg, administered to mice intraperitoneally was inactive vs tail pressure method[A03033]. Ethanol/water (50%) extract of flowers administered by gastric intubation to mice was inactive vs hot plate method and tail clip method[T16726].

Anthelmintic activity. Dried bark powder at a concentration of 1.0 ml was active on Ascaris lumbricoides[M28471]. Fresh leaf juice, at a concentration of 1 ml, was inactive on Ascaris lumbricoides[M28471]. Powdered dried root at a concentration of 1.0 ml was inactive on Ascaris lumbricoides[M28471]. Powdered dried leaves, at a concentration of 1.0 ml was inactive on Ascaris lumbricoides[M28471]. Dried plant taken orally by human adults of both sexes was active. IC$_{100}$ 2.0 gm. Equal

parts of a mixture containing Butea frondosa, Moringa pterygosperma, Piper nigrum, Azadirachta indica and Embelia ribes was used. Dosing was three times daily for 4–8 weeks. 11 cases of Ascariasis; nine cases of Ancylostomiasis; nine cases of Hymenolepsis nana were treated. Stool specimens were found to be negative at end of treatment period[T02211]. Powdered dry seeds, at a concentration of 1.0 ml was inactive on Ascaris lumbricoids[M28471].

Antibacterial activity. Powdered dried bark, at a concentration of 100.0 microliters, on agar plate was inactive on Escherichia coli, Pseudomonas aeruginosa, Shigella flexneri, Staphylococcus aureus and Streptococcus pyogenes[M28471]. Ethanol (95%) extract of dried flowers, undiluted, on agar plate was active on Escherichia coli and Staphylococcus aureus[W03693]. Powdered dried root, at a concentration of 100.0 microliters on agar plate, was inactive on Escherichia coli, Pseudomonas aeruginosa, Shigella flexneri, Staphylococcus aureus, and Streptococcus pyogenes[M28471]. Ethanol (95%) extract of dried fruit, undiluted, on agar plate was active on Escherichia coli and Staphylococcus aureus[W03693]. Saline extract of leaves at a concentration of 1–20 on agar plate was active on Staphylococcus aureus, and inactive on Pasteurella pestis[W01047]. Powdered dried leaves at a concentration of 100.0 microliters on agar plate, was inactive on Shigella flexneri, Staphylococcus aureus, Streptococcus pyogenes, Escherichia coli and Pseudomonas aeruginosa[M28471]. Ethanol (95%) extract of dried leaves, undiluted, on agar plate was active on Escherichia coli, and Staphylococcus aureus[W03693]. Fresh leaf juice, at a concentration of 100.0 microliters on agar plate, was active on Pseudomonas aeruginosa and inactive on Escherichia coli, Shigella flexneri, Staphylococcus aureus and Streptococcus pyogenes[M28471]. Ethanol (95%) extract of dried root, undiluted on agar plate was active on Escherichia coli and Staphylococcus aureus[W03693]. Water, and hexane extracts of dried seeds, at doses of 10.0%, applied externally to mice, were active on *Staphylococcus aureus*[M30038] Powdered dried seeds, at a concentration of 100.0 microliters on an agar plate, was active on *Staphylococcus aureus*[M28471]. The powdered dried seeds, at 100.0 microliters on an agar plate, was inactive on *Escherichia coli, Pseudomonas aeruginosa, Shigella flexneri,* and *Streptococcus pyogenes*[M28471]. Water extract of dried seeds, at a concentration of 1:10, on agar plate, was active on *Bacillus cereus, Bacillus megaterium, Bacillus subtilis, Sarcina lutea,* and *Staphylococcus aureus.* The extract was equivocal on *Escherichia coli, Salmonella edinburgi,* and *Serratia marcesens;* inactive on *Klebsiella aerogenes* and produced weak activity on *Proteus mirabilis* and *Streptococcus faecalis*[T02717].

Anticonvulsant activity. Ethanol/water (1:1) extracts of dried leaves and dried stem, at a dose of 500.0 mg/kg, administered to mice intraperitoneally were inactive vs electroshock-induced convulsions[A03033]. Ethanol (70%) extract of fresh root, at variable dosage levels, given intraperitoneally to mice of both sexes, was active vs metrazole, and strychnine-induced convulsions[T06510].

Antifertility effect. Ethanol (95%), water, and petroleum ether extracts of bark administered to female mice were inactive[A02435].

Antifungal activity. Powdered dried bark, powdered dried root, powdered dried seeds, fresh leaves, and powdered dried leaves, at concentrations of 1.0 ml on agar plate, were inactive on *Epidermophyton floccosum, Microsporum canis, Microsporum gypseum, Trichophyton mentagrophytes,* and *Trichophyton rubrum*[M28471]. (Plant Pathogens) Water extract of dried seeds, at a concentration of 1:10 on an agar plate, was active on *Botrytis allii, Coniophora cerebella, Penicillium expansum, Phytophthora cactorum,* and *Polyporus versicolor.* The extract was equivocal on *Fusarium oxysporum* F. sp. Lycopersici; and inactive on *Aspergillus oryza*[T02717].

Antihemolytic activity. An entire dried plant at a concentration of 0.2 ml was active on red blood cells[T16412].

Antihepatotoxic activity. Ethanol (95%) extract of dried leaves at a dose of 300.0 mg/kg, administered to mice by gastric intubation was inactive vs CCl_4-induced hepatotoxicity[T08733].

Antihistamine activity. Ethanol/water (1:1) extract of dried root, at a concentration of 0.001 gm/ml, was active on guinea pig ileum[W3022A].

Anti-implantation effect. Ethanol (95%), water, and petroleum ether extracts of bark, administered orally to female rats were inactive[A02435]. Ethanol/water (1:1) extract of dried aerial parts, administered orally to hamsters was active. However, the extract was inactive when administered to rats[T02678]. Ethanol/water (50%) extract of entire plant, at a dose of 100.0 mg/kg, administered by gastric intubation to pregnant hamsters was inactive[T16726]. Water extract of dried leaves, at a dose of 750.0 mg/kg, administered to rats by intravenous infusion, was active vs carrageenin-induced pedal edema[K07497].

Anti-inflammatory activity. Hot water extract of bark administered orally to rats was inactive vs formalin-induced pedal edema[A04420]. Water extracts of dried flowers and dried stem, at doses of 1.0 g/kg, administered by Intravenous infusion to rats, were inactive vs carrageenin-induced pedal edema[K07497]. Water extract of dried root, at a dose of 750.0 mg/kg, administered to rats by intravenous infusion, was active vs carrageenin-induced pedal edema[K07497]. Water extract of dried seeds, at a concentration of 1 gm, administered to rats by intravenous infusion, was active vs carrageenin-induced pedal edema[K07497].

Antimalarial activity. Ethanol (95%) extract of dried leaves and twigs, produced weak activity on *Plasmodium falciparum.* IC_{50} 60.0 mcg/ml[M23556]. Water extract of the bark administered orally to chicken at a dose of

1.82 gm/kg was inactive on *Plasmodium gallinaceum*[A00785].

Antimycobacterial activity. An extract of the entire plant on agar plate was active on *Mycobacterium tuberculosis*[A05542]. Water extract of dried seeds, at a concentration of 1:10 on agar plate, was active on *Mycobacterium phlei*[T02717].

Antispasmodic activity (unspecified type). Water extract of dried flowers at a concentration of 1.0 gm was inactive on rat duodenum vs ACh-induced contractions[K07497]. Ethanol/water (1:1) extract of fruits was active on guinea pig ileum vs ACh and histamine-induced spasms[69]. Ethanol (95%), and water extracts of leaves were both active on guinea pig ileums vs ACh, and histamine-induced spasms. Water extract of dried leaves at a concentration of 1000 mg was inactive on rat duodenum vs ACh-induced contractions[K07497]. Ethanol/water (1:1) extracts of dried leaves and dried stem were inactive on guinea pig ileum vs ACh and histamine-induced spasms[A03033]. Water extract of dried root, and dried stem at concentrations of 1.0 gm were inactive on rat duodenum vs ACh-induced contractions[K07497]. Ethanol/water (1:1) extract of dried root, at a concentration of 0.001 gm/ml, was active on guinea pig ileum[W3022A]. Ethanol/water (1:1) extract of rootbark was active on guinea pig ileum vs ACh and histamine-induced spasms[A03033]. Ethanol/water (1:1) extract of rootwood was active on guinea pig ileum vs ACh and histamine-induced spasms[A03033]. Water extract of dried seeds, at a concentration of 1 gm, was active on rat duodenum. Contractions was inhibited 32.6% vs ACh-induced contractions[K07497].

Antitumor activity. Ethanol/water (1:1) extract of dried aerial parts administered intraperitoneally to mice was active on LEUK-P388[T02678]. Ethanol/water (1:1) extract of dried leaves, when administered to mice intraperitoneally was inactive on LEUK-P388 and LEUK-L1210[A03033]. Ethanol (95%) extract of dried leaves, at a dose of 100.0 mg/kg, administered intraperitoneally to mice was inactive on Sarcoma 180(ASC)[M23643].

Antiulcer activity. Methanol extract of dried flower buds, at a dose of 4.0 gm/kg, administered by gastric intubation to rats was active[K20618]. Methanol extract of dried leaves, at a dose of 2.0 gm/kg administered by gastric intubation to mice was inactive vs stress-induced ulcers (water-immersion)[M16948].

Antiviral activity. Ethanol/water (50%) extract of flowers at a concentration of 0.05 mg/ml in cell culture was inactive on Vaccinia virus[T16726]. Ethanol/water (50%) extract of leaves and twigs, at a concentration of 0.05 mg/ml in cell culture, was inactive on Vaccinia virus[T16726]. Ethanol/water (1:1) extract of rootbark, at a concentration of 50.0 mcg/ml in cell culture, produced weak activity on Vaccinia virus[A03335].

Antiyeast activity. Powdered dried leaves, powdered dried root, powdered dried bark, and powdered dried seeds, at concentrations of 100.0 microliters on agar plate, were inactive on *Candida albicans*[M28471]. Fresh leaf juice, at a concentration of 100.0 microliters, on agar plate was inactive on *Candida albicans*[M28471]. Water extract of dried seeds, at a concentration of 1:10 on agar plate, was active on *Candida pseudotropicalis, Candida reukaufii* and *Pyricularia oryza* and equivocal on *Saccharomyces carlsbergenesis*[T02717].

Barbiturate sleeping time decreased. Ethanol (95%) extract of dried leaves, at a dose of 300.0 mg/kg, administered to mice by gastric intubation, was inactive vs CCl_4-induced hepatotoxicity[T08733].

Carcinogenesis inhibition. Water extract of dried leaves, at a dose of 600.0 mg/per gm diet, in the ration of mice, was active vs benzo(A)pyrene-induced carcinogenesis, and 3-methyl-4-dimethylaminoazobenzene-induced carcinogenesis[K09214].

CNS depressant activity. Water and ethanol (95%) extracts of leaves administered intraperitoneally to dogs and mice were active in both animals[A03456]. Ethanol (70%) extract of fresh root, at variable dosage levels, administered intraperitoneally to mice of both sexes, produced strong activity[T06510].

Cytotoxic activity. Ethanol/water (1:1) extract of dried leaves in cell culture was inactive on CA-9KB. $ED_{50} > 20.0$ mcg/ml[A03033]. Ethanol/water (1:1) extract of fruits was inactive on CA-9KB in cell culture. $ED_{50} > 20$ mcg/ml[A03335]. Ethanol/water (1:1) extract of the aerial parts, in cell culture was active on CA-9KB. $ED_{50} < 20.0$ mcg/ml[T02678]. Ethanol/water (1:1) extract of root bark, in cell culture was inactive on CA-9KB. $ED_{50} > 20.0$ mcg/ml[A03335]. Ethanol/water (1:1) extract of rootwood, in cell culture, was inactive on CA-9KB. $ED_{50} > 20.0$ mcg/ml[A03335].

Diuretic activity. Ethanol/water (1:1) extracts of dried leaves, and dried stem at doses of 250.0 mg/kg, administered intraperitoneally to saline loaded male rats, were inactive. Urine was collected for four hours post-drug[A03033]. Water extract of dried leaves, dried stem, dried root, and dried seeds, at doses of 25.0 mg/kg, administered to rats by intravenous infusion were active[K07497].

Embryotoxic effect. Ethanol (70%) extract of bark at dosages of 200, 400, and 800 mg/kg, administered orally to female rats were inactive[T01112]. Ethanol/water (1:1) extract of root, at a dose of 200.0 mg/kg, administered orally to rats, was inactive[W01362]. Water extract of shade dried bark at a dose of 400 mg/kg, dosing on days 1–7, administered orally to rats was active[T14492]. Water extract of dried leaves at a dose of 175.0 mg/kg, administered intragastric to pregnant rats was active[K16006]. Water extract of shade dried root, at a dose of 200.0 mg/kg, given to rats orally was active. Dosing on days 1–7[T14492].

Estrogenic effect. Leaves in the ration of mice was inactive[A05972].

Hyperglycemic activity. 25% Aqueous, and 25% hot water extracts of dried fruits, at doses of 0.5 ml/animal, administered by gastric intubation produced a maximal change in blood sugar of 15.3% (increase) vs alloxan-induced hyperglycemia[M22673]. Ethanol/water (1:1) extract of dried leaves, at a dose of 250.0 mg/kg given administered orally to rats produced more than 30% drop in blood sugar level[A03033]. Ethanol/water (50%) extract of entire plant at a dose of 250.0 mg/kg, administered by gastric intubation to rats was active[T16726].

Hypoglycemic activity. Ethanol/water (50%) extract of flowers at a dose of 250.0 mg/kg administered by gastric intubation to rats was active[T16726].

Hypoproteinemia activity. Ethanol (95%) extract of fresh leaves, at a dose of 10.0 mg/kg, administered intravenously to rats was active[H15082].

Hypotensive activity. Ethanol (95%), and water extracts of leaves administered intravenously to dogs both active[A03456]. Ethanol/water (1:1) extracts of dried leaves and dried stem at doses of 50.0 mg/kg administered intravenously to dogs were inactive[A03033]. Ethanol/water (1:1) extract of dried root, administered intravenously to dogs, at variable dosage levels produced weak activity[W3022A]. Rootbark, at a dose of 0.01 mg/animal, administered to cats intravenously, was active. Duration was 20–30 minutes[A03335]. Water extract of dried stem bark, at a dose of 20.0 mg/kg, administered intravenously to dogs, was active[K21278].

Hypothermic activity. Methanol extract dried leaves at a dose of 2.0 gm/kg administer intragastric to mice was inactive[M16948]. Ethanol/water (1:1) extract of dried stem, at a dose of 500.0 mg/kg, administered intraperitoneally to mice was inactive[A03033].

Immunostimulant activity. Powdered root administered intravenously to female mice at a dose of 100.0 mg/kg, was inactive vs rate of clearance of colloidal carbon[T02434].

Inotropic effect. Water extract of dried stem bark, at concentrations of 1.0 mcg/ml and 10 ng/ml, produced negative and positive effect respectively, on frog hearts. Reported biological activity is highly dose-dependent[K21278].

Interferon induction stimulation. Ethanol/water (1:1) extract of dried aerial parts, at a concentration of 0.012 mg/ml in cell culture was active on Ranikhet virus but inactive on Vaccinia virus[T06590].

Mutagenic activity. Chloroform extract of roasted seeds, at a dose of 0.15 mg/gm, administered intraperitoneally to mice was inactive. Ethyl acetate extract, at a dose of 0.33 mg/kg, administered intraperitoneally to mice, was active. The effects were determined by the micronucleus test[HO5163].

Myocardial depressant activity. Water and 95% ethanol extracts of leaves were active on the hearts of rabbits[A03456].

Polygalacturonase inhibition. Hot water extract of bark was active[A07091].

Protopectinase inhibition. Hot water extract of bark was active[A07091].

Semen coagulation effect. Ethanol/water (1:1) extract of the dried aerial parts was inactive on the semen of rats[T02678].

Skeletal muscle relaxant activity. Ethanol (95%), and water extracts of the plant were active on the rectus abdominus muscle of frogs[A03456]. Water extract of dried stem bark, at a concentration of 10.0 mg/ml, was inactive on the rectus abdominus of frog[K21278].

Smooth muscle relaxant activity. Water extract of dried stem bark, at a concentration of 10.0 mg/ml, was inactive on guinea pig ileum and rat stomach[K21278].

Spermicidal effect. Ethanol/water (1:1) extract of the dried aerial parts was inactive on the sperm of rats[T02678].

Toxic effect. Leaves in the ration of rats on a 60 day feeding showed no toxicity[W02435]. Ethanol/water (1:1) extract of dried root, at a dose of 10.0 gm/kg (dose expressed as dry weight of plant), administered to mice by gastric intubation, and also subcutaneously, was inactive[R00001].

Toxicity assessment (Quantitative). Ethanol/water (1:1) extract of dried aerial parts, when administered intraperitoneally to mice of both sexes, the LD_{50} was 8.0 mg/kg[T02678]. Ethanol/water (1:1) extract of flowers administered to mice intraperitoneally produced a LD_{50} >1000 mg/kg[T16726]. Dried leaves fed to mice produced a LD_{50} 1850 mg/kg[T08733]. Ethanol/water (50%) extract administered to mice intraperitoneally, produced a maximum tolerated dose of 1.0 gm/kg[A03335]. Ethanol/water (1:1) extract of leaves and roasted seeds, when administered intraperitoneally to mice; for both extracts the LD_{50} >1.0 gm/kg[A03033].

Uterine stimulant effect. Ethanol/water (1:1) extract of dried aerial parts was active on the uterus of nonpregnant rat uterus[T02678]. Water extract of bark was inactive on the uterus of nonpregnant rats[A02600]. Water, and Ethanol (95%) extracts of leaves were inactive on the uterus of rats[A03456]. Water extract, at a concentration of 225.0 gm/liter, was active on guinea pig uterus[A04132].

Wound healing acceleration. Hexane extract of dried seeds, at a dose of 10.0%, applied externally to mice, was active on *Staphylococcus aureus* vs pyoderma induced by *Staphylococcus aureus*[M30038].

21 | Persea americana

P. mill

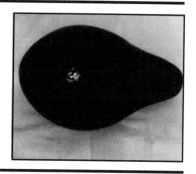

Common Names

A'aboca	West Indies	Avocado	Nicaragua
Abacateiro	Brazil	Avocado pear	Indonesia
Abacateiro	Cuba	Avocado pear	Israel
Afia	Guinea	Avocado pear	Jamaica
Aguacate	Argentina	Avocado pear	Jamaica
Aguacate	Belize	Avocado pear	South Africa
Aguacate	Brazil	Avocado	Sri Lanka
Aguacate	Colombia	Avocado	Trinidad
Aguacate	Cuba	Avocado	Turkey
Aguacate	Guatemala	Avocado	West Indies
Aguacate	Honduras	Avocat	Mauritius
Aguacate	Mexico	Avocat	Rodrigues Islands
Aguacate	Nicaragua	Buite	Colombia
Aguacate	Panama	Butter pear	Nicaragua
Aguacate	Paraguay	Cura	Cuba
Aguacate	Puerto Rico	Curo	Colombia
Aguacatero	Canary Islands	Hoja de palto	Easter Island
Aguacatillo	Mexico	Kukataj	Mexico
Aguate	Peru	Kuulup	Nicaragua
Agucatillo	Cuba	On	Belize
Ahuacaquahuitl	Mexico	Palta	Argentina
Alligator pear	West Indies	Palta	Cuba
Aquacate	Guatemala	Palta	Peru
Aquacate	Mexico	Palto	Peru
Auacatl	Mexico	Pear	Belize
Avocado	Argentina	Pear	Guyana
Avocado	Australia	Pear	Nicaragua
Avocado	Cuba	Sarin	Nicaragua
Avocado	Indonesia	Sikya	Nicaragua
Avocado	Israel	Wagadi	Nicaragua
Avocado	Jamaica	Zaboka	Haiti
Avocado	Japan	Zaboka	West Indies
Avocado	Mexico		

From: Medicinal Plants of the World *By: Ivan A. Ross Humana Press Inc., Totowa, NJ*

BOTANICAL DESCRIPTION

Tree of the LAURACEAE family with straggling-ascending branches, usually up to about 15 meters high, sometimes much taller. Leaves spirally arranged, often clustered near the branch ends, narrowly to broadly elliptical or obovate, usually pointed at the tip, up to 20 cm long and over 15 cm broad, with well developed petioles, glaucous beneath. Flowers in a much branched compact panicle shorter than the leaves, greenish-yellow. Fruits variable in size and shape according to the variety, usually shiny and green or brownish when ripe, often pear-shaped, up to about 15 cm long; flesh soft, greenish or yellow, oily, surrounding one large loose round seed.

ORIGIN AND DISTRIBUTION

Native of Mexico, now widespread in the tropics and subtropics. Avocado is cultivated commercially in Florida, California, and Hawaii in the USA, as well as in several South American countries, South Africa, Australia, and tropical Asia.

TRADITIONAL MEDICINAL USES

Belize. Hot water extract of dried leaves is taken orally for cough[T05011].

Bolivia. Hot water extract of dried fruits is taken orally for amenorrhea Hot water extract of dried leaves is taken orally as for amenorrhea[T15375].

Brazil. Hot water extract of buds is taken orally as an emmenagogue, and an antisyphiletic. Hot water extract of fresh leaves is taken orally to treat hypertension or induce diuresis[T10623]. Hot water extract of leaves is taken orally as a diuretic. Hot water extract of the fruit is taken orally as an aphrodisiac by males[W02290].

Canary Islands. Dried bark is taken as a food. Hot water extract of dried seeds is taken orally as a diuretic[T15880].

Colombia. Extract of the mesocarp is administered orally to cows as an abortifacient[A00710]. Hot water extract of dried

leaves is taken orally as an emmenagogue and as a treatment for sterility. Hot water extract of dried seeds is taken orally for sterility in women; and as an emmenagogue. Hot water extract of fruit is taken orally as an emmenagogue and as a treatment for sterility[T15375]. Hot water extract of leaves is used as an emmenagogue[A00710]. Hot water extract of the seeds are claimed to have antifertility properties[T02988].

Costa Rica. Infusion of young leaves is taken orally as an emmenagogue and as an abortifacient[M00695].

Cuba. Hot water extract of shoots is taken orally by pregnant females as an abortifacient[W02855].

Ecuador. Hot water extract of the plant is taken orally as a contraceptive[T15375].

Guatemala. Roasted seeds are eaten as a remedy for diarrhea[W01280].

Haiti. Decoction of dried bark is taken orally for amenorrhea. Dried fruit is eaten for liver troubles. Fresh seeds are eaten for hepatitis, for liver troubles and for amenorrhea. Juice from fresh seeds is applied to eye for eye problems[T13846].

Honduras. Hot water extract of the fruit is taken orally by male adults as a sexual stimulant[A04613].

Indonesia. Hot water extract of dried leaves is taken orally as an antihypertensive[T02774].

Jamaica. Fruits are considered "great provocatives," hence the Spaniards do not like their wives to indulge too much. Hot water extract of leaves is taken orally as a cure for high blood pressure[W01316].

Mauritius. Hot water extract of dried leaves is taken orally as an emmenagogue[T02146].

Mexico. Bark and leaves extract is taken as an emmenagogue[A00115]. Decoction of fresh branches is taken orally to treat infertility in female human adults[T09672]. Decoction of Corymbosa stem, plants of *Satureja brownei* or *Satureja xalapensis* and one seed of *Persea americana* are boiled or extracted in alcohol. The decoction is taken in the morning after breakfast for anemia[T08016]. Decoction of dried leaves is taken orally as a remedy for coughs and colds. Half a leaf of *Persea americana* is boiled with leaves of *Lippia dulcis*. Half a cup is taken[T08016]. To soften the body before childbirth, avocado pit, avocado leaves, and salt are used in a bath[T08771]. For premature contractions, avocado leaves and salt are used in a bath. The patients also take boiled water with 10 drops of "Esencia mara-vaillosa" (commercial preparation)[T08771]. Decoction of fresh leaves and seeds is taken orally for contraception, to speed birth, for dysmenorrhea and as an emmenagogue. Leaves and seeds, prepared with pine smoke and fat is used externally as a poultice for wounds and bruises[T09672]. Decoction of leaves is taken orally to treat diarrhea[K16948]. Hot water extract is taken as an emmena-gogue[W02855], and a diuretic[W02290]. Decoction of the fresh bark is used externally for skin blemishes; orally to prevent miscarriage, to speed up postpartum recovery, to treat hem-orrhage between menstrual periods, and to treat menorrhagia[T09672]. Fruit pulp is used as an aphrodisiac[W02855]. Hot water extract of bark, at a dose of two full soupspoons every two hours, is taken as an emmenagogue[M00695]. Hot water extract of buds is taken orally as an emmenagogue and an antisyphiletic[W02290]. Hot water extract of seeds, mixed with moneyworth, wood sorrel and spurge, is taken orally by women suffering from exces-sive bleeding after an abortion[L01490]. Hot water extract of the fruit is taken orally as an aphrodisiac[W02290], and as an ammena-gogue[A00115]. Hot water extract of trunk bark is taken orally as an emmenagogue[W02855]. Seed oil is used externally as an astringent, to treat sores and to remove scars[J01414].

Panama. Hot water extract of leaves is taken orally to treat hypertension, and as an emmenagogue[T01287].

Paraguay. Extract of the plant is taken orally as an abortifacient and as an emmenagogue[J01423]. Hot water extract of leaves, together with *Aristolochia triangularis* and *Jacaranda mimosifolia*, is taken orally for fertility regulation in females[A03499,L02293].

Peru. Hot water extract of dried seeds is taken orally for Amebic dysentery, as an antidiarrheal, antidiabetic and astringent. Externally the extract is used to wash wounds and for baldness[T15323]. Hot water extract of leaves is taken orally as an aborti-facient by the Kichos Indians[A04471].

South Africa. Fruit pulp is eaten as an aph-rodisiac, and as an emmenagogue[A05825].

Trinidad. Water extract of grated seeds is taken orally every other day as a remedy for diabetes[W01284].

West Africa. Hot water extract of leaves is taken orally as a diuretic[A07304].

West Indies. Hot water extract of leaves is taken orally as an antidiarrheal[T00701].

CHEMICAL CONSTITUENTS

(ppm unless otherwise indicated)

5-Dehydro-avenasterol, Sd Ol 1.6-6.8%
5-Hydroxy-tryptamine, Sd
7-Dehydro-avenasterol, Sd Ol 0.9-1.7%
24-Methylene cycloartenol, Pl
1,2,4-Trihydroxyheptadeca-16-ene, Pl
Abscisic acid, Fr; Sd; Fr
Alanine, Fr 960-4,625
Alpha carotene, Fr 0.19-1
Alpha cubebene, Lf EO
Alpha phellandrene, Lf EO
Alpha pinene, Lf EO
Alpha terpinene, Lf EO
Alpha tocopherol, Fr 13-49
Alpha tocopherol, Sd Ol
Anethole, Bk
Apigenin, Lf
Arginine, Fr 470-2,293
Ascorbic acid, Fr 65-994
Ash, Fr 0.6-5.6%
Aspartic acid, Fr 0.2-1.1%
Astragalin, Lf
Beta carotene, Fr 0.3-27
Beta myrcene, Lf EO
Beta ocimene, Lf EO
Beta pinene, Lf EO
Beta sitosterol, Lf
Biotin, Fr 0.1-0.4

Boron, Fr 5-13
Caffeic acid, Fr
Calcium, Fr 60-964
Campesterol, Sd Ol 4.9-6.3%
Camphene, Lf EO
Carbohydrate, Fr 0.8-62.9%
Carvone, Lf EO
Catechin, Sd
Chaviccol methyl ester, Lf EO 90.03%
Chlorogenic acid, Fr
Cholesterol, Sd Ol 1.1-2.3%
Cineol, Lf EO
Copper, Fr 2-11
Cryptoxanthin, Fr 0.38-2
Cyanidin, Lf
Cycloartenol, Pl
Cynaroside, Lf
Cystine, Fr 170-816
D-Arabinitol, Sd
D-Erythro-L-gluco-nonulose, Fr
D-Glycero-D-galacto-heptitol, Fr
D-Glycero-D-galacto-heptose, Fr
D-Glycero-D-galacto-octulose, Fr
D-Glycero-D-manno-octulose, Fr
D-Limonene, Lf EO
D-Mannoheptulose, Fr
D-Mannoketoheptose, Fr
D-Taloheptulose, Fr
Decan-1-ol acetate, Lf EO
Dihydro-phaseic acid, Fr
Dimethyl-sciadinonate, Lf
Dopamine, Fr
Epsilon carotene, Pl
Essential oils, Lf 0.5%
Estragole, Fr Pe 60-90%; Lf EO 90.03%
Fat, Fr 6.1-86.4%
Fiber, Fr 1.0-10.6
Folacin, Fr 0.5-2.8
Folic acid, Fr 0.3-2.4
Galactitol, Sd
Gamma terpinene, Lf EO
Glutamic acid, Fr 1,660-8,045
Glycerol, Fr
Glycine, Fr 660-3226
Hentriacosane, Fr
Heptacosane, Fr
Heptadecane-1-2-4-triol, Sd
Hex-cis-3-en-1-ol, Lf EO
Hexan-1-al, Lf EO
Histidine, Fr 230-1,127
Iron, Fr 6-61
Isoleucine, Fr 570-2759

Isolutein, Fr
Kilocalories, Fr 940-6700
Lecithin, Fr
Leucine, Fr 990-4780
Linoleic acid, Fr 2.4-50.5%
Linolenic acid, Fr 0.02-2.85%
Lutein, Fr 3.2-16
Luteolin, Lf
Lysine, Fr 750-3,653
Magnesium, Fr 370-1,740
Manganese, Fr 2-10
Mannoheptulose, Fr 0.6-3.1%
Methionine, Fr 290-1,438
Methyl-chavicol, Lf
MUFA, Fr 9.6-37.3%
Myoinositol, Fr
N-Hexadecane, Lf EO
N-Octane, Lf EO
Nerol acetate, Lf EO
Niacin, Fr 14-101
Nonacosane, Fr
Octan-1-ol, Lf EO
Oleic acid, Fr 2.7-69.1%
P-Coumaric acid, Fr
P-Coumarylquinic acid, Fr
Palmitic acid, Fr 0.4-26.6%
Palmitoleic acid, Fr 0.6-2.5
Pantothenic acid, Fr 8-37.7
Paraffin, Lf
Pentacosane, Fr
Pentan-1-ol, Lf EO
Perseitol, Sd 8.9%; Fr 0.4-3.8%
Phenylalanine, Fr 540-2,643
Phosphorus, Fr 260-3,030
Phytosterols, Fr
Pinene, Lf
Potassium, Fr 2,780-27,470
Procyanidins, Lf, Fr Pe
Proline, Fr 620-2,993
PUFA, Fr 1.9-7.6%
Pyridoxine, Fr 6-23
Quercetin, Lf
Quercetin-3-diglucoside, Lf
Riboflavin, Fr 1-7.7
Sabinene, Lf EO
Saturated fatty acids, Fr 2.4-9.4%
Sciadinonic acid dimethyl ester, Lf
Scopoletin, Lf
Serine, Fr 810-3,148
Serotonin, Fr
Sodium, Fr 20-520
Stearic acid, Fr 120-4,320

Stigmast-7-en-3-beta-ol, Sd oil
Stigmasterol, Sd oil
Tannin, Lf 4.7%
Tartaric acid, Fr 200
Thiamin, Fr 0.5-4.2
Threonine, Fr 530-2,565
Triacosane, Fr
Tryptophan, Fr 170-816
Tyramine, Fr
Tyrosine, Fr 390-1,904
Valine, Fr 970-3,770
Violaxanthin, Fr
Vitamin A Sd oil
Vitamin D, Sd oil; Fr 0.1
Vitamin B6, Fr 10.9
Volemitrol, Sd
Water, Fr 71.6-83.0%
Zinc, Fr 4-16

PHARMACOLOGICAL ACTIVITIES AND CLINICAL TRIALS

Allergenic activity. Fresh fruit eaten by human adults of both sexes was active. The effect was investigated by an immunoblotting technique in sera of allergenic patients[K20557]. Fruit taken by human adult was active. Skin prick tests produced positive IGE-mediated reactions with varying symptoms from rhinoconjunctivitis to anaphylactic shock[K18294].

Analgesic activity. Flavonoid fraction of dried seeds, at a dose of 80.0 mg/kg administered intraperitoneally to mice was active vs hot plate method[T02554].

Antibacterial activity. Methanol/water (1:1) extract of leaves in broth culture was inactive on *Bacillus subtilis*, *Escherichia coli*, *Proteus vulgaris*, *Pseudomonas aeruginosa*, *Staphylococcus albus*, and *Staphylococcus aureus*[J00209]. Petroleum ether extract of seeds, on agar plate was active on *Sarcina lutea* and *Staphylococcus aureus*, and inactive on *Bacillus subtilis*, *Escherichia coli* and *Salmonella typhosa*[W01662].

Anticlastogenic activity. Fruit juice, at a dose of 50.0 ml/kg, administered intraperitoneally to mice, was active on marrow cells vs mitomycin C, and dimethylnitrosamine-induced micronuclei[K17561].

Antiedema activity. Methanol extract of fruit, applied externally to mice at a dose of 2.0 mg/ear, was active. The inhibition ratio was eight vs 12-0-tetradecanoylphorbol-13-acetate (TPA)-induced ear inflammation[K11173].

Antifungal activity. Chloroform extract of freeze-dried fruit peel, on agar plate was active on *Cladosporium cladosporiodes*[H07994].

Antigiardiasis activity. Decoction of leaves and stem at a concentration of 4.0 mg/ml produced weak activity on *Giardia intestinalis*[K17990].

Antihypertensive activity. Water extract of dried leaves at a concentration of 0.1 ml/animal, administered intravenously to rats was active vs nicotine and norepinephrine-induced hypertension[T02774].

Antimalarial activity. Ethanol (95%), and hexane extracts of dried leaves and stem, at a dose of 100.0 mg/kg (daily dosing for four days), administered by gastric intubation to mice were inactive on *Plasmodium berghei*[K07977].

Antiyeast activity. Ethanol (60%) extract of dried leaves on agar plate was inactive on *Candida albicans*[M31296].

Barbiturate potentiation. Flavonoid fraction of dried seeds, at a dose of 80.0 mg/kg administered intraperitoneally to mice was active[T02554].

Cell proliferation inhibition. Water extract of dried leaves at a concentration of 200.0 mcg/ml was inactive on lymphocytes vs phytohemagglutinin-induced proliferation. The effect is reversible[K19547].

Chronotropic effect (positive). Ethanol/water (1:1) extract of fresh leaves at a dose of 40.0 ml/kg, administered by gastric intubation to rats was inactive[T10623].

Collagen synthesis inhibition. Seed oil, at a dose of 10% administered to rats by gastric intubation was active. Weanling animals were fed on a diet supplemented with given oil for eight weeks, after which dorsal skin assay for moisture, protein total collagen and soluble collagen. Only the latter has increased, by 36% vs control[M27157].

Comutagenic activity. Fruit juice, at a dose of 50.0 ml/kg, administered intraperitoneally to mice was active on marrow cells vs tetracycline-induced micronuclei[K17561].

Death. Dried fruit administered orally to canary was active. One canary and three cockatiels died after eating avocado. necropsy of the canary revealed enlarged spleen, subcutaneous edema and phlebitis (judged unrelated to avocado ingestion). The cockatiels showed hydropericardium, possibly due to avocado. Deaths of all birds were attributed to avocado intoxication. Pulp, at a doses of 1.0 and 0.7 ml/animal, administered by gastric intubation to budgerigars and canaries were active. Birds were given doses of a mixture of 8.7 gm avocado pulp mixed with 2.0 ml water. Two of four budgerigars given two doses died, all budgerigars given four doses died and one canary given four doses died. Necropsy showed excess epicardial fluid, generalized lung congestion and nonsuppurative inflammation. Death was attributed to lung congestion caused by avocado[M18901].

Diuretic activity. Ethanol/water (1:1) extract of fresh leaves, at a dose of 40.0 ml/kg, administered to rats by gastric intubation, was active. Five parts fresh plant material in 100 parts water/ethanol[M17736].

Hypertensive activity. Fresh fruit eaten by human adults was active. Induction of a hypertensive crisis in a patient on monoamine-oxidase inhibitor therapy[N13077]. Ethanol (95%), and water extracts of dried leaves and stem at a doses of 0.1 ml/kg, administered intravenously to dogs were active[A03360]. Ethanol/water (1:1) extract of fresh leaves at a dose of 40.0 ml/kg, administered to rats by gastric intubation produced weak activity[T10623]. Flavonoid fraction of dried seeds, at a dose of 2.0 mg/kg administered intravenously to male rats produced weak activity[T02554].

Larvicidal activity. Leaves (undiluted) in the ration of *Bombyx mori* larvae was active[T00295].

Lysyl oxidase inhibition. Seed oil, at a dose of 10.0% administered by gastric intubation to rats was active. Weanling animals were fed on a diet supplemented with given oil for eight weeks, after which dorsal skin assayed for given activity. 56% decrease in activity observed[57]. Unsaponifiable fraction at a concentration of 0.5% was active on the skin of rats. Enzyme activity was decreased by 30%[M25183].

Molluscicidal activity. Ethanol (95%) extract of dried leaves at a concentration of 100.0 ppm was inactive on *Biomphalaria glabrata* versus eggs and adults. The hexane-ethyl acetate extract was inactive vs both eggs and adults[M25853]. Ethanol (95%), and hot water extracts of seeds at a concentration of 10,000 ppm, were active on *Biomphalaria straminea*[W00500]. Ethanol (95%), and water extracts of dried seeds, at concentrations of 10,000 ppm were inactive on *Biomphalaria glabrata* and *Biomphalaria straminea*[W02949]. Homogenate of fresh entire plant was inactive on *Lymnaea columella* and *Lymnaea cubensis*. Fruits, leaves and roots were tested[T04621].

Phagocytosis stimulation. Unsaponifiable fraction of dried fruit, at a dose of 0.5 ml/animal, administered intraperitoneally to male mice was active[T07238].

Pharmacokinetic study. Seed oil applied to the skin is rapidly absorbed[M05179].

Smooth muscle relaxant activity. Ethanol (95%) extract of dried leaves and stem, at a concentration of 33 ml/liter was active on rabbit duodenum[A03360].

Smooth muscle stimulant activity. Flavonoid fraction of dried seeds produced weak activity on guinea pig ileum[T02554].

Spasmogenic activity. Ethanol (95%) extract at a concentration of 3.3 ml/liter, and water extract at a concentration of 0.33 ml/liter, administered to guinea pigs intraperitoneally at were active on the ileum[A03360].

Toxic effect. Powdered freeze-dried fruit, at a concentration of 1.0 ml, administered to budgerigar by gastric intubation was active[K11884]. Seed oil, at variable concentrations was inactive. Various tests involving creams and other beauty care products with avocado oil concentrations as high as 10% showed little or no irritation. Undiluted seed oil applied by patches was inactive. Patches remained on subject for 48 hours and test was repeated in 14 days. No sensitization occurred. Seed oil, at a dose of 0.25 ml/animal administered subcutaneously to rats was inactive. Given daily for 30 days, no gross pathological effects were seen. Seed coat, at a dose of 625.0 mg/kg taken orally by human adult was inactive[M05179].

Toxicity assessment (quantitative). Ethanol (95%) extract of dried leaves and stem produced a minimum toxic dose of 1.0 ml/animal, when administered intraperitoneally to mice. The water extract a minimum toxic dose of 0.5 ml/animal[A03360].

Flavonoid fraction of dried seeds when administered intraperitoneally to mice produced a LD_{50} 340.0 mg/kg[T02554].

Tumor promotion inhibition. Methanol extract of fresh fruits at a concentration of 200.0 mcg in cell culture was active on Epstein-Barr virus vs 12-0-hexadecanoyl-phorbol-13-acetate-induced Epstein-Barr virus activation[T15279].

Uterine stimulant effect. Ethanol (95%) of leaves and stem, at a concentration of 0.33 ml/liter was active on rat uterus. The water extract at a concentration of 0.033 ml/liter produced strong activity on rat uterus[A03360].

WBC-macrophage stimulant. Water extract of freeze-dried fruit at a concentration of 2.0 mg/ml was inactive. Nitrite formation was used as an index of the macrophage stimulating activity to screen effective foods[M27208].

22 | Phyllanthus niruri

L.

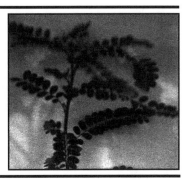

Common Names

Bhoomi amalaki	India	Gale-wind grass	West Indies
Bhui amla	Bangladesh	Graine en bas fievre	French Guiana
Bhui-amla	India	Hurricane weed	West Indies
Bhuianvalah	India	Jar amla	Fiji
Bhuimy-amli	East Indies	Jar-amla	India
Bhuin-amla	Pakistan	Kizha nelli	India
Bhumyamalaki	India	Mapatan	Papua-New Guinea
Cane peas senna	West Indies	Mimosa	West Indies
Carry-me seed	Fiji	Niruri	Pakistan
Carry-me seed	West Indies	Para-parai mi	Paraguay
Chamber bitters	West Indies	Pei	Admiralty Islands
Chancapiedra	Peru	Phyllanto	Brazil
Chickweed	West Indies	Pombinha	East Indies
Creole senna	Virgin Islands	Querba pedra	Brazil
Daun marisan	East Indies	Quinine weed	West Indies
Derriere-dos	Haiti	Sampa-sampalukan	Philippines
Deye do	Haiti	Sasi	Papua-NewGuinea
Elrageig	Sudan	Se	Papua-New Guinea
En bas	West Indies	Shka-nin-du	Mexico
Eruption plant	Papua-New Guinea	Viernes santo	Puerto Rico
Gale wind grass	Fiji	Ya-tai-bai	Thailand
Gale-o-wind	Bimini	Yerba de san pablo	Philippines

BOTANICAL DESCRIPTION

A herb of the EUPHORBIACEAE family that grows up to 60 cm. The plant is bitter in taste, the leaves are small, green, and short-petioled with a thin and glaucous under surface. The flowers are unisexual, monoecious, minute, greenish, and inconspicuous, short-stalked and borne in pairs in the axils of the leaves. The fruit is a capsule, globose, slightly depressed at the top with six enervations. In the roots, the secondary growth starts very early and is well pronounced. There is a distinct cambium. No starch grains, mineral crystals or latex vessels are seen both in root and stem.

ORIGIN AND DISTRIBUTION

The plant originated in India, usually occurring as a winter weed throughout the hotter

From: Medicinal Plants of the World *By: Ivan A. Ross Humana Press Inc., Totowa, NJ*

parts. Now widespread throughout the tropics and subtropics in sandy regions during rainy seasons.

TRADITIONAL MEDICINAL USES

Admiralty Islands. Hot water extract of dried bark and leaves administered orally is used for acute venereal disease. Bark and leaves are boiled with water and the solution (500 ml) is taken twice daily for up to six months[T07369].

Argentina. The plant is used as an emmenagogue by the rural populace[J01423].

Bimini. Hot water extract of the entire plant is administered orally, to reduce fevers, and as a laxative[T00359].

Brazil. Decoction of dried root is taken orally for jaundice. Decoction of dried seeds is taken orally for diabetes. Hot water extract of dried fruit is administered orally for diabetes. Infusion of dried leaves and stems is taken orally to treat kidney and bladder calculi. Infusion of the dried entire plant administered orally, is used to dissolve kidney and bladder stones, and for renal diseases[T15975].

Dominican Republic. Hot water extract of leaves is administered orally as a popular fever remedy[W00673].

East Africa. Hot water extract of the aerial parts administered orally is used as a diuretic[W01586].

East Indies. Hot water extract of the entire plant is administered orally, for menstrual troubles/complaints, to treat diabetes, as a purgative, and as a tonic[W02290].

Fiji. Decoction of dried leaves and roots is taken orally for fever, and for good health. Dried entire plant, grounded in buttermilk is administered orally for jaundice. Fresh leaf juice is used externally for cuts and bruises. For eye diseases the juice is mixed with castor oil and applied to the eye. Infusion of dried leaves is administered orally for dysentery and diarrhea. Infusion of green root is taken orally to treat heavy menstrual periods[T10632].

French Guiana. Hot water extract of leaves is administered orally as a cholagogue[J10155].

Haiti. Decoction of dried leaves is taken orally for or used in bath for fever, and orally for indigestion[T13846]. Hot water extract of dried entire plant is administered orally as a spasmolytic and is also against fever[T04647].

India. Decoction of the dried aerial parts administered orally is used for diarrhea[K17122], and jaundice[T08388]. Fresh plant juice is taken orally for genito-urinary disorders[T10133]. The fruit is used externally for tubercular ulcers, scabies and ringworm[L02008]. Hot water extract of dried entire plant is administered orally for diabetes[A14379], as a diuretic[K08911], for gonorrhea and urogenital tract infections[M22721], for jaundice[M16717,T08282], for leucorrhea[M23826], and for asthma in Ayurvedic medicine[T09366]. Hot water extract of dried leaves is taken orally for diabetes. Hot water extract of fresh shoots is taken orally for dysentery, and for jaundice[M22721]. Hot water extract of leaves, administered orally is used as a stomachic[L02008], for menorrhagia[A06590], and for intermittent fever[W01145]. Water extract of roots is taken orally as a galactagogue[A04766].

Malaysia. Hot water extract of leaves administered orally, is used after a miscarriage and as an emmenagogue[A06590].

Mexico. Hot water extract of dried leaves is emetic when taken as a strong tea[W02493].

Papau-New Guinea. Fresh leaf juice is taken orally for venereal diseases. Fresh root juice is taken orally for venereal diseases. Decoction of dried entire plant is administered orally to treat venereal diseases[M23272]. For malaria the decoction is drunk and used to bathe patient, and for tuberculosis, a single dose of decoction is taken orally[T09033]. Decoction of dried leaf when taken orally is a treatment for diarrhea. A cupful of leaf decoction is drunk daily[K18559].

Peru. Hot water extract of dried entire plant is administered orally for gallstones, as a diuretic, and for renal calculi[T15323].

Philippines. Decoction of dried entire plant is used as a bath for newborns. Believed to remove disease-causing elements from the skin. Orally the decoction is used for coughs in infants[T10116]. Hot water extract of the entire plant is administered orally as an emmenagogue[A00115,A04508].

Puerto Rico. Hot water extract of leaf and stem is taken orally for fevers[A04418].

Sudan. Hot water extract of dried leaves is taken orally as an analgesic[A06766].

Tanzania. Hot water extract of fresh entire plant is administered orally for gonorrhea[T10354].

Thailand. Hot water extract of commercial sample of the entire plant, is administered orally as an antipyretic[W3022A]. Hot water extract of dried aerial parts administered orally is used as a diuretic, as an antipyretic, and for malaria[M18836]. Hot water extract of dried entire plant is administered orally as an antiinflammatory agent[W03804].

Virgin Islands. Hot water extract of the plant is taken orally to increase the appetite[W00903].

West Indies. Hot water extract of roots together with hot water extract of *Citrus aurantifolia* roots is taken orally to increase appetite. Hot water extract of the entire plant administered orally, is taken for malaria and malarial fever. The plant is boiled and the tea taken. Water extract of the leaves and roots is taken orally for diabetes, and as a diuretic[T00701,W01316].

CHEMICAL CONSTITUENTS

(ppm unless otherwise indicated)

(+)-Catechin, Rt Cult.
(+)-Gallocatechin, Rt Cult
(-)-Epi-catechin, Rt Cult
(-)-Epi-catechin-3-gallate, Rt Cult
(-)-Epi-gallocatechin-3-O-gallate, Rt
(-)-Limonene, Lf EO 4.5%
(-)-Nor-serurinine, Pl
(-)Epi-gallocatechin, Rt Cult
4-Hydroxy-lintetralin, Lf 200
4-Hydroxy-sesamin, Pl
4-Methoxy-nor-securinine, Aer, Rt, St.
2,3-dimethoxy-iso-lintetralin, Lf 2

24-Isopropyl cholesterol, Aer 18
Ascorbic acid, Lf 0.41%
Astragalin, Lf
Beta sitosterol, Lf
Corilagin, Pl 7
Cymene, Lf EO 11%
Demethylenedioxy niranthin, Lf 2
Dotriacontanoic acid, Aer 65
Ellagic acid, Pl 108-972
Eriodictyol-7-O-alpha-L-rhamnoside, Rt
Estradiol, Pl 3
Fisetin-41-O-beta-D-dlucoside, Pl 400
Gallic acid, Rt Cult 2.7-27
Geranin, Pl 0.23%
Hinokinin, Pl
Hydroxy niranthin, Lf 4
Hypophyllanthin, Lf 500, Aer 100
Hypophyllanthin, Pl 0.05-0.17%
Iso-lintetralin, Pl 3.4
Iso-quercitrin, Lf
Kaempferol-4-O-alpha-L-rhamnoside, Aer 0.9%, Rt
Linnanthin, Lf 2
Linoleic acid, SD Ol 21%
Linolenic acid, Sd Ol 51.4%
Lintetralin, Lf 5-15
Lupeol acetate, Rt
Lupeol, Rt
Niranthin, Lf 9-430
Nirphyllin, Aer 7
Nirtetralin, Pl, Lf 9-930
Nirurin, Pl 400
Nirurine, Aer 39.8
Nirurinetin, Pl
Nor-securinine, Rt
Phyllanthenol, Aer 20
Phyllanthenone, Aer 8
Phylantheol, Aer 15
Phyllanthin, Lf 400, Aer 1100-3250
Phyllanthine, Rt, Lf, St
Phyllanthus, Pl
Phyllester, Aer 12
Phyllnirurin, Aer 6
Phyllochrysine, Lf, St
Phylltetrin, Aer
Phyltetralin, Pl, Lf 0.14%
Quercetin, Lf, Pl
Quercitrin, Lf
Repandusinic acid A, Pl
Repandusinic acid, Pl 0.12%
Ricinoleic acid, Sd Ol 1.2%
Rutin, Pl, Lf

Salicylic acid methyl ester, Lf EO
Seco-4-hydroxy-lintetralin, Lf 20
Trans-phytol, Pl
Triacontan-1-al, Aer 60
Triancontan-1-ol, Aer 560

PHRMACOLOGICAL ACTIVITIES AND CLINICAL TRIALS

Aldose reductase inhibition. Ethanol (70%) extract of dried entire plant was active. IC_{50} 1.0 mcg/ml[M21373].

Analgesic activity. Methanol extract of dried callus tissue at a concentration of 10.0 mg/kg, administered intraperitoneally to mice was active vs. acetic acid-induced writhing, and vs. formalin-induced pedal edema. The extract, at 50.0 mg/kg was inactive vs. tail flick response to radiant heat[K17672]. Ethanol/water (1:1) extract of dried entire plant at a dose of 50 mg/kg, administered intragastric to male mice was active. The extract also administered intraperitoneally to male mice at a dose of 0.3 mg/kg was active. In both cases antinociceptive effects demonstrated using five different models of nociception[K19491].

Angiotensin-converting enzyme inhibition. Chromatographic fraction of dried entire plant at a concentration of 100.0 mcg/ml was active[M18866].

Antibacterial activity. Water extract of fresh entire plant at a concentration of 1.0% on agar plate was inactive on *Neisseria gonorrhea*[T10354]. Saline extract of leaves, at a concentration of 10% on agar plate was active on *Pasteurella pestis* and *Staphylococcus aureus*, and inactive on *Escherichia coli* [W01047]. Chloroform extract of dried leaves, at a concentration of 1.0 gm/ml on agar plate was inactive on *Bacillus subtilis, Escherichia coli, Pseudomonas aeruginosa* and *Staphylococcus aureus*. Methanol extract was active on *Staphylococcus aureus*, but inactive on *Bacillus subtilis, Escherichia coli,* and *Pseudomonas aeruginosa*[T06766].

Antidiarrheal activity. Ethanol/water (1:1) extract of dried aerial parts at a concentration of 300 mg was inactive for antidiarrheal activity on both guinea pig and rabbit ileums vs *E. Coli*-Inte Rotoxin-induced diarrhea[K17122].

Antifungal activity. Petroleum ether extract of whole plant showed antifungal activity against *Helminthosporium sativa*. The leaf extract showed antifungal activity against *Alternaria alternata*, while it had no activity against *Curvalaria lunata*[T00001].

Antihepatotoxic activity. Hexane extract of dried aerial parts at a concentration of 1.0 mg/ml, when tested for antihepatotoxic activity on rat liver cell in cell culture was active. Results significant at $P < 0.01$ level vs. CCl_4-Induced hepatotoxicity. The extract was inactive vs. galactosamine-induced toxicity[T11593]. Dried entire plant administered to sheep by gastric intubation at a dose of 1.0 gm/kg was active. Animals were dosed daily for 10 days after receiving hepatotoxic paracetamol. A mixture of *Andrographis paniculata, Phyllanthus niruri* and *Solanum nigrum* used. Changes induced by toxin were ameliorated by treatment. Changes include anemia, leukocytosis with neutrophilia and lymphopenia, increased coagulation, decreased glucose, cholesterolemia, hypotriglyceridemia jaundice and elevation of AST and ALT[K11808]. Powdered dried entire plant administered by gastric intubation to rats at a dose of 200.0 mg/kg was active on liver homogenate vs ethanol treated rats dosed for 45 days. Triglyceride, cholesterol and phospholipid contents in fatty liver were reduced to normal levels[M17464]. Water extract of dried leaves, at a concentration of 2.0 ml/kg, administered to rats by gastric intubation was active. Effective as pretreatment, vs CCl_4-induced hepatotoxic activity[T12115].

Antihypercholesterolemic activity. Dried entire plant in the ration of rats was active. Fatty liver was induced with alcohol. The plant material reduced the increased deposition of triglycerides, cholesterol and phospholipids in the liver, heart and kidney that resulted from alcohol treatment[T14998].

Antihyperglycemic activity. Water extract of dried entire plant when administered by gastric intubation to rats was active vs alloxan-induced hyperglycemia[M22721].

Antihyperlipemic activity. Water extract of dried entire plant fed to rats in the ration was active. Fatty liver was induced with alcohol. The plant material reduced the increased deposition of triglycerides, cholesterol and phospholipids in the liver, heart, and kidney that resulted from the alcohol treatment[T14998].

Antimutagenic activity. Water extract of dried leaves, at a dose of 10.0 ml/kg, administered by gastric intubation to mice was active vs nickle-induced clastogenicity[K07087].

Antipyretic activity. Ethanol/water (1:1) extract of commercial sample of the entire plant, variable dosage levels administered by gastric intubation to rabbits was inactive vs yeast-induced pyrexia[W3022A].

Antispasmodic activity. Ethanol/water (1:1) extract of the entire plant was active on guinea pig ileum vs ACh and histamine-induced spasms[A03335].

Antitumor activity. Ethanol/water (1:1) extract administered intraperitoneally to mice was active on LEUK (Friend Virus-Solid)[A03335]. Ethanol (95%) extract, and water extract of dried aerial parts, at doses of 100.0 mg/kg were both inactive on Sarcoma 180(ASC)[M23643].

Antiviral activity. Ethanol (95%) extract of dried aerial parts was active on hepatitis B virus. Antiviral activity was measured in serum of patients who were positive for the hepatitis B virus[N24831]. Water extract of the dried entire plant at a dose of 9.0 mg/animal administered to woodchuck was active vs hepatitis in long-term chronic carriers of woodchuck hepatitis. No effect was seen in either experimental or control animals. When experimental animals were later switched to intraperitoneal administration, two of them showed a drop in antigen titer (two others died of unrelated causes). No control animals showed any effects[M16717]. Water extract of the dried entire plant administered by gastric intubation to woodchuck was active on woodchuck hepatitis virus. Biological activity reported has been patented[M16072]. Water extract of the dried entire plant at a concentration of 9.0 mg/animal, administered intraperitoneally to woodchuck, was active vs hepatitis in recently infected woodchucks. Three out of four experimental animals showed elimination of woodchuck hepatitis surface antigen and woodchuck hepatitis DNA polymerase after 72 days. They remained negative for both for 300 days. Control animal did not show any change. Water extract of the dried entire plant at a concentration of 9.0 mg/animal, administered intraperitoneally to woodchuck, was active vs hepatitis in long-term chronic carriers of woodchuck hepatitis. Titer of woodchuck hepatitis surface antigen was lowered relative to untreated controls. 0.5 ml extract was given once a week[M16717]. Water extract of dried entire plant (plants cultivated in USA), when tested on hepatitis virus in cell culture was inactive vs Hepadnavirus DNA polymerase. IC_{50} 381.0 and 410.0 mcg/ml[M18866]. Ethanol (95%) extract of fresh entire plant tested on Tobacco Mosaic virus in cell culture was equivocal. The viral inhibitory activity was 7%[K09718]. Fresh leaf, and fresh root extract at a concentration of 4.0% was active on Peanut Mosaic virus, Tobacco Mosaic virus, and Tobacco Ring Spot virus[T10824].

Cardiotoxic activity. Ethanol/water (1:1) extract of a commercial sample of the entire plant at variable concentrations intravenously on dogs was inactive[W3022A].

Chromosome aberration inhibition. Water extract of dried fruit and leaf, at a dose of 685.0 mg/kg, administered to mice by gastric intubation was active vs chromosome damage induced by lead nitrate and aluminum sulphate in bone marrow chromosomes. Dosing was for seven days[M25745].

Chronotropic effect (positive). Ethanol/water (1:1) extract of a commercial sample of the entire plant, administered intravenously at variable dosages to dogs was inactive[W3022A].

Cytotoxic activity. Ethanol/water (1:1) extract of entire plant in cell culture was inactive on CA-9KB, ED_{50} >20.0 mcg/ml[A03335]. DNA polymerase inhibition. Water extract of dried entire plant at a concentration of 50.0 mg/ml was active vs activity of woodchuck hepatitis virus DNA polymerase, 50 mg/ml gave about 25% inhibition. Both methanol and water extracts, at variable dosages were also active. Biological activity reported in these studies have been patented[M17062].

Hepatitis B surface antigen inactivation. Water extract of dried entire plant at a concentration of 0.2 mg/ml was active on hepatitis virus vs reaction of woodchuck hepatitis surface antigen with hepatitis B (Human) antibody. At a concentration of 0.63 mg/ml the extract was active on hepatitis B virus vs reaction of hepatitis B surface antigen with hepatitis B antibody[M16717]. Both water and methanol extracts of the dried entire plant, at variable concentrations were active and the biological activity reported has been patented[M17062]. Water extract of dried leaves, was active. hepatitis B surface antigen inactivation was assayed. IC_{50} 650 ng/ml. The methanol extract was also active. IC_{50} 1.2 mcg/ml. Water extract of dried leaves, was active. Hepatitis B surface antigen inactivation was assayed. IC_{50} 3.30 mcg/ml[K10104]. Chloroform

extract[T06317] and water extract[M17007] of dried leaves, stem, and also of dried roots, at a concentration of 2.0% were active.

Hypoglycemic activity. Water extract of the dried entire plant at a dose of 10.0 mg/kg, administered orally to rabbits was inactive. Drop in blood sugar of 15 mg relative to inert-treated control indicated positive results[A14379].

Hypotensive activity. Ethanol/water (1:1) extract of a commercial sample of the entire plant, when administered to dogs intravenously at variable dosage levels was inactive[W3022A].

Molluscicidal activity. Ethanol (95%) extract of dried stem, at a concentration of 250.0 ppm was inactive on *Biomphalaria pfeifferi* and *Bulinus truncatus*. Petroleum ether extract at a concentration of 25.0 ppm was active on *Biomphalaria pfeifferi* and *Bulinus truncatus*[T07986].

Nematocidal activity. Decoction of commercial sample of bark, at a concentration of 1.0 mg/ml was active on *Toxacara canis*[M26175].

Reverse transcriptase inhibition. Water extract of the dried entire plant on HIV-1 virus was active. ID_{50} 50.0 mcg/ml[K08911].

Spasmolytic activity. Methanol extract of dried callus tissue at a concentration of 320.0 mcg/ml on guinea pig ileum was inactive vs ACh-induced contractions[K17672].

Toxicity assessment (quantitative). Ethanol/water (1:1) extract of the entire plant administered orally to mice tolerated a maximum dose of 1.0 gm/kg[A03335]. Water extract of the dried entire plant at a dose of 0.1 mcg/animal was inactive. No weight loss found seven days after treatment with the extract[M16717].

23 | Portulaca oleracea

L.

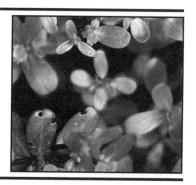

Common Names

Amloniya	Fiji	Olasiman	West Indies
Baldroegas	Madeira	Pappukura	India
Baraloniya	Fiji	Pigweed	Fiji
Barbin	Qatar	Portulaca	Italy
Barbir	Qatar	Posely	Nicaragua
Beldroega	Brazil	Pourpier	Dominica
Beldroegas	Madeira	Pourpier	West Indies
Bredo de porco	Brazil	Purchiacchella	Italy
Buklut-ul-hakima	India	Purslane	Dominica
Burra-lonia	India	Purslane	Europe
Common purslane	Madeira	Purslane	Jamaica
Common purslane	USA	Purslane	Netherlands
Coupie	Dominica	Purslane	USA
Coupie	West Indies	Purslane	West Indies
Croupier	French Guiana	Pusley	Europe
Demze	Guinea	Pusley	Guyana
Dorcellana	Italy	Pusley	Virgin Islands
Erba vasciulella	Italy	Pussley	West Indies
Farfena	Oman	Pussly	Jamaica
Goni	India	Pussly	West Indies
Khurfa	India	Rigia	Qatar
Khursa	Fiji	Rigla	Egypt
Khutura	India	Shoi-bee-reum	Egypt
Koolfa	India	Small purslain	India
Koupye	Haiti	Suvandacheera	India
Kulfa	India	Tarbari	India
Kupye	West Indies	Tokmakan	Turkey
Kurfa	India	Tukhm khurfa	Pakistan
Langiruh	Brunei	Verdolaga	Brazil
Lonika	India	Verdolaga	Canary Islands
Loonia	India	Verdolaga	Cuba
Lulimilwasenga	Tanganyika	Verdolaga	Nicaragua
Machixian	China	Verdolaga	Peru
Makabling	West Indies	Verdolaga	Puerto Rico
Mutunu	Tanganyika	Verdolaga	Spain
		Verdulaga	Spain

From: Medicinal Plants of the World *By: Ivan A. Ross Humana Press Inc., Totowa, NJ*

BOTANICAL DESCRIPTION

An annual, prostrate or spreading, succulent, branched herb of the PORTULACAEAE family; quite glabrous; 10–50 cm long. The stems are often purplish. Leaves are fleshy and flat, obtuse, oblong-obovate, base cuneate, 1 to 2.5 cm long. Flowers is sessile, axillary and terminal, few-flowered heads, the heads solitary or cymose, the buds compressed. Petals: five; yellow; about as long as the sepals. Stamens: 8–12.

ORIGIN AND DISTRIBUTION

A very common weed of cultivated and undisturbed land. Native of the Old World tropics. Now found in both temperate and tropical zones, from South Europe, where it is cultivated as a vegetable, to China.

TRADITIONAL MEDICINAL USES

Brazil. Seeds are taken orally and are said to be emmenagogic[W02855]. The wilted entire plant is said to cause death of cattle when ingested[A05311].

Canary Islands. Hot water extract of dried aerial parts is taken orally as a diuretic, calculolithic and for migraine[T15880].

China. Hot water extract of leaves is taken orally for arthritis. Hot water extract of stem is taken orally for arthritis[X00003].

Dominica. Leaves are employed as a plaster to ease pain of menstruation[W01267].

Europe. Aerial parts is eaten as a vegetable since early Roman times[W02033].

Fiji. Dried leaf and stem is taken orally for stomachache and paralysis[T10632].

French Guiana. Hot water extract of leaves is taken orally as a cholagogue[J10155].

Haiti. Decoction of dried leaves is taken orally for asthenia[T13846].

Hawaii. Water extract of plant is taken orally for asthma[K18991].

India. Hot water extract of dried leaves are taken orally as a diuretic and for lever diseases[T06767]. Leaves and shoot are cooked as a vegetable[K23485]. Leaves are used as a food[M25938]. Seeds are taken orally as a vermifuge[T06767].

Seeds steeped in wine are taken orally as an emmenagogue. In Ayurvedic and Unani medicine, the seeds are taken orally as a vermifuge[T05894]. Shoots are used as food[M25938].

Indo-China. Seeds are taken orally to provoke menses[A00115].

Italy. Decoction of dried leaves is taken orally as a diuretic and for gastronomic purposes[T16715].

Jamaica. Hot water extract of entire plant is taken orally as a vermifuge[W01270].

Malaysia. Hot water extract of dried entire plant is taken orally for chest pain[T08817].

New Caledonia. Seeds are taken orally to as an emmenagogue[A04174].

Nigeria. Hot water extract of fresh entire plant is taken orally as a sedative and heart tonic[T06510]. Hot water extract of fresh leaves and stem is taken orally for muscular aches and pains[T14146].

Peru. Hot water extract of dried seeds and of dried stems are taken orally as an antiscorbutic, antidysenteric, emmenagogue, vermifuge and against jaundice[T15323].

Sierra Leone. Infusion of dried leaves, taken orally, is used as an abortifacient. The infusion is taken with palm oil[T09679].

Tanzania. Decoction of hot water extract of entire plant is washed over the breasts as a galactagogue[A05550].

Virgin Islands. Hot water extract of aerial parts is taken orally for intestinal worms[W00903].

West Indies. Hot water extract of aerial parts is taken orally to provoke menses[A04610]. Hot water extract of leaves is taken orally for painful menstruation[T00701]. Seeds are taken orally to provoke menses[A00115].

CHEMICAL CONSTITUENTS
(ppm unless otherwise indicated)

3-(3,4-Dihydroxyphenyl)alanine docosahexaenoic acid, He
Alanine, Re 570-13,400
Alkaloids, Lf 300
Alpha linolenic acid, He 0.4-8.0%
Alpha tocopherol, Pl 82-2,309

Arabinose
Arginine, He 520-10,400
Ascorbate, Pl 224-5,230
Ascorbic acid, He 105-7,000
Ash, He 1.4-15.9%
Asparagic acid, Pl
Aspartic acid, He 770-19,600
Behenic acid, Sd 2,262
Beta amyrin, Aer
Beta carotene, He 11-4,650
Beta cyanin, He
Beta sitosterol, Sd
Caffeic acid, Pl
Calcium oxalate, He
Calcium, He 780-20,800
Campesterol, Aer
Capric acid
Carbohydrate, He 3.55-63.2%
Catechol
Cellulose, 10.5-13.2%
Chlorine, He 730-7,300
Chlorophyll, Pl
Cinnamic acid, Lf, St
Citric acid, Pl 5,100
Copper, He 2-19
Cystine, He 100-4,200
Digalactosyldiacyl glycerol, Lf; He
DNA, Pl
DOPA
Eicosapentaenoic acid, He 10
Fat, He 0.19-6.3%
Fat, Sd 17.4%
Fatty acids, Lf
Ferulic acid, Pl
Fiber, He 0.8-13.7%
Folacin, Pl
Fructose, Pl
Galactose, Pl
Glucose, He
Glutamic acid, He 0.15-3.38%
Glutathione, He 115-2,960
Glycine, He 460-11,000
HCN, Pl
Histidine, He 220-5,170
Iron, He 8-467
Isoleucine, He 530-11,400
Kaempferol, Aer
KCL, Pl
Kilocalories, He 260-2,955
Lauric acid, Sd Oil
Leucine, He 880-19,900
Linoleic acid, He 704-18,245

Linoleic acid, Sd 6.8%
Linolenic acid, He 0.32-6.43%
Linolenic acid, Sd 1.7%
Lysine, He 650-13,200
Magnesium, He 670-18,700
Malic acid, Pl 0.5%
Manganese, Pl
Methionine, He 90-2,814
Monogalactosyl-diactyl glycerol, Lf; He
Mucilage, Pl
Myristic acid, He 7-140
Niacin, He 5-79
Norepinephrine, Pl
Oleic acid, He 16-2,160
Oleic acid, Sd 5%
Oleracin-I, Pl
Oleracin-II, Pl
Omega-3's, Pl
Oxalates, Pl
Oxalic acid, Pl 0.17-1.7%
Palmitic acid, He 616-18,966
Palmitoleic acid, He 140-2,940
Pantothenic acid, Pl
Phenylalanine, He 580-11,500
Phorbic acid, Lf
Phosphatidyl choline, Lf
Phosphatidyl glycerol, Lf
Phosphatidyl inositol, Lf
Phosphatidyl serine, Lf
Phosphatidyl ethanolamine, Pl
Phosphorus, He 320-7,740
Phytin-P, Pl
Potassium, He 0.49-8.1%
Proline, He 540-13,200
Protein, He 1.3-26.0%
Quercetin, Lf, St
Resin, Pl 2.4%
Riboflavin, He 1-23
RNA, Seedling
Saponin, Pl
Serine, He 450-8,440
Sinapic acid, Pl
Sodium, He 440-7,400
Stearic acid, Sd 6,438
Stigmasterol, Aer
Sucrose, Pl
Sulfolipids, Pl
Sulfur, Pl
Tannin, Pl
Thiamin, He 1-10
Threonine, He 470-9,400
Tryptophan, He 160-3,400

Tyrosine, He 220-4,400
Valine, He 660-13,200
Vitamin A, Aer
Vitamin B6, Pl
Water, He 91.2-95.0%
Zinc, Sh 3-60

PHARMACOLOGICAL ACTIVITIES AND CLINICAL TRIALS

Aldose reductase inhibition. Hot water extract of dried aerial parts at a concentration of 0.01 mg/ml was inactive. The effect was tested on bovine lens aldase reductase[K11985].

Analgesic activity. Ethanol (95%) extract of fresh leaves, administered intragastric to mice at a dose of 1.0 gm/kg was active vs benzoyl peroxide-induced writhing and inactive vs tail flick response to hot water[T15876].

Antiandrogenic effect. Ethanol (95%) extract of dried seeds, administered subcutaneously to mice at a dose of 50.0 mg/animal was active[T07026].

Antibacterial activity. Acetone extract of dried leaves, undiluted on agar plate was active on *Pseudomonas aeruginosa* and *Salmonella* B, and inactive on *Salmonella newport*, *Escherichia coli*, *Salmonella typhi*, *Sarcina lutea*, *Serratia marcescens*, *Shigella flexneri*, *Staphylococcus albus* and *Staphylococcus aureus*. Ethanol (95%) extract was active on *Escherichia coli*, *Pseudomonas aeruginosa*, *Salmonella typhi*, *Sarcina lutea*, *Serratia marcescens*, *Shigella flexneri*, *Staphylococcus albus* and *Staphylococcus aureus*; and inactive on *Salmonella* B and *Salmonella newport*. Water extract was active on *Escherichia coli*, *Pseudomonas aeruginosa*, *Serratia marcescens* and *Shigella flexneri*; inactive on *Salmonella* B, *Salmonella newport*, *Salmonella typhi*, *Sarcina lutea*, *Staphylococcus albus*, and *Staphylococcus aureus*. Acetone extract of dried stem undiluted on agar plate was active on *Salmonella* B, *Salmonella typhi*, *Serratia marcescens* and *Staphylococcus albus*; inactive on *Escherichia coli*, *Pseudomonas aeruginosa*, *Salmonella newport*, *Sarcina lutea*, *Shigella flexneri*, and *Staphylococcus aureus*.

Ethanol (95%) extract was active on *Escherichia coli*, *Pseudomonas aeruginosa*, *Salmonella* B, *Salmonella typhi*, *Sarcina lutea*, *Serratia marcescens*, *Shigella flexneri*, *Staphylococcus albus*, and *Staphylococcus aureus*; inactive on *Salmonella newport*. Water extract was active on *Escherichia coli*, *Salmonella newport*, *Salmonella typhi*, *Serratia marcescens*, *Shigella flexneri*, and *Staphylococcus aureus*; inactive on *Pseudomonas aeruginosa*, *Salmonella* B, *Sarcina lutea*, and *Staphylococcus albus*[T16262]. Hot water and methanol extracts of the aerial parts at concentrations of 1.2 mg/disc on agar plate were inactive on *Streptococcus mutans* strains MT5091 and OMZ176[T15019]. Hot water extract of entire plant on agar plate was inactive on *Alcaligenes calcoaceticus*, *Escherichia coli*, *Klebsiella pneumonia*, *Proteus vulgaris*, *Pseudomonas aeruginosa*, *Salmonella typhimurium*, *Staphylococcus aureus*, and *Streptococcus faecalis*. MIC > 1600 mcg/ml[T11055].

Anticonvulsant activity. Ethanol (70%) extract of fresh entire plant administered intraperitoneally to mice of both sexes at variable dosage levels was inactive vs metrazole- and strychnine-induced convulsions[T06510].

Antifertility effect. Hot water extract of entire plant administered subcutaneously to female mice was inactive[A03483].

Antifungal activity. Acetone, ether, ethanol (95%), and chloroform extracts of dried aerial parts on agar plate were inactive on *Trichophyton rubrum*[W04249]. Water extract of fresh shoots undiluted on agar plate was equivocal on *Helminthosporium turcicum*[W01223].

Antihyperglycemic activity. Dried entire plant administered intragastric to rabbit at a dose of 2.0 gm/kg was inactive vs alloxan-induced hyperglycemia[M23340].

Antimycobacterial activity. Hot water extract of entire plant on agar plate was inactive on *Mycobacterium smegmatis*[T11055]. Leaf juice on agar plate produced weak activity on *Mycobacterium tuberculosis* MIC <1:40[A03634].

Antinematodal activity. Ethanol (95%) extract of entire plant was active on *Meloidogyne incognita*[A06630].

Antiparasitic activity. Ingestion of either juice or tablets made from pusley has been effective in the treatment of hookworm. In one study of 192 subjects, approximately 80% had negative stool after one month of treatment.

Antispermatogenic effect. Ethanol (95%) extract of dried seeds, administered subcutaneously to mice at a dose of 50.0 mg/animal was active[T07026].

Antitumor activity. Ethanol/chloroform extract of fresh entire plant, administered intraperitoneally to mice at a dose of 360.0 mg/kg was inactive on CA-755 and Leuk-L1210. A dose of 450.0 mg/kg was inactive on Sarcoma 180(ASC)[W01723]. Water extract of dried entire plant, administered intraperitoneally to mice at a dose of 150.0 mg/kg on days five, six, and seven, was active on CA-Ehrlich-ascites, methanol extract produced weak activity[H01040].

Antiulcer activity. Methanol extract of dried aerial parts, administered intragastric to mice at a dose of 2.0 gm/kg was inactive vs stress-induced ulcers (water-immersions)[M16948].

Antiviral activity. Hot water extract of dried aerial parts at a concentration of 0.5 mg/ml in VERO cell cultures was inactive on Herpes Simplex 1 virus, Measles virus, and Polio virus[K16835].

Antiyeast activity. Hot water extract of entire plant on agar plate was inactive on *Candida albicans*[T11055].

Chronotropic effect (negative). Water extract of fresh leaves and stem at a concentration of 0.55 mg/ml was active on rabbit atrium. The effect was not inhibited by atropine. Affected both spontaneously beating and electrically-paced atria. Effect reversed by addition of calcium[T15054].

CNS Depressant activity. Ethanol (defatted with petroleum ether) extract of entire plant, administered intraperitoneally to mice at a dose of 1.0 gm/kg produced weak activity[A02970].

Cytotoxic activity. Methanol extract of dried leaves at a concentration of 100.0 mcg/ml in cell culture was inactive on cells of Chinese hamster V79[K17316].

Hypertensive activity. Water extract of fresh leaves and stem, administered intravenously to rats at a dose of 1.4 mg/kg was active. Effect abolished by phentolamine, reduced by propranolol and unaffected by atropine[T15054].

Hypoglycemic activity. Dried entire plant administered intragastric to rabbits at doses of 0.5 and 1.0 gm/kg produced no effect after four, eight, and 25 hours. At doses of 1.5 and 2.0 gm/kg significant effect was observed after eight and 12 hours[M23340]. Seeds in mixture with seven other plants, administered orally to male rats at a dose of 4.0 gm/animal was active[J07575].

Hypotensive activity. Ethanol (95%) and water extracts of leaves and stem, administered intravenously to dogs at doses of 0.1 ml/kg were active[A03360].

Hypothermic activity. Methanol extract of dried aerial parts, administered intragastric to mice at a dose of 2.0 gm/kg was inactive[M16948].

Inotropic effect (negative). Water extract of fresh leaves and stem at a concentration of 0.55 mg/ml was active on rabbit atrium. Not inhibited by atropine; affected both spontaneously beating and electrically-paced atria. Effect reversed by addition of calcium[T15054].

Molluscicidal activity. Aqueous slurry (homogenate) of fresh fruit, fresh leaves and fresh roots were inactive on *Lymnaea columella* and *Lymnaea cubensis* LD$_{100}$ > 1000 ppm.

Paralyzing activity. Ethanol (95%) extract of frozen leaves at a concentration of 2.0 mg/ml was active on chicken nerve-muscle preparation. Augmentation was followed by blockade. Effect simulated by K[+], which appears to be the active species[K16940].

Plaque formation suppressant. Water and methanol/water (1:1) extracts of dried aerial parts at concentrations of 0.1 mg/ml produced weak activity on *Streptococcus mutans* and the methanol extract was active[T10387].

Platelet activating factor binding inhibition. Methanol extract of dried entire plant at a dose of 400.0 mcg/ml produced weak activity on rabbit platelets[K16653].

Skeletal muscle relaxant activity. Aqueous (dialyzed) fresh leaf and stem at a concentrations of 2.0 and 1.81 mg/ml were active on rat phrenic nerve (diaphragm) vs K[+]- and electrically-induced contractions, respectively. A dose of 30.0 mg/animal administered intravenously to chicks was active vs electrically induced contractions. Ether extract at concentration of 5.0 mg/ml was active vs K[+], caffeine, and electrically induced contractions[T15467]. Water extract at a concentration of 3.0 mg/ml was active on frog sciatic nerve, sartorius muscle, rat rectus abdominus and phrenic nerve (diaphragm)[T14146]. Methanol extract at a dose of 3.0 mg/ml was active on rat phrenic nerve (diaphragm) vs caffeine and electrically induced contractions. IC$_{50}$ 2.16 mg/ml was obtained when tested on phrenic nerve (diaphragm) vs electrically induced contractions[T15467]. Water extract administered intraperitoneally to rat at a dose of 200 mg/kg was active, at 5.0 gm/kg administered orally to rat produced weak activity[T13374]. A dose of 70.0 mg/person used externally on human adults was active vs resting and partially contracted muscles in healthy subjects and maximally contracted muscle in healthy subjects[T15468]. Hot water extract of fresh leaves at a concentration 3.0 mg/ml was active on frog rectus abdominus and rat phrenic nerve (diaphragm). Methanol extract at a concentration of 2.2 mg/ml was active on frog rectus abdominus and rat phrenic nerve (diaphragm)[T14745].

Skeletal muscle stimulant activity. Aqueous (dialyzed) fresh leaf and stem at a concentration of 0.82 mg/ml was active on rat phrenic nerve (diaphragm). A concentration of 1.2 mg/ml was active on rat rectus abdominus. Ether extract at a concentration of 1.66 mg/ml was active on rat phrenic nerve (diaphragm), and a concentration of 8.2 mg/ml was active on rat rectus abdominus. Water extract at a concentration of 2.5 mg/ml and methanol extract at a concentration of 1.03 mg/ml were active on rat phrenic nerve (diaphragm). Methanol extract at a concentration of 5.8 mg/ml was active on rat rectus abdominus. Twitch tension occurred before relaxation in each cases vs electrically induced contractions[T15466].

Smooth muscle relaxant activity. Ethanol (95%) and water extracts of leaves and stem, at concentrations of 0.33 ml/liter were active on rabbit duodenum[A03360]. Water extract of fresh leaves and stem at a concentration of 0.03 mg/ml was active on guinea pig taenia coli, a concentration of 0.05 mg/ml was active of guinea pig fundus (stomach). The activities were reduced by phentolamine, further reduced with the addition of propranolol. A concentration of 0.025 mg/ml was active on rabbit jejunum. The activity was reduced by phentolamine, further reduced with the addition of propranolol and unaffected by guanethidine or tetrodoxin[T15468]. A concentration of 0.02 mg/ml was active on rabbit aorta. Attenuated or inhibited by phentolamine and unaffected by guanethidine or tetrodoxin[T15054]. When applied externally at a dose of 70.0 mg/person the extract was active vs maximally contracted muscle in patients with spasticity[T15468].

Spasmogenic activity. Ethanol (95%) and water extracts of leaves and stem, at a concentration of 33.0 ml/liter, administered intraperitoneally to guinea pigs were active on the ileum[A03360].

Spasmolytic activity. Water extract of fresh leaves and stem at a concentration of 2.0 mg/ml was active on rat diaphragm vs electrically induced contractions[T16898].

Toxic effect (general). Fresh leaves administered orally to cows at a dose of 48.0 gm/kg was inactive[A05311].

Toxicity assessment (quantitative). Water extract of leaves and stem when administered intraperitoneally to mice the minimum toxic dose was 1.0 ml/animal[A03360]. Water extract of fresh leaves and stem, when administered intraperitoneally to mice LD$_{50}$ 1040 mg/kg[T13374].

Treatment of appendicitis. A decoction made of equal parts of pusley and *Taraxaci mongolici cum radice* was used in treating 31 cases of clinically diagnosed appendicitis. Of these, only one needed surgery; all the others recovered uneventfully.

Uterine stimulant effect. Ethanol (95%) and water extracts of leaves and stem at concentrations of 0.33 ml/liter were active on the rat uterus[A03360]. Water extract of leaves was active on the uterus of pregnant and nonpregnant rats and mice[A05606].

Vasoconstrictor activity. Ethanol (95%) extract of leaves and stem at a concentration of 0.33 ml/liter was active on rat hind quarters (isolated)[A03360].

24 | Psidium guajava
L.

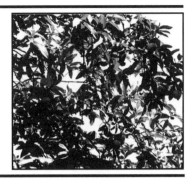

Common Names

Abas	Guam	Guayaba	Paraguay
Amba	Nepal	Guayaba	Puerto Rico
Amrood	India	Guayabe	Guatemala
Amrud	Fiji	Guayabero	Canary Islands
Amrut	Fiji	Guayabo	Canary Islands
Arasa	Paraguay	Guayabo	Mexico
Banjiro	Brazil	Guayabo	Peru
Banziro	Brazil	Guayava	Guatemala
Bilauti	Nepal	Guega	Papua-New Guinea
Borimak	Nicaragua	Gwawa	Papua
Bugoyab	Senegal	Ipera	Rwanda
Djambu bidji	Indonesia	Jaama	India
Djambu klutuk	Indonesia	Jambu biji	Indonesia
Fa-rang	Thailand	Kautonga	Indonesia
Goavy	Madagascar	Kiswahili	Tanzania
Goejaba	Surinam	Krue	Nicaragua
Goiabeira	Brazil	Ku'ava	Nicaragua
Goyav	Haiti	Kuabas	Nicaragua
Guava	Fiji	Kuava	Nicaragua
Guava	Ghana	Kuawa	Nicaragua
Guava	Guam	Kuiaba	Papua-New Guinea
Guava	Guyana	Kuliabas	Malaysia
Guava	Indonesia	Mabera	Tanzania
Guava	Mexico	Maduriam	India
Guava	Nepal	Mansala	India
Guava	Nicaragua	Motiram	India
Guava	Papua-New Guinea	Mpera	Tanzania
Guava	Sierra Leone	Mugwavha	Venda
Guava	Sri Lanka	Ngoaba	Guinea
Guava	Tanzania	Psidiium	Taiwan
Guava	USA	Quwawa	Taiwan
Guyaba	Cuba	Sigra	Nicaragua
Guayaba	Guatemala	Sikra	Nicaragua
Guayaba	Nicaragua	Tuava	Cook Islands

From: Medicinal Plants of the World *By: Ivan A. Ross Humana Press Inc., Totowa, NJ*

Tuava	Easter Island	Xalxocotyl	Mexico
Tuava	Rarotonga	Xalxoctl	Mexico
Wariafa	Nicaragua		

BOTANICAL DESCRIPTION

A spreading tree of the MYRTACEAE family which may grow up to as high as 15 meters, with bark peeling in large thin flakes. Leaves are simple, opposite, oblong, elliptic or ovate, in pairs on four-angled twigs, elliptical or oblong, 7–14 cm long, and 4–6 cm wide; consisting of obtuse or micronulate apex; margin entire or slightly curved; with broadly cuneate or obtuse base. blade with more or less hairy beneath; the veins parallel and conspicuously raised below; petiole 5–10 mm long. Flowers are white, axillary, solitary or two to three together on slender peduncles, about three cm in diameter; consisting of calyx-tube campanulate, deeply divided into 4–5 lobes above the ovary; petals are large and broad, spreading; stamens are numerous, about length of petals, free, inserted on disk. Fruit globose or pear-shaped, tipped with remnants of the calyx lobes, the pulp is white or pink, juicy, containing many small, hard, seeds. It is propagated either by seeds, grafting or cutting.

ORIGIN AND DISTRIBUTION

A native of Central America, sometimes cultivated but also very common as an adventive in pastures and wayside thickets throughout the tropics and subtropics.

TRADITIONAL MEDICINAL USES

Andaman Islands. Ripe fruit is eaten as a food[K23301].

Bolivia. A few drops of liquid from boiled leaves of *Psidium guajava* is mixed with a tablespoon of *Orbignya martiana* fruit oil and taken orally four times a day for coughs[T08478].

Brazil. Dried fruit is taken orally to treat diarrhea, stomachache, and diabetes[H11158].

Canary Islands. Hot water extract of dried fruit is used as an antihemorrhoidal[T15880].

China. Extract of roots is taken orally by monks in south China to suppress libido[W01996].

Cook Islands. Dried leaves of *Psidium guajava* and *Citrus aurantium* are crushed together and taken orally for pain around the navel. Infusion of dried leaves is taken orally to relieve postpartum pain and rid the body of residual stale blood. For sores, dried leaves are chewed with or without coconut oil and then applied to the sores[T09553].

Fiji. Dried fruit is taken orally for constipation. Infusion of dried leaves and root is taken orally for diarrhea and indigestion. Fresh leaf juice is taken orally for dysentery and upset stomach[T10632].

Ghana. Peeled twig is used as a chewing stick[T03316].

Guam. Hot water extract of leaves is administered intravaginal to treat vaginitis and to promote conception[A01962].

Guatemala. Decoction of dried bark and leaves is taken orally to treat fevers, respiratory ailments and skin infections[K19264]. Dried fruit is powdered and eaten for stomach cramps[W01280]. Infusion of dried leaves is taken orally to treat infections[K16364]. The hot water extract is applied externally for dermatomucosal lesions and ringworm[M27151].

Haiti. Decoction of dried leaves is taken orally for diarrhea. Fresh fruit juice is taken orally for diarrhea[T13846].

India. Crushed fresh flowers together with the juice from buds, squeezed through muslin cloth, is taken orally as an anthelmintic. Decoction of dried leaves is taken orally for diarrhea and as an antiemetic[M23219]. Hot water extract of dried leaves is used in bath for high fever and headache[T07374]. Dried fruit is used for jaundice. One dose consists of the juice of one fruit of *Psidium guajava*, 0.25 liter goat's milk and a 1 to 1/2 inch root of an unidentified herb, possibly Sida. One dose is taken on alternate days. Three doses give significant relief[T10321]. Hot water extract of dried bark is taken orally as a remedy for stomachache[T07374].

Indonesia. Hot water extract of leaves is taken orally as an emmenagogue[A04162].

Ivory Coast. Dried stem is used as a chewing stick[M21947].

Japan. Extract of roots is taken orally by Japanese Monks as a suppressant of libido[W01996].

Madagascar. Hot water extract of young leaves is taken orally for diarrhea[M22964].

Malaysia. Hot water extract of bark is taken orally to expel the placenta and as an emmenagogue. Hot water extract of leaves is taken orally to expel the placenta and as an emmenagogue[A06590]. Water extract of dried bark and leaves is taken orally for after-birth disorders[T08817].

Mexico. Hot water extract of bark is taken orally for dysentery. Hot water extract of fruit is taken orally as a digestive. Hot water extract of leaves is used externally as a treatment for mange[J01414]; the extract is taken orally for diarrhea[K16948]. Infusion of dried leaves is taken orally for diarrhea[K19396].

Nigeria. Water extract of dried root is taken orally for diarrhea[K12864].

Panama. Hot water extract of flowers and fruits is taken orally as an emmenagogue. Hot water extract of fresh bark is taken orally for diarrhea. The decoction is taken as one dose. Hot water extract of fruit is taken orally for diarrhea. For this purpose, decoction of fruits is taken in water as one dose[T01287].

Papua-New Guinea. Fresh leaf juice is taken orally for diarrhea. Young top leaves are squeezed and the juice drunk with water[T09033].

Peru. Hot water extract of dried bark is taken orally as an astringent, antihemorrhagic, antidiarrheal and for stomach pain. Hot water extract of dried leaves is taken orally for stomach pain, as an astringent, antihemorrhagic and antidiarrheal.

Hot water extract of dried roots is taken orally as an astringent, antihemorrhagic, antidiarrheal and for stomach pain[T15323].

Philippines. Hot water extract of dried bark is used in steam baths postpartum. *Psidium guajava*, *Commiphora myrrha* and incense are added to the bath[T10116].

Rarotonga. Fresh leaf juice is taken orally for dysentery[K08575].

Rwanda. Hot water extract of dried leaves is taken orally for dysentery[T15786].

Senegal. Dried stem is used to brush teeth. Hot water extract of dried leaves is taken orally for diarrhea. Hot water extract of green fruit is taken orally for dysentery. Hot water extract of young shoots is taken orally for diarrhea[M21947].

Sierra Leone. Decoction of dried leaves is taken orally for diarrhea during pregnancy[T08806].

Taiwan.. Fresh fruit juice is taken orally to treat diabetes mellitus[K07622]. Hot water extract of dried branches is taken orally for liver diseases[T14999].

Tanzania. Decoction of dried leaves is taken orally to treat malaria[K15971]. Hot water extract of fresh leaves is taken orally for skin diseases[T10354].

Thailand. Hot water extract of dried leaves is taken orally for diabetes[W01792].

Venda. Decoction of dried roots is taken orally for venereal diseases. Decoction of *Opuntia vulgaris* and *Psidium guajava* is drunk twice a day[T08732].

CHEMICAL CONSTITUENTS
(ppm unless otherwise indicated)

1-8-Cineol, Lf EO; Fr; EO
2-3-4-6-Tetra-0-galloyl glucose, Rt
2-Alpha-hydroxy ursolic acid, Lf; Fr
2-Ethyl thiophene, Fr
2-Methyl propan-2-Ol, Fr1.0%
2-Methyl propane-1-thiol, Fr
2-Methyl propyl acetate, Fr 0.5%
2-Methyl thiophene, Fr
2-Phenethyl acetate, Fr 0.2%
2 Furfural, Fr
2 Methyl furfural, Fr

2Alpha hydroxyursolic acid beta-ionone, Fr
3-0-Methyl ellagic acid, Bk
3-3-Di-O-methyl ellagic acid, Bk
3-Methyl butan-1-ol, Fr 0.3%
3-Methyl thiophene, Fr
5-Ethoxy thiazole, Fr
6 Mercapto hexan-1-ol, Fr
Acetaldehyde, Fr 0.2%
Acetone, Fr 0.8%
Acetyl furan, Fr
Acutissimin A, Bk 0.086%
Acutissimin B, Bk 3.7
Alanine, Fr 410-2,952
Alpha amyrin, Fr
Alpha copaene, Fr 0.1%
Alpha humulene, Fr 0.6%
Alpha pinene, Fr; Lf EO
Alpha terpineol, Fr
Alpha linolenic acid, Fr 0.0 71-0.511%
Alpha selinene, Fr
Amritoside, St Bk 40; Lf 850; Wd
Araban, Fr
Arabinose, Fr (unripe)
Arabinose hexahydroxydiphenyl acid ester,
    Fr 0.1%
Arginine, Fr 210-1,512
Arjunolic acid, Rt 0.01%; Fr
Aromadendrene, Fr Pe EO
Ascorbic acid, Fr 200-14,300
Ascorbigen, Fr 253-2,145
Ash, Sd 30,000; Fr 6,000-43,200
Asiatic acid, Fr
Aspartic acid, Fr 520-3,744
Aviculatin, Lf
Benzaldehyde, Fr 0.1%
Benzene, Fr
Benzothiazole, Fr
Beta amyrin, Fr
Beta bisabolene, Fr 0.2%
Beta carotene, Fr 3-46
Beta caryophyllene, Fr 0.45%
Beta copaene, Fr
Beta farnesene, Fr
Beta humulene, Fr
Beta pinene, Fr; Lf EO
Beta silinene, Fr
Beta sitosterol, Lf
Brahmic acid, Fr
Butanal, Fr
Butanedione, Fr 2.0%
Butanoic acid ethyl ester, Fr 8.7%
Butanone, Fr 2.2%

Butyl acetate, 3-methyl, Fr 0.1%
Butyl acetate, Fr 0.1%
Butyraldehyde, Fr
Calamenene, Fr
Calcium, Fr 180-1,582
Calcium oxalate, Lf, Fr
Camphene, Fr
Carbohydrates, Fr 11.88-85.54%
Carophyllene oxide, EO; Fr
Caryophyllene, EO; Fr
Castalagin, Bk 0.17%
Casuarinin, Lf 0.021%; Bk 0.004%
Catechin (+), Bk 0.029%
Catechol-tannins, Lf 4.0-7.5%
Chlorine, Fr 40
Cineol, EO
Cinnamyl acetate, Fr
Cis-beta ocimene, Fr
Citral, Fr
Citric acid, Fr
Copper, Fr 1-9
Crataegolic acid, Lf
Curcumene, Fr
D-Galactose, Fr
D-Galacturonic acid, Fr
Daucosterol, Fr
Decanoic acid ethyl ester, Fr 0.1%
Delta elemene, EO
Delta cadinene, Fr
Diisopropyl disulfide, Fr
Dimethyl disulfide, Fr
Dimethyl sulfone, Fr
Dimethyl trisulfide, Fr
Dodecanoic acid ethyl ester, Fr
Ellagic acid, Bk 0.8%; Fr
Ellagic acid, Fr (unripe); Fl; St Bk 40; Lf 150
Essential oils, Lf 0.26-0.36%
Ethanol, Fr 25.8%
Ethyl acetate, Fr 26.2%
Ethyl butyrate, Fr
Eugenigrandin A, Bk 0.08%
Eugenol, EO
Farnesene, Fr
Fat, Fr 0.6-4.32%; Lf 6%; Sd 10-14.3%
Fiber, Fr 5.6-40.3; Sd 42.4%
Foeniculin, Lf
Fructose, Fr
Gallic acid ethyl ester, Rt
Gallic acid, Fr(unripe); Rt
Gallocatechin (+), Lf; Bk 0.057%
Galloyl-tannin, Rt
Gamma muurolene, Fr

Gentisic acid, Lf
Glucose, Sd 0.1%; Fr
Glucuronic acid, Fr
Glutamic acid, Fr 0.107-0.770%
Glycine, Fr 0.041-0.295
Grandinin, Bk 0.037%
Guafine, Bk 2%
Guaijavarin, Lf
Guaijaverin, Lf 0.035%; Fl; Fr
Guajavin B, Bk 211
Guajavin, Bk 24.5
Guajiverine, Lf
Guajivolic acid, Lf
Guavin A, Lf
Guavin B, Lf
Guavin C, Lf
Guavin D, Lf
Heptan-1-al, Fr
Hex-3-En-1-ol acetate, Fr
Hex-cis-3-en-1-ol acetate, Fr 0.5%
Hex-cis-3-en-1-ol, Fr1.0%
Hex-cis-3-enoic acid, Fr Pu 0.2
Hexadecanoic acid ethyl ester, Fr
Hexagalloyl glucose, Rt
Hexan-1-al, Fr 3.2%
Hexan-1-ol acetate, Fr
Hexanoic acid ethyl ester, Fr 15.5%
Hexanoic acid methyl ester, Fr 0.3%
Hexyl acetate, Fr 0.3%
Histidine, Fr 70-504
Hyperoside, Lf
Iron, Fr 3-24
Iso-quercetin, Lf
Iso-strictinin, Lf 30
Isoleucine, Fr 0.03-0.216
Kilocalories, Fr 0.051-0.367%
L-Malic acid, Fr
Lactic acid, Fr
Leucine, Fr 0.055-0.396%
Leucoanthocyanin, Bk
Leucocyanidins, Fr 0.1%
Leucocyanidins, Lf 0.4%
Limonene, Fr
Linalool, EO
Linoleic acid, Fr 0.182-1.31%
Linoleic acid, Sd 1.39%
Linolenic acid, Sd 200
Lupeol, Fr
Luteic acid, Bk
Lysine, Fr 230-1,656
Magnesium, Fr 98-735
Manganese, Fr 1-12

Maslinic acid, Lf
Mecocyanin, Fr
Menthol, Lf EO
Methanol, Fr
Methionine, Fr 50-360
Methyl ethyl ketone, Fr
Methylcinnamate, Fr
Methylisopropylketone, Fr
Mongolicain A, Bk
Myicetin, Bk
Myrcene, EO; Fr
Myristic acid, Fr 120-864
N-Octane, Fr
Nerolidiol, Lf
Niacin, Fr 12-86
Nonan-1-al, Fr
Octan-1-al, Fr
Octan-1-ol, Fr
Octanoic acid ethyl ester, Fr
Octyl acetate, Fr
Oleanolic acid, Lf; Fl; Wd
Oleic acid, Fr 520-3,744
Oleic acid, Sd 2.79%
Oxalic acid, Fr 140
Palmitic acid, Fr 0.144-1.037%
Palmitoleic acid, Fr 30-216
Pantothenic acid, Fr 2-11
Para cymene, Fr
Para-methyl styrene, Fr0.3%
Pectin, Fr 0.3-1.6%
Pedunculagin, Lf 0.06%; Bk 27
Pendunculagin, Lf
Pentane-2-thiol, Fr
Phenylalanine, Fr 20-144
Phosphorus, Fr 235-1,905
Phytin phosphorus, Fr 127-1,029
Potassium, Fr 0.2672-2.1658%
Procyanidin B-1, Lf; Bk 4.5
Procyanidin B-2, Lf
Procyanidin B-3, Lf
Prodelphinidin B-1, Bk
Proline, Fr 250-1,800
Protein, Fr 0.82-5.9%
Protein, Sd 15.2%
Psidinin A, Bk 0.016%
Psidinin B, Bk 24.5
Psidinin C, Bk 23.4
Psidiolic acid, Lf
Psiguavin, Bk 38.2
Pyrogallol tannins, Bk 13.5%
Pyrogallol tannins, Lf 4.0-7.8%
Quercetin, Lf

Quercetin-3-0-gentiobioside, Lf
Rhamnose, Fr
Riboflavin, Fr 1-4
Sel-11-en-4 alpha-ol, Lf
Serine, Fr 240-1,728
Sesquiguavene, Pl
Sodium, Fr 26-246
Stachyurin, Lf 15
Starch, Sd 13.2%
Stearic acid, Fr 160-1,152
Strictinin, Lf 62.5
Sucrose, Fr
Sugar, Lf
Sulfur, Fr 140
Tannin, Bk 11-30%
Tannin, Lf 9.0-10.0%
Tannin, Rt
Tannin, Sd 1.4%
Tellimagrandin 1, Lf 237.5
Tetradecanoic acid ethyl ester, Fr 0.2%
Thiamin, Fr 1-4
Threonine, Fr 310-2,232
Toluene, Fr0.2%
Trans-cinnamic acid, Fr Pu 0.4
Tryptophan, Fr 70-504
Tyrosine, Fr 100-720
Ursolic acid, Lf
Valeraldehyde, Fr
Valine, Fr 280-2,016
Valolaginic acid, Bk 114
Vescalagin carboxylic acid, Bk 20.5
Vitamin B6, Fr 1-10
Water, Fr 85.4-86.8%
Water, Sd 10.3%
Wax, Lf
Xanthophyll, Lf
Xylose, Fr
Zeatin nucleotide, Fr
Zeatin riboside, Fr
Zeatin, Fr
Zinc, Fr 2-20

PHARMACOLOGICAL ACTIVITIES AND CLINICAL TRIALS

ACh release inhibition. Methanol extract of dried leaves at a concentration of 800.0 mcg/ml was active on guinea pigs' ileum[M20821].

Analgesic activity. Dried fruits administered intraperitoneally to male rats at a dose of 50.0 mg/kg was active vs acetic acid-induced writhing[K20607]. Ethanol/water (1:1) extract of the aerial parts, administered intraperitoneally to mice at a dose of 0.094 mg/kg was inactive vs tail pressure method[W00374].

Anti-HCG activity. Ethanol (60%) extract of roots, administered subcutaneously to immature female rats was active[A04353].

Anti-PMS activity. Ethanol (60%) extract of roots, administered subcutaneously to immature female rats was active[A04353].

Antibacterial activity. Acetone extract of dried bark and leaves, at a concentration of 50.0 mg/disc was active on *Staphylococcus aureus*; produced weak activity on *Streptococcus pneumonia*. The extract was active on *Streptococcus pyogenes* MIC 10.0 mg/disc. Hexane extract at a concentration of 50.0 mg/disc, on agar plate produced weak activity on *Staphylococcus aureus*, *Streptococcus pneumonia*, and *Streptococcus pyogenes*. Methanol extract at a concentration of 50.0 mg/disc, on agar plate was active on *Streptococcus pneumonia* and *Streptococcus pyogenesi*; active on *Staphylococcus aureus* MIC 5.0 mg/disc[K19264]. Acetone extract of dried leaves, undiluted on agar plate was active on *Escherichia coli, Pseudomonas aeruginosa, Salmonella B, Salmonella newport, Salmonella typhi, Sarcina lutea, Serratia marcescens, Shigella flexneri, Staphylococcus albus*, and *Staphylococcus aureus*. Ethanol (95%) extract was active on *E. coli, P. aeruginosa, S. B, S. newport, S. typhi, S. flexneri*, and *S. albus*, and inactive on *S. lutea, Serratia marcescens*, and *S. aureus*. Water extract was active on *P. aeruginosa, S. lutea, S. marcescens, S. flexneri, S. albus*, and *S. aureus*, and inactive on *Salmonella B, S. newport*, and *S. typhi*[T16330]. Acetone extract of dried stem, undiluted on agar plate was inactive on *Escherichia coli, Pseudomonas aeruginosa, Salmonella B, Salmonella newport, Salmonella typhi, Sarcina lutea, Serratia marcescens, Shigella flexneri, Staphylococcus albus*, and *Staphylococcus aureus*. The ethanol (95%) extract was active on *E. coli, P. aeruginosa, S. newport, S. typhi, Sarcina lutea, Serratia marcescens, Shigella flexneri,* and *S. albus* and inactive on *Salmonella* B and *S. aureus*. The water extract was active on *Escherichia coli*, *P. aeruginosa*, *S. marcescens*, *S. flexneri*, *S. albus*, and *S. aureus*, and inactive on *Salmonella* B, *S. newport*, *S. typhi*, and *Sarcina lutea*[T16330]. Ethanol (95%) extract of dried bark, at a concentration of 5.0 mg/ml on agar plate was active on *Staphylococcus aureus* and *Bacillus subtilis*;and inactive on *Escherichia coli* and *Pseudomonas aeruginosa*. From extract of 10 ml/gm plant material, 0.1 ml of extract was placed in the well on the plate[T14756]. Ethanol (95%) extract of dried leaves, at a concentration of 1000 mcg/ml on agar plate was active on *Salmonella* D, *Shigella dysenteriae* 1, *Shigella flexneri* 2A, and *Shigella flexneri* 4A. The extract was inactive on *Salmonella* B, *Salmonella typhi* Type 2, *Shigella boydii*, *Shigella boydii* 5, *Shigella dysenteriae* 2, *Shigella flexneri* 3A, and *Shigella sonnei*[T15786]. Ethanol/water (1:1) extract of the aerial parts, at a concentration of >25.0 mcg/ml on agar plate was inactive on *Bacillus subtilis*, *Escherichia coli*, *Salmonella typhosa*, *Staphylococcus aureus*, and *Agrobacterium tumefaciens*[W00374]. Hot water extract of dried leaves undiluted, on agar plate was active on *Staphylococcus aureus* and *Sarcina lutea*[W01818]. Saline extract of leaves, at a concentration of 1–40 on agar plate was active on *Staphylococcus aureus* and inactive on *Escherichia coli*[W01047]. Tannin fraction of dried leaves at a concentration of 100.0 mcg/ml on agar plate was active on *Escherichia piracoli*; 110 mcg/ml active on *Escherichia coli*; 60.0 mcg/ml active on *Citrobacter diversus*; 85.0 mcg/ml active on *Klebsiella pneumonia* and *Shigella flexneri*; 95.0 mcg/ml active on *Salmonella enteritidis* and *Staphylococcus aureus*[K21572]. Water extract of fresh leaves, at a concentration of 1.0% on agar plate was active on *Neisseria gonorrhea*[T10354].

Anticholinergic activity. Water extract of dried fruits was active on rats' ileum vs ACh-induced contractions[P00142].

Anticonvulsant activity. Ethanol/water (1:1) extract of aerial parts, administered to mice at a dose of 0.094 mg/kg was inactive vs electroshock-induced convulsions[W00374].

Antidiarrheal activity. Decoction of dried leaves, administered to rats by gastric intubation at a dose of 10.0 ml/kg was active vs microlax-induced diarrhea[K11287]. Ethanol (95%) extract of dried leaves, administered by gastric intubation to mice at a dose of 750.0 mg/kg produced weak activity. 0.5 ml per 20 kg of castor oil was given to induce diarrhea[T15786].

Antiedema activity. Dried fruits administered intraperitoneally to male rats at a dose of 100.0 mg/kg was active vs acetic acid-induced peritoneal proteinexudation[K20607].

Antifungal activity. Acetone, Ethanol (95%), and water extracts of dried stem, at a concentration of 50% on agar plate was inactive on *Neurospora crassa*. Acetone, water and ethanol (95%) extracts of dried leaves, at a concentration of 50% on agar plate were inactive on *Neurospora crassa*,[T08589]. Hot water extract of dried leaves at a concentration of 1.0 ml in broth culture was active on *Epidermophyton floccosum*, and inactive on *Microsporum canis*, *Microsporum gypseum*, *Trichophyton mentagrophytes* var. algodonosa, and *Trichophyton rubrum*. Ethanol (95%) extract of dried bark, at a concentration of 50.0 mg/ml on agar plate was inactive on *Aspergillus niger*. From extract of 10 ml/g plant material, 0.1 ml was placed in the well of the plate[T14756]. Ethanol/water (1:1) extract of the aerial parts, at a concentration of >25.0 mcg/ml on agar plate was inactive on *Microsporum canis*, *Trichophyton mentagrophytes*, and *Aspergillus niger*[W00374]. Hot water extract of dried leaves undiluted, on agar plate was inactive on *Aspergillus niger*[W01818]. Water extract of fresh leaves, at a concentration of 1:1 on agar plate was active on *Fusarium oxysporum* F. sp. Lentis. The extract represented 1 gm dried leaves in 1.0 ml of water[K18143].

Antigonadotrophin effect. Ethanol/water (1:1) extract of roots, at a dose of 600.0 mg/animal in the ration of male rats was inactive; at a dose of 15.0 mg/animal administered subcutaneously to male rats, both water and ethanol/water (1:1) extracts induced sex organ atrophy[W01996].

Antihyperglycemic activity. Ethanol/water (50%) extract dried leaves, administered to rats by gastric intubation at a dose of 200.0 mg/kg was active vs alloxan-induced hyperglycemia[T10776]. Water extract of fresh fruits, administered by gastric intubation to rats at a doses of 5.0 and 8.0 gm/kg were active vs streptozotocin-induced hyperglycemia[K07622]. Fresh fruit juice administered intraperitoneally to mice at a dose of 1.0 gm/kg was active vs alloxan-induced hyperglycemia; the juice taken orally by human adults at a dose of 1.0 gm/kg was active. Results significant at $P < 0.05$ level[T07304].

Anti-inflammatory activity. Dried fruits, administered intraperitoneally to male rats at a dose of 100.0 mg/kg was active vs formaldehyde-induced arthritis and at a dose of 25.0 mg/kg vs carrageenin-induced pedal edema[K20607]. Ethanol/water (1:1) extract of the aerial parts, administered to rats at a dose of 0.094 mg/kg was inactive, vs carrageenin-induced pedal edema. Animals were dosed one hour before carrageenin injections[W00374].

Antilipolytic activity. Ethanol/water (50%) extract of dried leaves at a concentration of 100.0 mcg/ml was active on the adipocytes-epidermal fat pad of rats. The N-butanol soluble portion of 50% ethanol extract was used, vs epinephrine-induced lipolysis. At a concentration of 200.0 mcg/ml, the aqueous soluble portion of ethanol extract was active vs epinephrine-induced lipolysis. Results significant at $P < 0.01$ level. At a concentration of 500.0 mcg/ml the extract was active on the adipocytes-epididimal fat pad of rats vs epinephrine-induced lipolysis. Results significant at $P < 0.01$ level[T10776].

Antimalarial activity. Acetic acid, ethanol (95%), and water extracts of dried leaves were active on *Plasmodium falciparum*, with ED_{50} 10.0 mcg/ml, 36.0 mcg/ml, and 80.0 mcg/ml respectively[K15971]. Chloroform extract of dried leaves was inactive on *Plasmodium falciparum* vs hypoxanthine uptake by Plasmodia. IC_{50} 499.0 mcg/ml. Petroleum ether extract of dried leaves was weakly active on *Plasmodium falciparum* vs hypoxanthine uptake by Plasmodia. IC_{50} 49.0 mcg/ml[M25016].

Antimutagenic activity. Chloroform extract of fresh fruit, at a concentration of 100.0% on agar plate was active on *Salmonella typhimurium* TA97 vs 2-aminofluorene-induced mutagenesis and 4-nitro-o-phenylenediamine-induced mutagenesis. The extract was inactive on *Salmonella typhimurium* TA100 and TA1535 vs sodium azide-induced mutagenesis; *Salmonella typhimurium* TA98 vs 2-aminofluorene-induced mutagenesis and 4-nitro-o-phenylenediamine-induced mutagenesis. The water extract at a concentration of 100.0% on agar plate was active on *Salmonella typhimurium* TA100 vs 2-aminofluorene-induced mutagenesis and sodium azide-induced mutagenesis and *Salmonella typhimurium* TA97 and TA98 vs 2-amino-fluorene- and 4-nitro-o-phenylene-diamine-induced mutagenesis[K11473]. Chromatographic fraction of fresh leaves, at a concentration of 1.0 mg/plate on agar plate was active on *Escherichia coli* vs UV-induced mutation[K17280]. Methanol extract of dried fruits at a concentration of 50.0 microliters/disc on agar plate was inactive on *Bacillus subtilis* NIG-1125 HIS MET and *Escherichia coli* B/R-WP2-TRP. Methanol extract of dried leaves, at a concentration of 50.0 microliters/disc on agar plate was inactive on *Bacillus subtilis* NIG-1125 HIS MET and produced weak activity on *Escherichia coli* B/R-WP2-TRP[T08867]. Methanol extract of freeze-dried leaves, at a concentration of 5.0 mg/plate on agar plate was active on *Escherichia coli* WP-2 vs MNNG-induced mutation and UV-induced mutagenicity[M18291].

Antimycobacterial activity. Hot water extract of dried leaves undiluted, on agar plate was active on *Mycobacterium phlei*[W01818].

Antipyretic activity. Dried fruits, administered intraperitoneally to male rats at a dose of 50.0 mg/kg was active vs yeast-induced pyrexia[K20607].

Antispasmodic activity. Ethanol/water (1:1) extract of the aerial parts was inactive on guinea pig ileum vs ACh- and histamine-induced spasms[W00374]. Water extract of dried fruits was active on rat ileum vs ACh-induced contractions[P00142].

Antiviral activity. Ethanol/water (1:1) extract of the aerial parts, at a concentration of 50.0 mcg/ml in cell culture was inactive on Vaccinia virus[W00374].

Antiyeast activity. Ethanol (60%) extract of dried leaves on agar plate was active on *Candida albicans*[M31296]. Ethanol (95%) extract of dried bark, at a concentration of 50.0 mg/ml was inactive on *Candida albicans*. From the extract of 10 ml/g plant material, 0.1 ml was placed in the well of the plate[T14756]. Ethanol/water (1:1) extract of the aerial parts, at a concentration of 25.0 mg/ml was inactive on *Candida albicans* and *Cryptococcus neoformans*[W00374]. Hot water extract of dried leaves undiluted, on agar plate was inactive on *Saccharomyces cerevisiae*[W01818].

Carcinogenic activity. Water extract of unripe fruits, administered subcutaneously to female mice at a dose of 35.0 gm/animal weekly for 77 weeks was inactive. 0/15 rats developed tumors. When administered to male rats 2/15 developed tumors[M01250].

Cytotoxic activity. Chloroform extract of dried leaves in cell culture was active on CA-9KB, ED_{50} 7.9 mcg/ml. The Ethanol (95%) extract, was active on LEUK-P388, ED_{50} 7.6 mcg/ml, and inactive on CA-9KB-V1 (vinblastine resistant). ED_{50} >20.0 mcg/ml[K11652].

Diuretic activity. Ethanol/water (1:1) extract of the aerial parts, administered intraperitoneally to rats at a dose of 0.047 mg/kg was inactive vs saline-loaded animals. Urine was collected for four hours post-drug administration[W00374].

Estrous cycle disruption effect. Ethanol (95%) and hot water extracts of roots, administered subcutaneously to rats at a dose of 20.0 mg/animal, and ethanol/water (1:1) extract administered orally at a dose of 300.0 mg/animal daily were active[W01996].

Gastric emptying time increase. Water and methanol extracts of dried roots, administered intraperitoneally to rats at a dose of 250.0 mg/kg were active[K12864].

Glutamate-pyruvate-transaminase inhibition. Ethanol/water (1:1) extract of dried branches, at a concentration of 1.0 mg/ml in cell culture was active on rat liver cells vs CCl_4-induced hepatotoxicity and PGE-1-induced pedal edema[T14999].

Granuloma formation inhibition. Dried fruits, administered intraperitoneally to male rats at a dose of 25.0 mg/kg was active vs cotton pellet granuloma[K20607].

Hyperglycemic activity. Hot water extract of dried leaves, administered orally to mice at a dose of 5.0 gm/kg was active. A 16% rise in blood sugar was observed[W01792].

Hypoglycemic activity. Ethanol/water (1:1) extract of dried leaves, administered orally to mice and rabbits at a doses of 5.0 gm/kg were inactive[W01792]. Ethanol/water (1:1) extract of the aerial parts, administered orally to rats at a dose of 250 mg/kg was inactive. Less than 30% drop in blood sugar level was observed[W00374].

Hypothermic activity. Ethanol/water (1:1) extract of the aerial parts, administered intraperitoneally to mice at a dose of 0.094 mg/kg was inactive[W00374].

Insulin biosynthesis stimulation. Ethanol/water (50%) extract of dried leaves, administered to rats by gastric intubation at a dose of 200.0 mg/kg was inactive vs alloxan-induced hyperglycemia[T10776].

Intestinal motility inhibition. Water extract of dried roots, administered intraperitoneally to rats at a dose of 250.0 mg/kg was active[K12864].

Locomotor activity decrease. Decoction of dried leaves, administered by gastric intubation to rats at a dose of 10.0 ml/kg was active[K11287].

Molluscicidal activity. Aqueous slurry (homogenate) of fresh entire plant (fruits, roots and leaves) was inactive on *Lymnaea columella* and *Lymnaea cubensis*. LD_{100} >1M ppm[T04621]. Water extract of oven dried leaves was active on *Biomphalaria pfeifferi*[T14178]. Water saturated with fresh leaf essential oil, at a concentration of 1–10 was inactive on *Biomphalaria glabrata*[T07475].

Plant germination inhibition. Water extract of dried bark, at a concentration of 500.0 gm/liter produced weak activity on *Cuscuta reflexa* seeds after six days of exposure to the extract. Water extract of dried leaves, at a concentration of 500.0 gm/liter produced weak activity on *Cuscuta reflexa* seeds after six days of exposure to the extract. Water extract of dried stem at a concentration of 500.0 gm/liter was active on *Cuscuta reflexa* seeds after six days of exposure to the extract[M31053].

Plant growth inhibition. Water extract of dried leaves, at a concentration of 500.0 gm/liter produced weak activity. *Cuscuta reflexa* seedling length, weight and dry weight were measured after six days of exposure to the extract. Water extract of dried bark, at a concentration of 500.0 gm/liter produced weak activity on *Cuscuta reflexa* seedling length, weight and dry weight measured after six days of exposure to the extract. Water extract of dried stem at a concentration of 500.0 gm/liter was active on *Cuscuta reflexa* seedling length, weight and dry weight after six days of exposure to the extract[M31053].

Semen coagulation. Ethanol/water (1:1) extract of the aerial parts, at a concentration of 2.0% was inactive on rats' semen[W00374].

Smooth muscle relaxant activity. Methanol extract of dried leaves at variable concentration was active on guinea pigs' ileum[M20821]. Water extract of dried fruits was active on rat ileum[P00142].

Spasmogenic activity. Water extract of dried leaves, administered by gastric intubation to rats at a concentration of 20.0 ml/kg was active on the small intestine. Extract of paste made from fresh leaves was used[K11287].

Spasmolytic activity. Butanol extract of dried leaves at a concentration of 0.2 mg/ml was active on guinea pig ileum. There was 100.0% reduction in contraction vs ACh-induced contractions and 95.72% reduction in contraction vs KCl-induced contractions. The isopentyl alcohol extract at a concentration of 0.2 mg/ml was active on guinea pig ileum. There was a 83.60% reduction in contraction in contraction vs ACh-induced contractions and 77.80% reduction in contraction vs KCl-induced contractions. Butanol extract of dried stem bark at a concentration of 0.2 mg/ml was active on guinea pig ileum. 82.50% reduction in contraction was seen vs ACh-induced contractions and 52.70% reduction in contraction vs KCl-induced contractions. The isopentyl alcohol extract produced a 48.10% reduction in contraction on guinea pig ileum vs KCl-induced contractions and 67.40% reduction in contraction on pigeon ileum vs ACh-induced contractions[M27323]. Hexane extract of dried leaves at a concentration of 0.5 mg/ml, methanol and water extracts at concentrations of 1.0 mg/ml were active on guinea pig ileum, vs electrically-induced contractions[M26503].

Spermicidal effect. Ethanol/water (1:1) extract of the aerial parts was inactive in rats[W00374].

Spontaneous activity reduction. Methanol extract of dried leaves, administered by gastric intubation to mice at a dose of 3.3 mg/kg was active; when administered intraperitoneally to mice the ED_{90} was 4.1 mg/kg[M19413].

Toxicity assessment (quantitative). Ethanol/water (1:1) extract of the aerial parts, administered to intraperitoneally to mice produced a LD_{50} of 0.188 gm/kg[W00374].

Xanthine oxidase inhibition. Ethanol (70%) extract of dried leaves was active. IC_{50} 16.0 mcg/ml[M19490].

25 | Punica granatum

L.

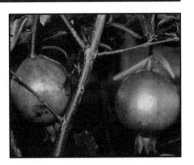

Common Names

Anar	Fiji	Pomegranate	Guyana
Anar	Fiji	Pomegranate	India
Anar	Nepal	Pomegranate	Madeira
Dadima	India	Pomegranate	Mexico
Darim	India	Pomegranate	Nepal
Darim	Nepal	Pomegranate	USA
Darinko bokra	Nepal	Pomegranate	West Indies
Delum	Japan	Posnar	India
Delun	Sri Lanka	Qsur roman	Morocco
Granada	Cuba	Qsur romman	Morocco
Granada	Guatemala	Ranato	Italy
Granada	Peru	Roma	Madeira
Granado	Canary Islands	Roman	Egypt
Granado	Mexico	Roman	Ethiopa
Granatum	India	Romeira	Madeira
Grenade	Rodrigues Islands	Romman	Jordan
Grenadier	Tunisia	Romman	Tunisia
Grenadillo	Belize	Romman amruj	Morocco
Gul armini	Pakistan	Ruman	Oman
Mathalanarakom	India	Seog-ryu	Oman
Melograno	Italy	Sham-al-rumman	Arabic countries
Mkoma manga	East Africa	Shih liu pi	China
Nar	Turkey	Shiliupi	China
Pomegranate	Turkey	Thab thim	Thailand
Pomegranate	Egypt	Thapthim	Thailand
Pomegranate	England	Zakuro	Thailand
Pomegranate	Greece		

BOTANICAL DESCRIPTION

The plant is an erect shrub of the PUNICACEAE family up to three meters high, much branched from the base, having branchlets slender, often ending in a spine. Leaves are simple; oblong-lanceolate; 1–9 by 0.5–2.5 cm; consisting of obtuse or marginate apex; base acute, shiny, glabrous. Flowers are showy, orange red, about three centimeters in diameter; 1–5 borned at

From: Medicinal Plants of the World *By: Ivan A. Ross Humana Press Inc., Totowa, NJ*

branch tips, the others solitary in the highest leaf-axils, sessile or subsessile; consisting of calyx 2–3 cm long, tubular, lobes erect to recurved, 5–9, thick, coriaceous; petals the same numbers as the calyx lobes, rounded or very obtuse; from edge hypanthium; filament free; inferior ovary, ovules numerous; style 1, stigma capitate. Fruit is globose berry, crowded by persistent calyx-lobes, having leathery pericarp filled with numerous seeds, which are surrounded by pink and red, transparent, juicy, acidic, pleasant tasting pulp. They are propagated by seeds or layering, in ordinary garden soil, with regular watering.

ORIGIN AND DISTRIBUTION

Pomegranate is one of the oldest drugs known. It is mentioned in the Ebers papyrus of Egypt written in about 1550 BC and is also included in many Ayurvedic texts. Pomegranate is native of Iran and is extensively cultivated as a fruit-tree or ornamental or for medicinal purposes in Mediterranean region such as Spain, Morocco, Egypt, Afghanistan, and Iran. It is commonly found in the tropics and subtropics.

TRADITIONAL MEDICINAL USES

Arabic Countries. Dried fruit peel is used as a contraceptive in the form of a pessary in Unani medicine[T06813].

Argentina. Decoction of dried pericarp is taken orally for diarrhea and to treat respiratory and urinary tract infections[K17523].

Belize. Hot water extract of dried leaves is used externally for "women's problems." Leaves are boiled and the liquid is used for washing[T05011].

Canary Islands. Hot water extract of fresh root bark is taken orally as an anthelmintic[T15880].

China. Dried entire plant is used externally for burns and to promote eschar formation in burn treatment[T14221].

Europe. Hot water extract of root bark is taken orally as an emmenagogue[A05825].

East Africa. Hot water extract of pounded or soaked root is taken orally for tapeworm infestations[K04594].

Ethiopia. Extract of dried fruit is used for skin lesions[K21091]. Leaves crushed in water is taken orally to expel tapeworms[T01868]. Hot water extract of root bark is taken orally as an emmenagogue[A05825].

Fiji. Fresh juice of *Punica granatum* and *Cynodon dactylon* leaf juice is taken orally for cold and running nose. Fresh fruit juice is taken orally for jaundice and for diarrhea[T10632]. Water extract of dried fruit peel is taken orally for diabetes. Rind is ground with water and taken first thing in the morning. Decoction of dried seed is taken orally for syphilis[T10632].

Greece. Water extract of fruit peel is used a vaginal suppository with or without oak gall to be applied for some hours and removed immediately after coitus[A04545]. Decoction of dried fruit peel is taken orally to treat tracheobronchitis. The dried peel is boiled in water[K19150].

Guatemala. Hot water extract of dried fruit is used externally for wounds, ulcers, bruises and sores, mouth lesions, stomatitis, leucorrhea, and vaginitis. For conjunctivitis the extract is applied ophthalmically[T15445].

India. Dried root is used as an abortifacient. three parts *Allium cepa* seeds; three parts of *punica granatum* root; two parts of *Cajanus cajan* and red lead oxide are taken with honey orally[T11208]. Fresh entire plant made into a paste is used for snake bite. The paste is applied to the bite; juice is dropped into the nostrils, ears, and navel[T09390]. Fresh plant juice is used for snakebite. Plant is made into a paste and applied to bite, juice is dropped into the nostrils, ears, and navel[T09390]. Hot water extract of dried bark and fruit is taken orally for leprosy, leucorrhea, and menorrhagia[T15475]. Hot water extract of root bark is taken orally as an anthelmintic[W00667]. Olive oil extract of dried fruit is used externally to prevent premature graying of hair. The mixture contains *Terminalia arjuna, Aglaia roxburghiana, Jasminum officianales, Indigofera tinctoria, Tinospora cordifolia, Pterocarpus marsupium, Eclipta alba, Pandanus tectorius, Oroxylum indicum, Valeriana hardwickii, Terminalia chebula, Terminalia bellerica, Emblica officinales, Punica granatum, Nelumbium speciosum,* and *Sesamum indicum*[T16239]. Powdered immature fruit is taken orally for peptic ulcers. A half teaspoon of powder is added to soft porridge and taken every morning[M27166]. Dried unripe fruit is taken orally for dysentery. Tender fruits or rinds of mature fruits are boiled in milk and made into a paste that is given internally[T08282]. Fruit juice is taken orally for high fever with loss of senses[K23824]. Water extract of dried fruit peel is taken orally for diarrhea[K10142]. Poultice of fruit peel and *Tamarix gallicai* bark is applied twice in 24 hours to the breasts to abate flaccidity. Hot water extract of dried fruit peel, mixed with aromatics is taken orally for treating diarrhea and dysentery[T09984].

Indonesia. Hot water extract of dried fruit peel is taken orally as an abortifacient[T09984]. Hot water extract of root bark is taken orally as an abortifacient[A05825].

Italy. Hot water extract of dried fruit peel is used for inflammations[M17807].

Malaysia. Extract of dried fruit is taken orally by pregnant human for childbirth disorders[T08817]. Hot water extract of leaves is taken orally for irregular menses[A06590].

Mexico. Hot water extract of fruit peel is taken orally to stop excessive bleeding during menses[L01490].

Peru. Hot water extract of dried bark is taken orally by pregnant human to prevent abortion; for bloody dysentery and as an antidiarrheal[T15323]. Hot water extract of dried root is taken orally to use against abortion, as an antidiarrheal and for bloody dysentery[T15323].

Sri Lanka. Hot water extract of fresh fruit is taken orally as a cooling agent and for dysentery[T09394].

Thailand. Hot water extract of dried root is taken orally as an anthelmintic[W03804]. Hot water extract of dried fruit peel is taken orally for diarrhea and dysentery[W03804].

Tunisia. Extract of the dried bark is taken orally to treat ulcers[T08514].

USA. Hot water extract of dried root bark is used as a vaginal douche. For diarrhea, steep a teaspoon of bark in a cup of boiling water, cool and drink one cup a day; taken orally as a remedy for tapeworm

West Indies. Fruit peel mixed and dry, ground fowl gizzard and white flour is eaten as a porridge for tapeworm[T00701].

CHEMICAL CONSTITUENTS

(ppm unless otherwise indicated)

2-(2-Propenyl)-delta-piperideine
2-O-Galloylpunicalin, Lf
1,2,4,6-Tetra-O-galloyl-beta-D-glucose, Lf
1,2,3,4,6-Penta-O-galloyl-beta-D-glucose, Lf
Alkaloids, Rt, Bk 0.1-0.7%
Apigenin-4'-O-beta-D-glucoside, Lf
Arachidic acid, Sd
Ascorbic acid, Fr 40-636
Ash, Fr 0.5000-3.5858%
Asiatic acid, Fl
Beta sitosterol, Bk
Betulinic acid, Bk, Lf
Boric acid, Fr 50
Calcium oxalate, Rind, Fr 4.0%
Calcium, Fr 30-650
Callistephin, Sd Coat, Ft Pe
Carbohydrates, Fr 16.2-92.7%
Carotene, Fr 0-2
Casuariin, Bk 940, Pl
Casuarinin, Bk 0.32%, PC 3.8
Cerebroside, Sd
Chlorine, Fr 20
Chlorogenic acid, Fr
Chrysanthemin, Sd Ct, Fr Pe
Cis-9,trans-11,cis-13-triene acid, Sd
Citric acid, Fr Ju 0.81-1.23%
Coniine, Pl
Copper, Fr 0-2
Corilagin, Lf 473.7, PC 4
Coumestrol, Sd
Cyanidin, Fl, Lf
Cyanidin-3,5-diglucoside, Sd Ct
Cyanidin-3-glucoside, Fr

Cyanin, Sd Ct, Fr Pe
D-Mannitol, Sd, Lf, St, Rt, Bk
Daidzein, Sd
Delphin, Sd Ct
Delphinidin, Fl, Lf
Delphinidin-3,5-diglucoside, PC
Delphinidin-3-0-beta-D-glucoside, Sd Ct
Delphinidin-3-glucoside, Sd Ct
Elaidic acid, PC 0.55%
Ellagic acid, Bk, Lf, PC, Fr Pe
Ellagic acid,3'-0-methyl-3-4-methyl, Bk
Ellagic acid,3-3'-4-tri-0-methyl, Bk
Ellagic acid,3-3'-di-0-methyl, Bk
Ellagitannin, Bk
Enedioxy, Bk
Estradiol, Sd
Estrone, Sd 4.0 mcg/kg-17.0 mg/kg
Fat, Sd 5-205; Fr 0.1-3.8%
Fiber, Fr 0.2-23.2%; Sd 22.4%
Flavogallol, PC
Fluoride, Cortex 5.8
Friedelin, Bk
Fructose, Fr
Gallagyldilactone, PC
Gallic acid, PC 0.09-4.00%
Genistein, Sd
Genistin, Sd
Glucose, Fr
Granatin A, PC, Lf 1.3%
Granatin B, Fr Pe, PC, Lf 1.72%
Granatins, Lf 1.5%
Gums, Rind, Fr 3.2%
Heneicosanoic acid, Sd Ol 5.0%
Hygrine, Bk 2.0%
Inulin, Rind, Fr 1.0%
Iron, Fr 3-16
Isopelletierine, Bk
Isoquercetrin, PC
Lauric acid, 4-methyl, Sd Ol 0.5%
Linoleic acid, Sd
Lureolin-3'-0-beta-D-glucoside, Lf
Luteolin-3'-0-beta-D-xylopyranoside, Lf
Luteolin-4'-0-beta-D-glucoside, Lf
Magnesium, Fr 0.012%
Malic acid, Fr
Maltose, Fr
Malvidin, Fr
Malvidin pentose glycoside, Fr
Mannitol, PC 1.8%, Lf 0.547%
Maslinic acid, Fl
Methyl pelletierine, Rt Bk
Methyl isopelletierine, Bk

Mucilage, Rind 0.6-34.0%
Neochlorogenic acid, Fr
Niacin, Fr 3-50
Nonadecanoic acid, Sd Ol 5.9%
Nor-hygrine, Bk 0.7%
Oleic acid, Sd
Oxalic acid, Fr 140
P-Coumarinic acid, Fr
Palmitic acid, Sd Ol 10.4%
Pantothenic acid, Fr 6-31
Pectin, PC 2-4%; Fr Pe 0.27%
Pedunculagin, Bk 82.4, PC 4
Pelargonidin-3,5-diglucoside, Fl
Pelargonidin-3-glucoside, Sd
Pelargonin, Sd Ct, Fr Pe
Pelletierine, Bk 21.6%, St 48.7%, Br 49.6%
Phosphatidylcholine, Sd
Phosphatidylinositol, Sd
Phosphatidylserine, Sd
Phosphorus, Fr 80-3,182
Phytosterols, Fr 170-892
Polyphenols, Fr Pe 0.22-1.05%
Potassium, Fr 0.133-1.895%
Protein, Fr 0.77-7.30%; Sd 2.5%
Protocatechuic acid, Fr
Pseudopelletierine, Bk 44.3%
Punicacortein A, Bk 28
Punicacortein B, Bk 27
Punicacortein C, Bk 1100
Punicacortein D, Bk 62
Punicafolin, Lf 137
Punicalagin, PC, Fr Pe, Bk 0.14%
Punicalin, PC, Fr Pe, Bk 880
Punicic acid, Sd Ol 33.3%
Punigluconin, Bk 140
Pyridine,N-(2'-5'-dihydroxy-phenyl), Lf
Resin, PC 4.5%
Riboflavin, Fr 0-4
Sedridine, Bk 0.3%
Sodium, Fr 9-350
Sorbitol, Fr
Starch, Sd 0
Stearic acid, Sd Ol 5.9%
Stearic acid,13-methyl, Sd Ol 1.5%
Strictinin, Lf 63
Styptic acid, Fl
Sulfur, Fr 0.012%
Tannin, Fr Ju 0.17%; PC 10.4-33.6%; St, Bk
    10-25%; Rt 28%; Lf 11%
Tellimagrandin 1, PC 26
Thiamin, Fr 0-4
Tricosanoic acid, Sd Ol 4.9%

Unicalin, PC
Ursolic acid, Lf, Fr
Vitamin B6, Fr 1-5
Water, Sd 35.0; Fr 78.00-82.32%
Wax, PC 0.8%
Xanthoxylin, Lf

PHARMACOLOGICAL ACTIVITIES AND CLINICAL TRIALS

Abortifacient effect. Ethanol (95%) extract of fruit administered orally rats at a dose of 200.0 mg/kg was inactive[W01362].

Allergenic activity. Fruit eaten by human adult was active. Case report of tongue angioedema following ingestion of the fruit. An IGE-mediated mechanism could not be demonstrated[M27829].

Analgesic activity. Ethanol/water (1:1) extract of the aerial parts, administered to mice intraperitoneally at a dose of 0.125 mg/kg was inactive vs tail pressure method[W00374].

Anthelmintic activity. Chloroform extract of dried root and stem, administered to mice by gastric intubation at a dose of 250.0 mg/kg for three days was active on *Hymenolepsis nana* and inactive on *Nippostrongylus brasiliense* and *Syphacia obvelata*[T12072]. Methanol extract of fruit peel administered orally to mice at a dose of 120.0 mg/kg was active on *Hymenolepis diminuta*. Eighty seven percent clearance of worms in two days was observed[W00456]. Water extract of dried fruitpeel at a concentration of 10.0 ml/plate was active on *Ascaris galli*, *Pheritima posthuma*, and *Taenia solium*[K11484].

Antiamoebic activity. Alkaloid fraction of dried root at a concentration of 1.0 mg/ml in broth culture was inactive on *Entamoeba histolytica* and *Entamoeba invadens*. The water extract at a concentration of 2.0 ml was active on *Entamoeba histolytica* and *Entamoeba invadens*. One hundred percent of growth was inhibition. Tannin fraction at a concentration of 10.0 mcg/ml was active on *Entamoeba histolytica* and *Entamoeba invadens*. One hundred percent growth was inhibited[K07637].

Antiancylostomiasis activity. Hot water extract of root bark ingested by human adults was inactive. Two ounces of bark boiled in two pints water with boiling down to one pint. Four ounces are given in hourly doses of one ounce, with the last dose followed by magnesium sulfate. Thirteen patients were treated[W00667].

Antiascariasis activity. Ethanol (95%) extract of the epicarp was active on earthworm. Paralysis occurred in 18 hours with a death rate of 50%[J08904].

Antibacterial activity. Acid-ethanol extract of dried fruit at a dose of 0.20 ml/disc on agar plate was inactive on *Pseudomonas aeruginosa*. Dichloromethane extraction, methanol extraction, and washing in petroleum ether also done, and acidic extract made alkaline; then washed with dichloromethane. Inactive on *Salmonella gallinarum*; acid extract made alkaline, then washed with dichloromethane. Inactive on *Staphylococcus albus*. Dichloromethane extraction, methanol extraction, and washing in petroleum ether also done and acidic extract made alkaline, then washed with dichloromethane. Strong activity on *Escherichia coli*, *Klebsiella pneumoniae*, and *Proteus vulgaris*. Dichloromethane extraction, methanol extraction, and washing in petroleum ether; dichloromethane extraction, petroleum ether extraction, and washing in methanol were done and acidic extract made alkaline; then washed with dichloromethane. Water extract of dried fruit at a dose of 0.20 ml/disc on agar plate was inactive on *Escherichia coli*, *Salmonella gallinarum*, and *Pseudomonas aeruginosa*, and showed strong activity on *Klebsiella pneumoniae*, *Proteus vulgaris*, and *Staphylococcus albus*[K21091]. Decoction of dried pericarp on agar plate was active on *Pseudomonas aeruginosa*[K17523]. Ethanol (80%) extract of dried aerial parts at a concentration of 100.0 mcg/ml on agar plate was active on *Bacillus anthracis*, *Proteus vulgaris*, and *Salmonella* paratyphi A; inactive on *Escherichia coli,* *Klebsiella pneumoniae, Pseudomonas aeruginosa, Shigella sonnei, Staphylococcus aureus,* and *Vibrio cholera*[T09667]. Ethanol (95%) extract of dried fruitpeel at a concentration of 10.0 mg/ml on agar plate was inactive on *Corynebacterium diphtheriae,* and *Diplococcus pneumonia;* weak activity on *Staphylococcus aureus, Streptococcus pyogenes,* and *Streptococcus viridans.* Water extract was inactive on *Corynebacterium diptheriae* and *Diplococcus pneumonia;* weak activity on *Staphylococcus aureus, Streptococcus pyogenes,* and *Streptococcus viridans*[M29966]. Ethanol (95%) extract of dried fruitpeel at a concentration of 100.0 mg/disc on agar plate was active on *Bacillus subtilis, Salmonella typhosa,* and *Shigella dysenteriae;* inactive on *Escherichia coli* and strong activity on *Staphylococcus aureus.* Water extract at a concentration of 20.0 mg/disc on agar plate was inactive on *Bacillus subtilis, Escherichia coli, Salmonella typhosa, Shigella dysenteriae,* and *Staphylococcus aureus.* Dose expressed as dry weight of plant material[P00004]. Ethanol/water (1:1) extract of the aerial parts at a concentration of >25.0 mcg/ml on agar plate was inactive on *Bacillus subtilis, Escherichia coli, Salmonella typhosa, Staphylococcus aureus,* and *Agrobacterium tumefaciens*[W00374]. Hot water extract of dried entire plant at a concentration of 62.5 mg/ml on agar plate was active on *Escherichia coli* and *Staphyloococcus aureus*[K14683]. Saline extract of leaves at a concentration of 1–40 on agar plate was active on *Staphylococcus aureus* and inactive on *Pasteurella pestis*[W01047]. Acetone extract of dried leaves on agar plate was active on *Escherichia coli, Pseudomonas aeruginosa, Salmonella newport, Salmonella typhosa, Sarcina lutea, Serratia marcescens, Shigella flexneri, Shigella flexneri 3A, Staphylococcus albus,* and *Staphylococcus aureus.* Ethanol (95%) extract on agar plate was active on *Escherichia coli, Pseudomonas aeruginosa, Salmonella B, Salmonella newport, Salmonella typhosa,*

Sarcina lutea, Serratia marcescens, Shigella flexneri, Shigella flexneri 3A, Staphylococcus albus, and *Staphylococcus aureus.* Water extract on agar plate was active on *Escherichia coli, Pseudomonas aeruginosa, Salmonella B, Salmonella newport, Salmonella typhosa, Serratia marcescens, Shigella flexneri,* and *Staphylococcus albus;* inactive on *Sarcina lutea, Shigella flexneri 3A* and *Staphylococcus aureus*[K09159]. Seed oil on agar plate was active on *Klebsiella pneumonia, Salmonella paratyphi,* and *Shigella flexneri*[A05854]. Acetone extract of dried stem on agar plate was active on *Escherichia coli, Pseudomonas aeruginosa, Salmonella B, Salmonella newport, Salmonella typhosa, Sarcina lutea, Serratia marcescens, Shigella flexneri, Shigella flexneri 3A, Staphylococcus albus,* and *Staphylococcus aureus.* The water extract was active on *Escherichia coli, Pseudomonas aeruginosa, Salmonella B, Salmonella newport, Salmonella typhosa, Serratia marcescens, Shigella flexneri,* and *Staphylococcus albus;* inactive on *Sarcina lutea, Shigella flexneri 3A,* and *Staphylococcus aureus*[K09159]. Tincture of dried fruit at a concentration of 30.0 microliters/disc (extract of 10 gram plant material in 100 ml ethanol) on agar plate was inactive on *Escherichia coli, Pseudomonas aeruginosa,* and *Staphylococcus aureus*[T15445].

Anticonvulsant activity. Ethanol/water (1:1) extract of the aerial parts administered intraperitoneally to mice at a dose of 0.125 mg/kg was inactive vs electroshock-induced convulsions[W00374].

Antidiarrheal activity. Decoction of dried fruitpeel administered intragastric to rats at a dose of 500.0 mg/kg was active vs castor oil-induced diarrhea. Ethanol (95%) extract administered intragastric to rats at a dose of 50.0 mg/kg was active. The extract reduced fecal output. At a dose of 500.0 mg/kg weak activity was produced vs castor oil-induced diarrhea[K10142]. Decoction of fruitpeel administered orally to children was active. The infantile diarrhea was treated with Kexieding capsule composed of five herbs including roasted ginger, clove, and fruit peel of *Punica granatum*. Of the 234 infants and 71 children treated, 281 (92%) were cured in 1–3 days and nine (3%) were significantly improved. The total effective rate was 95%. Only nine of 79 severe cases were caused by bacteria; one of them whom manifested symptoms of bacterial dysentery and bloody-mucoid stools was ultimately cured with Baitouweng mixture[M29313].

Antifertility effect. Fruit peel in the ration of guinea pigs of both sexes, at a dose of 18.0 gm/kg and in female rats was active[A03127].

Antifungal activity. Ethanol/water (1:1) extract of aerial parts at a concentration of >25.0 mcg/ml on agar plate was inactive on *Microsporum canis*, *Trichophyton mentagrophytes*, and *Aspergillus niger*[W00374]. Hot water extract of dried entire plant at a concentration of 62.5 mg/ml on agar plate was active on *Aspergillus niger*[K14683].

Anti-inflammatory activity. Ethanol (80%) extract of dried fruit peel administered to male rats by gastric intubation at a dose of 100.0 mg/kg produced weak activity vs carrageenin-induced pedal edema. Twenty three percent inhibition of edema was observed[M17807]. Ethanol/water (1:1) extract of aerial parts administered orally to rats at a dose of 0.125 mg/kg was inactive vs carrageenin-induced pedal edema. Animals were dosed one hour before carrageenin injections[W00374].

Antimalarial activity. Methanol extract of dried leaves was inactive on *Plasmodium falciparum* MIC >25.0 mcg/ml[K11643].

Antimutagenic activity. Methanol extract of dried fruit at a concentration of 50.0 microliters/disc on agar plate was inactive on *Bacillus subtilis* NIG-1125, His Met, and *Escherichia coli* B/R-WP2-TRP[T08867].

Antimycobacterial activity. Ethanol (95%) extract of dried aerial parts at a concentration of 1–50 on agar plate produced weak activity on *Mycobacterium tuberculosis*[A15182].

Antinematodal activity. Water extract of a commercial sample of pericarp, at a concentration of 10.0 mg/ml was inactive on *Toxacara canis*. The methanol extract produced weak activity[M29965].

Antioxidant activity. Methanol extract of fruit at a concentration of 50.0 microliters was active[K23609].

Antispasmodic activity. Ethanol/water (1:1) extract of aerial parts was inactive on guinea pig ileum vs ACh- and histamine-induced spasms[W00374].

Antiuremic activity. Decoction of dried bark in the drinking water of rats at a dose of 150.0 mg/kg was active vs casein/adenine-induced renal failure. Urea, creatinine, methylguanidine, and guanidinosuccinic acid assayed[K20525].

Antiviral activity. Hot water extract of dried root bark at a concentration of 0.1 mg/ml in cell culture was active on Herpes Simplex 1 virus and measles virus; a concentration of 0.5 mg/ml was active on Poliovirus 1; when administered intragastric to mice at a dose of 5.0 mg/animal was active on Herpes Simplex 1 virus[K16835]. Water extract of fruit in cell culture was active on Coxsackie B5 virus, Herpes Simplex virus, Influenza virus (Lee), Poliovirus 1, and REO virus Type 1[K04780].

Antiyeast activity. Acid-ethanol extract of dried fruit at a concentration of 0.20 ml/disc on agar plate was inactive on *Candida albicans*. Dichloromethane extraction, methanol extraction, and washing in petroleum ether and acidic extract made alkaline, then washed with dichloromethane. Strong activity was shown with dichloromethane extraction and petroleum ether extraction; washing with methanol and acidic extract made alkaline, then extracted with dichloromethane[K21091]. Ethanol (95%) extract of dried fruitpeel at a concentration of 100.0 mg/disc on agar plate produced strong activity on *Candida albicans*. The water extract at a concentration of 20.0 mg/

disc was inactive. Dose expressed as dry weight of plant material[P00004]. Ethanol/water (1:1) extract of aerial parts at a concentration of >25.0 mcg/ml on agar plate was inactive on *Candida albicans* and *Cryptococcus neoformans*[W00374]. Tincture of dried fruit at a concentration of 30.0 microliters/disc (extract of 10 grams plant material in 100 ml ethanol) on agar plate was inactive on *Candida albicans*[T15445].

Barbiturate Potentiation. Ethanol/water (1:1) extract of aerial parts administered intraperitoneally to mice at a dose of 0.125 mg/kg was inactive[W00374].

Carbonic anhydrase inhibition. Acetone (90%) extract was active[K13751].

Cytotoxic activity. Acetone extract of dried bark at a concentration of 5.0% was equivocal by cylinder plate method on CA-Ehrlich ascites; 21 mm inhibition. Ether extract at a concentration of 5.0% was inactive by cylinder plate method on CA-Ehrlich ascites; 15 mm inhibition. Water extract at a concentration of 5.0% was inactive by cylinder plate method on CA-Ehrlich ascites; 0 mm inhibition[W03044]. Hot water extract of fruitpeel at a dose of 120.0 mcg/ml in cell culture was active on CA-JTC-26. The inhibition rate was 59%[M27219]. Methanol/water (1:1) extract of bark in cell culture was active on CA-9KB. ED_{50} < 20.0 mcg/ml[X00001]. Water extract of dried pericarp at a concentration of 120.0 mcg/ml in cell culture was active on CA-Mammary-Microalveolar and Cells-Human-Embryonic HE-1[M26592].

Diuretic activity. Ethanol/water (1:1) extract of serial parts administered intraperitoneally to saline-loaded male rats was active. Urine was collected for four hours postdrug[W00374].

Embryotoxic effect. Acetone, hot water, and methanol extracts of dried root administered by gastric intubation to pregnant rats at doses of 150.0 mg/kg were inactive. Rats were dosed on days 1–7[T11177]. Ethanol (95%) extract of fruit administered orally to female

rats at a dose of 200.0 mg/kg was inactive[W01362]. Methanol and Acetone extracts of dried entire plant administered by gastric intubation to pregnant rats at doses of 200.0 mg/kg were inactive. Dosing was done on days 1–7[T11279].

Estrogenic effect. Dried seed extract at variable dosage levels administered subcutaneously to ovariectomized mice was active. Activity 4.0–17.0 mcg oestrone/kg[T06788]. Seed oil administered intraperitoneally to mice at a dose of 0.4 ml/animal produced strong activity; at a dose of 0.5 ml/animal administered intraperitoneally to rabbit was active; and subcutaneously to ovariectomized rats was active. The unsaponifiable fraction administered intraperitoneally to female rabbits at a dose of 250.0 mg/animal was active[A05611].

Feeding deterrent (insect). Seed oil at a concentration of 1.0% in the ration was inactive on *Anthonomus grandis*[T15029].

Glutamate-pyruvate stimulation. Tannin fraction (hydrolyzable) of pericarp, administered intraperitoneally to mice at a dose of 20.0 ml/kg was active. Solutions equal to 0.5% gallotannin were injected daily dosing for two days followed by sacrifice and examination on days three, five, or nine[T00440].

Hepatotoxic activity. Tannin fraction (hydrolyzable) of pericarp, administered intraperitoneally to mice at a dose of 20.0 ml/kg was active. Solutions equal to 0.5% gallotannin were injected daily dosing for two days followed by sacrifice and examination on days three, five, or nine. Histological examination showed severely damaged liver parenchyma[T00440].

Hypoglycemic activity. Ethanol/water (1:1) extract of aerial parts administered orally to rats at a dose of 250.0 mg/kg was inactive. Less than 30% drop in blood sugar level was observed[W00374]. Flowers administered orally to male rats at a dose of 4.0 gm/animal was active[J07575].

Hypothermic activity. Ethanol/water (1:1) extract of aerial parts administered intraperitoneally to mice at a dose of 0.125 mg/kg was active[W00374].

Intestinal antisecretory activity. Decoction of dried fruitpeel administered intragastric to rats was active vs $MgSO_4$-induced enteropooling. The ethanol (95%) extract at a dose of 500.0 mg/kg was active vs $MgSO_4$-induced enteropooling[K10142].

Molluscicidal activity. Ethanol (95%) and water extracts of dried root at concentrations of 1000 ppm produced weak activity on *Biomphalaria glabrata* and *Biomphalaria straminea*[W02949].

Plant growth inhibitor. Hot water extract of bark at a concentration of 2.0 gm/liter was active. The number of fronds of *Lemna paucicostata* >1 mm in length was 57% of control[M26939].

Plant root growth stimulant. Hot water extract of bark at a concentration of 2.0 gm/liter was active. Root length in *Brassica rapa* was 121% of control and the number of roots >5 mm in length in *Cucumis sativus* was 554% of control[M26939].

Plaque formation suppressant. Water extract of a commercial sample of pericarp was inactive on *Streptococcus mutans* IC_{50} >1000 mcg/ml. Methanol extract was active IC_{50} 60.0 mcg/ml. Methanol/water (1:1) extract was active IC_{50} 370.0 mcg/ml[T11789]. Water, methanol, and methanol/water (1:1) extracts of dried bark at a concentrations of 1.0, 0.5, and 1.0 mg/ml respectively, were active on *Streptococcus mutans*[T10387].

Prostaglandin synthetase inhibition. Hot water extract of a commercial sample of pericarp at a concentration of 750.0 mcg/ml showed weak activity on rabbit microsomes[T08539].

Protease (HIV) inhibition. Water extract of dried pericarp at a concentration of 200.0 mcg/ml was equivocal. The methanol extract was inactive[K21241].

Semen coagulation. Ethanol/water (1:1) extract of aerial parts at a concentration of 2.0% was inactive on rat sperm[W00374].

Spermicidal effect. Ethanol/water (1:1) of aerial parts was inactive on rat sperm[W00374].

Toxicity assessment (quantitative). Ethanol/water (1:1) extract of aerial parts administered intraperitoneally to mice produced LD_{50} 0.25 gm/kg[W00374].

Tyrosinase inhibition. Methanol/water (1:1) extract of dried pericarp at a concentration of 330.0 mcg/ml produced weak activity. 35.3% inhibition[K23694]. Methanol/water (1:1) extract of dried root bark at a concentration of 330.0 mcg/ml produced weak activity, 29.7% inhibition[K23694].

Uterine relaxation effect. Seed oil administered intraperitoneally to mice at a dose of 0.2 ml/animal was active[A05606].

Uterine stimulant effect. Water extract of fruitpeel was active on the uterus of nonpregnant rats[A02600].

26 | Syzygium cumini

(Linn.) Skeels

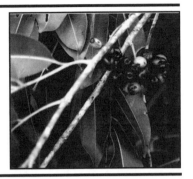

Common Names

Alla naeredu	India	Jamun	Nepal
Azeitona	Brazil	Java plum	Nepal
Jam	India	Java plum	Brazil
Jaman	India	Java plum	India
Jaman	Pakistan	Java plum	Nepal
Jamblon	Rodrigues Islands	Java plum	West Indies
Jambol	West Indies	Luk-wa	Thailand
Jambolan	Brazil	Madan	Japan
Jambolan	India	Malabar plum	Brazil
Jambolana	Nepal	Malak rose-apple	Brazil
Jambolao	Brazil	Naeredu	India
Jambu	India	Naval	India
Jambul	India	Negresse	India
Jambul	USA	Rotra	Madagascar
Jamdlan	India	Tete	West Indies
Jamoon	Guyana	Wa	Thailand
Jamoon	India	Waa	Thailand
Jamun	India		

BOTANICAL DESCRIPTION

A smooth tree of the MYRTACEAE family, Four to fifteen meters in height. Leaves leathery oblong-ovate to elliptic or obovate and 6 to 12 cm long, the tip being broad and shortly pointed. The panicles are borne mostly from the branchlets below the leaves, often being axillary or terminal, and are four to six cm long. The flowers are numerous, scented, pink or nearly white, without stalks, and borne in crowded fascicles on the ends of the branchlets. The calyx is funnel-shaped, about 4 mm long, and 4-toothed. The petals cohere and fall all together as a small disk. The stamens are very numerous and as long as the calyx. Fruit oval to elliptic; 1.5 to 3.5 cm long, dark purple or nearly black, luscious, fleshy and edible; it contains a single large seed.

ORIGIN AND DISTRIBUTION

The original home of *Syzygium cumini* is India or the East Indies. It is found in Thailand, Philippines, Madagascar, and some other countries. The plant has been successfully introduced into many other tropical countries such as the West Indies, East and

From: Medicinal Plants of the World *By:* Ivan A. Ross Humana Press Inc., Totowa, NJ

West Africa and some subtropical regions including Florida, California, Algeria, and Israel.

TRADITIONAL MEDICINAL USES

Brazil. Decoction of dried leaves is taken orally to treat diabetes[K09337].

India. Bark paste and curd is taken orally three times a day for two days to cure dysentery[K23156]. Decoction[A14429] and fluid extract[A14534] of dried bark is taken orally for diabetes. Ten grams of dried leaves of *Zanthoxylum armatum* boiled in eight liters of water along with 125 gm of mixture having equal parts of bark of *Acacia nilotica*, *Mangifera indica*, and *Syzygium cumini* until the quantity of water is reduced to two liters. Fifty mililiters of decoction is taken twice a day after meals[M24146]. Hot water extract of dried bark is taken orally for dysentery, indigestion, and as a blood purifier[T09230]. Decoction of dried bark is taken orally for venereal ulcers. *Terminalia arjuna*, *Pongamia pinnata*, *Vateria indica*, *Syzygium cumini*, *Ficus benghalensis*, *F. religiosa*, *F. racemosa*, *F. talbotii*, and *Azadirachta indica* are used[T16239]. Fruits are taken orally to cure gastro-intestinal complaints[K23171]. Hot water extract of dried fruits is used externally as an astringent and orally for stomach ulcers and to reduce acidity[T09230]. Hot water extract of dried fruits and seeds is taken orally for diabetes[A14379]. Leaves are taken orally for leucorrhea; two young leaves are chewed with cold water for 3–4 days[K23171]. Decoction of dried seeds is taken orally for diabetes[A14429]. The fluidextract is taken orally as an antiinflammatory[A14534] and the hot water extract is taken orally as an antipyretic[M19921], and for diabetes 100–250 mg seed powder is taken orally three times a day with water[M22542]. Decoction of dried seeds is taken orally for diarrhea; the seeds are taken together with *Cassia auriculata*[M23219]. Hot water extract of dried seeds taken orally is prescribed in Ayurvedic medicine for diabetes[T06838], it is also used as an astringent in dysentery and

diarrhea and to reduce urinary sugars in diabetes[T10448]. Leaf juice is taken orally to treat diabetes. The juice is taken mixed with milk every morning[K23365]. Fresh leaf juice is taken orally for stomach pain[T09486]. Seeds are taken orally for diabetes[K11282]. Stembark juice is taken orally for constipation and to stop blood discharge in the feces, mixed with buttermilk and taken every day[K23365].

Pakistan. Hot water extract of dried aerial parts is used for diabetes[T09984]. Seeds are taken orally for diarrhea, diabetes, dysentery, and blood pressure[J07469].

Thailand. Dried stembark is taken orally as as a cardiotonic, as a CNS stimulant, and for fainting[R00001]. Hot water extract of dried bark is taken orally as an antipyretic[W3022A]. Hot water extract of dried seeds is taken orally for diabetes[W01792]. Leaf ash is used externally to relieve itching caused by centipede bite. Decoction of the root is taken orally as an antiemetic and to increase lactation in new mothers[T12027].

USA. Fluidextract of seeds is reputed valuable for diabetes[A05638].

West Indies. Seeds are used for diabetes[T00701].

CHEMICAL CONSTITUENTS
(ppm unless otherwise indicated)

1-Galloyl glucose, Sd
3-6-Hexahydroxy-diphenoyl glucose, Sd
3-Galloyl glucose, Sd
4-6-Hexahydroxy-diphenoyl glucose, Sd
6-Galloyl glucose, Sd
Acetophenone,2-6-dihydroxy-4-methoxy, Fl
Alanine, Lf
Alpha copanene, St EO 2.15%
Alpha humulene, Lf EO 2.80%; St EO 6.51%; Fr EO 2.30%
Alpha pinene, Lf EO 30.10%; St EO 18.56%; Fr EO 30.89
Alpha terpineol, Lf EO
Astragalin, St Bk
Beta caryophyllene, Lf EO 2.50%; Fr EO 0.40%
Beta phellandrene, Lf EO
Beta pinene, Lf EO 20.50%; St EO 12.61%; Fr EO 10.81%
Beta sitosterol, Lf; St Bk 600

Betulinic acid, Lf; St Bk 0.11%
Borneol acetate, Lf EO 2.20%; Lf EO
   1.46%; Fr EO 0.32%
Borneol, Lf EO
Bornylene, Lf EO
Camphene, St EO 1.31%; Fr EO 1.0%
Cinnamic acid methyl ester, Lf EO
Cis ocimene, Lf EO 9.0%; St EO 14.83%;
   Fr EO 18.50%
Citric acid, Fr; Lf
Clycolic acid, Lf
Corilagin, Sd
Cuminaldehyde, Lf EO
Cyanin, Fr
Daucosterol, St Bk
Delphinidin-3-0-beta-D-gentiobioside, Fr
Delta cadinene, St EO 1.46%
Dotriacontan-1-ol, Lf
Ellagic acid, Sd; St Bk
Ellagic acid,3-3-3-tri-o-methyl, Sd; Bk
Ellagic acid,3-3-di-o-methyl, Sd; Bk
Epi friedelanol, St Bk 600
Eugenin, St Bk 20
Eugenol, Lf EO
Friedelanol, St Bk
Friedelin, St Bk 800
Fructose, Fr; Lf
Gallic acid, Sd; Bk
Gamma cadiene, St EO 0.64%
Gamma terpinene, St EO 0.65%
Glucose, Fr
Glycine, Lf
Hentriacontan-1-ol, Lf
Heptacosan-1-ol, Lf
Hexahydroxy diphenic acid, Sd
Iso rhamnetin 3-0-rutinoside, Rt
Jambolin, Sd
Kaempferol, St Bk
Leucine, Lf
Limonene, Lf EO 8.50%; St EO 6.48%; Fr
   EO 4.50%
Malic acid, Fr
Malvidin-3-0-beta-D-laminaribioside, Fr
Mannose, Fr
Maslinic acid, Lf
Methyl xanthoxylin, Fl
Montanyl alcohol, Lf
Myrcene, St EO 4.28%
Myricetin-3-0-beta-D-glucoside, Rt
Myricetin-3-0-robinoside, Rt
N-dotriacontane, Lf
N-Hentriacontane, Lf

N-Heptacosane, Lf
N-Hexacosane, Lf
N-Nonacosane, Lf
N-Octacosane, Lf
N-Tetratriacontane, Lf
N-Triacontane, Lf
N-Tritriacontane, Lf
Octacosan-1-ol, Lf
Oleanolic acid, Fl 0.5%; Sd
Oxalic acid, Lf
Petunidin-3-0-beta-D-gentibioside, Fr
Quercetin, Sd; St Bk
Rutin, Lf 1.5%
Sucrose, St Bk
Taxifolin, Sd
Terpinolene, Lf EO; St EO 0.96%
Tetratriacontan-1-ol, Lf
Trans ocimene, Lf EO 9.50%; St EO
   12.24%; Fr EO 12.10%
Triacontan-1-ol, Lf
Tritriancontan-1-ol, Lf
Tyrosine, Lf

PHARMACOLOGICAL ACTIVITIES AND CLINICAL TRIALS

Abortifacient effect. Ethanol/water (1:1) extract of the aerial parts, administered orally to rats at a dose of 200.0 mg/kg was inactive[W00374].

Analgesic activity. Ethanol/water (1:1) extract of the aerial parts, administered intraperitoneally to mice at a dose of 0.375 mg/kg was inactive vs tail pressure method[W00374]. Methanol extract of dried seeds, administered intraperitoneally to mice at a dose of 25.0 mg/kg was active vs acetic acid-induced writhing. Results significant at $P < 0.001$ level[T10448].

Antiaggression effect. Methanol extract of dried seeds, administered intraperitoneally to mice at a dose of 150.0 mg/kg was active vs foot shock induced agression. Results significant at $P < 0.01$ level[T10448].

Antibacterial activity. Ethanol (95%) and water extracts of dried fruit at concentrations of 100.0 and 20 mg/disc respectively (expressed as dry weight of the fruit) on agar plate, were inactive on *Bacillus subtilis*, *Escherichia coli*, *Salmonella typhosa*, *Shigella* *dysenteriae*, and *Staphylococcus aureus*[P00004]. Ethanol/water (1:1) extract of of the aerial parts at a concentration >25.0 mcg/ml on agar plate was inactve on *Bacillus subtilis*, *Escherichia coli*, *Salmonella typhosa*, *Staphylococcus aureus*, and plant pathogen *Agrobacterium tumefaciens*[W00374]. Saline extract of leaves at a concentration of 1:80 on agar plate was active on *Staphylococcus aureus*[W01047].

Antibradykinin activity. Methanol extract of dried seeds administered intraperitoneally to mice was active vs bradykinin-induced pedal edema[M19921].

Anticlastogenic activity. Fruit juice administered intraperitoneally to mice at a dose of 50.0 ml/kg was active on mice marrow cells vs mitomycin C-, tetracycline and dimethylnitrosamine-induced micronuclei[K17561].

Anticonvulsant activity. Ethanol/water (1:1) Ethanol/water (1:1) extract of the aerial parts, administered intraperitoneally to mice at a dose of 0.375 mg/ml was inactive vs electroshock-induced convulsions[W00374]. Methanol extract of dried seeds, administered intraperitoneally to mice at a dose of 150.0 mg/kg was inactive vs strychnine-induced convulsions[T10448].

Antifungal activity. Ethanol/water (1:1) extract of the aerial parts at a concentration >25.0 mcg/ml on agar plate was inactive on *Microsporum canis*, *Trichophyton mentagrophytes*, and *Aspergillus niger*[W00374].

Antihistamine activity. Ethanol/water (1:1) extract of dried bark at a concentration of 0.01 gm/ml was active on guinea pig ileum[W3022A]. Methanol extract of dried seeds administered intraperitoneally to rats was active vs histamine-induced pedal edema[M19921].

Antihyperglycemic activity. Decoction of the aerial parts taken orally by human adults at a dose 500.0 mg/person was active; also produced oliguria, and patients complained of pain in the loins. Symptoms cleared up after one week[A14458]. Powdered commercial of seeds, administered by gastric intubation

to rats at a dose of 53.2 mg/kg was active. Effect seen in streptozotocin-induced diabetic animals challenged with glucose after having received daily dose of extract for one week. This dose was inactive vs glucose-induced hyperglycemia[M27423]. Ethanol (95%) and hot water extracts of dried seeds, administered orally and intravenously to human adults at variable dosage levels were active[A14331]. When administered intragastric to rats at a dose of 50.0 mg/kg the extract was active vs alloxan-induced hyperglycemia[A14413]. Ethanol (95%) extract of dried seeds, administered intraperitoneally to rats at a dose of 75.0 mg/animal was inactive vs streptozotocin-induced hyperglycemia[T12220]. The hot water extract, administered intragastric to rabbits at a dose of 10.0 gm/kg (dry weight of seeds) was active vs alloxan-induced hyperglycemia[W01792]. Seeds administered by gastric intubation to rabbits at a dose of 1.0 gm/kg was active[T06838]. Seeds administered orally to human adults at a dose of 4–24 gm/person was active when administered to 28 diabetic patients. Results significant at $P < 0.05$ level[M06777]. Hot water extracts of dried fruit pulp, administered by gastric intubation to dogs at a dose of 150.0 gm/kg (expressed as dry weight of the fruit) and to rabbits at a dose of 50.0 gm/kg were inactive vs alloxan-induced hyperglycemia[A14333].

Anti-implantation effect. Ethanol/water (1:1) extract of the aerial parts, administered orally to rats at a dose of 100.0 mg/kg was inactive[W00374].

Anti-inflammatory activity. Chloroform extract of dried seeds, administered intrapaw to rats at a dose of 2.5 mg/paw was active vs carrageenin-induced pedal edema. The extract at 100.0 mg/kg administered intraperitoneally to rats was active vs turpentine-induced joint edema, carrageenin-, PGE-1-, histamine-, sertonin-, bradykinin-, and hyaluronidase-induced pedal edema. A dose of 25.0 mg/kg was active vs formalin-, carrageenin-, and kaolin-induced pedal edema; adjuvant- and formaldehyde-induced arthritis[M19921]. Ethanol/water (1:1) extract of the aerial parts, administered orally to rats at a dose of 0.375 mg/kg was inactive vs carrageenin-induced pedal edema. Animals were dosed one hour before carrageenin injections[W00374].

Antipyretic activity. Chloroform[M23489] and methanol[M19921] extracts of dried seeds, administered intraperitoneally to rats at doses of 50.0 mg/kg were active vs yeast-induced pyrexia.

Antispasmodic acitivity. Ethanol/water (1:1) extract of the aerial parts was inactive on guinea pig ileum vs ACh- and histamine-induced spasms[W00374]. Ethanol/water (1:1) extract of dried bark at a concentration of 0.01 gm/ml was active on guinea pig ileum[W3022A].

Antitoxic activity. Methanol extract of dried seeds, administered intraperitoneally to mice at a dose of 50.0 mg/kg was active. Antagonized amphetamine toxicity[T10448].

Antiviral activity. Ethanol/water (1:1) extract of dried entire plant at a concentration of 0.1 mg/ml in cell culture was inactive on Ranikhet virus and Vaccinia virus. For Ranikhet virus, infected chorioallantoic membrane viral titre decreased 10% and for Vaccinia virus, 0%[K13748]. The extract when injected into chick embryo at a dose of 1.0 mg/animal, was inactive on Ranikhet virus and Vaccinia virus. Infected chick embryo viral titre decreased 10% and 0% respectively[K13748]. Ethanol/water (1:1) extract of the aerial parts at a concentration of 50.0 mcg/ml in cell culture was inactive on Ranikhet virus and Vaccinia virus[W00374]. Water extract of the bark was active on Potato X virus[A03478].

Antiyeast activity. Ethanol (95%) and water extracts of dried fruit at concentrations of 100.0 and 20.0 mg/disc respectively (expressed as dry weight of the fruit) on agar plate, were inactive on *Candida albicans*[P00004]. Ethanol/water (1:1) extract of the aerial parts at a concentration >25.0 mcg/ml on agar plate was inactive on *Candida albicans* and *Cryptococcus neoformans*[W00374].

Barbiturate potentiation. Methanol extract of dried seeds, administered intraperitoneally to mice at a dose of 25.0 mg/kg was active. Results significant at $P < 0.001$ level[T10448].

Capillary permeability decrease. Chloroform extract of dried seeds, administered intraperitoneally to rats at a dose of 50.0 mg/kg was active[M23489].

Cathepsin B induction. Seeds administered by gastric intubation to Rhesus monkeys at a dose of 240.0 mg/animal daily for 15 days was active. When administered to rats at a dose of 170.0 mg/animal showed weak activity and active at a dose of 510.0 mg/animal[N14164].

CNS depressant activity. Methanol extract of dried seeds, administered intraperitoneally to mice at a dose of 25.0 mg/kg was active[T10448].

Conditioning avoidance response decrease. Methanol extract of dried seeds, administered intraperitoneally to mice at a dose of 150.0 mg/kg was active. Results significant at $P < 0.001$ level[T10448].

Death. Methanol extract, administered intraperitoneally to mice at a dose of 400.0 mg/kg was inactive[T10448].

Diuretic activity. Ethanol/water (1:1) extract of the aerial parts, administered intraperitoneally to rats at a dose of 0.187 mg/kg was inactive. Urine was collected for four hours postdrug from saline-loaded animals[W00374]. Water extract of dried leaves, administered by gastric intubation to rats at a concentration of 2.5% was active. Animals were given water or 2.5% solution of *Syzygium cumini*. Quantity of solution equalled five percent of body weight. Urinary excretion was 59% for controls, and 68% for 2.5% group. No changes in sodium or potassium excretion were found[M21409].

Estrogenic effect. Methanol extract of leaves administered subcutaneously to mice was active[A05970].

Fish poison. Water extract of fresh bark was active, LD_{50} 0.18%[T14676].

Hypoglycemic activity. Ethanol (95%) and water extracts of dried seeds, administered intragastric to rabbits at variable dosage levels were active. Hot water extract administered intragastric to dogs at a dose of 20.0 gm/kg (dry weight of seed) was inactive. At 10.0 gm/kg administered intragastric to rabbits, the extract was active[A14333]. Seeds administered by gastric intubation to rats at doses of 170.0, 240.0, and 510.0 mg/animal daily for fifteen days were active[N14164]. Ethanol/water (1:1) extract of the aerial parts, administered orally to rats at a dose of 250.0 mg/kg was inactive. Less than 30% drop in blood sugar level was observed[W00374]. Hot water extract of dried fruit pulp, administered by gastric intubation to dogs at a dose of 200.0 gm/kg (expressed as dry weight of fruit pulp) was inactive, to rabbits at 50.0 gm/kg was active[A14333]. Water extract of dried fruit and seeds, administered orally to rabbits at a dose of 10.0 mg/kg was active. Drop in blood sugar of 15 mg relative to inert-treated controls indicated positive results[A14379].

Hypotensive activity. Ethanol/water (1:1) extract of dried bark, administered intravenously to dogs at variable dosage levels was inactive[W3022A].

Hypothermic activity. Ethanol/water (1:1) extract of the aerial parts, administered intraperitoneally to mice at a dose of 0.375 mg/kg was inactive[W00374]. Methanol extract of dried seeds, administered intraperitoneally to mice at a dose of 50.0 mg/kg was active. Results significant at $P < 0.001$ level[T10448].

Leukocyte migration inhibition. Chloroform extract of dried seeds, administered intraperitoneally to rats at a dose of 50.0 mg/kg was active vs carrageenin-induced pleurisy[M23489].

Molluscicidal activity. Ethanol (95%) and water extracts at concentrations of 10,000 ppm were inactive on *Biomphalaria glabrata* and *Biomphalaria straminea*[W02949]. Water saturated with essential oil of fresh leaves at a concentration of 1:10 was inactive on *Biomphalaria glabrata*[T07475].

Natriuretic activity. Water extract of dried leaves, administered by gastric intubation to rats at a concentration of 2.5% was inactive. Animals were given water or 2.5% solution of *Syzygium cumini*. Quantity of solution equalled 5% of body weight. Urinary excretion was 59% for controls and 68% for 2.5% group. No changes in sodium or potassium excretion were found[M21409].

Nematocidal activity. Decoction of a commercial sample of bark at a concentration of 10.0 mg/ml was inactive on *Toxocara canis*[M26175]. Water and methanol extracts of dried seeds at concentrations of 5.0 and 1.0 mg/ml, respectively, were inactive on *Toxacara canis*[M28316].

Plaque formation suppressant. Water, methanol and methanol/water (1:1) extracts of a commercial sample of bark were active on *Streptococcus mutans* with IC_{50} of 260.0, 120.0 and 380.0 mcg/ml respectively[T11789].

Polygalacturonase inhibition. Hot water extract of bark showed weak activity. Hot water extract of leaves was active[A07091].

Prostaglandin inhibition. Meth-anol extract of dried seeds administered intraperitoneally to rats was active vs PGE-1-induced pedal edema[M19921].

Protease (HIV) inhibition. Water extract of dried bark at a dose of 200.0 mcg/ml showed weak activity, the methanol extract was active[K21241].

Protopectinase inhibition. Hot water extract of bark was inactive. Hot water extract of leaves was active[A07091].

Semen coagulation. Ethanol/water (1:1) extract of the aerial parts at a concentration of 2.0% was inactive on rat semen[W00374].

Skeletal muscle relaxant effect. Methanol extract of dried seeds, administered intraperitoneally to mice at a dose of 100.0 mg/kg was active vs Rotarod test. Results significant at $P < 0.02$ level[T10448].

Spermicidal effect. Ethanol/water (1:1) extract of the aerial parts was inactive on rat sperm[W00374].

Spontaneous activity reduction. Methanol extract of dried seeds, administered intraperitoneally to mice at a dose of 25.0 mg/kg was active. Results significant at $P < 0.001$ level[T10448].

Toxic effect. Ethanol/water (1:1) extract of dried stembark, administered by gastric intubation and subcutaneously to mice at doses of 10.0 gm/kg (dry weight of stembark) were inactive[R00001].

Toxicity assessment. Ethanol (95%) extract of dried seeds, when administered intravenously to mice LD_{50} was 0.4 gm/kg and 4.0 gm/kg with intragastric administration[A14331]. Ethanol/water (1:1) extract of the aerial parts, administered intraperitoneally to mice showed a LD_{50} of 0.75 gm/kg[W00374].

Weight increase. Powdered commercial sample of seeds, administered by gastric intubation to rats at a dose of 53.2 mg/kg was active. Animals were dosed daily for one week[M27423].

27 | Tamarindus indica

L.

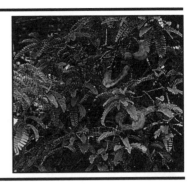

Common Names

Ajagbon	Nigeria	Tamarind	Bangladesh
Ambliki	India	Tamarind	Guyana
Amli	Fiji	Tamarind	India
Ambali	India	Tamarind	Indonesia
Asam jawa	Indonesia	Tamarind	Japan
Asam jawa	Malaysia	Tamarind	West Indies
Asem	Indonesia	Tame tamarind	West Indies
Cheench	India	Tamarinde	Guinea
Cinca	India	Tamarindo	Canary Islands
Dakhar	Senegal	Tamarindo	Cuba
Hamer	Saudi Arabia	tamarindo	Guatemala
Icheku oyibo	Nigeria	Tamarindo	Indonesia
Imli	Fiji	Tamarindo	Madagascar
Imli	India	Tamarindo	Nicaragua
Kaju asam	Indonesia	Tamarindo	Peru
Ma khaam	Thailand	Tamarindo	Puerto Rico
Makham	Thailand	Tamarindo	Brazil
Manhan	China	Tamarini	Guinea
Mkwaju	Tanzania	Tamparanu	Nicaragua
Ntemi	Guinea	Tamrand	Nicaragua
Ntomi	Guinea	Tateli	India
Pokok asam jawa	Malaysia	Tetul	India
Slim	Nicaragua	Timer hendi	Morocco
Tamarin	Rodrigues Islands	Tombi	Guinea
Tamarin des indes	West Indies	Tombinyi	Guinea
Tamarind	West Indies	Tsaniya	Nigeria

BOTANICAL DESCRIPTION

A large tree of the LEGUMINOSAE family, up to 30 meters high, having spreading branches; bark brownish-gray; flaked. Leaves are even-pinnate, consisting of 10–18 pairs of small leaflets, rather closed together; petioles and rachis 5–12 cm long; leaflets oblong; 8–30 by 3–9 mm; opposite, pink or reddish when young, membranous, glabrous, apex obtuse or rounded, base unequal. Inflorescence is in terminal raceme, yellowish-orange or pale green;

From: Medicinal Plants of the World *By: Ivan A. Ross Humana Press Inc., Totowa, NJ*

consisting of calyx-tube narrow turbinate, with four imbricate segments, one cm long; petals three, unequal, upper cordate, about one cm long, two lateral ones, narrowed towards the base; fertile stamens three, base connate; ovary linear, about seven mm long, pubescent, on a stalk adnate to the calyx-tube. Pods are oblong, slightly curved, 5–15 by 1–2.5 cm, reddish brown. Seed is glossy, dark brown, embedded in a thick, sticky and acid brown pulp.

ORIGIN AND DISTRIBUTION

Native of tropical Africa, at present pan-tropic. It is cultivated for the edible fruits and as ornamental and shade tree.

TRADITIONAL MEDICINAL USES

Brazil. Decoction of dried fruit is taken orally for fevers[K07977].

Canary Islands. Dried fruit is eaten as a choleretic[T15880].

China. Fresh fruit is used as a food[T09391].

Colombia. Hot water extract of dried fruit is taken orally as an abortive[T15375].

Dominican Republic. water extract of dried leaves is taken orally to treat liver complaints[K23019].

Fiji. Dried fruit pulp is taken orally for sore throat and diarrhea. Dried leaves in a poultice with mustard oil is applied on the affected area for sprains. For eye troubles, leaves soaked in water is applied as a poultice. Infusion of dried bark, fruit and leaves is taken orally for piles. Infusion of dried fruit is taken orally to invoke vomiting[T10632].

Guatemala. Hot water extract of dried fruit is taken orally as a sudorofic, febrifuge, for urinary tract infections and infections of the skin and mucosa; externally for skin eruptions and erysipelas[T15445]. Hot water extract of dried fruit pulp is used for ringworm and skin fungal diseases[M27151].

Guinea. Water extract of bark is taken orally by women after childbirth, and together with the bark of *Afzelia africana*, as a remedy for troubles during pregnancy[A00708].

India. Externally bark is used as an astringent. Orally it is used as a tonic, febrifuge and the ash obtained by heating the bark with salt in an earthen pot is mixed with water and taken orally for colic, indigestion, as a gargle for sore throat, and as a mouthwash for apthous sores[K23896]. Hot water extract of dried bark is taken orally for paralysis and as a tonic[T09230]. Fruit juice mixed with *Calotropis gigantea* latex is taken orally to relieve menstrual pains[M27166]. Hot water extract of dried leaves is taken orally for inflammatory swellings and for urinary discharges[T09230]. Leaf juice is taken orally to treat encephalitis. four drops of leaf juice with three drops of latex from *Caltropis gigantea* are taken once a day for eight days. For rheumatic arthritis, leaf juice, latex of *Calotropis gigantea*, goat milk, and sesame oil is applied externally[K11282].

Indonesia. Water extract of fruit is taken orally as an abortifacient[A00710].

Ivory Coast. Hot water extract of leaf and root is taken orally to treat sleeping sickness. Decoction together with leaves and roots of *Afzelia africana* and ficus species is drunk and used as a vapor bath[W00799].

Madagascar. Hot water extract of trunk bark is taken orally for amenorrhea[W02855].

Malaysia. Hot water extract of root mixed with several other plants is taken orally for amenorrhea[A04587].

Nigeria. Fresh leaves ground along with those of *Prosopis africana* in equal proportions is taken with water orally to treat malaria fever. Cold water and 1.5 teaspoonful of crushed potash are added to 1–2 handfuls of leaves and left until an extract is obtained. The extract is used as a laxative[K08933]. Hot water extract of the dried bark an husk of the pods together with the leaves and bark of *Diospyros mespiliformis* is drunk for leprosy[T01679].

Peru. Hot water extract of dried fruitpeel is taken orally as a laxative[T15323].

Saudi Arabia. Dried fruit is taken orally medicinally[W04179].

Senegal. Hot water extract of dried stem bark is taken orally medicinally[T09739]. Externally, it is used as a cicatrizant[T12145].

Sudan. Dried fruit pulp is taken orally as a purgative, for malaria and for bacterial infections[H11898].

Tanzania. Decoction of dried leaves is taken orally to treat malaria[K15971]. Decoction of hot water extract of dried bark and root is drunk together with that of *Stereospermum kunthianum* for the treatment of leprosy[T01679]. Decoction of root is taken orally for distended painful abdomen and for dysentery. Juice from fresh leaves is taken for bloody diarrhea[T16181].

Thailand. Hot water extract of dried fruit pulp is taken orally as an expectorant. Hot water extract of dried leaves is taken orally as a cathartic. Hot water extract of dried seed is taken orally as an anthelmintic[W03804].

West Indies. Fruit pulp is taken orally as a laxative[T00701].

CHEMICAL CONSTITUENTS

(ppm unless otherwise indicated)

3-4-Dihydroxy phenyl acetate, Sd
Acetic acid, Fr
Alkylthiazoles, Fr
Alpha humulene, Fr Pu 2.0%
Alpha murolene, Fr Pu
Alpha Pinene, Fr Pu
Alpha copaene, Fr Pu 0.6%
Alpha oxo-glutaric acid, Fr, Lf, Fl
Alpha terpineol, Fr
Arabinose, Fr
Arachidic acid, Sd Ol
Aromadendrene, Fr Pu 90%
Ascorbic acid, Fr 24-585
Ascorbic acid, Lf 600
Ash, Fl 3.5%; Sd 2.5-3.2%
Ash, Lf 2.6-7.3%; Fr 2.7-3.94%
Behenic acid, Sd Ol
Benzoic acid,3-4-dihydroxy methyl ester, Sd
Beta caryophyllene, Fr Pu 0.5%
Beta pinene, Fr Pu
Beta carotene, Fl 10
Beta carotene, Fr 0-1
Beta carotene, Lf 2-110
Beta elemene, Fr Pu 0.3%; Sd

Calcium pectate, Fr
Calcium tartrate, Fr
Calcium, Fl 2,650
Calcium, Fr 698-2,829
Calcium, Lf 0.1-2.3%
Calcium, Sd 1,210
Carbohydrate, Fl 75%
Carbohydrate, Fr 62.5-92.5%
Carbohydrate, Lf 70.6-75.0%
Carbohydrate, Sd 65.1-74.0%
Carvacrol, Fr Pu 0.5%
Cellulose, Fr 1.8-3.2%
Chlorine, Lf 940
Cinnamaldehyde, Fr
Citric acid, Fr
Copper, Lf 21
D-Arabinose, Sd
D-Galactose, Sd
D-Glucose, Sd
D-Xylose, Sd
Epi-catechin, Sd
Ethyl-cinnamate, Fr
Fat, Fl 9%
Fat, Fr 0.3-0.9%
Fat, Lf 3.6-4.4%
Fat, Sd 6.0-7.4%
Fiber, Fl 6%
Fiber, Fr 3.1-7.4%
Fiber, Lf 5.7-18.6%
Fiber, Sd 0.7-4.3%
Fructose, Fr 9-12%
Furfural, Fr Pu 3.0%
Galactose, Fr
Galacturonic acid, Fr
Gamma cadinene, Fr Pu 0.4%
Geranial, EO
Geraniol, EO
Glucose, Fr 21-28%
Glyoxylic acid, Fr, Lf, Fl
HCN, Pl
Hordenine, Bk
Invert sugars, Fr 30-40%
Iron, Fl 70
Iron, Fr 13-109
Iron, Lf 52-88
Isoorientin, Lf 10
Isovitexin, Lf 5
Lactic acid, Fr
Lauric acid, Sd Ol
Lignoceric acid, Sd Ol
Limonene, Fr
Linalool, Fr Pu 0.10%

Linoleic acid, Fr 590-860
Linoleic acid, Sd Ol 2.7-3.4%
Linolenic acid, Sd Ol
Lysine, Fr 1,390-2,026
Magnesium, Fr 920-1,341
Magnesium, Lf 710
Malic acid, Fr 1%
Malic acid, Lf 1.5%
Methionine, Fr 140-204
Methoxyl, Fr
Methyl glutamic acid, Sp
Methyl salicylate, Fr
Methyleneglutamic acid, Sp
Methyleneglutamine, Sp
Mucilage, Sd
MUFA, Fr 1,810-2,640
Myrcene, Fr Pu
Myristic acid, Fr 70-102
N-Octadecane, Fr Pu 0.15%
Niacin, Fl 60
Niacin, Fr 16-33
Niacin, Lf 66
Oleic acid, Fr 1,810-2,638
Oleic acid, Sd 1.6-2.0%
Orientin, Lf 12.5
Oxalic acid, Fr
Oxalic acid, Lf 1,960
Oxaloacetic acid, Fr, Lf, Fl
Oxalosuccinic acid, Fr, Lf, Fl
P-Cresol, Fr
Palmitic acid, Fr 1,680-2,449; Sd Ol
Pantothenic acid, Fr 1-2
Pectin, Fr 2.0-2.5%; Sd
Pentosan, Fr 4.2-4.8%
Phenol, Fr
Phlobotannin, Sd
Phosphorus, Fl 2,200
Phosphorus, Fr 1,130-1,647
Phosphorus, Lf 1,000-2,281
Phosphorus, Sd 2,370
Pipecolinic acid, Fr
Piperitone, Fr
Potassium , Fl 1.27%
Potassium, Fr 0.6-1.5%
Potassium, Lf 1.197%
Potassium oxide, Fr 1,032-7,654
Proline, Fr
Protein, Fl 12.5%
Protein, Fr 2.8-11.7%
Protein, Lf 14.1-22.4%
Protein, Sd 17.1-20.1%
PUFA, Fr 590-860

Pyridoxine, Fr 1-2
Quinic acid, Fr
Riboflavin, Fl 6
Riboflavin, Fr 1-3
Riboflavin, Lf 1-5
Safrole, Fr
SFA, Fr 2,720-3,965
Sodium, Fl 250
Sodium, Fr 49-743
Sodium, Lf 351
Stearic acid, Fr 600-874; Sd Ol
Succinic acid, Fr
Sulfur, Lf 630
Tamarind xyloglucan, Fr
Tamarindienal, Fr Pu
Tamarindus galactoxyloglucan, Sd
Tannin, Bk 7%
Tannin, Sd
Tartaric acid, Fr 8-18%
Tartaric acid, Lf 12-28%
Thiamin, Fl 4; Lf 4; Fr 2-9
Tryptophan, Fr 180-262
Uronic acid, Fr
Vitexin, Lf 28.5
Water, Fr 31.4%

PHARMACOLOGICAL ACTIVITIES AND CLINICAL TRIALS

Allergenic activity. Powder of a commercial sample of fruit showed weak activity. Reactions to patch tests occurred most commonly in patients who were regularly exposed to the substance, or who had already had dermatitis on the fingertips. Previously unexposed patients has few reactions, i.e., no irritant reactions[M17058].

Antibacterial activity. Acetone extract of commercial sample of fruit on agar plate was active on *Salmonella typhimurium*. The ethanol (70%) extract was active on *Bacillus cereus, Bacillus megaterium, Escherichia coli, Pseudomonas aeruginosa, Salmonella typhimurium, Staphylococcus albus*, and *Staphylococcus aureus*[T06729]. Tincture of dried fruit at a concentration of 30.0 microliters/disc on agar plate was active on *Escherichia coli*. Extract of 10 gm dried fruit in 100 ml ethanol was used[T15445]. Ethanol (95%) and hot water extracts of dried rootbark on agar plate were inactive on *Escherichia coli* and *Staphylococcus aureus*[W03693]. Ethanol (95%) extract of fruit on agar plate was active on *Bacillus subtilis, Escherichia coli, Salmonella typhosa, Staphylococcus aureus*, and *Vibrio cholera*[W00232]. Ethanol (95%) extract of dried fruit on agar plate was active on *Escherichia coli* and inactive on *Staphylococcus aureus*. The hot water extract was active on *Escherichia coli* and equivocal on *Staphylococcus aureus*. Ethanol (95%) extract of dried leaves on agar plate was active on *Staphylococcus aureus* and inactive on *Escherichia coli*; hot water extract was active on *Staphylococcus aureus* and *Escherichia coli*[W03693]. Methanol extract of dried stem bark at a concentration of 10.0 mg/ml was active on several gram negative organisms and inactive on several gram positive organisms. A concentration of 15.0 mg/ml was active on *Sarcina lutea*[T09739].

Antifungal activity. Acetone and ethanol (95%) extracts of dried leaves at concentrations of 50% on agar plate were inactive on *Neurospora crassa*; the water extract was active. Acetone and water extracts of dried bark at concentrations of 50% on agar plate were inactive, and ethanol (95%) at a concentration of 50% extract was active on *Neurospora crassa*. Acetone and water extracts of dried stem at a concentration of 50% were inactive and ethanol (95%) extract at a concentration of 50% on agar plate was active on *Neurospora crassa*[T08589]. Ethanol (70%) extract of commercial sample of fruit on agar plate was active on several fungi[T06729]. Ethanol (95%) extract of fruit on agar plate was active on *Trichophyton mentagrophytes* and *Trichophyton rubrum*[W00232]. Ethanol/water (1:1) extract of dried fruit at a concentration of 333.0 mg/ml (expressed as dry weight of plant) on agar plate was active on *Aspergillus fumigatus, Aspergillus niger, Penicillium digitatum, Rhizopus nigricans*, and *Trichophyton mentagrophytes*. At concentrations of 333.0 and 500

mg/ml the extract was inactive on *Aspergillus niger, Botrytis cinerea*[T16238]. At 500 mg/ml the extract was active on *Aspergillus fumigatus, Fusarium oxysporum, Penicillium digitatum, Rhizopus nigricans, Trichophyton mentagrophytes*, and inactive on *Botrytis cinerea*[T12725]. Hot water extract of dried fruit pulp at a concentration of 1.0 ml in broth culture was active on *Microsporum canis, Epidermophyton floccosum, Trichophyton mentagrophytes* var. granulare and inactive on *Microsporum gypseum* and *Trichophyton mentagrophytes* var. algodonosa[M27151]. Water extract of fresh leaves on agar plate produced strong activity on *Ustilago nuda*[T08889].

Antihepatotoxic effect. Hot water extract of dried leaves at a concentration of 1.0 mg/plate in cell culture was active on hepatocytes when measured by leakage of LDH and ASAT[K23019].

Antilithic activity. Dried fruit pulp ingested by human adults at a dose of 3.0 gm/day was inactive. Tamarind intake did not affect crystallization rates of calcium or oxalate in urine samples from normal or stone-forming subjects[M20685].

Antimalarial activity. Ethyl acetate and petroleum ether extracts of dried leaves were active on *Plasmodium falciparum*. ED_{50} 70.0 and 90.0 mcg/ml, respectively. The ethanol (95%) and water extracts were inactive ED_{50} >500 mcg/ml[K15971]. Methanol extract of dried fruit was inactive on *Plasmodium falciparum* vs hypoxanthine uptake by Plasmodia. IC_{50} >499 mcg/ml[M25016].

Antinematodal activity. Water extract of commercial sample of pulp at a concentration of 10.0 mg/ml was inactive, and methanol extract produced weak activity on *Toxacara canis*[M29965].

Antioxidant activity. Methanol extract of fresh seed at a concentration of 0.2 mg/well produced strong activity by thiocyanate assay[K16969].

Antischistosomal activity. Water extract at a concentration of 100.0 ppm was active on *Schistosoma mansoni*[M26095].

Antiviral activity. Ethanol (80%) extract of freeze dried fruit, at variable concentration in cell culture, was equivocal on Herpes virus Type 1; inactive on Adenovirus, Coxsackie B2 virus, Measles virus, Polio virus I and Semlicki-forest virus vs plaque inhibition[T06435]. Ethanol/water (1:1) extract of flowers at a concentration of 50.0 mcg/ml in cell culture produced weak activity on Ranikhet virus[A03335]. Water extract of bark was active on Potato X virus[A03479].

Antiyeast activity. Ethanol/water (1:1) extract of dried fruit at a concentration of 333.0 mg/ml (expressed as dry weight of plant) on agar plate was inactive on *Candida albicans*, *Saccharomyces pastorianus*, and *Candida albicans*[T12725]. Tincture of dried fruit at a concentration of 30.0 microliters/disc on agar plate was inactive on *Candida albicans*. Extract of 10 gm dried fruit in 100 ml ethanol was used[T15445].

Cytotoxic activity. Ethanol/water (1:1) extract of flowers in cell culture was inactive on CA-9KB. ED_{50} >20.0 mcg/ml[A03335].

Diuretic activity. Decoction of dried fruit administered via nasogastric to rats at a dose of 1.0 gm/kg produced strong activity[T15295].

Embryotoxic effect. Ethanol/water (1:1) extract of dried fruit administered to rats by gastric intubation at a dose 100.0 mg/kg was inactive[T05679].

Hepatic mixed function oxidase inhibition. Dried fruit in the ration of rats at a dose of 2.5 mg% was active[M22818].

Hypotensive activity. Hot water extract of dried root, administered intravenously to rats at a dose of 1.0 ml/animal was inactive[M29843].

Juvenile hormone activity. Acetone extract of stem was active[J08616].

Lipid peroxide formation inhibition. Hot water extract of dried leaves at a concentration 1.0 mg/plate in cell culture was active on hepatocytes when monitored by reduction of malonaldehyde[K23019].

Molluscicidal activity. Aqueous slurry (homogenate) of fresh entire plant (fruits, leaves and roots) was inactive on *Lymnaea columella* and *Lymnaea cubensis*. LD_{100} >1M ppm[T04621]. Methanol extract of dried seeds at a concentration of 100.0 ppm was equivocal on *Bulinus globosus*. 10% mortality was observed[T04176]. Water and methanol extracts of dried fruit pulp were active (assayed after 24 hours exposure) on *Bulinus truncatus*. LC_{50} 400.0 ppm and 300.0 ppm, respectively[K07796].

Mutagenic activity. Dried fruit at a concentration of 0.1 mg/plate on agar plate was active on *Salmonella typhimurium* TA1535 and inactive on *S. typhimurium* TA1537, TA1538, and TA98[T16468].

Plant germination inhibition. Chloroform extract of dried leaves produced weak activity vs *Amaranthus spinosus* (20% inhibition). Ethanol (95%) extract at a concentration of 8000 ppm was active vs Allium roots[W02544]. Chloroform extract of dried seeds was active vs *Amaranthus spinosus* (36% inhibition)[T03367].

Polygalacturonase inhibition. Hot water extract of bark was active. Hot water extract of leaves was active[A07091].

Protopectinase inhibition. Hot water extract of bark was inactive[A07091]. Hot water extract of leaves was active[A07091].

Radical scavenging effect. Hot water extract of dried leaves at a concentration of 250.0 mg/liter was active. When measured by decoloration of diphenylpicryl hydroxyl radical solution 57% decoloration was observed[K23019].

Spasmolytic activity. Ethanol (95%) extract of fresh leaves and stem at a concentration of 3.3 ml/liter was active on guinea pig ileum. Water extract, administered intraperitoneally to guinea pig at a concentration of 33.0 ml/liter was active on the ileum[A03360].

Toxicity assessment (quantitative). Ethanol/water (1:1) extract of flowers, when administered orally to mice the maximum tolerated dose was 1.0 gm/kg[A03335].

Vasodilator activity. Ethanol (95%) extract of fresh leaves and stem, at a concentration of 0.33 ml/liter was active on the isolated hind quarter of rat[A03360].

Cross Reference

Common name	Country	Latin binomial
A'aboca	West Indies	*Persea americana*
Aainud-dik	India	*Abrus precatorius*
Aaku pero	Buka Island	*Cassia alata*
Aam	Fiji	*Mangifera indica*
Aam	India	*Mangifera indica*
Aamp	Nepal	*Mangifera indica*
Aanabahe-hindi	India	*Carica papaya*
Aanp	Nepal	*Mangifera indica*
Ababau	Nicaragua	*Carica papaya*
Abacateiro	Brazil	*Persea americana*
Abacateiro	Cuba	*Persea americana*
Abas	Guam	*Psidium guajava*
Abuya	Congo-Brazzaville	*Hibiscus sabdariffa*
Acafrao	Brazil	*Curcuma longa*
Ach man	Guatemala	*Lantana camara*
Acibar	Argentina	*Aloe vera*
Afia	Guinea	*Persea americana*
African cucumber	USA	*Momordica charantia*
Agin ghas	Fiji	*Cymbopogon citratus*
Aglio	Italy	*Allium sativum*
Aguacate	Argentina	*Persea americana*
Aguacate	Belize	*Persea americana*
Aguacate	Brazil	*Persea americana*
Aguacate	Colombia	*Persea americana*
Aguacate	Cuba	*Persea americana*
Aguacate	Guatemala	*Persea americana*
Aguacate	Honduras	*Persea americana*
Aguacate	Mexico	*Persea americana*
Aguacate	Nicaragua	*Persea americana*
Aguacate	Panama	*Persea americana*
Aguacate	Paraguay	*Persea americana*

From: Medicinal Plants of the World *By: Ivan A. Ross Humana Press Inc., Totowa, NJ*

Common name	Country	Latin binomial
Aguacate	Puerto Rico	*Persea americana*
Aguacatero	Canary Islands	*Persea americana*
Aguacatillo	Mexico	*Persea americana*
Aguate	Peru	*Persea americana*
Agucatillo	Cuba	*Persea americana*
Agya ghas	Fiji	*Cymbopogon citratus*
Ahuacaquahuitl	Mexico	*Persea americana*
Aie	France	*Allium sativum*
Aikavitu	Nicaragua	*Manihot esculenta*
Ail	France	*Allium sativum*
Ail	Rodrigues Islands	*Allium sativum*
Ail	Tunisia	*Allium sativum*
Ainskati	India	*Catharanthus roseus*
Ajagbon	Nigeria	*Syzygium cumini*
Ajo	Guatemala	*Allium sativum*
Ajo	Nicaragua	*Allium sativum*
Ajo	Peru	*Allium sativum*
Akapulko	Philippines	*Cassia alata*
Akapulko	West Africa	*Cassia alata*
Akashneem	India	*Allium sativum*
Akoria	West Africa	*Cassia alata*
Alfonso mango	India	*Mangifera indica*
Alkushi	Pakistan	*Macuna pruriens*
Alkusi	India	*Macuna pruriens*
Alla naeredu	India	*Syzygium cumini*
Alligator pear	West Indies	*Persea americana*
Aloe	Argentina	*Aloe vera*
Aloe	Bimini	*Aloe vera*
Aloe	Rodrigues Islands	*Aloe vera*
Aloe	USA	*Aloe vera*
Aloe	Venezuela	*Aloe vera*
Aloe cactus	Cook Islands	*Aloe vera*
Aloes	Argentina	*Aloe vera*
Aloes	Trinidad	*Aloe vera*
Aloes	West Indies	*Aloe vera*
Aloes vrai	Tunisia	*Aloe vera*
Alovis	West Indies	*Aloe vera*
Alubosa elewe	Nigeria	*Allium sativum*
Am	India	*Mangifera indica*
Am	Pakistan	*Mangifera indica*
Amapolo	Nicaragua	*Hibiscus rosa-sinensis*
Amargoso	Philippines	*Momordica charantia*
Amba	Nepal	*Psidium guajava*
Amba	Oman	*Mangifera indica*
Ambliki	India	*Syzygium cumini*

Common name	Country	Latin binomial
American avocado	Mexico	*Persea americana*
American purging nut	South Africa	*Jatropa curcas*
Amita	India	*Carica papaya*
Amli	Fiji	*Syzygium cumini*
Amloniya	Fiji	*Portulaca oleracea*
Amm	India	*Mangifera indica*
Amp	Nepal	*Mangifera indica*
Ampalaya	Philippines	*Momordica charantia*
Ampalaya	USA	*Momordica charantia*
Amra	India	*Mangifera indica*
Amrood	India	*Psidium guajava*
Amrud	Fiji	*Psidium guajava*
Amrut	Fiji	*Psidium guajava*
Amva	India	*Mangifera indica*
Anaha	Nicaragua	*Manihot esculenta*
Anar	Fiji	*Punica granatum*
Anar	India	*Punica granatum*
Anar	Nepal	*Punica granatum*
Anbali	India	*Syzygium cumini*
Andok-ntang	Guinea	*Mangifera indica*
Ango	Brazil	*Curcuma longa*
Ango hina	Brazil	*Curcuma longa*
Antolanagan	Philippines	*Hibiscus rosa-sinensis*
Anyigli	Togo	*Annona muricata*
Apele	Togo	*Annona muricata*
Apple leaf	West Indies	*Annona muricata*
Aquacate	Mexico	*Persea americana*
Aquate	Guatemala	*Persea americana*
Arasa	Paraguay	*Psidium guajava*
Ardhol	Fiji	*Hibiscus rosa-sinensis*
Areglisse	West Indies	*Abrus precatorius*
Aroganan	China	*Hibiscus rosa-sinensis*
Art pumpkin	West Indies	*Momordica charantia*
Aruppu	India	*Lantana camara*
Asabi-e-safr	Arab Country	*Curcuma longa*
Asam jawa	Indonesia	*Syzygium cumini*
Asam jawa	Malaysia	*Syzygium cumini*
Asem	Indonesia	*Syzygium cumini*
Asm	India	*Mangifera indica*
Asorosi	Haiti	*Momordica charantia*
Assorossi	Haiti	*Momordica charantia*
Atay biya	Philippines	*Catharanthus roseus*
Atmagupta	India	*Macuna pruriens*
Auacatl	Mexico	*Persea americana*
Avacado pear	Jamaica	*Persea americana*

Common name	*Country*	*Latin binomial*
Avea	Arab Countries	*Curcuma longa*
Avispa	Nicaragua	*Hibiscus rosa-sinensis*
Avocado	Argentina	*Persea americana*
Avocado	Australia	*Persea americana*
Avocado	Cuba	*Persea americana*
Avocado	Indonesia	*Persea americana*
Avocado	Israel	*Persea americana*
Avocado	Jamaica	*Persea americana*
Avocado	Japan	*Persea americana*
Avocado	Mexico	*Persea americana*
Avocado	Nicaragua	*Persea americana*
Avocado	Sri Lanka	*Persea americana*
Avocado	Trinidad	*Persea americana*
Avocado	Turkey	*Persea americana*
Avocado	West Indies	*Persea americana*
Avocado pear	Indonesia	*Persea americana*
Avocado pear	Israel	*Persea americana*
Avocado pear	Jamaica	*Persea americana*
Avocado pear	South Africa	*Persea americana*
Avocat	Mauritius	*Persea americana*
Avocat	Rodrigues Islands	*Persea americana*
Awaqa'pi l'ta	Argentina	*Cymbopogon citratus*
Awunwon	West Africa	*Cassia alata*
Ayengogo	Guinea	*Cassia alata*
Azeitonia	Brazil	*Syzygium cumini*
Ba dau dai	Indonesia	*Moringa pterygosperma*
Ba dau me	Vietnam	*Jatropa curcas*
Badie	Ivory Coast	*Carica papaya*
Bagbherenda	Fiji	*Jatropa curcas*
Bai nicagi	Guinea	*Cassia alata*
Baidhok	India	*Macuna pruriens*
Bake	Ivory Coast	*Carica papaya*
Bakua	Guinea	*Cassia alata*
Baldroegas	Madeira	*Portulaca oleracea*
Balilang	Malaysia	*Cassia alata*
Balsam pear	Australia	*Momordica charantia*
Balsam pear	Thailand	*Momordica charantia*
Balsam pear	USA	*Momordica charantia*
Balsam spple	West Indies	*Momordica charantia*
Balsambirne	Bahamas	*Momordica charantia*
Balsamina	India	*Momordica charantia*
Balsamina	Peru	*Momordica charantia*
Balsamino	Panama	*Momordica charantia*
Ban kareli	India	*Momordica charantia*
Banban	Papua-New Guinea	*Hibiscus rosa-sinensis*

Common name	Country	Latin binomial
Banjiro	Brazil	*Psidium guajava*
Banlasun	Nepal	*Allium sativum*
Banziro	Brazil	*Psidium guajava*
Baquitche	Guinea-Bissau	*Hibiscus sabdariffa*
Barajo	Guatemala	*Cassia alata*
Baraloniya	Fiji	*Portulaca oleracea*
Baramasiya	India	*Momordica charantia*
Barbados aloe	Nepal	*Aloe vera*
Barbados aloe	USA	*Aloe vera*
Barbados aloe	West Indies	*Aloe vera*
Barbados purging nut	South Africa	*Jatropa curcas*
Barbin	Qatar	*Portulaca oleracea*
Barbir	Qatar	*Portulaca oleracea*
Barbof	Senegal	*Momordica charantia*
Basap	Senegal	*Hibiscus sabdariffa*
Bedon-al-babo	Guinea-Bissau	*Carica papaya*
Belaselika	Nicaragua	*Manihot esculenta*
Beldroega	Brazil	*Portulaca oleracea*
Beldroegas	Madeira	*Portulaca oleracea*
Beleda	Borneo	*Annona muricata*
Belki	India	*Macuna pruriens*
Ben aile	New Caledonia	*Moringa pterygosperma*
Ben aile	Senegal	*Moringa pterygosperma*
Ben nut tree	Mauritius	*Moringa pterygosperma*
Ben nut tree	West Indies	*Moringa pterygosperma*
Benambo	Guinea-Bissau	*Abrus precatorius*
Bepaia	Guinea-Bissau	*Carica papaya*
Besar	Nepal	*Curcuma longa*
Bhada	India	*Cyperus rotundus*
Bhoomi amalaki	India	*Phyllanthus niruri*
Bhoostrina	India	*Cymbopogon citratus*
Bhui amla	Bangladesh	*Phyllanthus niruri*
Bhui-amla	India	*Phyllanthus niruri*
Bhuianvalah	India	*Phyllanthus niruri*
Bhuimy-amali	East Indies	*Phyllanthus niruri*
Bhuin-amla	Pakistan	*Phyllanthus niruri*
Bhumyamalaki	India	*Phyllanthus niruri*
Bi ni da zugu	Nigeria	*Jatropa curcas*
Big purging nut	South Africa	*Jatropa curcas*
Big sage	West Indies	*Lantana camara*
Bilauti	Nepal	*Psidium guajava*
Billaganneru	India	*Catharanthus roseus*
Bisap	Senegal	*Hibiscus sabdariffa*
Bitter cucumber	Thailand	*Momordica charantia*
Bitter gourd	Fiji	*Momordica charantia*

Common name	Country	Latin binomial
Bitter gourd	India	*Momordica charantia*
Bitter gourd	Thailand	*Momordica charantia*
Bitter gourd	USA	*Momordica charantia*
Bitter melon	USA	*Momordica charantia*
Bitter pear melon	Taiwan	*Momordica charantia*
Black reed	USA	*Cymbopogon citratus*
Black vomit nut	South Africa	*Jatropa curcas*
Bo-amb	India	*Mangifera indica*
Boa noite	Brazil	*Catharanthus roseus*
Bobobo	Ivory Coast	*Momordica charantia*
Bofre	Ivory Coast	*Carica papaya*
Bonboye	West Indies	*Lantana camara*
Bondio	Senegal	*Hibiscus sabdariffa*
Boppai	India	*Carica papaya*
Boppayi	India	*Carica papaya*
Borimak	Nicaragua	*Psidium guajava*
Botuje	Nigeria	*Jatropa curcas*
Bowen mango	USA	*Mangifera indica*
Brede mourounge	Rodrigues Islands	*Moringa pterygosperma*
Bredo de porco	Brazil	*Portulaca oleracea*
Broomweed	Nicaragua	*Momordica charantia*
Brown man's fancy	West Indies	*Catharanthus roseus*
Buah betek	Malaysia	*Carica papaya*
Buah ketela	Malaysia	*Carica papaya*
Buah papaya	Malaysia	*Carica papaya*
Buckbead	Guyana	*Abrus precatorius*
Budibaga	Senegal	*Carica papaya*
Bugoyab	Senegal	*Psidium guajava*
Buite	Colombia	*Persea americana*
Buklut-ul-hakima	India	*Portulaca oleracea*
Bumango	Senegal	*Mangifera indica*
Bumpapa	Senegal	*Carica papaya*
Bunchberry	India	*Lantana camara*
Bunga raya	Malaysia	*Hibiscus rosa-sinensis*
Bunga taya ayam	Guatemala	*Lantana camara*
Bunja raja raja	Malaysia	*Aloe vera*
Bupapay	Senegal	*Carica papaya*
Burra-lonia	India	*Portulaca oleracea*
Butter pear	Nicaragua	*Persea americana*
Caca poule	Dominica	*Catharanthus roseus*
Cago	Nepal	*Curcuma longa*
Camara	Brazil	*Lantana camara*
Camara	Canary Islands	*Lantana camara*
Cambara de espinto	Guatemala	*Lantana camara*
Cana limon	Canary Islands	*Cymbopogon citratus*

Common name	Country	Latin binomial
Candelabra bush	Thailand	*Cassia alata*
Candle tree	Malaysia	*Cassia alata*
Cane peas senna	West Indies	*Phyllanthus niruri*
Cantal muluumg	Somalia	*Jatropa curcas*
Capii cedron	Paraguay	*Cymbopogon citratus*
Capim cidrao	Brazil	*Cymbopogon citratus*
Capim santo	Brazil	*Cymbopogon citratus*
Caprika	West Indies	*Momordica charantia*
Carailla	Guyana	*Momordica charantia*
Cariaquita	Colombia	*Lantana camara*
Cariaquito	West Indies	*Lantana camara*
Carilla	India	*Momordica charantia*
Carilla	USA	*Momordica charantia*
Carilla	West Indies	*Momordica charantia*
Carraquillo	Colombia	*Lantana camara*
Carry-me seed	Fiji	*Phyllanthus niruri*
Carry-me seed	West Indies	*Phyllanthus niruri*
Cassava	Brazil	*Manihot esculenta*
Cassava	Nicaragua	*Manihot esculenta*
Cassava	Nigeria	*Manihot esculenta*
Cassava	Tanzania	*Manihot esculenta*
Cassava	Thailand	*Manihot esculenta*
Cassava	Venezuela	*Manihot esculenta*
Cassava	West Indies	*Manihot esculenta*
Cassava	Zaire	*Manihot esculenta*
Cebilhoums	France	*Allium sativum*
Cerasee	Bahamas	*Momordica charantia*
Cerasee	Bimini	*Momordica charantia*
Cerasee	Jamaica	*Momordica charantia*
Cerasee	Trinidad	*Momordica charantia*
Cerasee	West Indies	*Momordica charantia*
Chamber bitters	West Indies	*Phyllanthus niruri*
Chamorro	Guam	*Mangifera indica*
Chancapiedra	Peru	*Phyllanthus niruri*
Chanoti	Pakistan	*Abrus precatorius*
Chashm-i-kharosh	Pakistan	*Abrus precatorius*
Chatilla	Guatemala	*Catharanthus roseus*
Chavelita	Peru	*Catharanthus roseus*
Chaywala ghas	Fiji	*Cymbopogon citratus*
Cheench	India	*Syzygium cumini*
Chemparathy	India	*Hibiscus rosa-sinensis*
Chibda	India	*Carica papaya*
Chichihualxochitl	Mexico	*Carica papaya*
Chickweed	West Indies	*Phyllanthus niruri*
Chido	India	*Cyperus rotundus*

Common name	Country	Latin binomial
China rosa	Kuwait	*Hibiscus rosa-sinensis*
China rose	India	*Hibiscus rosa-sinensis*
China rose plant	India	*Hibiscus rosa-sinensis*
Chinese hibiscus	Nepal	*Hibiscus rosa-sinensis*
Chirbhita	India	*Carica papaya*
Chirmu	India	*Abrus precatorius*
Chirukattli	India	*Aloe vera*
Choon kin phee	Malaysia	*Hibiscus rosa-sinensis*
Chou blak	Haiti	*Hibiscus rosa-sinensis*
Christmas blossom	Nicaragua	*Cassia alata*
Chuan chin pi	Malaysia	*Hibiscus rosa-sinensis*
Chuan chin pi	Vietnam	*Hibiscus rosa-sinensis*
Chuen kan pi	Malaysia	*Hibiscus rosa-sinensis*
Chum het thet	Thailand	*Cassia alata*
Chum ngay	Indonesia	*Moringa pterygosperma*
Chumhet thai	Thailand	*Cassia alata*
Chumhet thet	Thailand	*Cassia alata*
Chumhet yai	Thailand	*Cassia alata*
Chunhati	India	*Abrus precatorius*
Cidreirarana	Brazil	*Lantana camara*
Cigu	Thailand	*Macuna pruriens*
Cinca	India	*Syzygium cumini*
Citronella	India	*Cymbopogon citratus*
Citronella	USA	*Cymbopogon citratus*
Citronelle	Rodrigues Islands	*Cymbopogon citratus*
Co cu	Malaysia	*Cyperus rotundus*
Coci	Zaire	*Manihot esculenta*
Common lantana	China	*Lantana camara*
Common papaw	India	*Carica papaya*
Common purslane	Madeira	*Portulaca oleracea*
Common purslane	USA	*Portulaca oleracea*
Concombre-coolis	West Indies	*Momordica charantia*
Condiamor	Belize	*Momordica charantia*
Condiamor	Guatemala	*Momordica charantia*
Congorca	Brazil	*Catharanthus roseus*
Consumption bush	West Indies	*Catharanthus roseus*
Coquinho	Madeira	*Cyperus rotundus*
Coraillie	West Indies	*Momordica charantia*
Corosol	West Indies	*Annona muricata*
Corossol	Dominica	*Annona muricata*
Corossol	Rodrigues Islands	*Annona muricata*
Cortalinde	Guinea-Bissau	*Cassia alata*
Coupie	Dominica	*Portulaca oleracea*
Coupie	West Indies	*Portulaca oleracea*
Cowhage	India	*Macuna pruriens*

Common name	Country	Latin binomial
Cowhage	Nepal	*Macuna pruriens*
Cowitch	Guyana	*Macuna pruriens*
Cowitch	Trinidad	*Macuna pruriens*
Cowitch vine	Virgin Islands	*Macuna pruriens*
Crab's eye	India	*Abrus precatorius*
Crab's eye vine	Thailand	*Abrus precatorius*
Crab's stone	India	*Abrus precatorius*
Crab-eye berries	India	*Abrus precatorius*
Crabs eyes	India	*Abrus precatorius*
Creole senna	Virgin Islands	*Phyllanthus niruri*
Croupier	French Guiana	*Portulaca oleracea*
Cu gau	Malaysia	*Cyperus rotundus*
Cu gau	Vietnam	*Cyperus rotundus*
Cuasquito	Guatemala	*Lantana camara*
Cucarda	Peru	*Hibiscus rosa-sinensis*
Cuencas de oro	Puerto Rico	*Lantana camara*
Cun de amor	Puerto Rico	*Momordica charantia*
Cundeamor	Brazil	*Momordica charantia*
Cundeamor	Cuba	*Momordica charantia*
Cundeamor	Mexico	*Momordica charantia*
Cundeamor	Puerto Rico	*Momordica charantia*
Cundeamor	USA	*Momordica charantia*
Cura	Cuba	*Persea americana*
Curacao aloe	West Indies	*Aloe vera*
Curcuma	Iran	*Curcuma longa*
Curcuma	Nepal	*Curcuma longa*
Curo	Colombia	*Persea americana*
Cussu	India	*Macuna pruriens*
Custard apple	Rodrigues Islands	*Annona muricata*
Cuta	Mexico	*Jatropa curcas*
Cutcha	Guinea-Bissau	*Hibiscus sabdariffa*
Da-tha-lwon	India	*Moringa pterygosperma*
Dadima	India	*Punica granatum*
Dadmardan	India	*Cassia alata*
Dadmurdan	Fiji	*Cassia alata*
Dadrughna	India	*Cassia alata*
Daintha	India	*Moringa pterygosperma*
Dakhar	Senegal	*Syzygium cumini*
Dakouma	Senegal	*Hibiscus sabdariffa*
Dam but	Vietnam	*Hibiscus rosa-sinensis*
Damabo	Ivory Coast	*Abrus precatorius*
Dandalonbin	India	*Moringa pterygosperma*
Danthalons	India	*Moringa pterygosperma*
Darim	India	*Punica granatum*
Darim	Nepal	*Punica granatum*

Common name	Country	Latin binomial
Darinko bokra	Nepal	*Punica granatum*
Dasani	India	*Hibiscus rosa-sinensis*
Dasuan	China	*Allium sativum*
Datiwam	Nepal	*Jatropa curcas*
Daun marisan	East Indies	*Phyllanthus niruri*
Delum	Japan	*Punica granatum*
Delun	Sri Lanka	*Punica granatum*
Demar pirkok	Panama	*Macuna pruriens*
Demze	Guinea	*Portulaca oleracea*
Derriere-dos	Haiti	*Phyllanthus niruri*
Deye do	Haiti	*Phyllanthus niruri*
Dhak I houm	Indonesia	*Moringa pterygosperma*
Diaboy	Senegal	*Moringa pterygosperma*
Dian	Borneo	*Annona muricata*
Dickwar	India	*Aloe vera*
Dilau	India	*Curcuma longa*
Dilaw	Philippines	*Curcuma longa*
Dinon	Puerto Rico	*Jatropa curcas*
Djambu bidji	Indonesia	*Psidium guajava*
Djambu klutuk	Indonesia	*Psidium guajava*
Dok mai	Vietnam	*Hibiscus rosa-sinensis*
Dorcellana	Italy	*Portulaca oleracea*
Double hibiscus	Trinidad	*Hibiscus rosa-sinensis*
Dra thiam	Thailand	*Allium sativum*
Drum stick	Nepal	*Moringa pterygosperma*
Drum stick tree	India	*Moringa pterygosperma*
Drumstick	India	*Moringa pterygosperma*
Drumstick	Sri Lanka	*Moringa pterygosperma*
Drumstick tree	Fiji	*Moringa pterygosperma*
Du du	Vietnam	*Carica papaya*
Dua can	Vietnam	*Catharanthus roseus*
Dulagondi	India	*Macuna pruriens*
Ebabayo	Tanzania	*Carica papaya*
Ehi	Tanzania	*Carica papaya*
Eldeis	Sudan	*Cyperus rotundus*
Elrageig	Sudan	*Phyllanthus niruri*
Elrigeg	Sudan	*Phyllanthus niruri*
Embe	Tanzania	*Mangifera indica*
Embusabusu	Congo	*Momordica charantia*
En bas	West Indies	*Phyllanthus niruri*
Eranda-kakdi	India	*Carica papaya*
Erba vasciulella	Italy	*Portulaca oleracea*
Eruption plant	Mexico	*Phyllanthus niruri*
Erva cidreira	Brazil	*Cymbopogon citratus*
Erva cidreira capim	Brazil	*Cymbopogon citratus*

Common name	Country	Latin binomial
Esi	India	*Carica papaya*
Eso botuje	Nigeria	*Jatropa curcas*
Etamanane	Senegal	*Jatropa curcas*
Evatbimi	Papua-New Guinea	*Phyllanthus niruri*
Eyezom	Guinea	*Momordica charantia*
Fa-rang	Thailand	*Psidium guajava*
Fafy	Oman	*Carica papaya*
Fakai	Sierra Leone	*Carica papaya*
Fakai laa	Sierra Leone	*Carica papaya*
Farfena	Oman	*Portulaca oleracea*
Fasab	Senegal	*Hibiscus sabdariffa*
Fencing flower	Trinidad	*Hibiscus rosa-sinensis*
Fever grass	Belize	*Cymbopogon citratus*
Fever grass	Guyana	*Cymbopogon citratus*
Fever grass	Nicaragua	*Cymbopogon citratus*
Fiki	Tonga	*Jatropa curcas*
Fla baya	Trinidad	*Hibiscus rosa-sinensis*
Fleur barriere	Trinidad	*Hibiscus rosa-sinensis*
Flores rosa	Guam	*Hibiscus rosa-sinensis*
Folere	Guinea-Bissau	*Hibiscus sabdariffa*
Foulsepatte	Rodrigues Islands	*Hibiscus rosa-sinensis*
Fruta bomba	Cuba	*Carica papaya*
Frutilla	Mexico	*Lantana camara*
Fruto bomba	Cuba	*Carica papaya*
Fu yong pi	China	*Hibiscus rosa-sinensis*
Futoreishi	Japan	*Momordica charantia*
Gale wind grass	Fiji	*Phyllanthus niruri*
Gale-o-wind	Bimini	*Phyllanthus niruri*
Gale-wind grass	West Indies	*Phyllanthus niruri*
Galingale	Madeira	*Cyperus rotundus*
Galinggang hutan	Indonesia	*Cassia alata*
Gandheriya	India	*Lantana camara*
Ganhoma	Guinea-Bissau	*Macuna pruriens*
Garlic	Brazil	*Allium sativum*
Garlic	China	*Allium sativum*
Garlic	Cuba	*Allium sativum*
Garlic	Europe	*Allium sativum*
Garlic	Guyana	*Allium sativum*
Garlic	India	*Allium sativum*
Garlic	Indonesia	*Allium sativum*
Garlic	Iran	*Allium sativum*
Garlic	Japan	*Allium sativum*
Garlic	Kuwait	*Allium sativum*
Garlic	Libya	*Allium sativum*
Garlic	Mexico	*Allium sativum*

Common name	*Country*	*Latin binomial*
Garlic	Nicaragua	*Allium sativum*
Garlic	Poland	*Allium sativum*
Garlic	Taiwan	*Allium sativum*
Garlic	Thailand	*Allium sativum*
Garlic	USA	*Allium sativum*
Garlic	West Indies	*Allium sativum*
Garlic clove	Nicaragua	*Allium sativum*
Gati ma nya	Ecuador	*Cymbopogon citratus*
Gaungchi	India	*Abrus precatorius*
Gchi	India	*Abrus precatorius*
Gelenggang	Malaysia	*Cassia alata*
Gelenngang	Indonesia	*Cassia alata*
Getha	Saudi Arabia	*Moringa pterygosperma*
Ghai kunwar	India	*Aloe vera*
Ghanti phul	Nepal	*Hibiscus rosa-sinensis*
Ghee kanwar	India	*Aloe vera*
Gheekuar	India	*Aloe vera*
Ghikanvar	India	*Aloe vera*
Ghikuar	India	*Aloe vera*
Ghikumar	India	*Aloe vera*
Ghikumari	India	*Aloe vera*
Ghikwar	India	*Aloe vera*
Ghiu kumari	Nepal	*Aloe vera*
Ghongchi	India	*Abrus precatorius*
Ghrit kumari	India	*Aloe vera*
Ghrita kumari	India	*Aloe vera*
Ghughchi	India	*Abrus precatorius*
Ghumchi	India	*Abrus precatorius*
Ghun	India	*Abrus precatorius*
Ginger grass	Ecuador	*Cymbopogon citratus*
Goassien	Guam	*Abrus precatorius*
Goassien	Ivory Coast	*Abrus precatorius*
Goavy	Madagascar	*Psidium guajava*
Goejaba	Surinam	*Psidium guajava*
Goeratji	Indonesia	*Curcuma longa*
Gogu	India	*Hibiscus sabdariffa*
Goiabeira	Brazil	*Psidium guajava*
Goncha	Pakistan	*Macuna pruriens*
Goncha	Pakistan	*Macuna pruriens*
Goni	India	*Portulaca oleracea*
Goppe	India	*Carica papaya*
Goyav	Haiti	*Psidium guajava*
Grahakanya	India	*Aloe vera*
Graine en bas fievre	French Guiana	*Phyllanthus niruri*
Granada	Cuba	*Punica granatum*

Common name	Country	Latin binomial
Granada	Guatemala	*Punica granatum*
Granada	Peru	*Punica granatum*
Granado	Canary Islands	*Punica granatum*
Granado	Mexico	*Punica granatum*
Granatum	India	*Punica granatum*
Grenade	Rodrigues Islands	*Punica granatum*
Grenadier	Tunisia	*Punica granatum*
Grenadillo	Belize	*Punica granatum*
Grili	Papua-New Guinea	*Cassia alata*
Gros rose	French Guiana	*Hibiscus rosa-sinensis*
Guanabana	Barbados	*Annona muricata*
Guanabana	Cuba	*Annona muricata*
Guanabana	Dominican Republic	*Annona muricata*
Guanabana	Panama	*Annona muricata*
Guarka patha	India	*Aloe vera*
Guarpatha	India	*Aloe vera*
Guava	Fiji	*Psidium guajava*
Guava	Ghana	*Psidium guajava*
Guava	Guam	*Psidium guajava*
Guava	Guyana	*Psidium guajava*
Guava	Indonesia	*Psidium guajava*
Guava	Mexico	*Psidium guajava*
Guava	Nepal	*Psidium guajava*
Guava	Nicaragua	*Psidium guajava*
Guava	Papua-New Guinea	*Psidium guajava*
Guava	Sierra Leone	*Psidium guajava*
Guava	Sri Lanka	*Psidium guajava*
Guava	Tanzania	*Psidium guajava*
Guava	USA	*Psidium guajava*
Guayaba	Cuba	*Psidium guajava*
Guayaba	Guatemala	*Psidium guajava*
Guayaba	Nicaragua	*Psidium guajava*
Guayaba	Paraguay	*Psidium guajava*
Guayaba	Puerto Rico	*Psidium guajava*
Guayabe	Guatemala	*Psidium guajava*
Guayabero	Canary Islands	*Psidium guajava*
Guayabo	Canary Islands	*Psidium guajava*
Guayabo	Mexico	*Psidium guajava*
Guayabo	Peru	*Psidium guajava*
Guayava	Guatemala	*Psidium guajava*
Gudhal	India	*Hibiscus rosa-sinensis*
Guega	Papua-New Guinea	*Psidium guajava*
Guinea pea	India	*Abrus precatorius*
Guinea sorrel	Senegal	*Hibiscus sabdariffa*
Gul armini	Pakistan	*Punica granatum*

Common name	Country	Latin binomial
Gumamila	Philippines	*Hibiscus rosa-sinensis*
Gunch	India	*Abrus precatorius*
Gunchi	Pakistan	*Abrus precatorius*
Gunja	India	*Abrus precatorius*
Gurhal	India	*Hibiscus rosa-sinensis*
Guri-ginja	India	*Abrus precatorius*
Gurivinda	India	*Abrus precatorius*
Gurje-tiga	India	*Abrus precatorius*
Gurupacha	Colombia	*Lantana camara*
Gwana	Papua	*Psidium guajava*
Gwanda	Nigeria	*Carica papaya*
Gwo fla bays	Trinidad	*Hibiscus rosa-sinensis*
Gwo waz baya	Trinidad	*Hibiscus rosa-sinensis*
Habat al arus	Sudan	*Abrus precatorius*
Habat elmlock	India	*Abrus precatorius*
Habat elmlock	Sudan	*Abrus precatorius*
Habb el meluk	Mexico	*Jatropa curcas*
Habb el meluk	Sudan	*Jatropa curcas*
Haeo muu	Thailand	*Cyperus rotundus*
Haldi	Fiji	*Curcuma longa*
Haledo	Nepal	*Curcuma longa*
Halodhi	India	*Curcuma longa*
Hama suge	Japan	*Cyperus rotundus*
Hamaiga	Nicaragua	*Hibiscus sabdariffa*
Hamer	Saudi Arabia	*Syzygium cumini*
Hardi	Fiji	*Curcuma longa*
Haridra	India	*Curcuma longa*
Hedge flower	Thailand	*Lantana camara*
Herbe a oignons	New Caledonia	*Cyperus rotundus*
Hibiscus	Easter Island	*Hibiscus rosa-sinensis*
Hibiscus	Guyana	*Hibiscus rosa-sinensis*
Hibiscus	West Indies	*Hibiscus rosa-sinensis*
Hibiscus	Vietnam	*Hibiscus rosa-sinensis*
Hierba de limon	Costa Rica	*Cymbopogon citratus*
Hierba luisa	Ecuador	*Cymbopogon citratus*
Hierba luisa	Peru	*Cymbopogon citratus*
Hindu ma pangi	Bangladesh	*Hibiscus rosa-sinensis*
Hoja de palto	Easter Island	*Persea americana*
Hong can	Vietnam	*Hibiscus rosa-sinensis*
Horseeye bean	Thailand	*Macuna pruriens*
Horseradish	India	*Moringa pterygosperma*
Horseradish tree	Fiji	*Moringa pterygosperma*
Horseradish tree	Guam	*Moringa pterygosperma*
Horseradish tree	India	*Moringa pterygosperma*
Horseradish tree	Indonesia	*Moringa pterygosperma*

Common name	Country	Latin binomial
Horseradish tree	Malaysia	*Moringa pterygosperma*
Horseradish tree	Mauritius	*Moringa pterygosperma*
Horseradish tree	Nepal	*Moringa pterygosperma*
Horseradish tree	Nigeria	*Moringa pterygosperma*
Horseradish tree	USA	*Moringa pterygosperma*
Horseradish tree	West Indies	*Moringa pterygosperma*
Hsiang fu	China	*Cyperus rotundus*
Hsiang fu	Vietnam	*Cyperus rotundus*
Hsiang fu tzu	China	*Cyperus rotundus*
Huai mao ts'ao	China	*Cyperus rotundus*
Huang chiang	Malaysia	*Curcuma longa*
Hui t'ou ch'ing	China	*Cyperus rotundus*
Huong phu	Malaysia	*Cyperus rotundus*
Hurricane weed	West Indies	*Phyllanthus niruri*
Hyang boo ja	Malaysia	*Cyperus rotundus*
I'ita	Nigeria	*Carica papaya*
Ibepe	Nigeria	*Carica papaya*
Ibuya	Congo-Brazzaville	*Hibiscus sabdariffa*
Icheku oyibo	Nigeria	*Syzygium cumini*
Imli	Fiji	*Syzygium cumini*
Imli	India	*Syzygium cumini*
Indian aloe	Nepal	*Aloe vera*
Indian licorice	India	*Abrus precatorius*
Indian sorrel	Senegal	*Hibiscus sabdariffa*
Inkulu	Congo-Brazzaville	*Hibiscus sabdariffa*
Ipera	Rwanda	*Psidium guajava*
Ipi	Papua-New Guinea	*Carica papaya*
Itk	Nicaragua	*Manihot esculenta*
Jaama	India	*Psidium guajava*
Jaba	India	*Hibiscus rosa-sinensis*
Jabaphool	India	*Hibiscus rosa-sinensis*
Jam	India	*Syzygium cumini*
Jaman	India	*Syzygium cumini*
Jaman	Pakistan	*Syzygium cumini*
Jamblon	Rodrigues Islands	*Syzygium cumini*
Jambol	West Indies	*Syzygium cumini*
Jambolan	Brazil	*Syzygium cumini*
Jambolan	India	*Syzygium cumini*
Jambolana	Nepal	*Syzygium cumini*
Jambolao	Brazil	*Syzygium cumini*
Jambu	India	*Syzygium cumini*
Jambu Biji	Indonesia	*Psidium guajava*
Jambul	India	*Syzygium cumini*
Jambul	USA	*Syzygium cumini*
Jamdlan	India	*Syzygium cumini*

Common name	Country	Latin binomial
Jamoon	Guyana	Syzygium cumini
Jamoon	India	Syzygium cumini
Jamun	India	Syzygium cumini
Jamun	Nepal	Syzygium cumini
Japa	India	Hibiscus rosa-sinensis
Japa puspi	Nepal	Hibiscus rosa-sinensis
Japakusum	India	Hibiscus rosa-sinensis
Japanese nutgrass	Japan	Cyperus rotundus
Jar amla	Fiji	Phyllanthus niruri
Jar-amla	India	Phyllanthus niruri
Jarak pagar	Indonesia	Jatropa curcas
Jasum	Fiji	Hibiscus rosa-sinensis
Jasum	India	Hibiscus rosa-sinensis
Jasunt	India	Hibiscus rosa-sinensis
Jaswand	India	Hibiscus rosa-sinensis
Java plum	Brazil	Syzygium cumini
Java plum	India	Syzygium cumini
Java plum	Nepal	Syzygium cumini
Javanese turmeric	Indonesia	Curcuma longa
Jequiriti bean	Taiwan	Abrus precatorius
Jequirity	Taiwan	Abrus precatorius
Jequirity plant	Philippines	Abrus precatorius
Jericho rose	Germany	Hibiscus sabdariffa
Jhad-chibhadi	India	Carica papaya
Jia pushpa	India	Hibiscus rosa-sinensis
Jiquiriti	Brazil	Abrus precatorius
Joba	India	Hibiscus rosa-sinensis
Jumbee bead	Virgin Islands	Abrus precatorius
Jumble beads	Virgin Islands	Abrus precatorius
Jumble beads	West Indies	Abrus precatorius
Kabaiura	Papua-New Guinea	Cassia alata
Kaju asam	Indonesia	Syzygium cumini
Kaka pul	West Indies	Catharanthus roseus
Kakara	India	Momordica charantia
Kakayi	Nigeria	Momordica charantia
Kakiral	India	Momordica charantia
Kakle	East Africa	Momordica charantia
Kakoenji	Indonesia	Curcuma longa
Kakral	India	Momordica charantia
Kalo haledo	Nepal	Curcuma longa
Kalyani	India	Abrus precatorius
Kalyani	Kenya	Abrus precatorius
Kananeranda	India	Jatropa curcas
Kantotan	Philippines	Catharanthus roseus
Kaocho	Nepal	Macuna pruriens

Common name	Country	Latin binomial
Kapikachchhu	India	Macuna pruriens
Karala	India	Momordica charantia
Karawila	Sri Lanka	Momordica charantia
Karela	Fiji	Momordica charantia
Karela	India	Momordica charantia
Karela	Nepal	Momordica charantia
Karela	USA	Momordica charantia
Karela	West Indies	Momordica charantia
Karimuthan	India	Cyperus rotundus
Karkade	Egypt	Hibiscus sabdariffa
Karkade	Germany	Hibiscus sabdariffa
Karkade	Italy	Hibiscus sabdariffa
Karkade	Somaliland	Hibiscus sabdariffa
Karkadeh	Sudan	Hibiscus sabdariffa
Karkadesh	Egypt	Hibiscus sabdariffa
Karumusa	India	Carica papaya
Karutha kapalam	India	Carica papaya
Kasaleka	Nicaragua	Manihot esculenta
Kasera	Fiji	Manihot esculenta
Kasera	Nicaragua	Manihot esculenta
Kasla	Philippines	Jatropa curcas
Katafaga	Fiji	Manihot esculenta
Katara ara tara	Cook Islands	Annona muricata
Kath	India	Carica papaya
Kathazhai	India	Aloe vera
Kauso	Nepal	Macuna pruriens
Kausva	Nepal	Macuna pruriens
Kaute	India	Hibiscus rosa-sinensis
Kaute'enua	Cook Islands	Hibiscus rosa-sinensis
Kaute'enua	Rarotonga	Hibiscus rosa-sinensis
Kauti	Rarotonga	Hibiscus rosa-sinensis
Kautonga	Indonesia	Psidium guajava
Kavach	India	Macuna pruriens
Kavanch	India	Macuna pruriens
Kawach	India	Macuna pruriens
Kawanch	India	Macuna pruriens
Kawanch	Pakistan	Macuna pruriens
Kawanh	India	Macuna pruriens
Kayaga	China	Hibiscus rosa-sinensis
Kayakit	West Indies	Lantana camara
Kelor	Indonesia	Moringa pterygosperma
Kelor	Malaysia	Moringa pterygosperma
Kelor pea	Malaysia	Moringa pterygosperma
Kembang sepatu	Indonesia	Hibiscus rosa-sinensis
Kerainch	India	Macuna pruriens

Common name	Country	Latin binomial
Kerqum	Morocco	*Curcuma longa*
Ketapeng	Indonesia	*Cassia alata*
Ketepeng	Indonesia	*Cassia alata*
Kewanch	India	*Macuna pruriens*
Khamin chan	Thailand	*Curcuma longa*
Khurfa	India	*Portulaca oleracea*
Khursa	Fiji	*Portulaca oleracea*
Khutura	India	*Portulaca oleracea*
Kikerewe	Tanzania	*Abrus precatorius*
Kiko eka	Marquesas Island	*Curcuma longa*
King of the forest	Jamaica	*Cassia alata*
Kinkeliba	Gabon	*Cassia alata*
Kislin	Nicaragua	*Cassia alata*
Kiswahili	Tanzania	*Psidium guajava*
Kiwepe	Tanzania	*Lantana camara*
Kizha nelli	India	*Phyllanthus niruri*
Ko bushi	Japan	*Cyperus rotundus*
Koening	Indonesia	*Curcuma longa*
Koenir	Indonesia	*Curcuma longa*
Koenjet	Indonesia	*Curcuma longa*
Kolales halomtanto	Guam	*Abrus precatorius*
Konch	India	*Macuna pruriens*
Konchkari	Pakistan	*Macuna pruriens*
Kondin	Indonesia	*Curcuma longa*
Koolfa	India	*Portulaca oleracea*
Koonch	India	*Abrus precatorius*
Koraikizhangu	India	*Cyperus rotundus*
Korchijhan	India	*Cyperus rotundus*
Korosol	Haiti	*Annona muricata*
Korphad	India	*Aloe vera*
Koupye	Haiti	*Portulaca oleracea*
Koute	Indonesia	*Hibiscus rosa-sinensis*
Kowez	India	*Macuna pruriens*
Kowosol	West Indies	*Annona muricata*
Kra thiam	Thailand	*Allium sativum*
Krachiap daeng	Thailand	*Hibiscus sabdariffa*
Kraval chruk	Malaysia	*Cyperus rotundus*
Kravanh chruk	Malaysia	*Cyperus rotundus*
Krikpe	Ivory Coast	*Abrus precatorius*
Krue	Nicaragua	*Psidium guajava*
Ku'ava	Nicaragua	*Psidium guajava*
Kuabas	Nicaragua	*Psidium guajava*
Kuava	Nicaragua	*Psidium guajava*
Kuawa	Nicaragua	*Psidium guajava*
Kuges	Senegal	*Hibiscus sabdariffa*

Common name	**Country**	**Latin binomial**
Kuguazi	West Indies	*Momordica charantia*
Kuiaba	Papua-New Guinea	*Psidium guajava*
Kukataj	Mexico	*Persea americana*
Kulfa	India	*Portulaca oleracea*
Kuliabas	Malaysia	*Psidium guajava*
Kumari	India	*Aloe vera*
Kumaro	India	*Aloe vera*
Kunam-paran popo	Admiralty Islands	*Carica papaya*
Kunch	India	*Abrus precatorius*
Kunni	India	*Abrus precatorius*
Kunvar pata	India	*Aloe vera*
Kunwar	India	*Aloe vera*
Kupye	West Indies	*Portulaca oleracea*
Kurcum	Oman	*Curcuma longa*
Kurfa	India	*Portulaca oleracea*
Kuulup	Nicaragua	*Persea americana*
L'ail	West Indies	*Allium sativum*
La'au fai lafa	Nicaragua	*Cassia alata*
Laboma	Ivory Coast	*Abrus precatorius*
Lagitua	New Britain (East)	*Hibiscus rosa-sinensis*
Laguana	Guam	*Annona muricata*
Lahsun	Fiji	*Allium sativum*
Lai	Nicaragua	*Allium sativum*
Lai	West Indies	*Allium sativum*
Lal ambari	India	*Hibiscus sabdariffa*
Laloi	Haiti	*Aloe vera*
Laloi	India	*Aloe vera*
Laluwe	Trinidad	*Aloe vera*
Laluwe	West Indies	*Aloe vera*
Langiruh	Brunei	*Portulaca oleracea*
Lantana	Australia	*Lantana camara*
Lantana	India	*Lantana camara*
Lapalapa	Nigeria	*Jatropa curcas*
Large leaf lantana	Guatemala	*Lantana camara*
Lasan	Fiji	*Allium sativum*
Lasan	India	*Allium sativum*
Lashun	India	*Allium sativum*
Lasun	Fiji	*Allium sativum*
Lasun	India	*Allium sativum*
Lasun	Nepal	*Allium sativum*
Lasuna	India	*Allium sativum*
Latora moa	Guatemala	*Lantana camara*
Latuwani	India	*Abrus precatorius*
Lay	Haiti	*Allium sativum*
Lelegurua	New Britain (East)	*Hibiscus rosa-sinensis*

Common name	Country	Latin binomial
Lemon grass	Ecuador	*Cymbopogon citratus*
Lemon grass	Guyana	*Cymbopogon citratus*
Lemon grass	India	*Cymbopogon citratus*
Lemon grass	Argentina	*Cymbopogon citratus*
Lemon grass	Brazil	*Cymbopogon citratus*
Lemon grass	Egypt	*Cymbopogon citratus*
Lemon grass	Nicaragua	*Cymbopogon citratus*
Lemon grass	Sierra Leone	*Cymbopogon citratus*
Lemon grass	Thailand	*Cymbopogon citratus*
Lemon grass	USA	*Cymbopogon citratus*
Lenzaa	Congo	*Momordica charantia*
Lesi	Admiralty Islands	*Carica papaya*
Lesi tangata	Tonga	*Carica papaya*
Lesun	Fiji	*Allium sativum*
Licorice	West Indies	*Abrus precatorius*
Liluvha	Venda	*Catharanthus roseus*
Lingiruh	Brunei	*Portulaca oleracea*
Lo Hoei	Vietnam	*Aloe vera*
Lo hong phle	Vietnam	*Carica papaya*
Lohong	Vietnam	*Jatropa curcas*
Loloru	New Britain (East)	*Hibiscus rosa-sinensis*
Lonika	India	*Portulaca oleracea*
Loonia	India	*Portulaca oleracea*
Lou houey	Vietnam	*Aloe vera*
Love bean	USA	*Abrus precatorius*
Lu chuy	Vietnam	*Aloe vera*
Lufyambo	East Africa	*Abrus precatorius*
Luk-wa	Thailand	*Syzygium cumini*
Lulimilwasenga	Tanganyika	*Portulaca oleracea*
Lumba-lumba	East Africa	*Momordica charantia*
Lumbuzi	Congo	*Momordica charantia*
Luvambo	Tanzania	*Abrus precatorius*
Lyann legliz	Haiti	*Abrus precatorius*
Ma feng shu	Indonesia	*Jatropa curcas*
Ma khaam	Thailand	*Syzygium cumini*
Ma klam taanuu	Thailand	*Abrus precatorius*
Ma ra	Thailand	*Momordica charantia*
Ma-rum	Thailand	*Moringa pterygosperma*
Maamidi	India	*Mangifera indica*
Mabera	Tanzania	*Psidium guajava*
Machete	Puerto Rico	*Momordica charantia*
Machixian	China	*Portulaca oleracea*
Madagascar periwinkle	Madagascar	*Catharanthus roseus*
Madan	Japan	*Syzygium cumini*
Maduriam	India	*Psidium guajava*

Common name	Country	Latin binomial
Maiden apple	USA	*Momordica charantia*
Maiden apple	Virgin Islands	*Momordica charantia*
Maiden's blush	USA	*Momordica charantia*
Majo	Mexico	*Allium sativum*
Mak hung	Vietnam	*Carica papaya*
Makabling	West Indies	*Portulaca oleracea*
Makalalaska	Nicaragua	*Momordica charantia*
Makham	Thailand	*Syzygium cumini*
Malabar plum	Brazil	*Syzygium cumini*
Malak rose-apple	Brazil	*Syzygium cumini*
Malako	Thailand	*Carica papaya*
Maliof	Papua-New Guinea	*Cassia alata*
Malungai	Guam	*Moringa pterygosperma*
Malungal	Philippines	*Moringa pterygosperma*
Malunggay	Philippines	*Moringa pterygosperma*
Mam-maram	India	*Mangifera indica*
Mama	Angola	*Carica papaya*
Mamioko	Bougainville	*Carica papaya*
Mamoeiro	Paraguay	*Carica papaya*
Manamat	East Africa	*Momordica charantia*
Mandaar	India	*Hibiscus rosa-sinensis*
Mandara	India	*Hibiscus rosa-sinensis*
Mande	Ghana	*Carica papaya*
Mande	Senegal	*Carica papaya*
Manga	Brazil	*Mangifera indica*
Mangai	India	*Moringa pterygosperma*
Mange kuli	West Indies	*Momordica charantia*
Mangga	Guam	*Mangifera indica*
Mangguo	China	*Mangifera indica*
Mango	Brazil	*Mangifera indica*
Mango	Canary Islands	*Mangifera indica*
Mango	China	*Mangifera indica*
Mango	Curacao	*Mangifera indica*
Mango	Egypt	*Mangifera indica*
Mango	Fiji	*Mangifera indica*
Mango	Guam	*Mangifera indica*
Mango	Guatemala	*Mangifera indica*
Mango	Guyana	*Mangifera indica*
Mango	Haiti	*Mangifera indica*
Mango	India	*Mangifera indica*
Mango	Ivory Coast	*Mangifera indica*
Mango	Mexico	*Mangifera indica*
Mango	Nepal	*Mangifera indica*
Mango	Nicaragua	*Mangifera indica*
Mango	Pakistan	*Mangifera indica*

Common name	Country	Latin binomial
Mango	Peru	*Mangifera indica*
Mango	Puerto Rico	*Mangifera indica*
Mango	Sudan	*Mangifera indica*
Mango	Tanzania	*Mangifera indica*
Mango	Tonga	*Mangifera indica*
Mango	Venezuela	*Mangifera indica*
Mango	West Indies	*Mangifera indica*
Mango dusa	Nicaragua	*Mangifera indica*
Mango tree	India	*Mangifera indica*
Mangofruit	India	*Mangifera indica*
Mangu	Nicaragua	*Mangifera indica*
Mangue	Rodrigues Islands	*Mangifera indica*
Mangueira	Brazil	*Mangifera indica*
Manhan	China	*Syzygium cumini*
Manioc	Central Africa	*Manihot esculenta*
Manioc	Rodrigues Islands	*Manihot esculenta*
Manioc	Sri Lanka	*Manihot esculenta*
Manioka	Samoa	*Manihot esculenta*
Maniota	Venezuela	*Manihot esculenta*
Manjan	Borneo	*Carica papaya*
Manjikattali	India	*Aloe vera*
Mankro	Nicaragua	*Mangifera indica*
Mannyok	Venezuela	*Manihot esculenta*
Mansala	India	*Psidium guajava*
Mapatan	Papua-New Guinea	*Phyllanthus niruri*
Mara khee nok	Thailand	*Momordica charantia*
Maranga	Mauritius	*Moringa pterygosperma*
Margoze	Rodrigues Islands	*Momordica charantia*
Marum	Malaysia	*Moringa pterygosperma*
Marum	Thailand	*Moringa pterygosperma*
Mata pasto	Brazil	*Cassia alata*
Mathalanarakom	India	*Punica granatum*
Mathe	India	*Cyperus rotundus*
Maua	Kenya	*Catharanthus roseus*
Mave	India	*Mangifera indica*
Maviyakuku	Rwanda	*Lantana camara*
Mbosa	Congo	*Momordica charantia*
Mbum	Senegal	*Moringa pterygosperma*
Mbunbulu	Congo	*Momordica charantia*
Mchingu	Tanzania	*Cassia alata*
Medisiyen blen	West Indies	*Jatropa curcas*
Mediterranean aloe	West Indies	*Aloe vera*
Meetho sirgavo	India	*Moringa pterygosperma*
Melao de sao caetano	Brazil	*Momordica charantia*
Meleni	Brazil	*Momordica charantia*

Common name	Country	Latin binomial
Melograno	Italy	*Punica granatum*
Melon tree	India	*Carica papaya*
Melon tree	Nigeria	*Carica papaya*
Mena	Rotuma	*Curcuma longa*
Merelesita	Venezuela	*Manihot esculenta*
Merunggai	Malaysia	*Moringa pterygosperma*
Mesta	Bangladesh	*Hibiscus sabdariffa*
Metaftum	Guinea-Bissau	*Macuna pruriens*
Mewa	Nepal	*Carica papaya*
Mexicaine	West Indies	*Momordica charantia*
Mijeh	Thailand	*Macuna pruriens*
Mikana	Hawaii	*Carica papaya*
Mille fleurs	West Indies	*Lantana camara*
Mimosa	West Indies	*Phyllanthus niruri*
Mini mal	Sri Lanka	*Catharanthus roseus*
Miniklalasni	Nicaragua	*Momordica charantia*
Minimini	Mozambique	*Abrus precatorius*
Mishquina	Peru	*Abrus precatorius*
Miski miski	Peru	*Abrus precatorius*
Mkinda	Tanzania	*Lantana camara*
Mkoma manga	East Africa	*Punica granatum*
Mkwaju	Tanzania	*Syzygium cumini*
Mokka	Japan	*Carica papaya*
Momotica	Curacao	*Momordica charantia*
Mongrang jangtong	India	*Cassia alata*
Moothoo	India	*Cyperus rotundus*
Moringa	India	*Moringa pterygosperma*
Moringa	West Indies	*Moringa pterygosperma*
Moringa tree	West Indies	*Moringa pterygosperma*
Moringue	Angola	*Moringa pterygosperma*
Moth	India	*Cyperus rotundus*
Motha	India	*Cyperus rotundus*
Motha sedge	India	*Cyperus rotundus*
Mothe	Nepal	*Cyperus rotundus*
Motipitipi	East Africa	*Abrus precatorius*
Motiram	India	*Psidium guajava*
Moudie-bi-titi	Ivory Coast	*Abrus precatorius*
Mpera	Tanzania	*Psidium guajava*
Mugwavha	Venda	*Psidium guajava*
Muhoko	Tanzania	*Manihot esculenta*
Mula mula	India	*Cassia alata*
Mulu mulu	Papua-New Guinea	*Cassia alata*
Munaga	India	*Moringa pterygosperma*
Munga	India	*Moringa pterygosperma*
Mungay	India	*Moringa pterygosperma*

Common name	Country	Latin binomial
Munigha	India	*Moringa pterygosperma*
Mupapawe	Venda	*Carica papaya*
Mupfure donga	Venda	*Jatropa curcas*
Muringa	India	*Moringa pterygosperma*
Murr sbarr	Tunisia	*Aloe vera*
Murunga	Sri Lanka	*Moringa pterygosperma*
Murungai	India	*Moringa pterygosperma*
Musabar	India	*Aloe vera*
Musing	India	*Moringa pterygosperma*
Musta	India	*Cyperus rotundus*
Mustaka	India	*Cyperus rotundus*
Mustha	India	*Cyperus rotundus*
Mutha	India	*Cyperus rotundus*
Muthanga	India	*Cyperus rotundus*
Mutunu	Tanganyika	*Portulaca oleracea*
Mvuti	Tanzania	*Lantana camara*
Mwang-la-nyuki	East Africa	*Abrus precatorius*
Mwangaruchi	Tanzania	*Abrus precatorius*
Mwembe	Tanzania	*Mangifera indica*
Naeredu	India	*Syzygium cumini*
Nagareishi	Japan	*Momordica charantia*
Namugolokoma	Mozambique	*Abrus precatorius*
Nania nania	Ivory Coast	*Momordica charantia*
Nao harnaka	Papua-New Guinea	*Manihot esculenta*
Nar	Turkey	*Punica granatum*
Nara cheen	Thailand	*Momordica charantia*
Naval	India	*Syzygium cumini*
Nayantara	Bangladesh	*Catharanthus roseus*
Nayantara	India	*Catharanthus roseus*
Ndebie ni	Guinea	*Abrus precatorius*
Ndebie ni	Nepal	*Abrus precatorius*
Ndebie ni	Nigeria	*Abrus precatorius*
Nebeday	Senegal	*Moringa pterygosperma*
Neboday	Senegal	*Moringa pterygosperma*
Nebreday	Senegal	*Moringa pterygosperma*
Negresse	West Indies	*Syzygium cumini*
Nepalamu	India	*Jatropa curcas*
Neveday	Senegal	*Moringa pterygosperma*
Nevorday	Senegal	*Moringa pterygosperma*
Nevredie	Senegal	*Moringa pterygosperma*
Nghe	Vietnam	*Curcuma longa*
Ngoaba	Guinea	*Psidium guajava*
Nguene	Ivory Coast	*Momordica charantia*
Nichinichi so	Japan	*Catharanthus roseus*
Ninfa	Mexico	*Catharanthus roseus*

Common name	Country	Latin binomial
Nipay	Philippines	*Macuna pruriens*
Niruri	Pakistan	*Phyllanthus niruri*
Nisha	India	*Curcuma longa*
Nita	Cook Islands	*Carica papaya*
Nityakalyani	India	*Catharanthus roseus*
Njepaa	Sierra Leone	*Cassia alata*
Noboday	Senegal	*Moringa pterygosperma*
Nobody	Senegal	*Moringa pterygosperma*
Noumeh	Papua-New Guinea	*Manihot esculenta*
Nsa	Congo-Brazzaville	*Hibiscus sabdariffa*
Ntemi	Guinea	*Syzygium cumini*
Ntomi	Guinea	*Syzygium cumini*
Nutgrass	Brazil	*Cyperus rotundus*
Nutgrass	Guyana	*Cyperus rotundus*
Nutgrass	Hawaii	*Cyperus rotundus*
Nutgrass	India	*Cyperus rotundus*
Nutgrass	Iran	*Cyperus rotundus*
Nutgrass	Japan	*Cyperus rotundus*
Nutgrass	Nepal	*Cyperus rotundus*
Nutgrass	West Indies	*Cyperus rotundus*
Nutsedge	Hawaii	*Cyperus rotundus*
Nyanyra	Togo	*Momordica charantia*
Nyinya	East Africa	*Momordica charantia*
O rababa	Senegal	*Carica papaya*
Oegkoti-tong	India	*Mangifera indica*
Oendre	Indonesia	*Curcuma longa*
Ojo-mgbimgbi	Nigeria	*Carica papaya*
Okookoo	Nigeria	*Momordica charantia*
Okpo ndichi	Sierra Leone	*Cassia alata*
Olasiman	West Indies	*Portulaca oleracea*
Old maid	West Indies	*Catharanthus roseus*
Olesi	Nigeria	*Carica papaya*
Olho de pombo	Brazil	*Abrus precatorius*
Olinda	India	*Abrus precatorius*
Ombulu	East Africa	*Abrus precatorius*
Omita	India	*Carica papaya*
Ommal	India	*Carica papaya*
On	Belize	*Persea americana*
Ondwa	Guinea	*Mangifera indica*
Oniani tita	Cook Islands	*Cyperus rotundus*
Onion	India	*Allium sativum*
Orozus	Mexico	*Lantana camara*
Orozuz	Mexico	*Lantana camara*
Orututi	Tanzania	*Abrus precatorius*
Osang	Guinea	*Cymbopogon citratus*

Common name	*Country*	*Latin binomial*
Osito	East Africa	*Abrus precatorius*
Osito	Pakistan	*Abrus precatorius*
Otesse	Guinea-Bissau	*Hibiscus sabdariffa*
Owulo idu	Nigeria	*Jatropa curcas*
Pace	Guinea-Bissau	*Carica papaya*
Paja de limon	Costa Rica	*Cymbopogon citratus*
Palotsina	Philippines	*Cassia alata*
Palta	Argentina	*Persea americana*
Palta	Cuba	*Persea americana*
Palta	Peru	*Persea americana*
Palto	Peru	*Persea americana*
Panaminik	Nicaragua	*Momordica charantia*
Panini	India	*Aloe vera*
Panj phuli	India	*Lantana camara*
Papae	Guinea-Bissau	*Carica papaya*
Papai	India	*Carica papaya*
Papai	West Indies	*Carica papaya*
Papaia	Guinea-Bissau	*Carica papaya*
Papapa	Fiji	*Carica papaya*
Papaw	Jamaica	*Carica papaya*
Papaw	Malaysia	*Carica papaya*
Papaw	Myanmar	*Carica papaya*
Papaw	USA	*Carica papaya*
Papaw	West Indies	*Carica papaya*
Papay	Haiti	*Carica papaya*
Papay	India	*Carica papaya*
Papaya	Brazil	*Carica papaya*
Papaya	Fiji	*Carica papaya*
Papaya	Gold Coast	*Carica papaya*
Papaya	Guatemala	*Carica papaya*
Papaya	Guyana	*Carica papaya*
Papaya	India	*Carica papaya*
Papaya	Indonesia	*Carica papaya*
Papaya	Japan	*Carica papaya*
Papaya	Malaysia	*Carica papaya*
Papaya	Nepal	*Carica papaya*
Papaya	Papua-New Guinea	*Carica papaya*
Papaya	Peru	*Carica papaya*
Papaya	Tanzania	*Carica papaya*
Papaya	USA	*Carica papaya*
Papaya tree	India	*Carica papaya*
Papaye	Guadeloupe	*Carica papaya*
Papaye	Rodrigues Islands	*Carica papaya*
Papayer	Ivory Coast	*Carica papaya*
Papayer	Vietnam	*Carica papaya*

Common name	Country	Latin binomial
Papayer	Zaire	*Carica papaya*
Papayi	Guadeloupe	*Carica papaya*
Papayilla	Peru	*Momordica charantia*
Papayo	Mexico	*Carica papaya*
Papayu	India	*Carica papaya*
Papeeta	Pakistan	*Carica papaya*
Papeta	India	*Carica papaya*
Papeya	India	*Carica papaya*
Papia	Senegal	*Carica papaya*
Papita	Fiji	*Carica papaya*
Papita	India	*Carica papaya*
Papitha	India	*Carica papaya*
Papoia	Guinea-Bissau	*Carica papaya*
Pappukura	India	*Portulaca oleracea*
Paprika	West Indies	*Momordica charantia*
Para-parai mi	Paraguay	*Phyllanthus niruri*
Parimi	India	*Carica papaya*
Parindakaya	India	*Carica papaya*
Paroka	Guadeloupe	*Momordica charantia*
Pasarin	Panama	*Lantana camara*
Pasarrion	Panama	*Lantana camara*
Pasupu	India	*Curcuma longa*
Patti poo	Sri Lanka	*Catharanthus roseus*
Patwa	India	*Hibiscus sabdariffa*
Pauh	Indonesia	*Mangifera indica*
Paupau	India	*Carica papaya*
Pavakkachedi	India	*Momordica charantia*
Paw paw	Nigeria	*Carica papaya*
Pawpaw	East Africa	*Carica papaya*
Pawpaw	England	*Carica papaya*
Pawpaw	Fiji	*Carica papaya*
Pawpaw	Malaysia	*Carica papaya*
Pawpaw	Oman	*Carica papaya*
Pawpaw	Papua-New Guinea	*Carica papaya*
Pawpaw	Philippines	*Carica papaya*
Pe fo tze	Vietnam	*Jatropa curcas*
Pear	Belize	*Persea americana*
Pear	Nicaragua	*Persea americana*
Pear	West Indies	*Persea americana*
Pei	Admiralty Islands	*Phyllanthus niruri*
Pepino montero	Nicaragua	*Momordica charantia*
Perchnut	West Indies	*Jatropa curcas*
Periwinkle	Guyana	*Catharanthus roseus*
Periwinkle	India	*Catharanthus roseus*
Periwinkle	Jamaica	*Catharanthus roseus*

Common name	Country	Latin binomial
Periwinkle	Philippines	*Catharanthus roseus*
Periwinkle	USA	*Catharanthus roseus*
Periwinkle	West Indies	*Catharanthus roseus*
Periya laut	Malaysia	*Momordica charantia*
Pervenche de madagascar	French Guiana	*Catharanthus roseus*
Pha-ka-krong	Guatemala	*Lantana camara*
Phaeng phoi farang	Thailand	*Catharanthus roseus*
Phaka drong	Thailand	*Lantana camara*
Phakas krong	Thailand	*Lantana camara*
Phyllanto	Brazil	*Phyllanthus niruri*
Physic nut	Ghana	*Jatropa curcas*
Physic nut	Guam	*Jatropa curcas*
Physic nut	Nepal	*Jatropa curcas*
Physic nut	Thailand	*Jatropa curcas*
Physic nut	Guyana	*Jatropa curcas*
Physic nut	Nigeria	*Jatropa curcas*
Physic nut	South Africa	*Jatropa curcas*
Physic nut	Virgin Islands	*Jatropa curcas*
Physic nut bush	Fiji	*Jatropa curcas*
Piao branco	Brazil	*Jatropa curcas*
Pignon d'inde	Rodrigues Islands	*Jatropa curcas*
Pigweed	Fiji	*Portulaca oleracea*
Pindi	India	*Jatropa curcas*
Pink flower	West Indies	*Catharanthus roseus*
Pink-edge red lantana	Australia	*Lantana camara*
Pinnao de purga	Brazil	*Jatropa curcas*
Pinon	Guatemala	*Jatropa curcas*
Pinon	Mexico	*Jatropa curcas*
Pinon	Peru	*Jatropa curcas*
Pinon botija	Cape Verde Islands	*Jatropa curcas*
Pinoncillo	Mexico	*Jatropa curcas*
Poi poi	Kenya	*Carica papaya*
Pois a gratter	Trinidad	*Macuna pruriens*
Pokok asam jawa	Malaysia	*Syzygium cumini*
Pom kouli	Guadeloupe	*Momordica charantia*
Pombinha	East Indies	*Phyllanthus niruri*
Pomegranate	Egypt	*Punica granatum*
Pomegranate	England	*Punica granatum*
Pomegranate	Greece	*Punica granatum*
Pomegranate	Guyana	*Punica granatum*
Pomegranate	India	*Punica granatum*
Pomegranate	Madeira	*Punica granatum*
Pomegranate	Mexico	*Punica granatum*
Pomegranate	Nepal	*Punica granatum*
Pomegranate	Turkey	*Punica granatum*

Common name	Country	Latin binomial
Pomegranate	USA	*Punica granatum*
Pomegranate	West Indies	*Punica granatum*
Pomme nerveille	West Indies	*Momordica charantia*
Pomme Z'Indiens	West Indies	*Momordica charantia*
Pomme-coolie	Guadeloupe	*Momordica charantia*
Poop man's treacle	Iran	*Allium sativum*
Popai	India	*Carica papaya*
Portulaca	Italy	*Portulaca oleracea*
Posely	Nicaragua	*Portulaca oleracea*
Posnar	India	*Punica granatum*
Poua grate	Guadeloupe	*Macuna pruriens*
Pourpier	Dominica	*Portulaca oleracea*
Pourpier	West Indies	*Portulaca oleracea*
Poyam	Admiralty Islands	*Carica papaya*
Prayer beads	India	*Abrus precatorius*
Precatory beads	West Indies	*Abrus precatorius*
Prickly lantana	Guatemala	*Lantana camara*
Psidium	Taiwan	*Psidium guajava*
Pui chi	Bangladesh	*Cassia alata*
Pumo	Nicaragua	*Annona muricata*
Punnetang	India	*Jatropa curcas*
Puntar waithia	Nicaragua	*Annona muricata*
Puppai	India	*Carica papaya*
Purchiacchella	Italy	*Portulaca oleracea*
Purge nut bush	West Indies	*Jatropa curcas*
Purging physic	Nicaragua	*Jatropa curcas*
Purgueira	Guinea-Bissau	*Jatropa curcas*
Purple nutsedge	Hawaii	*Cyperus rotundus*
Purple nutsedge	Japan	*Cyperus rotundus*
Purslane	Dominica	*Portulaca oleracea*
Purslane	Europe	*Portulaca oleracea*
Purslane	Jamaica	*Portulaca oleracea*
Purslane	Netherlands	*Portulaca oleracea*
Purslane	USA	*Portulaca oleracea*
Purslane	West Indies	*Portulaca oleracea*
Pusley	Europe	*Portulaca oleracea*
Pusley	Virgin Islands	*Portulaca oleracea*
Pussley	Jamaica	*Portulaca oleracea*
Pussley	West Indies	*Portulaca oleracea*
Pwa grate	Haiti	*Macuna pruriens*
Pwa grate	Trinidad	*Macuna pruriens*
Qanabisi	Nicaragua	*Cassia alata*
Qisaul-barri	India	*Momordica charantia*
Qsur roman	Morocco	*Punica granatum*
Qsur romman	Morocco	*Punica granatum*

Common name	Country	Latin binomial
Quanabana	Nicaragua	*Annona muricata*
Querba pedra	Brazil	*Phyllanthus niruri*
Quinine weed	West Indies	*Phyllanthus niruri*
Quisaul-barri	Saudi Arabia	*Momordica charantia*
Quwawa	Taiwan	*Psidium guajava*
Rajani	India	*Curcuma longa*
Ram goat rose	West Indies	*Catharanthus roseus*
Ram joyti	Nepal	*Jatropa curcas*
Rame	Indonesia	*Curcuma longa*
Ramjeevan	Nepal	*Jatropa curcas*
Ramunggai	Malaysia	*Moringa pterygosperma*
Ranato	Italy	*Punica granatum*
Rantana	Guatemala	*Lantana camara*
Rapahoe	India	*Aloe vera*
Rashun	India	*Allium sativum*
Rason	India	*Allium sativum*
Rati	India	*Abrus precatorius*
Rati gedi	India	*Abrus precatorius*
Rattanjot	India	*Catharanthus roseus*
Ratti	India	*Abrus precatorius*
Ravinta	India	*Moringa pterygosperma*
Red flowered sage	Guatemala	*Lantana camara*
Red rose	West Indies	*Catharanthus roseus*
Red roselle	India	*Hibiscus sabdariffa*
Red sorrel	Egypt	*Hibiscus sabdariffa*
Red sorrel	Germany	*Hibiscus sabdariffa*
Red sorrel	India	*Hibiscus sabdariffa*
Red sorrel	Senegal	*Hibiscus sabdariffa*
Renga	Cook Islands	*Curcuma longa*
Rerenga	Cook Islands	*Curcuma longa*
Rhizoma cyperii	Taiwan	*Cyperus rotundus*
Rigia	Qatar	*Portulaca oleracea*
Rigla	Egypt	*Portulaca oleracea*
Ringworm bush	Fiji	*Cassia alata*
Ringworm bush	Guyana	*Cassia alata*
Ringworm bush	West Indies	*Cassia alata*
Ringworm cassia	Malaysia	*Cassia alata*
Ringworm shrub	Australia	*Cassia alata*
Roma	Madeira	*Punica granatum*
Roman	Egypt	*Punica granatum*
Roman	Ethiopia	*Punica granatum*
Roman candle tree	Fiji	*Cassia alata*
Romeira	Madeira	*Punica granatum*
Romman	Jordan	*Punica granatum*
Romman	Tunisia	*Punica granatum*

Common name	Country	Latin binomial
Romman amruj	Morocco	*Punica granatum*
Rosa de Jamaica	Guatemala	*Hibiscus sabdariffa*
Rosary bean	West Indies	*Abrus precatorius*
Rose cayene	Guadeloupe	*Hibiscus rosa-sinensis*
Rose ce chine	Vietnam	*Hibiscus rosa-sinensis*
Rose of China	China	*Hibiscus rosa-sinensis*
Rosella	Egypt	*Hibiscus sabdariffa*
Roselle	Egypt	*Hibiscus sabdariffa*
Roselle	India	*Hibiscus sabdariffa*
Roselle	Iraq	*Hibiscus sabdariffa*
Roselle	Japan	*Hibiscus sabdariffa*
Roselle	Mexico	*Hibiscus sabdariffa*
Roselle	Senegal	*Hibiscus sabdariffa*
Roselle hemp	Nicaragua	*Hibiscus sabdariffa*
Roselle hemp	Senegal	*Hibiscus sabdariffa*
Rotra	Madagascar	*Syzygium cumini*
Roxella red sorrel	Thailand	*Hibiscus sabdariffa*
Roz kaiyen	Guadeloupe	*Hibiscus rosa-sinensis*
Ruman	Oman	*Punica granatum*
S-s'ad	Morocco	*Cyperus rotundus*
Sabar	Saudi Arabia	*Aloe vera*
Saber	Jordan	*Aloe vera*
Sabila	Canary Islands	*Aloe vera*
Sabila	Cuba	*Aloe vera*
Sabila	Guatemala	*Aloe vera*
Sabila	Malaysia	*Aloe vera*
Sabila	Nicaragua	*Aloe vera*
Sabila	Puerto Rico	*Aloe vera*
Sabila	West Indies	*Aloe vera*
Sabr	Saudi Arabia	*Aloe vera*
Sabuu dam	Thailand	*Jatropa curcas*
Sada bahar	Pakistan	*Catharanthus roseus*
Sadabahar	India	*Catharanthus roseus*
Sadaphool	India	*Hibiscus rosa-sinensis*
Sadaphul	India	*Catharanthus roseus*
Safed chirami	India	*Abrus precatorius*
Safed gumchi	India	*Abrus precatorius*
Saffran vert	Mauritius	*Curcuma longa*
Safran	Mauritius	*Curcuma longa*
Safran	Rodrigues Islands	*Curcuma longa*
Saga	Indonesia	*Abrus precatorius*
Saga	Saudi Arabia	*Momordica charantia*
Saga saga	Philippines	*Abrus precatorius*
Sagadi	Nicaragua	*Cymbopogon citratus*
Sagadi abiruau	Nicaragua	*Cymbopogon citratus*

Common name	Country	Latin binomial
Sahajan	India	*Moringa pterygosperma*
Sahanjana	India	*Moringa pterygosperma*
Sahjan	India	*Moringa pterygosperm*
Sahjna	India	*Moringa pterygosperma*
Sahjna	Pakistan	*Moringa pterygosperma*
Saijan	Fiji	*Moringa pterygosperma*
Saijan	Guyana	*Moringa pterygosperma*
Saijan	West Indies	*Moringa pterygosperma*
Sailor's flower	West Indies	*Catharanthus roseus*
Saimal	Nepal	*Jatropa curcas*
Sainjan	India	*Moringa pterygosperma*
Sainjna	India	*Moringa pterygosperma*
Sajana	India	*Moringa pterygosperma*
Sajiba	Nepal	*Jatropa curcas*
Sajina	India	*Moringa pterygosperma*
Sajiwa	Nepal	*Jatropa curcas*
Sajiwan	Nepal	*Jatropa curcas*
Sajiyon	Nepal	*Jatropa curcas*
Sajna	Bangladesh	*Moringa pterygosperma*
Sajna	Fiji	*Moringa pterygosperma*
Sajna	India	*Moringa pterygosperma*
Sakarkanda	Fiji	*Manihot esculenta*
Sakarkanda	Papua-New Guinea	*Manihot esculenta*
Sakumau	Malaysia	*Cymbopogon citratus*
Salijan	India	*Moringa pterygosperma*
Sambathoochedi	India	*Hibiscus rosa-sinensis*
Sampa-sampalukan	Philippines	*Phyllanthus niruri*
Sanga	Ivory Coast	*Abrus precatorius*
Sanguinaria	Colombia	*Lantana camara*
Sanjna	India	*Moringa pterygosperma*
Saponaire	Rodrigues Islands	*Catharanthus roseus*
Sapsap	Senegal	*Moringa pterygosperma*
Saput	Nicaragua	*Annona muricata*
Saqal	Oman	*Aloe vera*
Saragavo	India	*Moringa pterygosperma*
Sarifa	Nicaragua	*Annona muricata*
Sarimsak	Turkey	*Allium sativum*
Sarin	Nicaragua	*Persea americana*
Sasi	Papua-New Guinea	*Phyllanthus niruri*
Satiman-G	Nepal	*Jatropa curcas*
Satui	Sierra Leone	*Hibiscus sabdariffa*
Savila	Mexico	*Aloe vera*
Savila	Peru	*Aloe vera*
Savilla	Bolivia	*Aloe vera*
Sawa sawa	Sierra Leone	*Hibiscus sabdariffa*

Common name	Country	Latin binomial
Sdatiwan	Nepal	*Jatropa curcas*
Se	Papua-New Guinea	*Phyllanthus niruri*
Se'd	Qatar	*Cyperus rotundus*
Seemanepaalam	India	*Jatropa curcas*
Seer	Iran	*Allium sativum*
Segat	India	*Moringa pterygosperma*
Segra	India	*Moringa pterygosperma*
Sehjan	India	*Moringa pterygosperma*
Semper vivum	West Indies	*Aloe vera*
Sengseng	India	*Cassia alata*
Senicikobia	India	*Hibiscus rosa-sinensis*
Senitoa yaloyalo	India	*Hibiscus rosa-sinensis*
Seog-ryu	Oman	*Punica granatum*
Seremaia	Nicaragua	*Annona muricata*
Serimentok	India	*Momordica charantia*
Seripupa	India	*Momordica charantia*
Serocontil	Nicaragua	*Cassia alata*
Sha ts'ao	China	*Cyperus rotundus*
Shahjnah	India	*Moringa pterygosperma*
Shajiwan	Nepal	*Moringa pterygosperma*
Shajmah	India	*Moringa pterygosperma*
Shajna	India	*Moringa pterygosperma*
Sham-al-rumman	Arab Countries	*Punica granatum*
Shejan	India	*Moringa pterygosperma*
Shigru	India	*Moringa pterygosperma*
Shih liu pi	China	*Punica granatum*
Shiliupi	China	*Punica granatum*
Shka-nin-du	Mexico	*Phyllanthus niruri*
Shobanjan	Nepal	*Moringa pterygosperma*
Shobhanjana	India	*Moringa pterygosperma*
Shoe black	Nicaragua	*Hibiscus rosa-sinensis*
Shoe flower	Indonesia	*Hibiscus rosa-sinensis*
Shoe flower	Nepal	*Hibiscus rosa-sinensis*
Shoe flower plant	Kuwait	*Hibiscus rosa-sinensis*
Shoi-bee-reum	Egypt	*Portulaca oleracea*
Siang tan	Vietnam	*Aloe vera*
Sibhanjanavriksha	India	*Moringa pterygosperma*
Siete negritos	Guatemala	*Lantana camara*
Sigra	Nicaragua	*Psidium guajava*
Sigru	India	*Moringa pterygosperma*
Sijeh	Thailand	*Macuna pruriens*
Sikra	Nicaragua	*Psidium guajava*
Sikya	Nicaragua	*Persea americana*
Sindjo el	Guinea-Bissau	*Cassia alata*
Siru	Nepal	*Cyperus rotundus*

Common name	Country	Latin binomial
Sitronel	Haiti	*Cymbopogon citratus*
Skastajat stuki	Mexico	*Lantana camara*
Skin mango	Brazil	*Mangifera indica*
Slim	Nicaragua	*Syzygium cumini*
Small purslain	India	*Portulaca oleracea*
Soanjna	Fiji	*Moringa pterygosperma*
Sobbar	Jordan	*Aloe vera*
Sobhanja	India	*Moringa pterygosperma*
Sobhanjan	India	*Moringa pterygosperma*
Sobhanjana	India	*Moringa pterygosperma*
Sohawjana	Pakistan	*Moringa pterygosperma*
Soijan	Nepal	*Moringa pterygosperma*
Sojna	India	*Moringa pterygosperma*
Sokobale	Fiji	*Manihot esculenta*
Sonkach	India	*Abrus precatorius*
Sonth	India	*Moringa pterygosperma*
Sorosi	Nicaragua	*Momordica charantia*
Sorrow see	Belize	*Momordica charantia*
Sorsaca	Curacao	*Annona muricata*
Souchet rond	Vietnam	*Cyperus rotundus*
Sour sop	Dominican Republic	*Annona muricata*
Sour sop	Puerto Rico	*Annona muricata*
Sour sop tree	USA	*Annona muricata*
Sour-sop	Jamaica	*Annona muricata*
Soursop	Barbados	*Annona muricata*
Soursop	Dominica	*Annona muricata*
Soursop	Guam	*Annona muricata*
Soursop	Guyana	*Annona muricata*
Soursop	Jamaica	*Annona muricata*
Soursop	Nicaragua	*Annona muricata*
Soursop	Virgin Islands	*Annona muricata*
Soursop	West Indies	*Annona muricata*
Soursop leaf	West Indies	*Annona muricata*
Sowasap	Nicaragua	*Annona muricata*
Sudan tea	East Africa	*Hibiscus sabdariffa*
Sujna	India	*Moringa pterygosperma*
Sunara	India	*Moringa pterygosperma*
Sundan	India	*Moringa pterygosperma*
Sus	Egypt	*Abrus precatorius*
Sus	USA	*Abrus precatorius*
Sus saika	Nicaragua	*Cassia alata*
Sus tara saika	Nicaragua	*Cassia alata*
Sus waha tara	Nicaragua	*Cassia alata*
Sushavi	India	*Momordica charantia*
Susur	Indonesia	*Hibiscus sabdariffa*

Common name	Country	Latin binomial
Suvandacheera	India	*Portulaca oleracea*
Sweet sage	Guyana	*Lantana camara*
T'ien t'ou ts'ao	China	*Cyperus rotundus*
Ta khrai	Thailand	*Cymbopogon citratus*
Ta-suan	China	*Allium sativum*
Taingilotra	Madagascar	*Macuna pruriens*
Takuragan	China	*Hibiscus rosa-sinensis*
Talatala	Guatemala	*Lantana camara*
Talcodja	Guinea-Bissau	*Macuna pruriens*
Tale'a	Rodrigues Islands	*Curcuma longa*
Tamarin	Rodrigues Islands	*Tamarindus indica*
Tamarin des indes	West Indies	*Tamarindus indica*
Tamarind	Bangladesh	*Tamarindus indica*
Tamarind	Guyana	*Tamarindus indica*
Tamarind	India	*Tamarindus indica*
Tamarind	Indonesia	*Tamarindus indica*
Tamarind	Japan	*Tamarindus indica*
Tamarind	West Indies	*Tamarindus indica*
Tamarinde	Guinea	*Tamarindus indica*
Tamarindo	Canary Islands	*Tamarindus indica*
Tamarindo	Cuba	*Tamarindus indica*
Tamarindo	Guatemala	*Tamarindus indica*
Tamarindo	Indonesia	*Tamarindus indica*
Tamarindo	Madagascar	*Tamarindus indica*
Tamarindo	Nicaragua	*Tamarindus indica*
Tamarindo	Peru	*Tamarindus indica*
Tamarindo	Puerto Rico	*Tamarindus indica*
Tamarinho	Brazil	*Tamarindus indica*
Tamarini	Guinea	*Tamarindus indica*
Tame tamarine	West Indies	*Tamarindus indica*
Tamparanu	Nicaragua	*Tamarindus indica*
Tamrand	Nicaragua	*Tamarindus indica*
Tamusayt	Morocco	*Cyperus rotundus*
Tanglad	Indonesia	*Cymbopogon citratus*
Tapioka	Samoa	*Manihot esculenta*
Tapioka	Venezuela	*Manihot esculenta*
Tapulaga	China	*Hibiscus rosa-sinensis*
Tarantan	West Indies	*Cassia alata*
Tarbari	India	*Portulaca oleracea*
Tartago	Puerto Rico	*Jatropa curcas*
Tasplira	Nicaragua	*Momordica charantia*
Tateli	India	*Syzygium cumini*
Tauj dub	USA	*Cymbopogon citratus*
Tauj qab	USA	*Cymbopogon citratus*
Tavioka	Venezuela	*Manihot esculenta*

Common name	Country	Latin binomial
Te de limon	Guatemala	Cymbopogon citratus
Te'elango	West Indies	Cassia alata
Tej sar	Ethiopia	Cymbopogon citratus
Tellagaddalu	India	Allium sativum
Tembelekan	Guatemala	Lantana camara
Temoe lawak	Rodrigues Islands	Curcuma longa
Temu kunyit	Malaysia	Curcuma longa
Temu-lawak	Indonesia	Curcuma longa
Tete	West Indies	Syzygium cumini
Tetul	India	Syzygium cumini
Thab thim	Thailand	Punica granatum
Thapthim	Thailand	Punica granatum
Thom	Oman	Allium sativum
Thoum	Jordan	Allium sativum
Thum	Arab Countries	Allium sativum
Thum	Saudi Arabia	Allium sativum
Ti-plomb	West Indies	Lantana camara
Tiao ma tsung	China	Cyperus rotundus
Tiare kalova kalova	Papua-New Guinea	Hibiscus rosa-sinensis
Tiare tupapaku kimo	Cook Islands	Catharanthus roseus
Tiwahiwa	Nicaragua	Cymbopogon citratus
Tmer hendi	Morocco	Syzygium cumini
Tokmakan	Turkey	Portulaca oleracea
Tombi	Guinea	Syzygium cumini
Tombinyi	Guinea	Syzygium cumini
Tong chou	Vietnam	Jatropa curcas
Totoncaxihuitl	Mexico	Cassia alata
Townsville lantana	Australia	Lantana camara
Tree melon	India	Carica papaya
Tsaniya	Nigeria	Syzygium cumini
Tshidzimbambule	Venda	Lantana camara
Tsitsirika	Philippines	Catharanthus roseus
Tuava	Cook Islands	Psidium guajava
Tuava	Easter Island	Psidium guajava
Tuava	Rarotonga	Psidium guajava
Tubang bakod	Cape Verde islands	Jatropa curcas
Tubang bakod	Philippines	Jatropa curcas
Tubatuba	Guam	Jatropa curcas
Tukhm khurfa	Pakistan	Portulaca oleracea
Tulipan	Mexico	Hibiscus rosa-sinensis
Tum	Tunisia	Allium sativum
Tuma	Morocco	Allium sativum
Tumeric	Japan	Curcuma longa
Tumeric	Nepal	Curcuma longa
Tumeric	Thailand	Curcuma longa

Common name	Country	Latin binomial
Tuna	Panama	*Aloe vera*
Tungamuste	India	*Cyperus rotundus*
Tungamuthalu	India	*Cyperus rotundus*
Turmeric	Brazil	*Curcuma longa*
Turmeric	India	*Curcuma longa*
Turmeric	Iran	*Curcuma longa*
Turmeric	Japan	*Curcuma longa*
Turmeric	Malaysia	*Curcuma longa*
Turmeric	Marquesas Island	*Curcuma longa*
Turmeric	Mauritius	*Curcuma longa*
Turmeric	Nepal	*Curcuma longa*
Turmeric	Sri Lanka	*Curcuma longa*
Turmeric	Taiwan	*Curcuma longa*
Turmeric	Thailand	*Curcuma longa*
Turmeric	USA	*Curcuma longa*
Tuunuk	Nicaragua	*Carica papaya*
Twas	Nicaragua	*Carica papaya*
Ualapana	Dominica	*Annona muricata*
Uchhe	India	*Momordica charantia*
Udukaju	Thailand	*Jatropa curcas*
Uhon	India	*Curcuma longa*
Ukon	Japan	*Curcuma longa*
Ukon	Taiwan	*Curcuma longa*
Ul gum	South Korea	*Curcuma longa*
Ulhimar	India	*Momordica charantia*
Ulmak	Nicaragua	*Carica papaya*
Ungume	Guinea-Bissau	*Jatropa curcas*
Ushamanjairi	India	*Catharanthus roseus*
Vatakumba	India	*Carica papaya*
Vatre	Ivory Coast	*Carica papaya*
Vattu pulle	India	*Cymbopogon citratus*
Vellulli	India	*Allium sativum*
Velvetbean	Japan	*Macuna pruriens*
Venturosa	Canary Islands	*Lantana camara*
Venturosa	Colombia	*Lantana camara*
Verdolaga	Brazil	*Portulaca oleracea*
Verdolaga	Canary Islands	*Portulaca oleracea*
Verdolaga	Cuba	*Portulaca oleracea*
Verdolaga	Nicaragua	*Portulaca oleracea*
Verdolaga	Peru	*Portulaca oleracea*
Verdolaga	Puerto Rico	*Portulaca oleracea*
Verdulaga	Spain	*Portulaca oleracea*
Verveine	West Indies	*Lantana camara*
Vi nita	Ivory Coast	*Carica papaya*
Vi papaa	Rarotonga	*Mangifera indica*

Common name	*Country*	*Latin binomial*
Vieille fille	Rodrigues Islands	*Lantana camara*
Viernes santo	Puerto Rico	*Phyllanthus niruri*
Vine licorice	Nepal	*Abrus precatorius*
Vula'tolu	Venezuela	*Manihot esculenta*
Wa	Thailand	*Syzygium cumini*
Waa	Thailand	*Syzygium cumini*
Waan haang charakhe	Thailand	*Aloe vera*
Wagadi	Nicaragua	*Persea americana*
Wan hangchorakhe	Thailand	*Aloe vera*
Wanduru-me	Sri Lanka	*Macuna pruriens*
Wariafa	Nicaragua	*Psidium guajava*
Warse	Oman	*Curcuma longa*
Wasemu	Papua	*Cassia alata*
Wavu wavu	Papua-New Guinea	*Hibiscus rosa-sinensis*
Wayoye	Papua	*Carica papaya*
Wedsiyen	Haiti	*Jatropa curcas*
Weglis	West Indies	*Abrus precatorius*
Weleti	Papua	*Carica papaya*
West Indian ben	India	*Moringa pterygosperma*
White physic nut bush	West Indies	*Jatropa curcas*
White sage	Guatemala	*Lantana camara*
White sage	West Indies	*Lantana camara*
White tulip	West Indies	*Catharanthus roseus*
Wi	Papua	*Carica papaya*
Wild balsam pear	Bahamas	*Momordica charantia*
Wild sage	India	*Lantana camara*
Wild sage	West Indies	*Lantana camara*
Wild senna	West Indies	*Cassia alata*
Wiriwiri	Fiji	*Jatropa curcas*
Wolof	Senegal	*Moringa pterygosperma*
Wong keong	Malaysia	*Curcuma longa*
Wong Keung	Malaysia	*Curcuma longa*
Woz baya	Trinidad	*Hibiscus rosa-sinensis*
Xalxocotl	Mexico	*Psidium guajava*
Xiang fu	China	*Cyperus rotundus*
Ya-ta-bai	Thailand	*Phyllanthus niruri*
Yaa dam	Thailand	*Aloe vera*
Yabia	Venezuela	*Manihot esculenta*
Yabia damu	Venezuela	*Manihot esculenta*
Yadam	Thailand	*Aloe vera*
Yauhra	Nicaragua	*Manihot esculenta*
Yellow sage	Guatemala	*Lantana camara*
Yerba de san pablo	Philippines	*Phyllanthus niruri*
Yerba luisa	Easter Island	*Cymbopogon citratus*
Yesquin	Haiti	*Momordica charantia*

Common name	Country	Latin binomial
Yovoviti	Togo	*Moringa pterygosperma*
Yuca	Guatemala	*Manihot esculenta*
Yuca	Nicaragua	*Manihot esculenta*
Yuca	Puerto Rico	*Manihot esculenta*
Zabila	Canary Islands	*Aloe vera*
Zabila	Mexico	*Aloe vera*
Zabila	Panama	*Aloe vera*
Zabila	Venezuela	*Aloe vera*
Zaboka	Haiti	*Persea americana*
Zaboka	West Indies	*Persea americana*
Zacate de limon	Nicaragua	*Cymbopogon citratus*
Zacate limon	Belize	*Cymbopogon citratus*
Zacate limon	Guatemala	*Cymbopogon citratus*
Zacate limon	Mexico	*Cymbopogon citratus*
Zague zrou	Ivory Coast	*Momordica charantia*
Zakuro	Thailand	*Punica granatum*
Zardchoobeh	Iran	*Curcuma longa*
Zoliv	Haiti	*Moringa pterygosperma*

Glossary

Abortifacient Anything used to cause abortion.

Acaulescent More or less stemless, the stem often subterranean.

Accessory Fruit formed from the expanded dome-like receptacle of a single flower, covered with numerous achenes, known only in the strawberry.

Achene Seed and pericarp attached only at the funiculus, the seed usually tightly enclosed by the fruit wall.

Acicular Needle-shaped.

Acuminate An acute apex in which the sides are concave and taper to an extended point.

Acute Apex formed by two straight margins, meeting at less than 90 degrees.

Aggregate Fruit formed from the many separate dry or fleshy fruits of a single flower, as in the raspberry.

Alkaloid A basic organic nitrogenous compound of plant origin that is pharmacologically active and bitter tasting; certain alkaloids, such quinine, atropine, codeine, and scopolamine, are used in medicine.

Allergenic A substance capable of inducing an allergic response.

Alternate One leaf at a node.

Alveolate Resembles the surface of a honeycomb.

Amblyopia Impaired vision.

Amenorrhea An abnormal suppression or nonoccurrence of menstruation.

Amoebicidal A substance that destroys amoebas.

Analgesic Pain reliever that does not induce loss of consciousness.

Angina Disease of the heart signaled by acute constricting pains in the chest.

Angiosperm Flower-bearing plants; ovules are enclosed in an ovary that forms the fruit after fertilization.

Ankylostomiasis A hookworm disease, common in tropical countries.

Anodyne A soothing pain-easing agent.

Anthelmintic Causes removal or death of worms in the body.

Anthers The pollen-bearing part of a stamen.

Anthrax A carbuncle.

Anti-inflammatory Reduces inflammation

Antidiabetic A medicine counteracting or checking diabetes.

Antidote Remedy counteracting the effects of a poison.

Antifebrile A substance that reduces fever.

Antileukemic Acts against a disorder and generally fatal condition of the blood and blood making tissues, characterized by a persistent excess of leukocytes.

Antinephritic Counteracts kidney disease.

Antipyretic Agent that relieves or reduces fever.

From: Medicinal Plants of the World *By:* Ivan A. Ross Humana Press Inc., Totowa, NJ

Antiscorbutic A remedy for scurvy.

Antiseptic Prevents infection or putrefaction; a disinfecting agent.

Antispasmodic Prevents or cures spasms, as in epilepsy.

Antitumor Refers to tumor growth-inhibiting properties, usually referred to in connection with cancer.

Aperient A mild laxative.

Apetalous Without petals.

Aphrodisiac Agents that stimulate sexual desire.

Aphtha (plural, aphthae) An ulcer of the mucous membrane, usually oral.

Apiculate Terminates in a short sharp flexible point.

Arachnoid Slender white loosely tangled hairs; cobwebby.

Arboreous Trees with well-developed trunk.

Arcuate An uncommon pattern in which the major veins curve gently upward.

Aristate An abrupt hard bristle-like point.

Astringent A substance that checks the discharge of mucus, serum etc., by causing contraction of the tissue.

Athlete's Foot A fungal infection of the foot, causing itching, blisters, and cracking of the skin.

Attenuate The apex drawn out into a long gradual taper.

Auriculate Has a pair of rounded lobes that somewhat resemble the human ear.

Axils The cavity or angle formed by the junction of the upper side of a leaf stalk or branch with a stem or branch.

Bactericide Anything that destroys bacteria.

Barbellate Hairs with barbs down the sides.

Berry Entire soft pericarp, as in the tomato or grape.

Biliousness Popular term used to describe conditions marked by general malaise, giddiness, vomiting, headache, indigestion, constipation, and so forth.

Blade Lamina, the flattened expanded portion; a few leaves are bladeless.

Bract A leaf much reduced in size, particularly if it is associated with a flower or inflorescence.

Bronchiectasias A chronic inflammation or degenerative condition of one or more bronchioles.

Bronchitis An inflammation of the tubes in the lungs.

Bulb An upright series of overlapping leaf bases attached to a small basal stem, as in the onion.

Caespitose Growing in tufts, mats, or clumps.

Calceolate Slipper-shaped.

Calculus Stone concretion in some part of the body

Calyx The outermost series of leaf-like parts of a flower, individually called sepals.

Canescent With a dense mat of gray-white hairs.

Carbuncle An extensive dangerous form of boil having a flat surface that discharges pus from multiple points and occupies several inches of skin surface.

Carcinogen A substance which causes cancer.

Cardiac Products that have an effect upon the heart.

Carminative A substance that prevents formation of or promotes expulsion of gas from the alimentary tract; relieves flatulence.

Catarrh Excessive secretion from an inflamed mucous membrane, especially of the air passages of the throat and head.

Cathartic Producing evacuation of the bowels.

Caudate The apex tail-like.

Caulescent Aerial stem or stems evident.

Cercaricidal Affected by a larval parasitic trematode worm.

Cholalogue A drug that stimulates the flow of bile by the liver.

Chronic Diseases that are of long duration, either mild or acute.

Ciliate Hairs along the margins only.

Ciliate With fine hairs on the margin.

Clambering Spreads over undergrowth or objects, usually without the aid of twinning stems or tendrils.

Clasping The bases partly to completely surrounding the stem.

Claw A long narrow stalk-like base of a petal or sepal.

Cleft Indented about halfway to the midrib or base of the blade.

Climbing Ascends upon other plants or objects by means of special structures.

Colic Pain resulting from excessive or sudden abdominal spasmodic contractions of muscles in the intestine walls, bile ducts, ureter, or any obstruction, twisting, or distention of any of the hollow organs or tubes following the stretching of the walls by gas or solid substances.

Coma Stupor; abnormally deep sleep.

Comose With a tuft of hairs at the apex of a seed or at the base of a floret in a grass spikelet.

Complete A flower that has all four series.

Conjunctivitis Inflammation of the mucous membrane lining of the eyelids and covering of the anterior part of the eyeball.

Constipation A morbid inactivity of the bowels.

Consumption A general term used to describe the wasting of tissues, including but not limited to, tuberculosis.

Contact dermatitis Local allergic reaction provoked by skin contact with chemical substances that act as antigens or haptens.

Contraceptive Prevents conception by chemical or physical means.

Cordate Of the shape of the stylized heart with the petiole attached between the basal lobes.

Corm An upright, hard, or fleshy stem surrounded by dry scaly leaves, as in the gladiolus bulb.

Corniculate Bears a small horn-like protuberance, as in the milkweed flower.

Corona Any outgrowth situated between the corolla and the androecium, as in milkweeds.

Crenate Scalloped, with blunt teeth.

Cruciform Cross-shaped, as in the sepals and petals of the mustard family.

Cuneate Wedge-shaped.

Cupule A series of fused bracts that form a cup beneath the true fruit, as in the acorn.

Cuspidate A sharp-pointed tip formed by abruptly and sharply concave sides.

Cyanogenic Capable of producing hydrocyanic acid (HCN).

Cystitis Inflammation of the urinary bladder.

Decoction A liquid preparation obtained by boiling medicinal plant substances in water and extracting drugs by straining the preparation.

Decumbent Stems lying upon the ground with their ends turned up.

Decussate Opposite leaves that alternate at right angles to one another at successive nodes, thereby forming four rows of leaves.

Dehiscent A fruit that opens by sutures, pores, or caps.

Deltoid Of the shape of an equilateral triangle.

Demulcent Substances used for their soothing and protective action; allays irritation of surfaces, especially mucous membranes.

Dengue Infective eruptive fever causing acute pains in joints.

Dentate Has coarse angular teeth directed outward at right angles to the margin.

Denticulate Finely dentate.

Depilatory Removes hair.

Diabetes Metabolic disorder affecting insulin production and resulting in faulty carbohydrate metabolism.

Diaphoretic Drugs that promote perspiration as a result of stimulation of the sweat glands.

Diarrhea Abnormal frequency and fluidity of stool discharges.

Dicotyledon An angiosperm having two cotyledons (seed leaves); usually the leaves are net-veined, and floral parts are in fours or fives.

Didymous A strongly lobed fruit, thus appearing as a pair.

Dioecious A species in which any particular plant bears either staminate or pistillate flowers, but not both; the species is composed of separate staminate and pistillate plants.

Diuretic Agent that increases urine flow by acting on the kidneys.

Divaricate Extremely divergent, more or less at a right angle.

Divergent Broadly spreading.

Divided Indented to the midrib or base of the blade.

Doubly serrate The serrations themselves serrate.

Dropsy A leakage of the watery part of the blood into any of the tissues or cavities of the body.

Drupe Exocarp and mesocarp fleshy, endocarp bony; the seed and endocarp constitute a **pyrene**; mango.

Dull Not shining; lacking luster.

Dysentery Inflammation of the bowel with evacuation of mucous and blood in the stool.

Dysmenorrhea Abnormal pains during the menstruation period. The pain may be either spasmodic or continuous.

Dyspepsia Difficult or painful digestion, generally chronic.

Dysuria Difficult, painful, or incomplete urination.

Ecbolic Causing contraction of the uterus and thus inducing abortion or promoting parturition.

Echinate With straight, often comparatively large, prickle-like hairs.

Eczema Noncontagious itching; inflammatory skin eruption characterized by papules, vesicles, and pustules that may also be associated with edema, scaling, or exudation.

Elephantiasis A chronic enlargement of the cutaneous and subcutaneous tissues. It is most common in the tropics and results from obstruction of the lymphatics.

Elliptic Oval, the ends rounded and is widest at the middle.

Emarginate With a shallow notch at the apex.

Emetic A drug or an agent having the power to empty the stomach by vomiting.

Emmenagogue Applied to drugs which have the power of stimulating the menstrual discharge.

Emollient A substance applied externally to soften the skin, or internally, to soothe an irritated or inflamed surface.

Empacho An infant disease resulting in diarrhea, pale stools, and sour vomit, attributed to diet of mother during pregnancy.

Emphysema Enlargement of air vesicles in the lungs; swelling of connective tissues of the body caused by to the presence of air.

Endocarp The innermost layer of the fruit wall; it may be soft, papery, or bony.

Endosperm The albumin of a seed.

Enema A liquid preparation injected into the rectum, resulting in complete emptying of the large bowel in minutes.

Enteritis Acute or chronic intestinal inflammation.

Entire Not in any way indented, the margin featureless.

Epidermis True skin of a plant below the cuticle.

Epilepsy A chronic nervous affliction characterized by loss of consciousness and/or muscular convulsions, sometimes accompanied by paroxysmic seizures.

Epiphyte A plant growing nonparasitically upon another.

Erose Gnawed, as if chewed upon.

Erysipelas An acute inflammation disease of the skin caused by infection by various strains of *Streptococcus* and accompanied by fever.

Erythrasma A chronic contagious dermatitis caused by an actinomycete and affecting warm moist areas.

Erythrocytes Red blood cells formed in red bone marrow.

Essential Applied to volatile oils of plants, marked by characteristic odor; also applied to fatty acids believed by nutritionists to be necessary for health.

Estrogenic effect The effect of female steroidal hormones in promoting ovulation and secondary sexual characteristics.

Evacuant A medicine or purgative that empties an organ, especially the bowel.

Exanthema A disease accompanied by eruptions of the skin, such as measles or scarlet fever.

Exocarp The outermost layer of the fruit wall; it may be the "skin" of the fruit, a leathery or hard rind.

Expectorant A medicine promoting secretion of bronchial mucus and facilitating the ejection of phlegm from the lungs by coughing.

Extract A pharmaceutical preparation obtained by dissolving the active constituents of a drug with a suitable solvent, evaporating the solvent, and adjusting to proscribe standards.

Falcate Sickle-shaped.

Fascicled Clustered.

Febrifuge A drug tending to reduce fever.

Fibrosis Morbid increase of fibrous tissue in the body; fibroid degeneration of blood capillaries.

Fibrositis Inflammation of fibrous tissue.

Filariasis A disease caused by parasitic worms.

Filiform Thread-like.

Fimbriate As in ciliate, but coarser and longer.

Fimbriate Fringed, the hairs coarser than in ciliate.

Flatulence The presence of an excessive amount of gas in stomach and intestine.

Flavonoid A group of organic compounds responsible for a great number of colors in fruits and flowers. In the past, they were often used in conjunction with mordants for the dyeing of fabrics.

Floccose With tufts of soft hairs that rub off easily.

Fruticose Shrubby, with more than one major stem.

Fumigate Applying smoke or vapor to affected part.

Funiculus The seed stalk.

Galactogogue An agent that induces or increases the secretion of milk.

Gastritis Inflammation of the stomach.

Gastrointestinal Pertaining to the stomach and intestines.

Genito-urinary Relating to the genital and the urinary organs or functions.

Germicidal A substance that kills germs and microorganisms in general.

Gingivitis Inflammation of the gums.

Glabrate Hairy at first, but then glabrous.

Glabrous Without hairs.

Glandular Hairs with swollen tips; gland-bearing.

Glaucoma Group of diseases characterized by increasing intraocular pressures causing defects in vision.

Glaucous Covered with a whitish waxy bloom.

Glochidiate Hairs barbed at the tip only, as in the hairs of certain cacti.

Glossitis Inflammation of the tongue.

Glycoside Naturally occurring substance consisting of sugars combined with nonsugars such as a flavonoid, coumarine, steroid, terpene, and so forth (aglycones).

Gonorrhea A venereal disease that causes inflammation of the mucous membranes of the urethra and adjacent cavities.

Gout A condition or uric acid metabolism. It occurs in paroxysms and is characterized by painful inflammation of parts of the joints and an excessive amount of uric acid in the blood.

Hastate More or less arrowhead-shaped, but with the basal lobes divergent.

Haustoria Roots or suckers found in parasitic plants.

Head Capitulum, a dense spherical or rounded inflorescence of sessile flowers, as in the Compositae family.

Helicoid cyme A one-sided coiled inflorescence resembling a fiddlehead, as in most members of the *Boraginaceae* family.

Hemolytic An agent capable of destroying blood cells.

Hemorrhoids An enlarged and often dilated blood vessel or vein of the anal canal or the lower portion of the alimentary tract.

Hemostatic An agent that arrests hemorrhage.

Hepatitis Inflammation of the liver.

Hernia Protrusion of an organ through its containing wall. It may occur in any part of the body, but is especially associated with the abdominal cavity.

Herpes Skin disease with patches of distinct vesicles.

Hesperidium Ovary superior; septations conspicuous, these lined with fleshy hairs, restricted to the citrus fruits.

Hip A vase-like leathery hypanthium containing several achenes; restricted to the rose.

Hirsute With rough or coarse, more or less erect hairs.

Hirtellous Minutely hirsute.

Hispid With long rigid bristly hairs.

Hives Any of various skin diseases, especially urticaria.

Hydrocele An accumulation of fluid in bag-like cavities in the body.

Hydrolysis The addition of water of a molecule of water to a chemical compound accompanied by a splitting of that compound into usually two fragments; hydrolysis is normally facilitated by the presence of small amounts of acids; for example, the degradation of starch into simple sugars achieved by prolonged heating of an acidified starch slurry in water.

Hypertension Abnormally high constrictive tension in blood vessels, usually revealed as high blood pressure.

Hypoglycemia Deficiency of normal glucose levels in the body; low blood sugar.

Imbricate Overlapping.

Incised Deeply and sharply cut.

Inflorescence Axes along which all the buds are flower buds.

Infusion The extract obtained from steeping of plant material in water, for example, tea.

Integument (Bot.) The skin of a seed.

Involucre A set of separate or fused bracts associated with a fruit, as in the walnut.

Jaundice Yellowness of the skin, mucus membranes and secretions, as a result of bile pigments in the blood.

Keel A structure resembling the bottom of a boat, as in the two fused lower petals of many legume flowers.

Laciniate Slashed into narrow pointed segments.

Lacrimation The excessive secretion of tears.

Lactagogue An agent that induces the secretion and flow of milk.

Lactation The formation and secretion of milk.

Lanate Woolly or cottony.

Lanceolate Lance-shaped, several times longer than wide; the sides curved, with the blade broadest below the middle.

Laryngitis Inflammation of the larynx.

Laxative A gentle bowel stimulant.

Lectin Protein that effects agglutination, precipitation, or other phenomena resembling the action of a specific antibody.

Leprosy A chronic disease of the skin and nerves characterized by whitish pigmentation.

Leukopenia An abnormally low number of leukocytes (white blood cells) in the blood.

Leukorrhea A white or yellowish mucopurulent vaginal discharge.

Liana A twining or climbing plant with rope-like woody stems.

Lianas Woody plants with elongate flexible, nonsupporting stems.

Linear Several times longer than wide, the sides more or less parallel.

Liniment An agent or substance applied to the skin by gentle friction or by brisk rubbing, meant to relieve superficial pain.

Lobed Indented about one-fourth to almost half way to the midrib or base of the blade.

Loch A syrupy medication having a local action in the mucus membrane of the throat.

Lodicule The highly reduced perianth of the grasses.

Lumbago Muscular rheumatism; a general term for backache in the lumbar region.

Lustrous Shining.

Lyrate With a series of pinnate lobes and a larger terminal lobe.

Malaria An acute, usually chronic, disease caused by protozoa belonging to the genus *Plasmodium* and transmitted by *Anopheles* mosquito. It is characterized by intermittent fever, anemia, and debility, and in its acute form, by chills, high fever, and profuse sweating at regular intervals.

Mange A contagious skin disease characterized by itching and hair loss, caused by parasitic mites.

Marasmus A wasting away of the body, associated with inadequate food.

Masticatory A substance chewed to increase salivation.

Mealy Swollen hairs which collectively form a covering resembling cooking meal.

Meningitis A disease of the membranes enveloping the brain and spinal cord.

Menorrhagia Excessive menstrual flow.

Mesocarp The middle layer of the fruit wall, often the fleshy edible portion.

Metrorrhagia Bleeding between periods.

Migraine A recurring and intensely painful headache, often accompanied by vomiting, giddiness, and disturbance of the vision.

Molluscicidal An agent that destroys a variety of skin diseases.

Monocotyledon Angiosperms having one cotyledon (seed leaf); the leaves are usually parallel-veined, and floral parts are in threes.

Monoecious A species in which any plant bears both ataminate and pistillate flowers.

Mucronate Possessing a hard short abrupt point.

Multiple Fruit derived from the fusion of an entire inflorescence, as in the pineapple.

Net A complex venation pattern of major and minor veins that form a network or reticulum.

Neuralgia An acute paroxysmal pain along the course of and over the local distribution of a nerve.

Obcordate As in the cordate leaf, but the petiole attached at the point of the heart.

Oblanceolate As in the lanceolate leaf, but the petiole attached at the narrow end.

Oblique Asymmetrical; unequal-sided.

Oblong About two or three times longer than broad; rectangular with rounded corners.

Obovate As in ovate, but the petiole attached at the narrow end.

Obtuse Apex formed by two lines that meet at more than a right angle.

Oliguria A deficiency in the excretion of urine.

Ophthalmia Inflammation of the eyeball or the conjunctiva of the eye.

Opposite Two leaves at a node.

Orbicular Circular or nearly so.

Oval Broadly elliptic, the length less than twice the width.

Ovate The shape of the longitudinal section through a chicken's egg, with the petiole attached at the broad end.

Oxytocic Stimulating movements of the uterus.

Palmate The major veins radiating from a common point at the base of the blade, as in the maples.

Palpitation A rapid pulsation or throbbing of the heart.

Panicle A loose compound flower cluster produced by irregular branching.

Papillate Pimple-like hairs or pimple-like protuberance.

Parallel Several to many veins of about the same size (the midrib sometimes more conspicuous) and parallel to one another, as in many monocots.

Parasiticide Any agent that destroys parasites.

Parted Indented nearly all the way to the midrib or the base of the blade.

Parturient Applied to substances used during childbirth.

Parturition The act of childbirth

Pediculicide An agent for treatment of the feet.

Pediculosis The condition of being infected with lice.

Peduncle The stalk supporting a single flower in an inflorescence.

Pepo A berry with a leathery rind, derived from an inferior ovary; use is often restricted to the squash family.

Perfect A flower with both stamens and carpels, without regard to the state of the perianth.

Perfoliate The condition of a sessile leaf when the base completely encircles the stem.

Pericarp The fruit wall, made up of the endocarp, mesocarp, and exocarp; the wall of the ripened ovary of a flower.

Peristalsis Wavelike muscular contractions of the intestines.

Petioles The stalk that supports the lamina; if missing, the leaf is sessile.

Phagocytosis The destruction and absorption of bacteria or microorganisms by phagocytes.

Pharynx The throat; the joint opening of the gullet and windpipe.

Phthisis A wasting disease of the lungs; difficulty in breathing.

Phyllode A leaflike petiole of a bladeless leaf, as in some *Acacia*.

Phyllode A petiole that develops into a flattened expansion taking the place of a leaf.

Phytoalexin An antimicrobial compound produced in a plant in response to fungal infection.

Piles A synonym for hemorrhoids.

Pilose With sparse slender soft hairs.

Pinnae A single leaflet of a pinnate leaf.

Pinnate Having the shape or arrangement of a feather. Prominent midvein with a series of major veins arising at about 30–45 degrees angles along its length.

Pistillate A unisexual (female) flower in which only carpels are present, the stamens being rudimentary or suppressed.

Pitted Covered with small cavities.

Pityriasis A skin disease in which the epidermis sheds thin scales as dandruff.

Pleurisy Inflammation of the pleura membrane enveloping the lung.

Pneumonia Refers to a large number conditions that include the inflammation or passive congestion of the lungs, resulting in portions of the lung becoming solid.

Pome Ovary inferior, surrounded by fleshy tissue, usually interpreted as a hypanthium, as in the apple or pear.

Postpartum After childbirth.

Poultice A mass of material applied to sore or inflamed part of the body for the purpose of supplying heat and moisture or acting as a local stimulant.

Prickly Heat Heat rash; irritation of the skin caused by heat.

Prolapse The descent of an organ or viscus of the body from its natural position.

Prophylactic Operating to ward off or protect against a disease.

Prostrate Lying flat upon the ground; typically without adventitious roots.

Proteolytic Cause splitting of proteins into smaller products during digestion.

Prothallus The first or false thallus formed in the germination of the sexually produced spores in ferns; a delicate cellular structure bearing the sexual organs.

Pruritus Localized or generalized itching due to the irritation of sensory nerve endings.

Psoriasis A noncontagious inflammatory skin disease characterized by reddish patches and white scales.

Pterygium A triangular fleshy mass of thickened conjunctiva occurring at the inner side of the eyeball causing a disturbance to vision.

Puberulent Minutely canescent.

Pubescent Downy; the hairs short soft and erect.

Pulmonary Pertaining to or affecting the lungs.

Punctate Dotted with pinpoint impressions or translucent dots.

Purgative Drugs which evacuate the bowels; more drastic than a laxative.

Pyorrhea A purulent discharge that contains or consists of pus.

Quinones Organic compounds based on benzene where two hydrogen atoms have been replaced in the same ring by two oxygen atoms. Quinones are usually highly colored and are often responsible for the yellow and red colors of some seeds, bark and woods etc.

Rank A vertical row of leaves.

Reniform Kidney-shaped or bean-shaped.

Repent Trailing, stems prostrate, creeping or sprawling, and often rooting at the node.

Resolvent Medicine that reduces swelling or inflammation.

Restorative A remedy that is efficient in restoring health and strength.

Resupinate Inverted because of a 180 degrees twist in a petiole or pedicel.

Reticulate Netted with regular slightly elevated lines.

Revolute The margin rolled toward the lower side of the blade.

Rheumatism A general term for painful inflammation of muscle, tendon, joint, bone, or nerve, resulting in discomfort.

Rhizome Horizontal underground stem distinguished from a root by scale-like leaves and axillary buds. Horizontal stem with reduced scaly leaves, as in many grasses.

Ringworm A common contagious disease produced by fungi that affects the skin, hair, or nails.

Rosette A radiating leaf cluster at or near the base of the plant.

Rostulate In rosettes.

Rounded The apex gently curved.

Rubefacient Applied to counter irritants to the skin; substances that produce blisters or inflammation.

Rugose Wrinkled.

Runcinate Coarsely-toothed, the teeth pointing toward the base of the leaf, as in the dandelion.

Sagittate Arrowhead-shaped.

Saponin A substance characterized by the ability to form emulsions and soapy lathers.

Scabies A contagious skin disease caused by a mite that burrows in the horny layer of the skin.

Scabrous Rough to the touch because of coarse stiff ascending hairs.

Scapose Bearing a flower or inflorescence on a leafless flowering stem.

Scrofula A tuberculous condition of the lymphatic glands characterized by enlarged suppurating abscess and cheese-like degeneration.

Scurfy Covered with minute scales.

Scurvy A nutritional disorder caused by deficiency of vitamin C; characterized by extreme weakness, spongy gums, and a tendency to develop hemorrhages under the skin, from the mucus membranes, and under the periosteum.

Sedative An agent that quiets nervous excitement.

Septum An internal partition within the fruit.

Sericeous Silky; the hairs long, fine, and appressed.

Serrate With coarse saw-like teeth that point forward.

Serrulate Finely serrate.

Setaceous Bristly.

Sheath The basal portion of a leaf that surrounds the stem.

Shingles A virus that lives in the nerves and affects one specific part of the body.

Shrubs Woody perennials with more than one principal stem arising from the ground.

Sinate Wavy in and out, in the plane of the blade.

Soporific Inducing sleep.

Sori Clusters of spore cases in ferns.

Spadix A spike or head of flowers with a fleshy axis, usually enclosed within a bract.

Spasmodic Periodic sharp attacks marked by spasms.

Spatulate Spoon-shaped.

Spine A leaf or portion of a leaf that is sharp-pointed, the most common examples being paired stipular spines; not to be confused with **thorns**, which are modified stems or **prickles**, which are mere outgrowths of the epidermis, as in the cultivated rose.

Spinose With a spine at the tip.

Sporangium A spore case in which asexual spores are produced.

Spreading Oriented outward and more or less diverging from the point of origin.

Staminate A unisexual (male) flower in which stamens are present, the carpels being rudimentary or suppressed.

Steam-distillation The process of isolating the volatile principles from a material by passing steam through it (or boiling it with water) and condensing the steam to recover the usually insoluble volatile substance.

Stimulant Anything that quickens or promotes the activity of some physiological process.

Stipe A stalk or support.

Stipules A pair of appendages located at the base of the petiole where it joins the stem; often short-lived and seen only as stipule scars; if not formed, the leaf is exstipulate.

Stolon A trailing runner or rootstock by which grasses may propagate.

Stomachic Applied to drugs given for disorders of the stomach.

Striated Marked with longitudinal lines.

Stricture Abnormal narrowing of a tubular organ; sometimes a result of inflammation.

Strigose Hairs sharp, appressed, rigid, and often swollen at the base.

Style The stalk between the ovary and the stigma.

Styptic Substances that clot the blood and thus stop bleeding.

Subulate Slender and tapering to a point, as in the awl, a tool used to make holes in leather.

Sudorific Producing copious perspiration.

Suffruticose Plants woody at the base but herbaceous above.

Sulcate Furrowed with longitudinal lines.

Suppository A small solid medication that is inserted into a bodily orifice other than the mouth.

Syconium A hollow vase-like inflorescence with the flowers lining the inside; restricted to the fig.

Syphilis A venereal disease, characterized by a variety of lesions, caused by *Treponema pallidum*.

Tachycardia Abnormally rapid heart action as a disease.

Tannin Astringent principle of many plants.

Tapeworm A parasitic worm of the class Cestoidea; a segmented an ribbon-like flatworm. It develops in the alimentary canals or vertebrates.

Tendril A twining leaf or portion of a leaf, as in the leaflets of the sweet pea; tendrils may also be of stem origin.

Tetanus An acute infectious disease caused by a bacillus and characterized by rigid spasmodic contractions of various voluntary muscles especially of the jaw.

Thrush A mycotic disease of the upper digestive tract (mouth, lips, and throat) resulting from infection by the fungus *Candida albicans*. It occurs especially in children and is characterized by small whitish spots on the tip and sides of the tongue.

Tisane A medical decoction or tea of herbs drunk as a beverage or for its mildly medicinal effect.

Tomentose Densely and softly matted.

Tonic A drug or an agent given to improve the normal tone of an organ or of the patient generally.

Trachoma A contagious virus disease of the eye characterized by granular conjunctivitis.

Trees Woody perennials with a single main stem or trunk.

Truncate The apex appearing chopped off.

Tuber An enlarged fleshy tip of an underground stem, as in the Irish potato.

Tuberculate Warty.

Tuberculosis An infectious disease caused by the tubercle bacillus. It may affect any tissue of the body, but especially occurs in the lungs.

Tumor Generally any abnormal swelling of the body other than those caused by direct injury is considered a tumor.

Turion A swollen scaly offshoot of a rhizome.

Twining Coiling around plants or objects as a means of support.

Typhus An infectious disease caused by the *Rickettsia* microorganism, characterized by high fever and delirium.

Ulcer An interruption of continuity of a surface with an inflamed base. Any open sore other than a wound.

Umbel An indeterminate inflorescence in which a number of nearly equal peduncles radiate from a small area at the top of a very short axis, giving an umbrella-like appearance.

Uncinate Hooked hairs.

Undulate Wavy perpendicular to the plane of the blade.

Uremia Condition of the blood caused by retention of urinary matter normally eliminated by the kidneys.

Varicose Abnormally dilated or knotted blood vessels.

Velutinous Velvety; the hairs dense, firm, and straight.

Venereal Pertaining to, or produced by, sexual intercourse.

Vermicide Substance that kills worms.

Vermifuge Substance that kills or expels intestinal worms.

Verticel An axillary whorl of flowers radiating in many directions, as in several members of the mint family (*Labiatae*).

Vertigo Any of a group of disorders in which dizziness is experienced.

Vesicant A blistering agent; any agent or drug that produces blisters on the skin.

Vesicatory Any substance capable of causing blisters.

Villous Shaggy; the hairs long, slender, soft, but not matted.

Vine Herbaceous plants with elongate, flexible, nonself-supporting stems.

Viscera Internal organs of the body, especially in the abdomen and thorax.

Viscid Sticky.

Vitiligo A skin disease characterized by whitish nonpigmented areas surrounded by hyperpigmented borders.

Vulnerary A remedy used for treating wounds.

Wart A common skin tumor caused by a virus infection. It is contagious from case to case or from skin area to skin area in the same individual.

Whitlow An old general term for any suppurative inflammation on a finger or toe.

Whorled Three or more leaves at a node.

Yaws An infectious, nonvenereal tropical disease caused by *Treponema pertenus*. It is characterized by an initial lesion (the mother-yaw), followed by further multiple lesions of the skin. It is also known as *Framboesia*.

Yellow Fever A tropical epidemic disease caused by mosquito-borne viral infection.

Bibliography

A00020 Suwal, P. N. Medicinal plants of Nepal. Ministry of Forests, Department of Medicinal Plants, Thapathali, Kathmandu, Nepal, 1970.

A00041 Jain, S. K. and C. R. Tarafder. Medicinal Plant-Lore of the Santals. **Econ Bot** 1970; 24: 178–241.

A00115 Quisumbing, E. Medicinal plants of the Philippines. **Tech Bull 16**, Rep Philippines, Dept Agr Nat Resources, Manilla 1951; 1.

A00136 Jiu, J. A survey of some medicinal plants of Mexico for selected biological activities. **Lloydia** 1966; 29: 250–259.

A00368 Mc Cuddin, C. R. Samoan medicinal plants and their usage. Office of comprehensive health planning, Department of Medical Services. Government of American Samoan, 1974.

A00455 Alvaro Viera, R. Subsidio Para O Estudo Da Flora Medicinal Da Guinea Portuguesa. Agencia-Geral Do Ultramar, Lisboa, 1959.

A00456 Zaguirre, J. C. Guide notes of bed-size preparations of most common local (Philippines) medicinal plants, 1944.

A00468 Malhi, B. S. and V. P. Trivedi. Vegetable antifertility drugs of India. **Q J Crude Drug Res** 1972; 12: 19–22.

A00499 Velez-Salas, F. Additional note on the antimalarial cundeamor. **Rev Farm** (Buenos Aires) 1944; 86: 512–516.

A00614 Paijmans, K. P. New Guinea vegetation. Elsevier Scientific Publ. Co., New York, 1976.

A00637 Rivera, G. Preliminary Chemical and Pharmacological studies on "cundeamor", *Momordica charantia*. II. **Amer J Pharm** 1942; 114: 72.

A00682 Couvee. Compilation of herbs, plants, crops supposed to be effective in various complaints and illnesses. **J Sci Res** 1952; 1s.

A00693 Ghosh, S., R. N. Chopra and A. Dutta. Chemical examination of the bark of *Moringa pterygosperma*. **Indian J Med Res**. 1935; 22: 785.

A00706 West, M. E., G. H. Sidrak and S. P. W. Street. The anti-growth properties of extracts from *Momordica charantia*. **West Indian Med J** 1971; 20(1): 25–34.

A00708 Vasileva, B. Plantes Medicinales de Guinee. Conarky, Republique, 1969.

A00709 Garcia-Barriga, H. Flora Medicinal De Colombia. Vol. 2/3 Universidad Nacional, Bogota, 1975.

A00710 Garcia-Barriga, H. Flora Medicinal De Colombia. Vol 1. Universidad Nacional, Bogota, 1974.

From: Medicinal Plants of the World *By: Ivan A. Ross Humana Press Inc., Totowa, NJ*

A00785   Spencer, C. F., F. R. Koniuszy, E. F. Rogers et al. Survey of plants for Antimalarial activity. **Lloydia** 1947; 10: 145–174.

A01897   Kinel, F. A. and J. Gedeon. Products from *Moringa pterygosperma*. **Arch Pharm(Weinheim)** 1957; 290: 302.

A01908   Ahmad, Y. S. A note on the plants of medicinal value found in Pakistan. Government of Pakistan Press, Karachi, 1957.

A01947   Pons, J. A. and D. S. Stevenson. Effect of *Momordica charantia* (cundeamor) in diabetes mellitus. I. A test for hypoglycemic activity in an alcohol extract. **Puerto Rico J Pub Health Trop Med** 1943; 19: 196.

A01962   Haddock, R. L. Some Medicinal Plants of Guam including English and Guamanian Common Names. **Report Regional Tech Mtg Med Plants,** Papeete, Tahiti, Nov, 1973, South Pacific Commissioner, Noumea, New Claedonia 1974; 79.

A01966   Bouquet, A. and M. Debray. Medicinal Plants of the Ivory Coast. **Trav Doc Orstom** 1974; 32: 1.

A02006   Cordell, G. A., S. G. Weiss and N. R. Farnsworth. Structure elucidation and chemistry of Catharanthus alkaloids. XXX. Isolation and structure of vincarodine. **J Org Chem** 1974; 39(4): 431–434.

A02047   Han, B. H., H. J. Chi, Y. N. Han and K. S. Ryu. Screening of the anti-inflammatory activity of crude drugs. **Korean J Pharmacog** 1972; 4(3): 205-209.

A02176   Batta, S. K. and G. Santhakumari. The antifertility effect of *Ocimum santum* and *Hibiscus rosa-sinensis*. **Indian J Med Res** 1970; 59: 777.

A02269   Jain, S. K. Studies in Indian Ethnobotany. II. Plant Used in Medicine by the Tribals of Madhya Pradesh. **Bull Reg Res Lab (Jammu India)** 1963; 1: 126–128

A02296   Pardo De Tavera, T. H. Medicinal plants of the Philippines. Blakiston, Philadelphia, 1901.

A02376   Joshi, M. S. and R. Y. Ambaye. Effect of alkaloids from *Vinca rosea* on spermatogenesis in male rats. **Indian J Exp Biol** 1968; 6: 256,257.

A02434   Kholkute, S. D., S. Chatterjee, D. N. Srivastava and K. N. Udupa. Effect of *Hibiscus rosa-sinensis* on the reproductive organs of male rats. **J Reprod Fertil** 1974; 38: 233,234.

A02435   Bhaduri, B., C. R. Ghose, A. N. Bose, B. K. Moza and U. P. Basu. Antifertility Activity of some Medicinal Plants. **Indian J Exp Biol**. 1968; 6: 252,253.

A02478   Kapoor, M., S. K. Garg and V. S. Mathur. Antiovulatory activity of five indigenous plants in rabbits. **Indian J Med Res** 1974; 62: 1225–1227.

A02479   Noble, R. L., C. T. Beer and J. H. Cutts. Role of chance observations in chemotherapy: *Vinca rosea*. **Ann NY Acad Sci** 1958; 76: 882.

A02600   Dhawan, B. N. and P. N. Saxena. Evaluation of some indigenous drugs for stimulant effect on the rat uterus. A preliminary report. **Indian J Med Res**. 1958; 46(6): 808–811.

A02750   Meguro, M. Growth-regulating substances in *Cyperus rotundus* rhizome. ll. Nature and properties of the inhibitor. **Univ Sao Paulo Fac Fil Cienc Let Bol Bot** 1969; 24: 145.

A02761   Meguro, M. and M. V. Bonomi. Inhibitory action of *Cyperus rotundus* rhizome extracts on the development of some fungi. **Univ Sao Paulo Fac Fil Cienc Let Bol Bot** 1969; 24: 173.

A02820   Singh, S. P. Presence of a growth inhibitor in the tubers of Nutgrass. **Proc Indian Acad Sci Ser** 1968; 67B: 18.

A02970 Fong, H. H. S., N. R. Farnsworth, L. K. Henry, G. H. Svoboda and M. J. Yates. Biological and Phytochemical evaluation of plants. X. Test results from a third two-hundred accessions. **Lloydia** 1972; 35(1): 35–48.

A03021 Akperbekova, B. A. and R. A. Abdullaev. Diuretic effect of drug form and galenicals from the roots of *Cyperus rotundus* growing in Azerbaidzhan. **Izv Akad Nauk Az Ssr Ser Biol Nauk** 1966; 4: 98.

A03033 Dhar, M. L., M. M. Dhar, B. N. Dhawan, B. N. Mehrotra, R. C. Srimal and J. S. Tandon. Screening of Indian plants for biological activity. Part IV. **Indian J Exp Biol**. 1973; 11: 43,54.

A03087 Leclerc, H. Sida Sabdariffa (*Hibiscus sabdariffa*) **Presse Med** 1938; 46: 1060.

A03113 Ghosal, S., S. Singh and S. K. Bhattachary. **Plant Med.** 1971; 19: 279

A03127 Gujraj, M. L., D. R. Varma and K. N. Sareen. Oral contraceptives. Part 1. Preliminary observations on the antifertility effect of some indigenous drugs. **Indian J Med Res** 1960; 48: 46,51.

A03158 Leupin, K. Karkade. **Pharma Acta Helv** 1935; 10: 138.

A03170 Gupta, M. B., T. K. Palit and K. P. Bhargava. Pharmacological studies to isolate the active constituents from *Cyperus rotundus* processing anti-inflammatory, anti-pyretic and analgesic activities. **Indian J Med Res** 1971; 59: 76.

A03319 Agarwal, S. K. and P. R. Rastogi. Triperpenoids of *Hibiscus rosa-sinensis*. **Indian J Pharmacy** 1971; 33: 41.

A03335 Dhar, M. L., M. M. Dhar, B. N. Mehrotra and C. Ray. Screening of Indian plants for biological activity. Part 1. **Indian J Exp Biol**. 1968; 6: 232–247.

A03360 Feng, P. C., L. J. Haynes, K. E. Magnus, J. R. Plimmer and H. S.

A. Sherrat. Pharmacological screening of some West Indian Medicinal Plants. **J Pharm Pharmacol** 1962; 14: 556–561.

A03403 Asprey, G. F. and P. Thornton. Medicinal Plants of Jamaica. Part I. **West Indian Med J** 1953; 2(4): 233–252.

A03411 Anon. The atlas of commonly used Chinese traditional drugs, revolutionary committee of the Inst Materia Medica, Chinese Acad Sci, Peking,1970.

A03442 Suggs, R. C. Marquesan sexual behavior. Harcourt, Brace and World, Inc., New York,1966.

A03456 Siddiqu, S. and M. I. Khan. Pharmacological study of *Moringa pterygosperma*. **Pak J Sci Ind Res** 1968; 11: 268–272.

A03478 Singh, R. Inactivation of potato virus X by plant extracts. **Phytopathol Mediterr** 1971; 10: 211.

A03483 Matsui, A. D. S., J. Rogers, Y. K. Woo, W. C. Cutting. Effects of some natural products on fertility in mice. **Med Pharmacol Exp** 1967; 16: 414.

A03499 Hnatyszyn, O., P. Arenas, A. R. Moreno, R. V. D. Rondina and J. D. Coussio. Preliminary Phytochemical study of Paraguayan medicinal plants. 1. Plants regulating fertility from medicinal folklore. **Rev Soc Cient** 1974; 14: 23.

A03522 Agarwal, S. L. and S. Shinde. Studies on *Hibiscus rosa-sinensis*. II. Preliminary Pharmacological investigations. **Indian J Med Res** 1967; 55: 1007–1010.

A03531 Barros, G. S. G., F. J. A. Mathos, J. E. V. Vieira, M. P. Sousa and M. C. Medeiros. Pharmacological screening of some Brazilian plants. **J Pharm Pharmacol** 1970; 22: 116.

A03566 Goto, M., T. Noguchi, T. Watanabe, I. Ishikawa, M. Komatsu and Y. Aramaki. Uterus-contracting ingredients in plants. **Takeda Kenkyusho Nempo** 1957; 16: 21.

A03597 Sharaf, A. The pharmacological characteristics of *Hibiscus sabdariffa*. **Planta Med** 1962; 10: 48–52.

A03602   Gimlette, J. D. Malay poisons and charm cures. J & A Churchill, London, 3rd Edition, 1929.

A03634   Fitzpatrick, F. K. Plant substances active against *Mycobacterium tuberculosis*. **Antibiot Chemother** 1954; 4: 528.

A03648   Simpson, K. S. and P. C. Banerjee. Cases of poisoning in the horse with Ratti seeds (*Abrus precatorius*) by oral administration. **Indian J Vet Sci Anim Husb** 1932; 2: 59.

A03680   Khalmatov, K. K. and E. D. Bazhenova. The diuretic action of some wild plants of Uzbekistan. **Tr Tashk Farm Inst** 1966; 4: 5.

A03685   Akperbekova, B. A. and D. Y. Guseinov. Studies on the influence of pharmaceutic preparations from rhizomes of *Cyperus rotundus* growing in Azerbaidzhan on the heart and vascular system. **Azerb Med Zh** 1966; 43: 12.

A03687   Subba Reddy, V. V. and M. Sirsi. Effects of *Abrus precatorius* on experimental tumors. **Cancer Res** 1969; 29: 1447–1451.

A03690   Hikino, H., K. Aota and T. Takemoto. Structure and absolute configuration of cyperotundone. **Chem Pharm Bull** 1966; 14: 890.

A03910   Johnson, I. S., H. F. Wright, G. H. Svoboda and J. Vlantis. Antitumor principles derived from *Vinca rosea*. 1. Vincaleukblastine and leurosine. **Cancer Res** 1960; 20: 1016.

A03931   Chevalier, J. The dietetic use of the flowers of *Hibiscus sabdariffa*. **Bull Sci Pharmacol** 1937; 44: 195.

A03932   Rovesti, P. Therapeutic and dietetic properties of "Karkade" (*Hibiscus sabdariffa*) a new colonial pink tea. **Farmacista Ital** 1936; 3(1): 13.

A04132   Hikino, H., K. Aota and T. Takemoto. Structure and absolute configuration of cyperotundone. **Chem Pharm Bull** 1966; 14: 890.

A04153   Weeks, J. H. Among the primitive Bakongo. Seeley, Service & Co., Ltd. England, 1914; 108.

A04162   Steenis-Kruseman, M. J. Van. Select Indonesian Medicinal Plants. **Organiz Sci Res Indonesia Bull** 1953; 18: 1.

A04168   Farnsworth, N. R. The Pharmacognosy of the periwinkles: Vinca and Catharanthus. **Lloydia** 1961; 24(3): 105–138.

A04171   Bouquet, A. Feticheurs et medecines traditionelles du Congo (Brazzaville). Mem Orstom No. 36,282 P. Paris, 1969.

A04174   Rageau, J. Les Plantes Medicinales De La Nouvelle-Cal edonie. Trav & Doc De Lorstom No. 23. Paris, 1973.

A04179   Morton, J. F. The balsam pear - an edible, medical and toxic plant. **Econ Bot** 1967; 21: 57.

A04219   Kapur, R. D. Action of some indigenous drugs on uterus. A preliminary note. **Indian J Med Res** 1948; 36: 47.

A04237   Desai, R. V. and E. N. Rupawala. Antifertility activity of the steroidal oil of the seed of *Abrus precatorius*. **Indian J Pharmacy** 1967; 29: 235–237.

A04238   Agarwal, S. S., N. Ghatak and R. B. Arora. Antifertility activity of the roots of *Abrus precatorius*. **Pharmacol Res Commun** 1970; 2: 159–164.

A04241   Carboneschl, C. L. Chemistry and toxicology of *Abrus precatorius* or seed of Jequirity. **Semana Med (Buenos Aires)** 1947; 2: 275–281.

A04245   Genest, K., A. Lavalle and E. Nera. Comparative acute toxicity of *Abrus precatorius* and Ormosia seeds in animals. **Arzneim-Forsch** 1971; 21: 888.

A04246   Lalithakumari, H., V. V. S. Reddy, G. R. Rao and M. Sirsi. Purification of proteins from *Abrus precatorius* and their biological properties. **Indian J Biochem Biophys** 1971; 8: 321.

A04248 David, J. P. and C. T. Peter. Toxicity of *Abrus precatorius* in domestic fowl. **Kerala J Vet Sci** 1970; 1: 125.

A04249 Tokarnia, C. H., J. Dobereiner and M. Monteiro. Experimental poisoning in cattle by the seeds of *Abrus precatorius*. **Pesqui Agropecu Brasil Ser Vet** 1970; 5: 441.

A04250 Hart, M. Hazards to health. Jequirity-bean poisoning. **New England J Med** 1963; 268: 885.

A04277 Milne, L. Shans at home. John Murray, London, 1910; 181.

A04281 Maugham, R. C. F. Portuguese East Africa, the history, scenery and great game of Manica and Sofala. John Murray, London, 1906; 271.

A04287 Khanna, U., S. K. Garg, S. B. Vohra, H. B. Walia and R. R. Chaudhury. Antifertility screening of plants. Part 11. Effect of seix indigenous plants on early pregnancy in albino rats. **Indian J Med Res**. 1969; 57: 237–244.

A04296 Berhault, J. Flore illustree du Senegal II. Govt. Senegal, Min Rural Dev, Water and Forest Div. Dakar, **2.** 1974

A04300 Das, S. K. Medicinal, Economic and useful plants of India. Bally seed store, West Bengal, 1955.

A04306 Oliver-Bever, B. Selecting local drug plants in Nigeria. Botanical and Chemical relationship in three families. **Q J Crude Drug Res** 1968; 8(2): 1194.

A04351 Sareen, K. N., N. Misra, D. R. Varma, M. K. P. Amma and M. L. Gujral. Oral contraceptives. V. Anthelmintics as antifertility agents. **Indian J Physiol Pharmacol** 1961; 5: 125–135.

A04361 Hooper, D. On Chinese medicine. Drug of Chinese Pharmacies in Malaya. **Gard Bull STR Settlm** 1929; 6: 1.

A04407 El-Hamid, A. Drug plants of the Sudan Republic in Native medicine. **Planta Med** 1970; 18: 278.

A04418 Loustalot, A. J. and C. Pagan. Local "Fever" Plants tested for presence of Alkaloids. **El Crisol** (Puerto Rico) 1949; 3(5): 3.

A04420 Chaturvedi, G. N. and R. H. Singh. Experimental studies on the Antiarthritic Effect of Certain Indigenous Drugs. **Indian J Med Res** 1965; 53: 71.

A04471 Tessman, G. Die Indianer Nordost-Perus, Grundlegende Forschunger Fur Eine Systematischen, De Gruyter Co., Hamburg, Germany, 1930.

A04487 Chopra, R. N. Indigenous Drugs of India, 1933.

A04508 ANON, Description of the Philippines. Part I., Bureau of Public Printing, Manila, 1903.

A04511 Garg, S. K. and G. P. Garg. Antifertility screening of plants. Part VII. Effect of five indigenous plants on early pregnancy in albino rats. **Indian J Med Res** 1970; 59: 302.

A04537 Jochle, W. Menses-inducing drugs: their role in antique, medieval and renaissance gynecology and birth control. **Contraception** 1974; 10: 425–439.

A04545 Jochle, W. Biology and Pathology of Reproduction in Greek Mythology. **Contraception** 1971; 4: 1–13.

A04580 Baquar, S. R. and M. Tasnif. Medicinal plants of Southern West Pakistan. **Pak P C S I R Bull Monogr** 1967; 3.

A04581 Stuart, G. A. Chinese Materia Medica. Vegetable Kingdom. American Presbyterian Mission Press, Shanghai, 1911.

A04587 Gimlette, J. D. A Dictionary of Malayan Medicine, Oxford Univ. Press., New York, USA, 1939.

A04608 Niyogi, S. K. and F. Rieders. Toxicity studies with fractions from *Abrus precatorius* seed kernels. **Toxicon** 1969; 7: 211.

A04610 Murray, J. A. Plants and drugs of Sind. Richardson and Co., London, 1881.

A04611 Ichimura, T. Important medicinal plants of Japan. Kanazawa city, Tokyo, 1932.

A04613   Girard, R. The Medicine Chest of the Chorti Indians. **Bol Indigenista**. 1947; 7(4): 347.

A04618   Khurana, S. M. P. Studies on *Calotropis procera* latex as an inhibitor of tobacco mosaic virus. **Phytopathol** 1972; Z 73: 341.

A04621   Desai, V. B., M. Sirsi, M. Shankarappa and A. R. Kasturibai. Chemical and Pharmacological investigations on the seeds of *Abrus precatorius*: Effect of seeds on mitosis and meiosis in grasshopper *Poecilocera picta* and some Ciliates. **Indian J Exp Biol** 1971; 9: 369.

A04766   Petelot, A. Les Plantes Medicinales Du Cambodge, Du Laos Et Du Vietnam, vol. 1–4. Archives Des Recherches Agronomiques Et Pastorales Au Vietnam No. 23, 1954.

A04780   Tomita, M., T. Kurokawa, K. Onozaki, T. Osawa, Y. Sakurai and T. Ukita. The surface structure of murine ascites tumors 11. Difference in cytotoxicity of various phytoagglutinins toward Yoshida Sarcoma cells in vitro. **Int J Cancer** 1972; 10: 602.

A04781   Niyogi, S. K. The Toxicology of Abrus *precatorius*. **J of Forensic Sci.** 1970; 15: 529.

A04782   Finberg, J. Smoking compositions. **Patent-US-2,930,720**: 1960.

A04807   Sievers, A. F., W. A. Archer, R. H. Moore and B. R. Mc Gowan. Insecticidal tests of plants from tropical America. **J Econ Entomol** 1949; 42: 549.

A04819   Bhakuni, O. S., M. L. Dhar, M. M. Dhar, B. N. Dhawan and B. N. Mehrotra. Screening of Indian plants for biological activity. Part II. **Indian J Exp Biol** 1969; 7: 250-262.

A04839   Mameesh, M. S., L. M. El-Hakim and A. Hassan. Reproductive failure in female rats fed the fruit or seed of Jatropha curcas. **Planta Med** 1963; 11: 98.

A04884   Niyogi, S. K. *Abrus precatorius* Poisonining in Mice, Pathologi-cal Findings. **J of Forensic Sci.** 1969; 16: 130.

A04891   Chorpa, R. N., P. De and N. N. De. *Moringa pterygosperma*. **Indian J Med Res** 1932; 20: 533.

A04893   Khalsa, H. G., Y. C. Wal and P. N. Agarwal. Insecticidal properties of *Abrus precatorius* and *Neriun indicum*. **Indian J Entomol** 1964; 26: 113.

A04902   Saksena, S. K. Study of antifertility activity of the leaves of *Momordica* (Karela). **Indian J Physiol Pharmacol** 1971; 15: 79–80.

A04908   Desai, V. B. and M. Sirsi. Antimicrobial activity of *Abrus precatorius*. **Indian J Pharmacy** 1966; 28: 164.

A04909   Misra, D. S., B. K. Soni and D. Sharma. Fractionation and characterization of haemagglutinating principal of *Abrus precatorius*. **Indian J Exp Biol** 1968; 6: 108.

A04910   Misra, D. S., R. P. Sharma and B. K. Soni. Toxic and haemagglutinating properties of *Abrus precatorius*. **Indian J Exp Biol** 1966; 4: 161.

A04913   Khan, A. H., B. Gul and M. A. Rahman. The interactions of the erythrocytes of various species with agglutinins of *Abrus precatorius*. **J Immunol** 1966; 96: 554.

A04923   Heckel, E. Les Plantes Medicinales et Toxiques de Madagascar. A. Challamel, Paris, 1903.

A04941   Kerharo, J. and A. Bouquet. Plantes Medicinales et Toxiques de La Cote-D'Ivoire - Haute-Volta. Vigot Freres, Paris, 1950; 297 pp.

A04942   Perrot, E. and P. Hurrier. Matiere Medicale Et Pharmacopee Sino-Annamites. Vigot Freres, Edit., Paris, 1907; 292 pp.

A05104   Matsui, A. D. S., S. Hoskins, M. Kashiwagi, B. W. Aguda, B. E. Zebart, T. R. Norton, W. C. Cutting. A survey of natural products from Hawaii and other areas of the Pacific for an antifertility effect in mice. **Int Z Klin Pharmakol Ther Toxikol** 1971; 5(1): 65–69.

A05123   Nagaty, H. F., M. A. Rifatt and T. A. Morsy. Trials on the effect on dog ascaris *In vivo* produced by the latex of ficus carica and papaya carica growing in Cairo gardens. **Ann Trop Med Parasitol** 1959; 53: 215.

A05124   Pillai, N. C., C. S. Vaidyanathan and K. V. Giri. A blood anticoagulant factor from the latex of *Carica papaya*. II. Its nature of action on blood coagulation. **Proc Indian Acad Sci Ser B** 1956; 43: 46.

A05125   Pillai, N. C., C. S. Vaidyanathan and K. V. Giri. A blood anticoagulant factor from the latex of *Carica papaya*. I. Purification and general properties. **Proc Indian Acad Sci Ser B** 1955; 42: 316.

A05126   Bose, B. C., A. Q. Saifi, R. Vijayvargiya and A. W. Bhagwat. Pharmacological study of *Carica papaya* seeds, with special reference to its anthelmintic action: Preliminary report. **Indian J Med Sci** 1961; 15: 888.

A05138   Sosto-Peralta, F. Intestinal occlusion caused by *Carica papaya*. Report of one case. **Rev Med Coata Rica** 1968; 25: 347.

A05171   Trivedi, V. P. and A. S. Mann. Vegetable drugs regulating fat metabolism in Caraka (Lekhaniya Dravyas). **Q J Crude Drug Res** 1972; 12: 1988.

A05197   Brailski, K., K. Mao and K. Kuk. The action of certain tropical fruits on the gastric function. **VOPR Pitaniya** 1960; 19(4): 39.

A05311   Canella, C. F. C., C. H. Tokarnia and J. Dobereiner. Experiments with plants supposedly toxic to cattle in Northeastern Brazil, with negative results. **Pesqui Agropecu Brasil Ser Vet** 1966; 1: 345–352.

A05332   Morton, J. F. A survey of medicinal plants of Curacao. **Econ Bot** 1968; 22: 87.

A05408   Morton, J. F. Ornamental plants with toxic and/or irritant properties. II. **Proc Fla State Hort Soc** 1962; 75: 484.

A05418   Dar, R. N., L. C. Garg and R. D. Pathak. Anthelmintic activity of *Carica papaya* seeds. **Indian J Pharmacy** 1965; 27: 335.

A05423   Bischoff, F., M. L. Long and M. Sahyun. Investigations of the hypoglycemic properties of reglykol pancreatine and papaw. **J Pharmacol Exp Ther** 1929; 36: 311.

A05449   Morton, J. F. Folk-remedy plants and esophageal cancer in Coro, Venezuela. **Morris Arboretum Bull** 1974; 25: 24–34.

A05464   Chopra, I. C., K. S. Jamwal, C. L. Chopra, C. P. N. Nair and P. P. Pillay. Preliminary pharmacological investigations of total alkaloids of *Lochnera rosea* (Rattonjot). **Indian J Med Res** 1959; 47: 40.

A05524   Webb, L. J. Guide to the medicinal and poisonous plants of Queensland. CSIR Bull 232, Melbourne, 1948.

A05542   Schramm, G. Plant and animal drugs of the old Chinese Materia Medica in the therapy of pulmonary tuberculosis. **Planta Med** 1956; 4(4): 97–104.

A05550   Haerdi, F. Native medicinal plants of Ulanga district of Tanganyika (East Africa). Dissertation, Verlag Fur Recht Und Gesellschaft Ag, Basel. **Dissertation PH. D. Univ Basel** 1964.

A05570   Gupta, S. S., D. Chandra and N. Mishra. Anti-inflammatory and anti-hyaluronidase activity of volatile oil of *Curcuma longa*. **Indian J Physiol Pharmacol** 1972; 16: 263A.

A05591   Noble, I. G. Fruta bomba (*Carica papaya*) in hypertension. **An Acad Cienc Med Fis Nat Habana** 1947; 85: 198.

A05606   Sharaf, A. Food plants as a possible factor in fertility control. **Qual Plant Mater Veg** 1969; 17: 153.

A05611   Sharaf, A. and S. A. R. Nigm. The Oestrogenic activity of pomegranate seed oil. **J Endocrinol** 1964; 29: 91.

A05638   ANON. Lilly's hand book of pharmacy and therapeutics. 5th Rev, Eli Lilly and Co., Indianapolis, 1898.

A05657   Gunsolus, J. M. Toxicity of Jequirity beans. **Journal Amer Med Assoc** 1955; 157: 779.

A05675   Inman, N. Notes on some poisonous plants of Guam. **Micronesica** 1967; 3: 55.

A05682   Krishnakumari, M. K. and S. K. Majumder. Bioassay of piperazine & some plant products with earthworms. **J Sci Ind Res** 1960; C 19: 202.

A05705   Thorp, R. H. anfd T. R. Watson. A survey of the occurrence of cardio-active constituents in plants growing wild in Australia. 1. Families Apocynaceae and Asclepiadaceae. **Aust J Exp Biol** 1953; 31: 529.

A05806   Neogi, N. C. and M. C. Bhatia. Biological investigation of Vinca rosea. **Indian J Pharmacy** 1956; 18: 73.

A05825   Watt, J. M. and M. G. Breyer-Brandwijk. The medicinal and poisonous plants of Southern and Eastern Africa. 2nd Ed, E. S. Livingstone, Ltd., London, 1962.

A05854   Chopra, C. L., M. C. Bhatia and I. C. Chopra. In Vitro antibacterial activity of oils from Indian medicinal plants. **J Amer Pharm Assoc Sci Ed** 1960; 49: 780.

A05858   Buchanan, E. Grove man dies after eating rosary beans. **Miami Herald** April 18, 1976. Miami, Fla USA.

A05937   Paris, R. R. and H. Moyse-Mignon. A Sympatholytic Apocynaceae, Vinca rosea. **CR Acad Sci** 1953; 240: 1993.

A05940   Pernet, M., G. Meyer, J. M. Bosser and G. Ratsiandavana. The Catharanthus of Madagascar. **CR Acad Sci** 1956; 243: 1352.

A05953   Maruzzella, J. C. and J. Balter. The action of essential oils on phytopathogenic. **Plant Disease Reptr** 1959; 43: 1143–1147.

A05970   Ray, B. N. and A. K. Pal, Estrogenic activity of tree leaves as animal feed. **Indian J Physiol Allied Sci** 1967; 20: 6.

A05972   Agliout, F. B. and L. S. Castillo. Estrogen content of legumes in the Philippines. **Philippine Agr** 1963; 46: 673.

A06024   Kerharo, J. Le Pisap du Senegal (*Hibiscus sabdariffa* L.) Ou Oseille de Guinee, Ou Karkade de L'erythree. **Planta Med Phytother** 1971; 4: 227.

A06027   Stimson, W. R. Ethnobotanical notes from Puerto Rico. **Lloydia** 1971; 34: 165.

A06518   Sharaf, A. Estrogenicity in plants. **Arab Sci Congr 5th, Baghdad** 1966, 1967; 1: 281.

A06589   Burkhill, I. H. Dictionary of the economic products of the Malay peninsula. Ministry of Agriculture and Cooperatives, Kuala Lumpur, Malaysia. Vol. 1, 1966.

A06590   Burkhill, I. H. Dictionary of the economic products of the Malay Peninsula. Ministry of Agriculture and Cooperatives, Kuala Lumpur, Malaysia. Volume II, 1966.

A06630   Abivardi, C. Studies on the effects of nine Iranian anthelmintic plant extracts on the root-knot nematode *Meloidogyne incognita*. **Phytopathol** 1971; 71: 300–308.

A06732   Peckolt, G. Brazilian anthelmintic plants. **Rev Flora Med** 1942; 9(7): 333.

A06987   Rao, D. S. Insecticidal properties of several common plants of India. **Econ Bot** 1957; 11: 274.

A07091   Prasad, V. and S. C. Gupta. Inhibitory effect of bark and leaf decoction on the activity of pectic enzymes of Alternaria tennis. **Indian J Exp Biol** 1967; 5: 192.

A07232   Gupta, S. S. Pituitary diabetes. III. Effect of indigenous antidiabetic-drugs against the acute hyperglycemic response of anterior pituitary extract on glucose fed albino rats. **Indian J Med Res** 1963; 51: 716.

A07281 Chatterjee, K. P. On the presence of an antidiabetic principle in *Momordica charantia*. **Indian J Physiol Pharmacol** 1964; 7: 240.

A07304 Nogueira Prista, L. and A. Correia Alves. Phytochemical Study of the leaves of *Persea americana*. **Garcia Orta** 1961; 9: 501.

A14266 Hartzell, A. and F. Wilcoxon. A survey of plant products for insecticidal properties. **Contr Boyce Thompson Inst** 1941; 12: 127–141.

A14280 Rivera, G. Preliminary Chemical and Pharmacological Studies on "Cundeamor," *Momordica charantia* L. (Part 1). **Amer J Pharm** 1941; 113(7): 281–297.

A14305 Gupta, S. S. and C. B. Seth. Experimental studies on pituitary diabetes. Part 11. Comparison of blood sugar level in normal and anterior pituitary extract induced hyperglycaemic rats treated with a few Ayurvedic remedies. **Indian J Med Res** 1962; 50(5): 708–714.

A14310 Kulkarni, R. D. and B. B. Gaitonde. Potentiation of tolbutamide action by Jasad Bhasma and Karela (*Momordica charantia*). **Indian J Med Res** 1962; 50(5): 715–719.

A14322 Brahmachari, H. D. and K. T. Augusti. Hypoglycaemic agents from Indian indigenous plants. **J Pharm Pharmacol** 1961; 13: 381,382.

A14328 Sharma, V. N., R. K. Sogani and R. B. Arora. Some observations on hypoglycemic activity of *Momordica charantia*. **Indian J Med Res** 1960; 48(4): 471–477.

A14331 ANON. Hypoglycemic medicament based on *Syzygium jambolanum* (Java Plum). **Patent-Fr M-6114** 1968; 4 pp.

A14333 Shorti, D. S., M. Kelkar, V. K. Deshmukh and R. Aiman. Investigation of the hyperglycemic properties of *Vinca rosea, Cassia auriculata* and *Eugenia jambolana*. **Indian J Med Res** 1963; 51(3): 464-467.

A14339 Pant, M. C., I. Uddin, U. R. Bhardwaj and R. D. Tewari. Blood sugar and total cholesterol lowering effect of glycine soja (Sieb and Zucc.), *Macuna pruriens* (D.C.) and *Dolichos biflorus* (Linn.) seed diets in normal fasting albino rats. **Indian J Med Res** 1968; 56 12: 1808–1812.

A14379 Jain, S. R. and S. N. Sharma. Hypoglycaemic Drugs of Indian Indigenous Origin. **Planta Med** 1967; 15(4): 439–442.

A14413 Sigogneau-jagodzinski, M., P. Bibal-Prot, M. Chanez, P. Boiteau and A. R. Ratsimamanga. Contribution to a study of the hypoglycemic and antidiabetic extract of Madagascar Rotra (*Eugenia jambolana* Lamarck). **CR Acad Sci Ser D** 1967; 264(8): 1119–1123.

A14429 Steinmetz, E. F. A Botanical drug from the tropics used in the treatment of diabetes mellitus. **Acta Phytother** 1961; 7: 23–25.

A14458 Khan, A. H. and A. Burney. A Preliminary study of the hypoglycaemic properties of indigenous plants. **Pak J Med Res** 1962; 2: 100–116.

A14461 Ram, S. Karela and Diabetes. **J Indian Med Assoc** 1956; 19: 181.

A14494 Sigogneau-jagodzinski, M., P. Bibal-Prot, M. Chanez and P. Boiteau. Contribution to a study of the action of a principal extract of Rotra of Madagascar (*Eugenia jambolana*, Myrtaceae) on blood sugar. **CR Acad Sci Ser D** 1967; 264: 1223–1226.

A14525 Gupta, S. S. and C. B. Seth. Effect of *Momordica charantia* Linn. (Karela) on glucose tolerance in albino rats. **J Indian Med Assoc** 1962; 39: 581–584.

A14531 Arauio, A. On diuresis and its medications under the influence of various fluid extracts of Brazilian plants. **Thesis - Univ Sao Paulo** 1929.

A14534   Steinmetz, E. F. A botanical drug from the tropics used in the treatment of diabetes mellitus. **Acta Phytother** 1960; 7: 23–25.

A15182   Wang, V. F. L. In Vitro Antibacterial activity of some common Chinese herbs on *Mycobacterium tuberculosis*. **Chin Med J** 1950; 68: 169–172.

A15203   Sigogneau-Jagodzinski, P., M. M. Bibal-Prot, P. B. Marc Chanez, M. Albert and R. Ratsimamanga. Contribution to the study of the action of an extract of Rotra De Madagascar (*Eugenia jambolana*, Myrtaceae) on serum glucose of normal rats. **CR Acad Sci Paris** 1967; 264: 1223–1226.

B00011   Praditvarn, L. and C. Sambhandharaksa. A study of the volatile oil from Siam lemongrass. **J Pharm Assoc Siam** 1950; 3(2): 87–92.

H00669   ANON. Ayurvedic drug to fight cancer. **Probe** 1985; 24(4): 234.

H01040   Kosuge, T., M. Yokota, K. Sugiyama, T. Yamamoto, M. Y. Ni and S. C. Yan. Studies on antitumor activities and antitumor principles of Chinese herbs. 1. Antitumor activities of Chinese herbs. **Yakugaku Zasshi** 1985; 105(8): 791–795.

H01195   Kuttan, R., P. Bhanumathy, K. Nirmala and M. C. George. Potential anticancer activity of turmeric (*Curcuma longa*). **Cancer Lett** 1985; 29(2): 197–202.

H01446   Chang, C. L. and M. T. Peng. In vitro inactivation of gonadotropins by Psidium root extract. **Taiwan I Hsueh Hui Tsa Chih** 1973; 72: 379.

H04816   Hara, S., J. Makino and T. Ikenaka. Amino acid sequence and disulfide bridges of serine protinease inhibitors from bitter gourd (*Momordica charantia* Linn.) seeds. **J Biochem** (Tokyo) 1989; 105(1): 88–92.

H05163   Villasenor, I. M., P. Finch, C. Y. Lim-Sylianco and F. Dayrit. Structure of a Mutagen from roasted seeds of *Moringa oleifera*. **Carcinogenesis** 1989; 10(6); 1085–1087.

H05351   Gewali, M. B., M. Hattori, Y. Tezuka, T. Kikuchi and T. Namba. Four ingol type diterpenes from *Euphorbia antiquorum* L. **Chem Pharm Bull** 1989; 37(6): 1547–1549.

H06015   Tomoda, M., R. Gonda, N. Shimizu, M. Kanari and M. Kimura. A reticuloendothelial system activating glycan from the rhizomes of *Curcuma longa*. **Phytochemistry** 1990; 29(4): 1083–1086.

H07994   Adikaram, N. K. B., D. R. Ewing, A. M. Karunaratne and E. M. K Wijeratne. Antifungal compounds from immature avocado fruit peel. **Phytochemistry** 1992; 31(1): 93–96.

H11158   Tanaka, T., N. Ishida, M. Ishimatsu, G. I. Nonaka and I. Nishioka. Tannins and related compounds. CXVI. Six new complex tannins, Guajavins, Psidinins and Psiguavin from the bark of *Psidium guajava* L. **Chem Pharm Bull** 1992; 40(8): 2092–2098.

H11898   Imbabi, E. S., K. E. Ibrahim, B. M Ahmed, I. M. Abulefuthu and P. Hulbert. Chemical characterization of tamarind bitter principle, Tamarindineal. **Fitoterapia** 1992; 63(6): 537–538.

H12480   Shimizu, N., M. Tomoda, I. Suzuki and K. Takada. Plant mucilages. XLIII. A representative mucilage with biological activity from the leaves of *Hibiscus rosa-sinensis*. **Biol Pharm Bull** 1993; 16(8): 735–739.

H12627   Kiuchi, F., Y. Goto, N. Sugimoto, N. Akao, K. Kondo and Y. Tsuda. Nematocidal activity of turmeric: Synergistic action of curcuminoids. **Chem Pharm Bull** 1993; 41(9): 1640–1643.

H15082 Faizi, S., B. S. Siddiqui, Saleemr, S. Siddiqui, K. Aftab and A. H. Gilani. Isolation and structure elucidation of new nitrile and mustard oil glycosides from *Moringa oleifera* and their effect on blood pressure. **J Nat Prod** 1994; 57(9): 1256–1261.

H16454 Chukuo, S., S. C. Chen, L. H. Chen, J. B. Wu, J. P. Wang and C. M. Teng. Potent antiplatelet, antiinflammatory and antiallergic isoflavanquinones from the roots of *Abrus precatorius*. **Planta Med** 1995; 61 4: 307–312.

H16648 Thebtaranonth, C., Y. Thebtaranonth, S. Wanauppathamkul and Y. Yuthavong. Antimalarial sesquiterpenes from tubers of *Cyperus rotundus*. Structure of 10,12-Peroxycalamenene, a sesquiterpene endoperoxide. **Phytochemistry** 1995; 40(1): 125–128.

I00004 Zagari, A. Medicinal plants. Vol 4, 5th Ed., Tehran University Publications, No 1810/4, Tehran, Iran, 1992, 4: 969 pp.

J00209 Ogunlana, E. O. and E. Ramstad. Investigation into the Antibacterial Actvities of local plants. **Planta Med** 1975; 27: 354.

J01414 Ortiz De Montellano, B. Empirical Aztec Medicine. **Science** 1975; 188: 215–220.

J01423 Moreno, A. R. Two hundred sixty-eight medicinal plants used to regulate fertility in some countries of South America, 1975.

J02755 Maheshwari, M. L. and S. K. Mukerjee. Lipids and Phenolics of healthy and malformed panicles of *Mangifera indica*. **Phytochemistry** 1975; 14: 2083,2084.

J02774 Osman, A. M., M. El-Garby Younes and A. Mokhtar. Chemical examination of local plants. VIII. Comparative studies between constituents of different parts of Egyptian *Hibiscus sabdariffa*. **Indian J Chem** 1975; 13: 198.

J03642 Osman, A. M., M. El-Garby Younes and A. Mokhtar. Sito-sterol-Beta-D-Galactoside from *Hibiscus sabdariffa*. **Phytochemistry** 1975; 14: 829,830.

J03769 Olaniyi, A. A. A neutral constituent of *Momordica foetida*. **Lloydia** 1975; 38: 361,362.

J05633 Samad, F., A. Mukhtar, Z. A. Jan and Z. U. Khan. Effect of alcohol extract of Ratti seeds (*Abrus precatorius*) on the reproduction of female rats. **J Math Sci** 1974; 12: 157.

J05751 Bodhankar, S. L., S. K. Garg and V. S. Mathur. Antifertility screening of plants. Part IX. Effect of five indigenous plants on early pregnancy in female albino rats. **Indian J Med Res** 1974; 62: 831–837.

J07469 Bhatia, I. S. and K. L. Bajaj. Chemical constituents of the seeds and bark of *Syzygium cumini*. **Planta Med** 1975; 28: 346.

J07575 Kazmi, H., M. Aslan, Z. U. Khan and M. I. Bureny. A report on the trial of a Unani prescription for diabetes. **Rawal Med** 1974; 3(2): 67.

J08287 Yagashi, R. Papain for the control of termites. **Patent-Japan Kokai-74,125,520** 1974.

J08538 Garg, S. K. Antifertility effect of oil from few indigenous plants on female albino rats. **Planta Med** 1974; 26: 391–393.

J08548 Garg. S. K. Effect of *Curcuma longa* (rhizomes) on fertility in experimental animals. **Planta Med** 1974; 26: 225–227.

J08616 Prabhu, V. K. K. and M. John. Juvenile activity in some plants. **Experientia** 1975; 31: 913.

J08904 Kaleysa Raj, R. Screening of indigenous plants for anthelmintic action against human *Ascaris lumbricoides*: Part 11. **Indian J Physiol Pharmacol** 1975; 19: 47–49.

J09860 Weiss, S. G. Antitumor principles of *Linum album* and

Catharanthus roseus. **Diss Abstr Int** 1974; 35: 2669.

J10115   Duke, J. A. Ethnobotanical observations on the Cuna Indians. **Econ Bot** 1975; 29: 278.

J10155   Luu, C. Notes on the traditional pharmacopoeia of French Guyana. **Plant Med Phytother** 1975; 9: 125–135.

J10330   Keiser, I., E. J. Harris, D. H. Miyashita, M. Jacobson and R. E. Perdue. Attraction of ethyl ether extracts of 232 botanical to Oriental fruit flies, melon flies, and Mediterranean fruit flies. **Lloydia** 1975; 38(2): 141–152.

J10345   Schultes, R. E. De Plantes Toxicariie e Mundo Novo Tropicale commentationes. XIX. Biodynamic Apocynaceous plants of the Northwest Amazon. **J Ethnopharmacol** 1979; 1(2): 165–192.

J01423   Moreno, A. R. Two hundred sixty-eight medicinal plants used to regulate fertility in some countries of South America. Unpublished (Stenciled) Review in Spanish, 1975.

J09596   Morton, J. F. Renewed interest in roselle (*Hibiscus sabdariffa*), the long-forgotten "Florida Cranberry". **Proc Fla State Hort Soc** 1974; 87: 415.

K00040   GRAS status of foods and food additives. **Fed Regist** 1976; 41: 38,644.

K00334   Dermarderosian, A. H., F. B. Giller and F. C. Roia. Phytochemical and Toxicological screening of household ornamental plants potentially toxic to humans. 1. **J Toxicol Environ Health** 1976; 1: 939.

K01147   Kholkute, S. D. and K. N. Udupa. Effects of *Hibiscus rosa-sinensis* on pregnancy of rats. **Planta Med** 1976; 29: 321–329.

K01337   Yegnanarayana, R., A. P. Saraf and J. H. Balwani. Comparison of anti-inflammatory activity of various extracts of *Curcuma longa.* **Indian J Med Res** 1976; 64: 601.

K01497   Hikino, H. and K. Aota. Sesquiterpenoids. Part 52. 4A,5A-Oxidoeudesm-11-En-3A-Ol, Sesquitterpenoid of *Cyperus rotundus.* **Phytochemistry** 1976; 15: 1265–1266.

K01510   Khan, Z. U. Antifertility effects of two local medicinal plants. **Rawal Med J** 1976; 5 1: 21–26.

K01737   Khan, Z. U., A. Waiz and I. A. Jafari. Effect of non-saponified matter of *Abrus precatorius* and its sub fractions on the survival of Blastocyst in ovariectomized pregnant rats. **Rawal Med J** 1976; 5 (2): 82.

K02033   Kholkute, S. D., V. Mudgal and P. J. Deshpande. Screening of indigenous medicinal plants for antifertility potentiality. **Planta Med** 1976; 29: 151–155.

K03417   Akperbekova, B. A. Pharmacognostic study of *Cyperus rotundus* L. rhizome. **Farmatsiya** 1967; 16(1): 43–45.

K03517   Singhal, K. C. Anthelmintic activity of Berberine Hydrochloride against Syphacia obvelata in mice. **Indian J Exp Biol** 1976; 14: 345–347.

K03520   Lal, J., S. Chandra, V. Raviprakash and M. Sabir. In vitro anthelmintic action of some indigenous medicinal plants on *Ascardia galli* worms. **Indian J Physiol pharmacol** 1976; 20: 64.

K03660   Pass, M. A., A. A. Seawright and T. Heath. Effect of ingestion of *Lantana camara* on bile formation in sheep. **Biochem Pharmacol** 1976; 25: 2101.

K03661   Kong, Y. C., S. Y. Hu, F. K. Lau, C. T. Che, H. W. Yeung, S. Cheung and J. C. C. Hwang. Potential anti-fertility plants from Chinese medicine. **Amer J Chin Med** 1976; 4: 105–128.

K03665   Wong, W. Some folk medicinal plants from Trinidad. **Econ Bot** 1976; 30: 103–142.

K04296   Devereux, G. A study of abortion in primitive societies. The Julian Press, Inc, New York, 1976.

K04594   Kokwaro, J. O. Medicinal plants of East Africa. East Afr Literature Bureau, Niarobi, 1976.

K04641   Siegel, R. K. Herbal intoxication. Pscyhoactive effects from herbal cigarettes, tea, and capsules. **J Amer Med Assoc** 1976; 236(5): 473–476.

K04754   Woo, W. S. and E. B. Lee. The screening of biological active plants in Korea using isolated organ preparations. 1. Anticholinergic and oxytocic actions in the ileum and uterus. **Annu Rept Nat Prod Res Inst Seoul Natl Univ** 1976; 15: 138.

K04768   Keys, J. D. Chinese herbs, Botany, Chemistry and Pharmacodynamics. Charles E. Tuttle Co., Rutland, Vermont, USA, 1976.

K04780   Konowalchuk, J. and J. I. Speirs. Antiviral activity of fruit extracts. **J Food Sci** 1976; 41: 1013.

K07087   Agarwa, K., H. Dhir, A. Sharma and G. Taluker. The efficacy of two species of Phyllanthus in counteracting nickel clastogenicity. **Fitoterapia** 1992; 63(1): 49–54.

K07256   Brandao, M. G. L., T. S. M. Grandi, E. M. M. Rocha and D.R. Sawyer. Survey of medicinal plants used as antimalarials in the Amazon. **J Ethnopharmacol** 1992; 36(2): 175–182.

K07316   Mlingi, N., N. H. Poulter and H. Rosling. An outbreak of acute intoxications from consumption of insufficiently processed cassava in Tanzania. **Nutrition Research** 1992; 12(6): 677–687.

K07365   Atta-Ur-Rahman. Some approches to the study of indigenous medicinal plants. **Bull Islamic Med** 1982; 2: 562–568.

K07404   Giordani, R., M. Siepaio, J. Moulin-Traffort and P. Regli. Antifungal action of *Carica papaya* latex. Isolation of fungal cell wall hydrolysing enzymes. **Mycoses** 1991; 34(11/12): 469–477.

K07408   Azuine, M. A., J. J. Kayal and S. B. Bhide. Protective role of aqueous turmeric extract against mutagenicity of direct-acting carcinogens as well as benzo(a)pyrene-induced genotoxicity and carcinogenicity. **J Cancer Res Clin Oncol** 1992; 118(6): 447–452.

K07497   Caceres, A., A. Saravia, S. Rizzio, L. Zabala, E. DeLeon, and F. Nave. Pharmacological properties of *Moringa oleifera*. 2. Screening for antispasmodic, antiinflammatory an diuretic activity. **J Ethnopharmacol** 1992; 36(3): 233–237.

K07622   Hsu, F. L. and J T. Cheng. Investigation in rats of the antihyperglycaemic effect of plant extracts used in Taiwan for the treatment of diabetes mellitus. **Phytother Res** 1992; 6(2): 108–111.

K07637   Segura, J. J., L. H. Morales-Ramos and J. Verde-Star. Growth inhibition of *Entamoeba histolytica* and *E. invadens* produced by the root of Granade (*Punica granatum* L.) **Arch Invest Med (Mex)** 1990; 21(3): 235–239.

K07698   Charles, V. and S. X. Charles. The use and efficacy of *Azadirachta indica* (neem) and *Curcuma longa* (turmeric) in scabies. **Trop Geogr Med** 1992; 44: 178–181.

K07796   Imbabi, E. S. and I. M. Abu-Al-Futuh. Investigation of the molluscicidal activity of *Tamarindus indica*. **Indian J Pharmacy** 1992; 30(2): 157–160.

K07849   Setiodihardjo, S. H. Tests of antibacterial effect of ointment containing *Cassia alata* L. leaves. **Thesis-MS- Dept Pharm Fac Math & Sci Univ Padjadjaran, Indonesia** 1986.

K07953   Nagasawa, H., T. Iwabuchi and H. Inatomi. Protection by treepeony (*Paeonia suffruticosa*

Andr.) of obesity in (SLN x C3H/HE) F_1 obese mice. **In Vitro** 1991; 5(2): 115–118.

K07977　Brandao, M., M. Botelho and E. Krettli. Antimalarial Experimental Chemotherapy using Natural Products. **Cienc Cult** 1985; 37(7): 1152–1163.

K07998　Carvalho, L. H., M. G. L. Brandao, D. Santos-Filho, J. L. C. Lopes and A. U. Krettli. Antimalarial activity of crude extracts from Brazilian plants studies In Vivo in *Plasmodium berghei*-infected mice and In Vitro against *Plasmodium falciparum* in culture. **Braz J Med Biol Res** 1991; 24(11): 1113–1123.

K08041　Mahmoud, I., A. alkofahi and A. Abdelaziz. Mutagenic and toxic activities of several spices and some Jordanian medicinal plants. **Int J Pharmacog** 1992; 30(2): 81–85.

K08273　Kusumoto, I. T., N. Kakiuchi, M. Hattori, T. Namba, S. Sutardjo and K. Shimotohno. Screening of some Indonesian Medicinal plants for inhibitory effects on HIV-1 Protease. **Shoyahugaku Zasshi** 1992; 46(2): 190–193.

K08278　Gupta, O. P., N. Sharma and D. Chad. A sensitive and relevant model for evaluating anti-inflammatory activity, papaya latex-induced rat paw inflammation. **J Pharmacol Toxicol Meth** 1992; 28(1): 15–19.

K08332　El-Saadany, S. S., M. Z. Sithoy, S. M. Labib and R. El-Massry. Biochemical dynamics and Hypocholesterolemic action of *Hibiscus sabdariffa* (Karkade). **Nahrung** 1991; 35(6): 567–576.

K08492　Ferriera, L. A. F., O. B. Henriques, A. A. S. Anderoni, G. R. F. Vital, M. M. C. Campos, G. G. Habermehl and Y. L. G. De Morales. Antivenom and biological effects of Ar-turmerone isolated from *Curcuma longa*

(Zingiberaceae). **Toxicon** 1992; 30(10): 1211–1218.

K08575　Holdsworth, D. K. Traditional medicinal plants of Rarotonga, Cook Islands. Part II. **Int J Pharmacog** 1991; 29(1): 71–79.

K08673　Sharma, S. K.aand V. P. Singh. The antifungal activity of some essential oils. **Ind Drugs Pharm Ind** 1979; 14(1): 3–6.

K08691　Gorgue, C. M. P., M. M. J. Champ, Y. Lozano and J. Delort-Laval. Dietary fiber from mango byproducts. Characterization and hypoglycemic effects determined by in vitro methods. **J Agr Food Chem** 1992; 40(10): 1864–1868.

K08721　Kusumoto, I. T., I. Shimada, N. Kakiuchi, M. Hattori, T. Namba and S. Supriyatna. Inhibitory effect of Indonesian plant extracts on reverse transcriptase of an RNA tumour virus (1). **Phytother Res** 1992; 6(5): 241–244.

K08820　Misbra, A. K., N. Kishore, N. K. Dubey and J. P. N. Chansouria. An evaluation of the toxicity of the oils of *Cymbopogon citratus* and *Citrus medica* in rats. **Phytother Res** 1992; 6(5): 279–281.

K08911　Ogata, T., H. Higuchi, S. Mochida, H. Matsumoto, A. Kato, T. Endo, A. Kaji and H. Kaji. HIV-1 reverse transcriptase inhibitor from *Phyllanthus niruri.* **AIDS Res Human Retroviruses** 1992; 8: 1937–1944.

K08933　Bhat, R. B., E. O. Eterjere and V. T. Oladipo. Ethnobotanical studies from Central Nigeria. **Econ Bot** 1990; 44(3): 382-390.

K09096　Liu, Y. G. Hypolipemics and blood platelet aggregation inhibitors comprising fish oil and plant extracts. **Patent-US-4,842,859:** 1989; 6 pp

K09153　Bhakuni, D. S., A. K. Goel, S. Jain, B. N. Mehrotra, G. K. Patnaik and V. Prakash. Screening of Indian plants for biological activity: Part XIII. **Indian J Exp Biol** 1988; 26(11): 883–904.

K09159   Misas, C. A. J., N. M. R. Hernandez and A. M. L. Abraham. Contribution to the biological evaluation of Cuban plants. 1V. **Rev Cub Med Trop** 1979; 31(1): 29–35.

K09163   Misas, C. A. J., N. M. R. hernandez and A. M. L. Abraham. The biological assessment of Cuban plants. III. **Rev Cub Med Trop** 1979; 31(1): 21–27.

K09214   Aruna, K. and V. M. Sivaramakrishnan. Anticarcinogenic effects of some Indian plant products. **Food Chem Toxicol** 1992; 30(11): 953–956.

K09337   Teixeira, C. C., F. D. Fuchs, R. M. Blotta, A. P. Da Costa, D. G. Mussnich and G. G. Ranquetat. Plants employed in the treatment of diabetes mellitus. Results of an ethnopharmacological survey in Porto Alegre, Brazil. **Fitoterapia** 1992; 63(4): 320–322.

K09718   Khan, M., D. C. Jain, R. S. Bhakuni, M. Zaim and R. S. Thakur. Occurrence of some antiviral sterols in *Artemisa annua*. **Plant Sci** 1991; 75: 161–165.

K10069   Alam, M. K. Medicinal Ethnobotany of the Marma Tribe of Bangladesh. **Econ Bot** 1992; 46(3): 330–335.

K10104   Pousset, J. L., J. P. Levesque, P. Coursaget and F. X. Galen. Hepatitis B surface antigen (HBSAg) inactivation and antiotension-converting enzyme (ACE) inhibition In Vitro by Combretum glutinosum Perr. (Combretaceae) extract. **Phytother Res** 1993; 7(1): 101–102.

K10142   Pillai, N. R. Anti-diarrheal activity of *Punica granatum* in experimental animals. **Int J Pharmacog** 1992; 30(3): 201,204.

K10577   Omer, S. A., F. H. Ibrahim, S. A. Khalid and S. E. I. Adam. Toxicological interactions of *Abrus precatorius* and *Cassia senna* in the diet of Lohmann broiler chicks. **Vet Hum Toxicol** 1992; 34(4): 310–313.

K10612   Badwi, S. M. A., H. M. Mousa, S. Adam and H. Hapke. Response of brown hi-sex chicks to low levels of *Jatropha curcas*, *Ricinus communis* or their mixture. **Vet Hum Toxicol** 1992; 34(4): 304.

K10618   Samia, M., E. Badwi, S. Adam and H. J. Hapke. Toxic effects of low levels of dietary *Jatropha curcas* seed on brown hi-sex chicks. **Vet Hum Toxicol** 1992; 34(2): 112–115.

K10660   Mukundan, M. A., M. C. Chacko, V. V. Annapurna and K. Krishnaswamy. Effect of turmeric and curcumin on BP-DNA adducts. **Carcinogenesis** 1993; 14(3): 493–496.

K10998   Fuiji, Y., T. Shibuya and T. Yasuda. Allelopathy of velvetbean. Its discrimination and identification of L-DOPA as a candidate of allelopathic substances. **JARQ** 1992; 25(4): 238–247.

K11173   Yasukawa, K., A. Yamaguchi, J. Arita, S. Sakurai, A. Ikeda and M. Takido. Inhibitory effect of edible plant extracts on 12-0-Tetradecanoylphorbol-13-Acetate-induced ear oedema in mice. **Phytother Res** 1993; 7(2): 185–189.

K11282   Reddy, M. B., K. R. Reddy and M. N. Reddy. A survey of plant crude drugs of Anantapur District, Andhra Pradesh, India. **Int J Crude Drug Res** 1989; 27(3): 145–155.

K11287   Lutterodt, G. D. Inhibition of Microlax-induced experimental diarrhoea with narcotic-like extracts of *Psidium guajava* leaf in rats. **J Ethnopharmacol** 1992; 37(2): 151–157.

K11291   Chattopadhyay, R. R., R. N. Banerjee, S. K. Sarkar, S. Ganguly and T. K. Basu. Antiinflammatory and acute toxicity studies with the leaves of *Vinca rosea* Linn. in experimental animals. **Indian J**

Physiol Pharmacol 1992; 36(4): 291,292.

K11473   Grove, I. S. and S. Bala. Studies on antimutagenic effects of guava (*Psidium guajava*) in *Salmonella typhimurium*. **Mutat Res** 1993; 300(1): 1–3.

K11484   Hukkeri, V. I., G. A. Kalyani, B. C. Hatpaki and F. V. Manvi. In Vitro anthelmintic activity of aqueous extract of fruit rind of *Punica granatum*. **Fitoterapia** 1993; 64(1): 69,70.

K11513   Orafidiva, L. O. The effect of autoxidation of lemon-grass oil on its antibacterial activity. **Phytother Res** 1993; 7(3): 269–271.

K11565   Hasan, C. M., S. N. Islam, K. Begum, M. Ilias and A. Hussain. Antibacterial activities of the leaves and stem bark of *Cassia alata* L. **Bangdladesh J Bot** 1988; 17(2): 135–139.

K11576   Crockett, C. O., F. Guede-Guina, D. Pugh, M. Vangah-Manda, T. J. Robinson, J. O. Qlubadewo and R. F. Ochillo. *Cassia alata* and the preclinical search for therapeutic agents for the treatment of opportunistic infections in AIDS patients. **Cell Mol Biol** 1992; 38(5): 505–511.

K11643   Ayudhaya, T. D., W. Nutakul, U. Khunanek et al., Study on the in vitro antimalarial activity of some medicinal plants against *Plasmodium falciparum*. **Bull Dept Med Sci** 1987; 29: 22–38.

K11645   Consoli, R. A. G. B., N. M. Mendes, J. P. Pereira, B. D. S. Santos and M. A. Lamounier. Larvicidal properties of plant extracts against *Aedes fluviatilis* (Lutz) (Diptera: Culicidae) in the laboratory. **Mem Inst Oawaldo Cruz** (Rio De Janeiro) 1988; 83(1): 87–93.

K11652   Villarreal, M. L., D. Alonso and G. Melesio. Cytotoxic activity of some Mexican plants used in traditional medicine. **Fitoterapia** 1992; 63(6): 518–522.

K11808   Bhaumik, A. and M. C. Sharma. Therapeutic efficacy of two herbal preparations in induced hepatopathy in sheep. **J Res Indian Med** 1993; 12(1): 33–42.

K11849   Shibib, B. A., L. A. Khan and R. Rahman. Hypoglycemic activity of *Coccinia indica* and *Momordica charantia* in diabetic rats: Depression of the hepatic gluconeogenic enzymes glucose-6-phosphatase and fructose-1,6-bisphosphatase and elevation of both liver and red-cell shunt enzyme glucose-6-phosphatase. **Biochem J** 1993; 292(1): 267–270.

K11884   Shopshire, C. M., E. Stauber and M. Arai. Evaluation of selected plants for acute toxicosis in budgerigars. **J Amer Vet Assocn** 1992; 200(7): 936–939.

K11898   Yilkirim, O. F., B. S. Uydes, M. Ark, I. Kanzik and F. Akar. Investigation of the antiulcer effect of the fruits of *Momordica charantia* in rats. **Abstr 3rd Intern Symp Pharm Sci, Ankara Univ** 1993; Abstr-P85.

K11985   Shin, K. H., M. S. Chung, Y. I. Chae, K. Y. Yoon and T. S. Cho. A survey for Aldose Reductase Inhibition of Herbal Medicines. **Fitoterapia** 1993; 64(2): 130–133.

K12472   Perdue Jr, R. E. Cell Culture. 1. Role in dixcovery of antitumor agents from higher plants. **J Nat Prod** 1982; 45(4): 418–426.

K12860   Jauk, L., E. M. Galati, S. Kirjavainen, A. M. Forestieri and A. Trovato. Analgesic and antipyretic effect of *Macuna pruriens*. **Int J Pharmacog** 1993; 31(3): 213–216.

K12864   Obasi, B. N. B., C. A. Igboechi, D. C. Anuforo and K. N. Aimufua. Effects of extracts of *Newbouldia laevis*, *Psidium guajava* and *Phyllanthus amarus* on gastrointestinal tract. **Fitoterapia** 1993; 64(3): 235–238.

K12995 Srivastava, Y., H. Venkatakrishna-Bhatt, Y. Verma and K. Venkaiah. Antidiabetic and adaptogenic properties of *Momordica charantia* extract: An experimental and clinical evaluation. **Phytother Res** 1993; 7(4): 285–289.

K13111 Crockett, C. O., F. Guede-Guina, D. Pugh, M. Vangah-Manda, T. J. Robinson, J. O. Qlubadewo and R. F. Ochillo. *Cassia alata* and the preclinical search for therapeutic agents for the treatment of opportunistic infections in AIDS patients. **Cell Mol Biol** 1992; 38(7): 799–902.

K13253 Hikino, H. Antihepatotoxic activity of crude drugs. **Yakugaku Zasshi** 1985; 105(2): 109–118.

K13363 Kumar, A., V. K. Sharma, H. P. Singh, P. Prakash and S. P. Singh. Efficacy of some indigenous drugs in tissue repair in buffaloes. **Indian Vet J** 1993; 70(1): 42–44.

K13618 Apul, B. S. and J. K. Mali. Poisoning of livestock by some toxic plants. **Progressive Farming** 1982; 6,7.

K13748 Rana, N. S. and M. N. Ioshi. Investigation on the antiviral activity of ethanolic extracts of Syzygium species. **Fitoterapia** 1992; 63(3): 542–544.

K13751 Satomi, H., K. Umemura, A. Ueno, T. Hatano, T. Okuda and T. Noro. Carbonic anhydrase inhibitors from the pericarps of *Punica granatum* L. **Biol Pharm Bull** 1993; 16(8): 787–790.

K13947 Ali, L., A. K. A. Khan, M. I. R. Mamun, M. Mosihuzzaman, N. Nahar, M. Nur-E-Alam and B. Rokeya. Studies on hypoglycemic effects of fruit pulp, seed, and whole plant of *Momordica charantia* on normal and diabetic model rats. **Planta Med** 1993; 59(5): 408–412.

K14086 Azuine, M. A. and S. V. Bhide. Protective single/combines treatment with betel leaf and turmeric against methyl (acetoxymethyl) nitrosamine-induced hamster oral carcinogenesis. **Int J Cancer** 1992; 51: 412–415.

K14566 Nagabhushan, M. and S. V. Bhide. Nonmutagenicity of curcumin and its antimutagenic action versus chili and capsaicin. **Nutr Cancer** 1986; 8(3): 201–210.

K14611 Osato, J. A., L. A. Santiago, G. M. Reno, M. S. Cuadra and A. Mori. Antimicrobial and antioxidant activities of unripe papaya. **Life Sci** 1993; 53(17): 1383–1389.

K14672 Lin, C. C. Crude drugs used for the treatment of diabetes mellitus in Taiwan. **Amer J Chin Med** 1992; 20(3/4): 269–279.

K14683 Anesini, C. and C. Perez. Screening of plants used in Argentina folk medicine for antimicrobial activity. **J Ethnopharmacol** 1993; 39(2): 119–128.

K14899 Soudamini, K. K. and R. Kuttan. Chemoprotective effect of curcumin against cyclophosphamide toxicity. **Indian J Pharm Sci** 1992; 54(6): 213–217.

K14943 Abraham, S., S. K. Abraham and G. Radhamony. Mutagenic potential of the condiments, ginger and turmeric. **Cytologia** 1976; 41(3/4): 591–595.

K14946 Rahmani, M., H. B. M. Ismail, F. Ahmad, A. R. Manas and M. A. Sukari. Screening of tropical plants for the presence of Bioactive compounds. **Pertanika** 1992; 15(2): 131–135.

K15267 Soni, K. B., A. Rajan and R. Kuttan. Reversal of aflatoxin induced liver damage by turmeric and curcumin. **Cancer Lett** 1992; 66(2): 115–121.

K15932 Chungsamarnvart, N. and S. Jiwajinda. Acaricidal activity of volatile oil from lemon and cotronella grasses on tropical cattle ticks. **Kasetsart J Nat Sci** 1992; 26(5): 46–51.

K15971 Gessler, M. C., M. H. H. Nkunyak, L. B. Mwasumbi, M. heinrich and M. Tanner. Screening of Tanzanian medicinal plants for antimalarial activity. **Acta Tropica** 1994; 56(1): 65–77.

K16006   Nath, D., N. Sethi, R. K. Singh and A. K. Jain. Commonly used Indian abortifacient plants with special reference to their teratologic effects in rats. **J Ethnopharmacol** 1992; 36(2): 147–154.

K16061   Obiefuna, P., O. Owolabi, B. Adegunloye, I. Obiefuna and O. Sofola. The petal extract of *Hibiscus sabdariffa* produces relaxation of isolated rat aorta. **Int J Pharmacog** 1994; 32(1): 69–74.

K16191   Damodaran, S. and S. Venkataraman. A study of the therapeutic efficacy of *Cassia alata* Linn. Leaf extract against pityriasis versicolor. **J Ethnopharmacol** 1994; 42(1): 19–23.

K16225   Reddy, A. C. P. and B. R. Lokesh. Effect of dietary turmeric (*Curcuma longa*) on iron-induced lipid peroxidation in the rat liver. **Food Chem Toxicol** 1994; 32(3): 279–283.

K16262   Schultes, E. V. and R. F. Raffauf. De Plantis Toxicariis E Mundo Novo Tropicale Commentationes xxxix. Febrifuges of Northwest Amazonia. **Harvard Pap in Bot** 1994; 5: 50–68.

K16266   Mishra, A. and N. Dubey. Evaluation of some essential oils for their toxicity against fungi causing deterioration of stored food commodities. **Appl Environ Microbiol** 1994; 60(4): 1101–1105.

K16304   Kulkarni, R. and N. Ravindra. Resistance to *Pythium aphanidermatum* in diploids and induced autotetraploids of *Catharanthus roseus*. **Planta Med** 1988; 54(4): 356–359.

K16653   Son, K. H., S. H. Kim, K. Y. Jung and H. W. Chang. Screening of platelet activating factor (PAF) antagonists from medicinal plants. **Korean J Pharmacog** 1994; 25(2): 167–170.

K16654   Elisabethsky, E. and Z. C. Castilhos. Plants used as analgesics by Amazonian Caboclos as a basis for selecting plants for investigation. **Int J Crude Drug Res**. 1990; 28(4): 309–320.

K16835   Kurokawa, M., H, Ochiai, K. Nagasaka, M. Neki, H. X. Xu, S. Kadota, S. Sutardio, T. Matsumoto, T. Namba and K. Shiraki. Antiviral traditional medicines against Herpes Simplex Virus (HSV-1), Poliovirus, and Measles virus In Vitro and their therapeutic efficacies for HSV-1 infection in mice. **Antiviral Res** 1993; 22(2/3): 175–188.

K16898   Parry, O., J. A. Marks and F. K. Okwuasaba. The skeletal muscle relaxant action of *Portulaca oleracea*. Role of potassium ions. **J Ethnopharmacol** 1993; 40(3): 187–194.

K16940   Habtemariam, S., A. L. Harvey and P. G. Waterman. The muscle relaxant properties of *Portulaca oleraceai* are associated with high concentration of potassium ions. **J Ethnopharmacol** 1993; 40(3): 195–200.

K16948   Zamora-Martinez, M. C. and C. N. P. Pola. Medicinal plants used in some rural populations of Oaxaca, Puebla and Veracruz, Mexico. **J Ethnopharmacol** 1992; 35(3) 229–257.

K16969   Tsuda, T., Y. Makino, H. Kato, T. Osawa and S. Kawakishi. Screening for antioxidative activity of edible pulses. **Biosci Biotech Biochem** 1993; 57(9): 1606–1608.

K17092   Akperbekova, B. A. and D. Ya Guseinov. Studies on the influence of pharmaceutic preparations from rhizomes of *Cyperus rotundus* growing in Azerbaidzhan on the heart and vascular system. **Azerb Med Zh** 1966; 43(7): 12–17.

K17122   Gupta, S., J. N. S. Yadava and J. S. Tandon. Antisecretory (Antidiarrheal) activity of Indian medicinal plants against *Escherichia coli* enterotoxin-induced secretion in rabbit and guinea pig ileal loop models. **Int J Pharmacog** 1993; 31(3): 198–204.

K17144 Soni, K. B., A. Rajan, R. Kuttan. Inhibition of aflatoxin-induced liver damage in ducklings by food additives. **Mycotoxin Res** 1993; 9(1): 22–27.

K17215 Vu, V. D. and T. T. Mai. Study on analgesic effect of *Cyperus stoloniferus* Retz. **Tap Chi Duoc Hoc** 1994; 1: 16,17.

K17262 Ogunti, E. O. and A. A. Elujoba. Laxative activity of *Cassia alata*. **Fitoterapia** 1993; 64(5): 437–439.

K17280 Matsuo, T., N. Hanamure, K. Shimoi, Y. Nakamura and I. Tomita. Identification of (+)-Gallocatechin as a bio-antimutagenic compound in Psidium guava leaves. **Phytochemistry** 1994; 36(4): 1027–1029.

K17316 Hirobe, C., D. Palevitch, K. Takeya and H. Itokawa. Screening test for antitumor activity of crude drugs (IV). Studies on cytotoxic activity of Israeli medicinal plants. **Nat Med** 1994; 48(2): 168–170.

K17523 Perez, C. and C. Anesini. Inhibition of *Pseudomonas aerguinosa* by Argentinean medicinal plants. **Fitoterapia** 1994; 65(2): 169–172.

K17557 Alam, K., T. Agua, H. Maven, R. Taie, K. S. Rao, I. Burrows, M. E. Huber and T. Rali. Preliminary screening of seaweeds, seagrass adn lemongrass oil from Papua New Guinea for antimicrobial and antifungal activity. **Int J Pharmacog** 1994; 32(4): 396–399.

K17561 Lim-Sylianco, C. Y., J. A. Concha, A. P. Jocano and C. M. Lim. Antimutagenic effects of expressions from twelve medicinal plants. **Philippine J Sci** 1986; 115(1): 23–30.

K17562 Lim-Sylianco, C. Y., J. A. Concha, A. P. Jocano and C. M. Lim. Antimutagenic effects of eighteen Philippine plants. **Philippine J Sci** 1986; 115(4): 293–296.

K17672 Santo, A. R. S., V. C. Filho, R. Niero, A. M. Viana, F. N. Moreno, M. M. Campos, R. A. Yunes, J. B. Calixto. Analgesic effects of callus culture extracts from selected species of Phyllanthus in mice. **J Pharm Pharmacol** 1994; 46(9): 755–759.

K17723 Vinitketkummuen, U., R. Puatanachokchai, P. Kongtawelert, N. Lertprasetsuke and T. Matsushima. Antimutagenicity of lemon grass (*Cymbopogon citratus* Stapf) to various known mutagens in the Salmonella mutation assay. **Mutat Res** 1994; 341(1): 71–75.

K17876 Balboa, J. G. and C. Y. Lim-Sylianco. Antigenotoxic effects of drug preparations Akapulko and Ampalaya. **Philipp J Sci** 1992; 121(4): 399–411.

K17959 Tennekoon, K. H., S. Jeevathayaparan, P. Angunawala, E. H. Karunanayake and K. S. A. Jayasinghe. Effect of *Momordica charantia* on key hepatic enzymes. **J Ethnopharmacol** 1994; 44(2): 93–97.

K17990 Ponce-Macotela, M., I. Navarro-Alegria, M. N. Martinez-Gordillo and R. Alvarez-Chacon. In vitro antigiardiasic activity of plant extracts. **Rev Invest Clin** 1994; 46(5): 343–347.

K18012 Muanza, D. N., B. W. Kim, K. L. Euler and L. Williams. Antibacterial and Antifungal activities if nine medicinal plants from Zaire. **Int J Pharmacog** 1994; 32(4): 337–345.

K18109 Bourdy, G. and A. Walter. Maternity and medicinal plants in Vanuatu 1. The cycle of reproduction. **J Ethnopharmacol** 1992; 37(3): 179–196.

K18142 Holdsworth, D. Medicinal plants of the Gazelle peninsula, New

Britain Island, Papau New Guinea. Part 1. **Int J Pharmacog** 1992; 30(3): 185–190.

K18143 Singh, J., A. K. Dubey and N. N. Tripathi. Antifungal activity of Mentha spicata. **Int J Pharmacog** 1994; 32(4): 314–319.

K18219 Cakici, I., C. Hurmoglu, B. Tunctan, N. Abacioglu, I. Kanzik and B. Sener. hypoglycaemic effect of *Momordica charantia* extracts om normoglycaemic or cyproheptadine-induced hyperglycaemic mice. **J Ethnopharmacol** 1994; 44(2): 117–121.

K18294 Blanco, C., T. Carrillo, R. Castillo, J. Quiralte and M. Cuevas. Avocado Hypersensitivity. **Allergy** 1994; 49(6): 454–459.

K18448 Benjamin, B. D., S. M. Kelkar, M. S. Pote, G. S. Kakli, A. T. Sipahimalani and M. R. Heble. *Catharanthus roseus* cell cultures: Growth, alkaloid synthesis and antidiabetic activity. **Phytother Res** 1994; 8(3): 185–186.

K18559 Holdsworth, D and L. Balun. Medicinal plants of the East and West Sepik Privinces, Papau New Guinea. **Int J Pharmacog** 1992; 30(3): 218–222.

K18745 Azuine, M. A. and S. V. Bhide. Ajuvant chemoprevention of experimental cancer: catechin and dietary turmeric in forestomach and oral cancer models. **J Ethnopharmacol** 1994; 44(3): 211–217.

K18765 Schmeda-Hirschmann, G. and A. Rojas De Arias. A screening method for natural products on Triatomine bugs. **Phytother Res** 1992; 6(2): 68–73.

K18790 Kositchaiwat, C., S. Kositchaiwat and J. Havanondha. Ulcer comparison to liquid antacid: A controlled clinical trial. **J Med Assoc Thailand** 1993; 76(1): 601–605.

K18804 Kumazawa, N., S. Ohto, O. Ishizuka, N. Sakurai, A. Kamogawa and M. Shinoda. Protective effects of various methanol extracts of crude drugs on experimental hepatic injury induced by carbon tetrachloride in rats. **Yakugaku Zasshi** 1990; 110(12): 950–957.

K18991 Hope, B. E., D. G. Massey and G. Fournier-Massey. Hawaiian Materia Medica for Asthma. **Hawaii Med J** 1993; 52(6): 160–166.

K19150 Malamas, M. and M. Marselos. The tradition of medicinal plants in Zagori, Epirus (Northwestern Greece). **J Ethnopharmacol** 1992; 37(3): 197–203.

K19264 Caceres, A., L. Figueroa, A. M. Taracena and B. Samayoa. plants used in Guatemala for the treatment of respiratory diseases. 2. Evaluation of activity of 16 plants against Gram-positive bacteria. **J Ethnopharmacol** 1993; 39(1): 77–82.

K19323 Tanira, M. O. M., A. K. Bashir, R. Dib, C. S. Goodwin, I. A. Wasfi and N. R. Banna. Antimicrobial and phytochemical screening of medicinal **Ethnopharmacol** 1994; 41(3): 201–205.

K19396 Lozoya, X., M. Meckes, M. Abou-Aid, J. Tortoriello, C. Nozzolillo and J. T. Arnason. Quercetin glycosides in *Psidium guajava* L. leaves and determination of a spasmolytic principle. **Arch Med Res** 1994; 25(1): 11–15.

K19400 Diogenes, M. J. N., S. M. De Morias and F. F. Carvalho. Perioral contact dermatitis by cardol. **Int J Dermatol** 1995; 34(1): 72,73.

K19490 Kirdpon, S., S. N. Nakorn and W. Kirdpon. Changes in urinary chemical composition in healthy volunteers after consuming roselle (*Hibiscus sabdariffa* Linn.) juice. **J Med Assoc Thailand** 1994; 77(6): 314–321.

K19491 Santos, A. R. S., V. C. Filho, R. A. Yunes and J. B. Calixto. Further studies on the antinociceptive action of the hydroalcoholic extracts from plants on the genus Phyllanthus. **J Pharm Pharmacol** 1995; 47(1): 66–71.

K19502 Audicana, M. and G. Bernaola. Occupational contact dermititis from citrus fruits: Lemon essential oils. **Contact Dermatitis** 1994; 31(3): 183–185.

K19538 Sankaranarayanan, J. and C. I. Jolly. Phytochemical, antibacterial and pharmacological investigations on *Momordica charantia* Linn., *Emblica officinalis* Gaertn. and *Curcuma longa* linn. **Indian J Pharm Sci** 1993; 55(1): 6–13.

K19547 Moraes, V. L. G., L. F. M. Santos, S. B. Castro, L. H. Loureiro, O. A. Lima et al. Inhibition of lymphocyte activation by extracts and fractions of Kalanchoe, Alternathera, Paullinia and Mikania species. **Phytomedicine** 1994; 1(3): 199–204.

K19563 Cunnick, J. and D. Takemoto. Bitter melon (*Momordica charantia*). **J Naturopathic Med** 1993; 4(1): 16–21.

K19580 Ibrahim D. and H. Osman. Antimicrobial activity of *Cassia alata* from Malaysia. **J Ethnopharmacol** 1995; 45(3): 151–156.

K19791 Gladding, S. Lantana camara. **Aust J Med Herb** 1995; 7(1): 5–9.

K20147 Morton, J. F. Lantana, or Red Sage (Lantana camara L., Verbenaceae), notorious weed and popular garden flower; some cases of poisoning on Florida. **Econ Bot** 1994; 48(3): 259–270.

K20239 Shirota, S., K. Miyazaki, R. Aiyama, M. Ichioka and T. Yokikura. Tyrosinase inhibitors from crude drugs. **Biol Pharm Bull** 1994; 17(2): 266–269.

K20280 Morrison, E. Local remedies ... Yeh or Nay. **West Ind Med J Suppl** 1994; 2(43): 9 pp.

K20355 Vu, V. D. and X. S. Pham. On the difference between *Cyperus rotundus* L. and *Cyperus stoloniferus* Retz. **Tap Chi Duoc Hoc** 1993; 4: 90–91.

K20471 Holdsworth, D. K. Traditional medicinal plants of Rarotonga, Cook Islands Part 1. **Int J Crude Drug Res** 1990; 28(3): 209–218.

K20557 Lavaud, F., A. Prevost, C. Cossart, L. Guerin, J. Bernard and S. Kochman. Allergy to latex, avocado pear, and banana. Evidence for a 30 KD antigen in immunoblotting. **J Allergy Clin Immunol** 1995; 95(2): 557–564.

K20607 Hussam, T. S., S. H. Nasralla and A. K. N. Chaudhuri. Studies on the antiinflammatory and related pharmacological activities of *Psidium guajava*. A preliminary report. **Phytother Res** 1995; 9(2): 118–122.

K20618 Akhtar, A. H. and K. U. Ahmad. Antiulcerogenic evaluation of the methanolic extracts of some indigenous medicinal plants of Pakistan in aspirin-ulcerated rats. **J Ethnopharmacol** 1995; 46(1): 1–6.

K20642 Elisabetsky, E., W. Figueiro and G. Oliveria. Traditional Amazonian nerve tonics as antidepressant agents. *Chaunochiton kappleri*. A case study. **J Herbs Spices Med Plants** 1992; 1(1/2): 125–162.

K20893 Gandhi, V. M., K. M. Cherian and M. J. Mulky. Toxicological studies on Ratanjyot oil. **Food Chem Toxicol** 1995; 33(1): 39–42.

K20898 Houghton, P. J. and K. P. Skari. The effect on blood clotting of some West African plants used against snakebite. **J Ethnopharmacol** 1994; 44(2): 99–108.

K21091 Desta, B. Ethiopian traditional herbal drugs. Part ll: Antimicrobial activity of 63 medicinal plants. **J Ethnopharmacol** 1993; 39(2): 129–139.

K21149 De Blasi, V., S. Debrot, P. A. Menoud, L. Gendre and J. Schowing. Amoebicidal effect of essential oils in vitro. **J Toxicol Clin Exp** 1990; 10(6): 361–373.

K21173 Azuine, M. A. and S. V. Bhide. Protective single/combined treatment with betel leaf and turmeric against methyl (acetoxymethyl) initrosamine-induced hamster oral carcinogenesis. **Int J Cancer** 1992; 51(3): 412–415.

K21212 Yin, X. J., D. X. Liu, H. Wang and Y. Zhou. A study on the mutagenicity of 102 raw pharmaceuticals used in chinese traditional medicine. **Mutat Res** 1991; 260(1): 73–82.

K21223 Muanza, D. N., K. L. Euler, L. Williams and D. J. Newman. Screening for antitumor and anti-HIV activities of nine medicinal plants from Zaire. **Int J Pharmacog** 1995; 33(2): 98–106.

K21233 Ibrahim, A. M. Anthelmintic activity of some Sudanese Medicinal Plants. **Phytother Res** 1992; 6(3): 155–157.

K21241 Kusumoto, I. T., T. Nakabayashi, H. Kida, H. Miyashiro, M. Hattori, T. Namba and K. Shimotohno. Screening of various plant extracts used in Ayurvedic medicine for inhibitory effect on human immunodeficiency virus type 1 (HIV-1) protease. **Phytother Res** 1995; 9(3): 180–184.

K21278 Limaye, D. A., A. Y. Nimbkay, R. Jain and M. Ahmad. Cardiovascular effects of the aqueous extract of *Moringa pterygosperma*. **Phytother Res** 1995; 9(1): 37–90.

K21572 Lutete, T., K. Kambu, D. Ntondele, K. Cimanga and N. Luki. Antimicrobial activity of tannins. **Fitoterapia** 1994; 65(3): 276–278.

K21579 Otake, T., H. Mori, M. Morimoto, N. Ueba, S. Sutardio, I. Kusumoto, M. Hattori and T. Namba. Screening of Indonesian plant extracts for anti-human immunodeficiency virus-Type 1 (HIV-1) activity. **Phytother Res** 1995; 9(1): 6–10.

K21634 Selvam, R., L. Subramanian, R. Gayathri and N. Angayarkanni. The antioxidant activity of turmeric (*Curcuma longa*). **J Ethnopharmacol** 1995; 47(2): 59–67.

K21650 Masaki, H., S. Sakaki, T. Atsumi and H. Sakurai. Active-oxygen scavenging activity of plant extracts. **Biol Pharm Bull** 1995; 18(1): 162–166.

K21690 Dong, T. X., T. B. Ng, R. N. S. Wong, H. W. Yeung and G. J. Xu. Ribosome inactivating protein-like activity in seeds of diverse Cucurbitaceae plants. **Int J Biochem** 1993; 25(3): 415–419.

K22944 Han, B. H., O. K. Yang, Y. C. Kim and Y. N. Han. Screening of the platelet activating factor (PAF) antagonistic activities on herbal medicines. **Yakhak Hoe Chi** 1994; 38(4): 462–468.

K23019 Joyeux, M., F. Mortier and J. Fleurentin. Screening of anti-radical, antilipoperoxidant and hepatoprotective effects of nine plant extracts used in Caribbean folk medicine. **Phytother Res** 1995; 9(3): 228–230.

K23071 Park, S. Y. and J. W. Kim. Screening and isolation of the antitumor agents from medicinal plants. (1). **Korean J Pharmacog** 1992; 23(4): 264–267.

K23156 Singh, K. K. and J. K. Maheshwari. Traditional Phytotherapy of some medicinal plants used by the Tharus of the Nainital District, Uttar Pradesh, India. **Int J Pharmacog** 1994; 32(1): 51–58.

K23166 Ahmad, F. B. and D. K. Holdsworth. Traditional medicinal plants of Sabah, Malaysia Part 111. The Rungus people of Kudat. **Int J Pharmacog** 1995; 33(3): 262.

K23171 Anis, M. and M. Iqbal. Medicinal plantlore of Aligarh, India. **Int J Pharmacog** 1994; 32(1): 59–64.

K23172 Laferriere, J. E. Medicinal plants of the lowland Inga People of Colombia. **Int J Pharmacog** 1994; 32(1): 90–94.

K23191 Bhattarai, N. K. Folk herbal remedies for Gynaecological complaints in central Nepal. **Int J Pharmacog**. 1994; 32(1): 13–26.

K23294   Girach, R. D., Aminuddin, P. A. Siddioui and S. A. Khan. Traditional plant remedies among the Kondh of District Dhenkanal (Orissa). **Int J Pharmacog** 1994; 32(3): 274–283.

K23301   Awasthi, A. K. Ethnobotanical studies on the Negrito Islanders of Andaman islands, India - The Great Andamanese. **Econ Bot** 1991; 45(2): 274–280.

K23365   Bhandary, M. J., K. R. Chandrashekar and K. M. Kaveriappa. Medical Ethnobotany of the Siddis of Uttar Kannada district, Karnataka, India. **J Ethnopharmacol** 1995; 47(3): 149–158.

K23394   Deshpande, S. S. and G. B. Maru. Effects of curcumin on the formation of benzo(a)pyrene derived DNA adducts *In Vitro*. **Cancer Lett** 1995; 96(1): 71–80.

K23418   Owalbi, O. A., B. J. Adegunloye, O. P. Ajagbona, O. A. Sofola and P. C. M. Obiefuna. Mechanism if relaxant effect mediated by an aqueous extract of *Hibiscus sabdariffa* petals in isolated rat aorta. **Int J Pharmacog** 1995; 33(3): 210–214.

K23485   Maikhuri, R. K. and A. K. Gangwar. Ethnobiological notes on the Khasi and Garo tribes of Meghalaya, Northeast India. **Econ Bot** 1993; 47(4): 345–357.

K23694   Iida, K., K. Hase, K. Shimomura, S. Sudo, S. Kadota and T. Namba. Potent inhibitors of tyrosinase activity and melanin biosynthesis from *Rheum officinale*. **Planta Med** 1995; 61(5): 425–428.

K23824   Singh, V. K. adn Z. A. Ali. Folk medicines in primary health care: common plants used for the treatment of fevers in India. **Fitoterapia** 1994; 65(1): 68–74.

K23834   Filipoy, A. Medicinal plants of the Pilaga of Central Chaco. **J Ethnopharmacol** 1994; 44(3): 181–193.

K23896   Khan, M. A., T. Khan and Z. Ahmad. Barks used as source of medicine in Madhya Pradsh, India. **Fitoterapia** 1994; 65(5): 444–446.

K23904   Syed, M., M. R. Khalid and F. M. Chaudhary. Essential oils of Gramineae family having antibacterial activity Part 1. (*Cymbopogon citratus, C. martinii* and *C. jawarancusa* oils. **Pak J Sci Ind Res** 1990; 33(12): 529–531.

K24869   Bhide, S. V., D. Magnus, A. Azuine, M. Lahiri and N. T. Telang. Chemoprevention of mammary tumor virus-induced and chemical carcinogen-induced rodent mammary tumors by natural plant products. **Breast Cancer Res Treat** 1994; 30(3): 233–242.

K25126   Singh, A., S. P. Singhand R. Bamezai. Postnatal modulation of hepatic biotransformation system enzymes via translactational exposure of F1 mouse pups to turmeric and curcumin. **Chem Lett** 1995; 96: 87–93.

K25257   Bhattarai, N. K. Folk anthelmintic drugs of Central Nepal. **Int J Pharmacog** 1992; 30(2): 145-150.

K25332   Singh, A., S. P. Singh and R. Bamezai. Postnatal modulation of hepatic biotransformation system enzymes via translactational exposure of F1 mouse pups to turmeric and curcumin. **Cancer Lett** 1995; 96(1): 87–93.

K25491   Shirota, S., K. Myazaki, M. Ichioka and T. Yokokura. Skin-lightening cosmetics containing melanin inhibitors from plants. **Patent-Japan Kokai Tokkyo Koho-06,227,960** 1994; 4 pp.

K25671   Paek, S. H., G. J. Kim, H. S. Jeong and S. K. Yum. AR-tumerone and B-atlantone induced internucleosomal DNA fragmentation associated with programmed cell death in human myeloid leukemia HL-60 cells. **Arch Pharm Res** 1996; 19(2): 91–94.

K25892   Selvanayahgam, Z. E., S. G. Gnanevendhan, K. Balakrishna and R. B. Rao. Antisnake venom botanicals from ethnomedicine. **J Herbs Spices Medicinal Plants** 1994; 2(4): 45–100.

L00242   Kholkute, S. D. Effect of *Hibiscus rosa-sinensis* on spermatogenesis and accessory reproductive organs in rats. **Planta Med** 1977; 127–135.

L00302   Munsho, S. R., T. A. Shetye and R. K. Nair. Antifertility activity of three indigenous plant preparations. **Planta Med** 1977; 31: 73–75.

L00484   Khafagy, S. M., Y. A. Mohamed, N. A. Abdel Salam and Z. F. Mahmoud. Phytochemical study of Jatropha curcas. **Planta Med** 1977; 31: 274–277.

L01365   Pass, M. A. and T. Heath. Gallbladder paralysis in sheep during Lantana poisoning. **J Comp Pathol** 1977; 87: 301.

L01413   Kholkute, S. D., V. Mudgal and K. N. Udupa. Studies on the antifertility potentiality of *Hibiscus rosa-sinensis*. Parts of medicinal value. Selection of species and seasonal variation. **Planta Med** 1977; 31–35.

L01490   Latorre, D. L. and F. A. Latorre. Plants used by the Mexican Kickapoo Indians. **Econ Bot** 1977; 31: 340–357.

L01534   Morton, J. F. Medicinal and other plants used by peolpe on Morth Caicos (Turks and Caicos Islands, West Indies). **J Crude Drug Res** 1977; 15: 1–24.

L01543   Rouge, P., C. Chatelain and J. P. Gracis. Precipitation of human serum-glycoproteins by extracts of *Abrus precatorius* seeds. **Planta Med** 1977; 31: 7.

L01568   Amico, A. Medicinal plants of Southern Zambesia. **Fitoterapia** 1977; 48: 101–139.

L01679   Oso, B. A. Mushrooms in Yoruba and medicinal practices. **Econ Bot** 1977; 31: 367.

L02008   Chauhan, J. S., M. Sultan and S. K. Srivastava. Two new

           Glycoflavones from the roots of the *Phyllanthus niruri*. **Planta Med Suppl** 1977; 32: 217–222.

L02293   Arenas, P. and R. Moreno Azorero. Plants of common use in Paraguayan folk medicine for regulating fertility. **Econ Bot** 1977; 31: 298–301.

L02359   Dixit, V. P. Effects of chronically administered Malvaceae flower extract on the female genital tract. **Indian J Exp Biol** 1977; 15: 650–652.

L02255   Alami, R., A. Macksad and A. R. El-Gindy. Medicinal plants in Kuwait. Al-Assiriya Printing Press, Kuwait, 1976.

M00352   Pass, M. A., R. T. Gemmell and T. J. Heath. Effect of Lantana on the ultrastructure of the liver of sheep. **Toxicol Appl Pharmacol** 1978; 43: 589.

M00425   Vesely, D. L., W. R. Graves, T. M. Lo, M. A. Fletcher and G. S. Levey. Isolation of a Guanylate cyclase inhibition from the balsam pear (*Momordica charantia* Abreviata). **Biochem Biophys Res Commun** 1977; 77: 1294.

M00695   Morton, J. F. Some folk medicine plants of Central American markets. **Q J Crude Drug Res**. 1977; 15: 165.

M00721   Hufford, C. D. and B. O. Oguntimein. Non-polar constituents of *Jatropha curcas*. **Lloydia** 1978; 41: 161.

M00729   Holdsworth, D. K. Medicinal plants of Papua-New Guinea, Technical Paper No. 175, South Pacific Commission, Noumea, New Caledonia, 1977.

M01121   Kholkute, S. D., D. N. Srivastava, S, Chatterjee and K. N. Udupa. Effects of some compounds isolated from *Hibiscus rosa-sinensis* on pregnancy in rats. **J Res Indian Med Yoga Homeopathy** 1976; 11: 106–108.

M01152   Dixit, V. P., P. Khanna and S. K. Bhargava. Effects of *Momordica charantia* fruit extract on the testicular function of dog. **Planta Med** 1978; 34: 280–286.

M01250 Kapadia, G. J., E. B. Chung, B. Ghosh, Y. N. Shukla, S. P. Basak, J. F. Morton and S. N. Pradhan. Carcinogenicity of some folk medicinal herbs in rats. **J Nat Cancer Inst** 1978; 60: 683–686.

M01377 Boum, R., J. L. Pousset, F. Lemonnier and M. Hadchouel. Action of extracts of *Carica papaya* on experimental jaundice induced in the rat by saponins extracted from *Brenani brieyi*. **Toxicol Appl Pharmacol** 1978; 46: 353.

M05080 Sharma, O. P., H. P. S. Makkar and R. K. Dawra. Effects of Lantana Toxicity of lysosomal and cytosol enzymes in guinea pig liver. **Toxicol Lett** 1983; 16(1/2): 41–45.

M05179 ANON. Final report of the safety assessment for avocado oil. **J Environ Pathol Toxicol** 1980; 4: 93–103.

M05253 Rukmini, C. and M. Vijayaraghavan. Nutritional and Toxicological evaluation of mango kernel oil. **J Amer Oil Chem Soc** 1984; 61(4): 789–792.

M05256 Premakumari, K. and P. A. Kurup. Lipid metabolism in rats fed rice and tapioca. **Indian J Med Res** 1982; 76: 488–493.

M05465 Mc Sweeney, C. S. and M. A. Pass. The role of the rumen in absorption of Lantana toxins in sheep. **Toxicon Suppl** 1983; 3: 285–288.

M06777 Bhatt, H. V., O. P. Gupta and P. S. Gupta. Hypoglycaemia induced by *Syzygium cumini* Linn. seeds in diabetes mellitus. **Asian Med J** 1983; 26(7): 489–491.

M07274 Plowman, T. The Ethnobotany of Coca (Erythroxylum spp., Erythroxylaceae). Advances in economic botany ethnobotany in the Neotropics G. T. Prance and J. A. Kallunki (Eds) New York Botanical garden, Bronx NY. 1984; 1: 62–111.

M09083 Takeda, N. and Y. Yasui. Identification of mutagenic substances in roselle color, elderberry color and safflower yellow. **Agr Biol Chem** 1985; 49(6): 1851,1852.

M09284 Onawunmi, G. O., W. A. Yisak and E. O. Ogunlana. Antibacterial constituents in the essential oil of *Cymbopogon citratus* (DC.) Stapf. **J Ethnopharmacol** 1984; 12(3): 279–286.

M10590 Van Beek, T. A. and R. Verpoorte. Phytochemical investigation of *Tabernaemontana undulata* **Fitoterapia** 1985; 56(5): 304–307.

M11890 Ng, T. B., C. M. Wong, W. W. Li, H. W. Yeung. Insulin-like molecules in *Momordica charantia* seeds. **J Ethnopharmacol** 1986; 15(1): 107–117.

M13661 Obidoa, O. and V. O. S. Ngodo. Effect of prolonged consumption of gari (cassava, *Manihot utilissima*) in rat hepatic energy metabolism. 1. Mitochondrial respiratory control. **Qual Plant Foods Hum Nutr** 1984; 34(3): 159–168.

M16717 Venkateswaran, P. S., I. Millman and B. S. Blumberg. Effects of an extract from *Phyllanthus niruri* on Hepatitis B and woodchuck Hepatitis viruses. In vitro and In vivo Studies. **Proc Nat Acad Sci** 1987; 84(1): 274–278.

M16948 Yamazaki, M., Y. Maebayashi, N. Iwase and T. Kaneko. Studies on pharmacologically active principles from Indonesian crude drugs. I. Principle prolonging pentobarbital-induced sleeping time from Curcuma xanthorrhiza Roxb. **Chem Pharm Bull** 1988; 36(6): 2070–2074.

M17007 Thyagarajan, S. P., K. Thiruneelakantan, S. Subramanian and T. Sundaravelu. In Vitro inactivation of HBSAg by *Eclipta alba* Hassk. and *Phyllanthus niruri* Linn. **Indian J Med Res Suppl** 1982; 76S: 124–130.

M17058   Seetharam, K. A. and J. S. Pasricha. Condiments and contact dermatitis of the finger tips. **Indian J Dermatol Venereol Leprol** 1987; 53(6): 325–328.

M17062   Venkateswaran, P. S., I. Millman and B. S. Blumberg. Composition, Pharmaceutical preparation and method for treating viral hepatitis. **Patent-US-4,673,575** 1987; 10 pp.

M17379   Abdu-Aguye, I., A. Sannusi, R. A. Alafiya-Tayo and S. R. Bhusnurmath. **Human Toxicol** 1986; 5(4): 269–274.

M17464   Umarani, D., T. Devaki, P. Govindaraju and K. R. Shanmugasundaram. Ethanol induced metabolic alterations and the effect of *Phyllanthus niruri* in their reversal. **Ancient Sci Life** 1985; 4(3): 174–180.

M17600   Mendes, N. M., N. M. Pereira, C. P. De Souza and M. L. Lima De Oliveira. Preliminary laboratory studies for the verification of molluscicidal activity of several species from the Brazilian Flora. **Rev Saude Publ Sao Paulo** 1984; 18: 348–354.

M17655   Karunanayake, E. H. and J. Welihinda. Oral hypoglycaemic medicinal plants of Sri Lanka. **Abstr Princess Congress I Bangkok Thailand** 1987; Abstr-BP-37.

M17736   De A Ribeiro, R., F. Barros, M. Margarida, R. F. Melo, C. Muniz, S. Chieia, M. G. Wanderley, C. Gomes and G. Trolin. Acute diuretic effects in conscious rats produced by some medicinal plants used in the state of Sap Paulo, Brasil. **J Ethnopharmacol** 1988; 24(1): 19–29.

M17781   Sharma, O. P., R. K. Dawra and H. P. S. Makkar. Isolation and partial purification of Lantana (Lantana camara L.) toxins. **Toxicol Lett** 1987; 37(2): 165–172.

M17807   Mascolo, N., G. Autore, F. Capasso, A. Menghini and M. P. Fasulo. **Phytother Res** 1987; 1(1): 28–31.

M17846   Rao, M. V. Antifertility effects of alcoholic seeds extract of *Abrus precatorius* Linn. in male albino rats. **Acta Eur Fertil** 1987; 18(3): 217–220.

M18213   Nisteswar, K and V. K. Murthy. Aphrodisiac effect of indigenous drugs - a myth or reality. **Probe** 1989; 28(2): 89–92.

M18291   Jain, A. K., K. Shimoi, Y. Nakamura, I. Tomita and T. Kada. Preliminary study on the desmutagenic and antimutgenic effect of some natural products. **Curr Sci** 1987; 56(24): 1266–1269.

M18378   Forestieri, A. M., F. C. Pizzimenti, M. T. Monforte and G. Bisignano. Antibacterial activity of some African Medicinal Plants. **Pharmacol Res Commun Suppl** 1988; 20(5): 33–36.

M18836   Kitisin, T. Pharmacological Studies. 3. *Phyllanthus niruri*. **Siriraj Hospital Gaz** 1952; 4: 641–649.

M18866   Ueno, H., S. Horie, Y. Nishi, H. Shogawa, M. Kawasaki, S. Suzuki et al. Chemical and pharmaceutical studies on medicinal plants in Paraguay. Geraniin, an Angiotensin-converting enzyme inhibitor from "Paraparai Mi," *Phyllanthus niruri*. **J Nat Prod** 1988; 51(2): 357–359.

M18896   Shinde, S., S. Phadke, and A. W. Bhagwat. Effect of Nagarmotha (*Cyperus rotundus* Linn.) on Reserpine-induced emesis in pigeons. **Indian J Physiol Pharmacol** 1988; 32(3): 229–230.

M18901   Hargis, A. M., E. Stauber, S. Casteel and D. Eitner. Avocado (*Persea americana*) intoxication in caged birds. **J Amer Vet Med Assoc** 1989; 194(1): 64–66.

M19413   Lutterodt, G. D. and A. Maleque. Effects on mice locomotor activity of a narcotic-like principle from *Psidium guajava* leaves. **J Ethnopharmacol** 1988; 24(2/3): 219–231.

M19431 Shalini, V. K. and L. Srinivas. Lipid peroxide induced DNA damage: production by turmeric (*Curcuma longa*). **Mol Cell Biochem** 1987; 77(1): 3–10.

M19490 Theoduloz, C., L. Franco, E. Ferro and G. Schmeda Hirschmann. Xanthine oxidase inhibitory activity on Paraguayan Myrtaceae. **J Ethnopharmacol** 1988; 24(2/3): 179–183.

M19731 Evans, D. A. and R. K. Raj. Extracts of Indian Plants as mosquito larvicides. **Indian J Med Res** 1988; 88(1): 38–41.

M19777 Itokawa, H. Research on the antineoplastic drugs from natural sources, especially from higher plants. **Yakugaku Zasshi** 1988; 108(9): 824–841.

M19921 Mahapatra, P. K., D. Chakraborty and A. K. N. Chaudhuri. Antiinflammatory and antipyretic activities of *Syzygium cumini*. **Planta Med** 1986; 6: 540–A.

M20030 Carbajal, D., A. Casaco, L. Arruzazabala, R. Gonzalez and Z. Tolon. Pharmacological study of *Cymbopogon citratus* leaves. **J Ethnopharmacol** 1989; 25(1): 103–107.

M20141 Ozaki, Y. and O. B. Liang. Cholagogic action of the essential oil obtained from *Curcuma xanthorrhiza* Roxb. **Shoyakugaku Zasshi** 1988; 42(4): 257–263.

M20390 Satyanarayana, K. and K. Sukumar. Phytosterilants to control the cotton bug, *Dysdercus cingulatus* F. **Curr Sci** 1988; 57(16): 918–919.

M20450 Han, B. H., Y. N. Han and M. H. Park. Chemical and biochemical studies on antioxidant components of ginseng. Advances in Chinese medicinal materials Research. **World Scientific Press Philadelphia, PA.** 1984; 485–498.

M20550 Das, P. C., A. Das, S. Mandal, C. N. Islam, M. K. Dutta, B. B. Patra, S. Sikdar and P. K. Chakrabartty. Antiinflammatory and antimicrobial activities of the seed kernel of *Mangifera indica*. **Fitoterapia** 1989; 60(3): 235–240.

M20684 Ozaki, Y. and S. Soedigdo. Cholagogic effect of Zingiber plants obtained from Indonesia. **Shayakugaku Zasshi** 1988; 42(4): 333–336.

M20685 Singh, P. P., P. Hada, I. Narula and S. K. Gupta. In Vivo effect okf tamarind (*Tamarindus indica* L.) on urolith inhibitory activity in urine. **Indian J Exp Biol**. 1988; 25(12): 863–865.

M20727 Yu, L. A. and Q. L. Xu. Treatment of infectious hepatitis with an herbal decoction. **Phytother Res** 1989; 3(3): 13,14.

M20737 Onawunmi, G. O. Evaluation of the antifungal activity of lemon grass oil. **Int J Crude Drug Res** 1989; 27(2): 121–126.

M20781 Sharma, O. P., R. K. Dawra, L. Krishna and H. P. S. Makkar. Toxicity of Lantana (Lantana camara L.) leaves and isolated toxins to rabbits. **Vet Hum Toxicol** 1988; 30(3): 214–218.

M20801 Natake, M., K. Kanazawa, M. Mizuno, N. Ueno, T. Kobayashi, G. I. Danno and S. Minamoto. Herb water-extracts markedly suppress the mutagenicity of TRP-P-2. **Agr Biol Chem** 1989; 53(5): 1423–1425.

M20821 Lutterodt, G. D. Inhibition of gastrointestinal release of acetylcholine by quercetin as a possible mode of action of *Psidium guajava* leaf extracts in the treatment of acute diarrhoeal disease. **J Ethnopharmacol** 1989; 25(3): 235–247.

M20879 Patel, V. K. and H. Venkatakrishna-Bhatt. Folklore therapeutic indigenous plants in periodontal disorders in India (Review, experimental and clinical approach). **Int J Clin Pharmacol TherToxicol** 1988; 26(4): 176–184.

M20895 Sakai, K., Y. Miyazaki, T. Yamane, Y. Saitoh, C. Ikwaw and T. Nishihata. Effect of extracts of Zingiberaceae herbs on gastric secretion in rabbits. **Chem Pharm Bull** 1989; 37(1): 215–217.

M21093 Elson, C. E., G. L. Underbakke, P. Hanson, E. Shrago, R. H. Wainberg and A. A. Qureshi. Impact of lemongrass oil, an essential oil, on serum cholesterol. **Lipids** 1989; 24(8): 677–679.

M21237 Dixit. V. P., P. Jain and S. C. Joshi. Hypolipidaemic effects of *Curcuma longa* L. and *Nardostachys jatamansi* DC. in triton-induced hyperlipidaemic rats. **Indian J Physiol Pharmacol** 1988; 32(4): 299–304.

M21299 Choi, Y. H., R. A. Hussain, J. M. Pezzuto, A. D. Kinghorn and J. F. Morton. Abrososides A-D, four novel sweet-tasting triterpene glycosides from the leaves of *Abrus precatorius*. **J Nat Prod** 1989; 52(5): 1118–1127.

M21373 Shimizu, M., S. Horie, S. Terashima, H. Ueno, T. Hayashi, M. Arisawa, S. Suzuki, M. Yoshizaki and N. Morita. Studies on Aldose Reductase inhibitors from natural products. II. Active components of a Paraguayan crude drug "Para-Parai Mi", *Phyllanthus niruri.* **Chem Pharm Bull** 1989; 37(9): 2531–2532.

M21409 Silva-Netto, C. R., R. A. Lopes and G. L. Pozetti. Changes in urinary volume and sodium and potassium excretion in rats submitted to Jambolao (*Syzygium jambolanum*) solution load. **Rev Fac Odont Ribeirao Preto** 1989; 23(2): 213–215.

M21411 Rai, M. K. and S. Upadhyay. Screening of medicinal plants of Chhindwara district against *Trichophyton mentagrophytes*: A casual organism of *Tinea pedis*. **Hindustan Antibiot Bull** 1988; 30(1/2): 33–36.

M21419 Choe, T. Y. Antibacterial activities of some herb drugs. **Korean J Pharmacog** 1986; 17(4): 302–307.

M21425 Mohsin, A., A. H. Shah, M. A. Al-Yahya, M. Tariq, M. O. M. Tanira and A. M. Ageel. Analgesic antipyretic activity and phytochemical screening of some plants used in traditional Arab system of medicine. **Fitoterapia** 1989; 60(2): 174–177.

M21482 Asthana, A., H. V. Mall, K. Dixit and S. Gupta. Fungitoxic properties of latex of plants with special reference to that of croton Bonplandianus baill. **Int J Crude Drugs Res** 1989; 27(1): 25–58.

M21802 Welihinda, J., G. Arvidson, E. Gylfe, B. Hellman and E. Karlsson. The insulin-releasing activity of the tropical plant *Momordica charantia*. **Acta Biol Med Germ** 1982; 41(12): 1229–1240.

M21947 Le Grand, A. Anti-infectious phytotherapy of the tree-savannah, Senegal (Western Africa) III: A review of the phytochemical substances and antimicrobial activity of 43 species. **J Ethnopharmacol** 1989; 25(3): 315–338.

M22015 Lei, Q. J., X. M. Jiang, A. C. Luo, Z. F. Liu, X. C. He, X. D. Wang, F. Y. Cui and P. I. Chen. Influence of balsam pear (the fruit of *Momordica charantia*) on blood sugar level. **Chung I Tsa Chih (Engl Ed)** 1985; 5(2): 99–106.

M22028 Akhtar, M. S., M. A. Athar and M. Yaqub. Effect of *Momordica charantia* on blood glucose level of normal and alloxan-diabetic rabbits. **Planta Med** 1981; 42(3): 205–212.

M22031 Aslam, M. and I. H. Stockley. Interaction between curry ingredient (karela) and drug (chlorpropamide). **Lancet** 1979; 607.

M22106 Iauk, L., E. M. Galati, A. M. Forestiri, S. Kirjavainen and A. Trovato. *Macuna pruriens* decoction lowers cholesterol and total lipid plasma levels in the rat. **Phytother Res** 1989; 3(6): 263–264.

M22131 Venkanna Babu, B., R. Moorti, S. Pugazhenthi, K. M. Prabhu and P. Suryanarayana Murthy. Alloxan recovered rabbits and animal model for screening for hypoglycaemic activity of compounds. **Indian J Biochem Biophys** 1988; 25(6): 714–718.

M22196 Occhiuto, F., C. Circosta and R. Costa De Pasquale. **J Ethnopharmacol** 1989; 26(2): 205–210.

M22285 Chen, C. P., C. C. Lin and T. Namba. Screening of Taiwanese crude drugs for antibacterial activity against *Streptococcus mutans*. **J Ethnopharmacol** 1989; 27(3): 285–295.

M22542 Shah, G. L. and G. V. Gopal. Ethnomedical notes from the tribal inhabitants of the North Gujarat (India). **J Econ Taxon Botany** 1985; 6(1): 193–201.

M22633 Webman, E. J., G. Edling and H. F. Mower. Free radical scavenging activity of papaya juice. **Int J Rad Biol** 1989; 55(3): 347–351.

M22670 Chandrasekar, B., B. Mukherjee and S. K. Mukherjee. Blood sugar lowering potentiality of selected Cucurbitaceae plants of Indian origin. **Indian J Med Res** 1989; 90(4): 300–305.

M22671 Singh, N., S. D. Tyagi and S. C. Agarwal. Effects of long term feeding of acetone extract of *Momordica charantia* (whole fruit powder) on alloxan diabetic albino rats. **Indian J Physiol Pharmacol** 1989; 33(2): 97–100.

M22673 Mossa, J. S. A study on the crude antidiabetic drugs used in Arabian folk medicine. **Int J Crude Drug Res** 1985; 23(3): 137–145.

M22721 Hukeri, V. I., G. A. Kalyani and H. K. Kakrani. Hypoglycemic activity of flavonoids of *Phyllanthus fraternus* in rats. **Fitoterapia** 1988; 59(1): 68–70.

M22728 Cooles, P. Diabetes and cassava in Dominica. **Trop Geograph Med** 1988; 40(3): 272–273.

M22746 De Mello, J. F. Plants in traditional medicine in Brazil. **J Ethnopharmacol** 1980; 2(1): 49–55.

M22780 Awuah, R. T. Fungitoxic effects of extracts from some West African plants. **Ann Appl Biol** 1989; 115(3): 451–453.

M22787 Ahn, B. Z. and J. H. Lee. Cytotoxic and cytotoxicity-potentiating effects of the curcuma root on L1210 cell. **Korean J Pharmacog** 1989; 20(4): 223–226.

M22818 Sambaiah, K. and K. Srinivasan. Influence of spices and spice principles on hepatic mixed function oxygenase system in rats. **Indian J Biochem Biophys** 1989; 26(4): 254–258.

M22823 De Messter, C., B. Rollmann, K. Mupenda and Y. Mary. The mutagenicity of cassava (*Manihot esculenta* Crantz) preparations. **Food Add Contam** 1990; 7(1): 125–136.

M22964 Quansah, N. Ethnomedicine in the Maroantsetra region of Madagascar. **Econ Bot** 1988; 42(3): 370–375.

M23039 Jakinovich Jr, W., C. Moon, Y. H. Choi and A. D. Kinghorn. Evaluation of plant extracts for sweetness using the Mongolian gerbil. **J Nat Prod** 1990; 53(1): 190–195.

M23109 Bailey, C. J., C. Day and B. A. Leatherdale. Traditional plant remedies for diabetes. **Diabetic Med** 1986; 3(2): 185,186.

M23149 Dennis, P. A. Herbal medicine among the Miskito of Eastern Nicaragua. **Econ Bot** 1988; 42(1): 16–28.

M23163 Akanji, A. O., I. Adeyefa, M. Charles-Davies and B. O. Osotimehin. Plasma glucose and thiocyanate responses to different mixed cassava meals in nondiabetic Nigerians. **Eur J Clin Nutr** 1990; 44(1): 71–77.

M23178 Srivastava, Y., H. Venkatakrishna-Bhatt and Y. Verma. Effect of

Momordica charantia Linn. Pomous aqueous extract on cataractogenesis in murrin alloxan diabetics. **Pharmacol Res Commun** 1988; 20(3): 201–209.

M23219   Reddy, M. B., K. R. Reddy and M. N. Reddy. A survey of medicinal plants of Chenchu Tribes of Andhra Pradesh, India. **Int J Crude Drugs Res** 1988; 26(4): 189–196.

M23272   Holdsworth, D., O. Gideon and B. Pilokos. Traditional medicine of New Ireland, Papau New Guinea part III Konos, Central New Ireland. **Int J Crude Drug Res** 1989; 27(1): 55–61.

M23340   Akhtar, M. S., Q. M. Khan and T. Khaliq. Effects of *Portulaca oleracae* (Kulfa) and *Taraxacum officinale* (Dhudhal) in normoglycaemic and alloxan-treated hyperglycaemic rabbits. **J Pak Med Assoc** 1985; 35: 207–210.

M23489   Chaudhuri, A. K. N., S. Pal, A. Gomes and S. Bhattacharya. Anti-inflammatory and related actions of *Syzygium cumini* seed extract. **Phytother Res** 1990; 4(1): 5–10.

M23497   Rafatullah, S., M. Tariq, M. A. Al-Yahya, J. S. Mossa and A. M. Ageel. Evaluation of turmeric (*Curcuma longa*) for gastric and duodenal antiulcer activity in rats. **J Ethnopharmacol** 1990; 29(1): 25–34.

M23556   Greassor, M., A. Y. Kedjagni, K. Koumaglo, C. DeSouza, K. Agbo, K. Aklikokou and K. A. Amegbo. In vitro antimalarial activity of six medicinal plants. **Phytother Res** 1990; 4(3): 115–117.

M23565   Bailey, C. J., C. Day, S. L. Turner and B. A. Leatherdale. Cerasee, a traditional treatment for diabetes. Studies in normal and streptozotocin diabetic mice. **Diabetes Res** 1985; 2: 81–84.

M23617   Comley, J. C. W. New Macrofilaricidal leads from plants. **Trop Med Parasitol** 1990; 41(1): 1–9.

M23643   Itokawa, H., F. Hirayama, S. Tsuruoka, K. Mizuno, K. Takeya and A. Nitta. Screening test for antitumor activity of crude drugs (III). Studies on antitumor activity of Indonesian Medicinal Plants. **Shoyakugaku Zasshi** 1990; 44(1): 58–62.

M23819   Msonthi, J. D. and D. Magombo. Medicinal herbs in Malawi and their uses. **Hamdard** 1983; 26(2): 94–100.

M23826   Jain, S. P. Tribal remedies from Saranda Forest, Bihar, India. 1. **Int J Crude Drug Res** 1989; 27(1): 29–32.

M23954   Teixeira, C. C., F. D. Fuchs, R. M. Blotta et al. Effect of tea prepared from leaves of *Syzygium jambos* on glucose tolerance in nondiabetic subjects. **Diabetes Care** 1990; 13(8): 907–908.

M24038   Le Grand, A. and P. A. Wondergem. Antiinfective phytotherapy of the savannah forests of Senegal (West Africa). 1. An inventory. **J Ethnopharmacol** 1987; 21(2): 109–125.

M24146   Alam, M. M., M. B. Siddiqui and W. Husain. Treatment of diabetes through herbal drugs in rural India. **Fitoterapia** 1990; 61(3): 240–242.

M24272   Guevara, A. P., C. Lin-Sylianco, F. Dayrit and P. Finch. Antimutagens from *Momordica charantia*. **Mutat Res** 1990; 230(2): 121–126.

M24428   Gasperi-Campani, A., L. Barbieri, M. G. Battelli nd F. Stirpe. On the distribution of ribosome-inactivating proteins amongst plants. **J Anat Prod** 1985; 48(3): 446–454.

M24523   Lemos, T. L. G., F. J. A. Matos, J. W. Alencar, A. A. Craveiro, A. M. Clark and J. D. Mc Chesney. Antimicrobial activity of essential oils of Brazilian plants. **Phytother Res** 1990; 4(2): 82–84.

M24764   Fourie, N., J. J. Van Der Lugt, S. J. Newsholme and P. W. Nel.

Acute Lantana camara toxicity in cattle. **J South African Vet Assoc** 1990; 58(4): 173–178.

M24831 Mehrotra, R., S. Rawat, D. K. Kulshreshtha, G. K. Patnaik and B. N. Dhawan. **Indian J Med Res [B]** 1990; 92(2): 133–138.

M24874 Triratana, T., P. Pariyakanok, R. Suwannuraks and W. Naengchomnog. The study of medicinal herbs on coagulatin mechanism. **J Dent Assoc Thailand** 1988; 38(1): 25–30.

M25016 Weenen, H., M. H. H. Nkunya, D. H. Bray, et al. Antimalarial compounds containing an α,β-unsaturated carbonyl moiety from Tanzanian medicinal plants. **Planta Med** 1990; 56(4): 368–370.

M25031 Day, C., T. Cartwright, J. Provost and C. J. Bailey. Hypoglycemic effect of *Momordica charantia* extracts. **Planta Med** 1990; 56(5): 426–429.

M25120 Akhter, M. H., M. Mathur and N. K. Bhide. Skin and liver toxicity in experimental Lantana camara poisoning in albino rats. **Indian J Physiol Pharmacol** 1990; 34(1): 13–16.

M25183 Werman, M. J., S. Mokady and I. Neeman. Partial isolation and characterization of a new natural inhibitor of Lysyl Oxidase from avocado seed oil. **J Agr Food Chem** 1990; 38(12): 2164–2168.

M25236 Suresh, M. and R. K. Rai. Cardol: The antifilarial principle from *Anacardium occidentale*. **Curr Sci** 1990; 59(9): 477–479.

M25250 Pasricha, J. S., P. Bhaumik and A. Agarwal. Contact dermatitis due to Xanthium strumarium. **Indian J Dermatol Venereol Leprol** 1990; 56(4): 319–321.

M25317 Kamesaki, T., T. Omi, E. Kajii and S. Ikemoto. New method of detecting the lectin activity of *Momordica charantia*. **Vox Sang** 1990; 58(4): 307,308.

M25326 Thamlikitkul, V., T. Dechatiwongse et al. Randomized controlled trial of *Cassia alata* Linn. for constipation. **J Med Assoc Thailand** 1990; 73(4): 217–221.

M25594 Lee, J. S. and J. W. Kim. Screening of biological activity of crude drugs using brine shrimp bioassay. **Korean J Pharmacog** 1990; 21(1): 100–102.

M25607 Cai, D. F., J. L. Wang, D. Z. Xun, X. J. Meng and J. Ma. Antiviral and interferon-inducing effect of kangli powder. **Chung Hsi I Chieh Ho Tas Chih** 1988; 8(12): 731–733.

M25712 Biswas, A. R., S. Ramaswamy and J. S. Bapna. Analgesic effect of *Momordica charantia* seed extract in mice and rats. **J Ethnopharmacol** 1991; 31(1): 115–118.

M25745 Dhir, H., A. K. Roy, A. Shama and G. Talukder. Protection afforded by aqueous extracts of Phyllanthus species against cytotoxicity induced by lead and aluminum salts. **Phytother Res** 1990: 4(5): 172–176.

M25765 Manyam, B. V. Paralysis agitans and Levodopa in Ayurveda: Ancient Indian Medical Treatise. **Movement Disorders** 1990; 5(1): 47,48.

M25836 Chattopadhyay, S. P. and P. K. Das. Evaluation of *Vinca rosea* for the treatment of warts. **Indian J Dermatol Venereol Leprol** 1990; 56(2): 107–108.

M25853 De Souza, C. P., M. L. Lima De Azevedo, J. L. C. Lopes, J. Sarti, D. D. Santos Filho et al. Chemoprophylaxis of schistosomiasis. Molluscicidal activity of natural products. **An Acad Brasil Cienc** 1984; 56(3): 333–338.

M25859 Johns, T., J. O. Kokwaro and E. K. Kimanani. Herbal remedies of the Luo of Siaya District, Kenya. Establishing quantitative criteria for consensus. **Econ Bot** 1990; 44(3): 369–381.

M25938 Saklani, A. and S. K. Jain. Ethnobotanical observations on plants used in Northeastern India. **Int J Crude Drug Res** 1989; 27(2): 65–73.

M25960 Deshpande, S. G., B. A. Nagasampagi and R. N. Sharma. Synergistic oviposition deterrence activity of extracts of *Glycosmis pentaphyllum* (Rutaceae) and other plants for *Phthorimaea operculella* (Zell) control. **Curr Sci** 1990; 59(19): 932–933.

M26052 Arora, R. B., T. Khanna, M. Imran and D. K. Balani. Effect of lipotab on myocardial infarction induced by isoproterenol. **Fitoterapia** 1990; 61(4): 356–358.

M26095 Elsheikh, S. H., A. K. Bashir, S. M. Suliman and M. E. Wassila. Toxicity of certain Sudanese plant extracts on Cercariae and Miracidia of *Schistosoma mansoni*. **Int J Crude Drug Res** 1990; 28(4): 241–245.

M26126 Abdel-Aziz, A., K. Brain and A. K. Bashir. Screening of Sudanese plants for molluscicidal activity and identification of leaves of Tacca leontopetaloides (L.) O Ktze (Tacaceae) as a potential new exploitable resources. **Phytother Res** 1990; 4(2): 62–65.

M26175 Kiuchi, F., M. Hioki, N. Nakamura, N. Miyashita, Y. Tsuda and K. Kondo. Screening of crude drugs used in Sri Lanka for nematocidal activity on the larva of *Toxacaria canis*. **Shoyakugaku Zasshi** 1989; 43(4): 288–293.

M26285 Moon, Y. N., M. H. Chung, H. K. Jhoo, D. Y. Lim and H. J. Yoo. Influence of Sopung-tang on the blood pressure response of the rat. **Korean J Pharmacog** 1990; 21(2): 173–178.

M26310 Ali, M. B., W. M. Salih, A. H. Mohamed and A. M. Homeida. Investigation of the antispasmodic potential of *Hibiscus sabdariffa* calyces. **J Ethnopharmacol** 1991; 31(2): 249–257.

M26503 Lozoya, X., G. Becerril and M. Martinez. Intraluminal perfusion model of in vitro guinea pig's ileum as a model of study of the antidiarrheic properties of the guava (*Psidium guajava*) **Arch Invest Med (Mex)** 1990; 21: 155–162.

M26592 Sato, A. Studies on anti-tumor activity of crude drugs. 1. The effects of aqueous extracts of some crude drugs in short-term screening test. **Yakugaku Zasshi** 1989; 109(6): 407–423.

M26843 Abatan, M. O. A note of the anti-inflammatory action of plants of some Cassia species. **Fitoterapia** 1990; 61(4): 336–338.

M26939 Shimomura, H., Y. Sashida and H. Nakata. Plant growth regulating activities of crude drugs and medicinal plants. **Shoyakugaku Zasshi** 1981; 35(3): 173–179.

M27078 Zhu, Z. L., Z. C. Zhong, Z. Y. Luo and Z. Y. Xiao. Studies on the active constituents of *Momordica charantia* L. **Yao Hsueh Hsueh Pao** 1990; 25(12): 898–903.

M27150 Grange, M. and R. W. Davey. Detection of antituberculous activity in plant extracts. **J Appl Bacteriol** 1990; 68(6): 587–591.

M27151 Caceres, A., B. R. Lopez, M. A. Giron and H. Logemann. Plants used in Guatemala for the treatment of Dermatophytic infections. I. Screeening for antimycotic activity of 44 plant extracts. **J Ethnopharmacol** 1991; 31(3): 263–276.

M27157 Werman, M. J., S. Mokady, M. E. Nimni and I. Neeman. The effect of various avocado oils on skin collagen metabolism. **Conn Tiss Res** 1991; 26(1/2): 1–10.

M27166 Nagaraju, N. and K. N. Rao. A survey of Plant crude drugs of Rayalaseema, Andhra Pradesh, India. **J Ethnopharmacol** 1990; 29(2): 137–158.

M27208 Miwa, M., Z. L. Kong, K. Shinohara and M. Watanabee. Macrophage stimulating activity of foods. **Agr Biol Chem** 1990; 54(7): 1863–1866.

M27219 Sato, A. Cancer Chemotherapy with Oriental Medicine. l. Antitumor activity of crude drugs with human tissue cultures in *In vitro* screening. **Int J Orient Med** 1990: 15(4): 171–183.

M27323 Kambu, K., L. Tona, S. Kaba, K. Cimanga and N. Mukala. Antispasmodic activity of extracts proceeding of plant antidiarrheic traditional preparations used in Kinshasa, Zaire. **Ann Pharm Fr** 1990; 48(4): 200–208.

M27351 Fuji, Y., T. Shibuya and T. Yasuda. L-3,4-Dihydroxyphenylalanine as an allelochemical candidate from *Macuna pruriens* (L.) DC. Var. Utilis. **Agr Biol Chem** 1991; 55(2): 617,618.

M27387 Masood, A.and K. S. Ranjan. The effect of aqueous plant extracts on growth and aflatoxin production by Aspergillus flavus. **Lett Appl Microbiol** 1991; 13(1): 32–34.

M27423 Al-Zaid, M. M., M. A. M. Hassan, N. Badir and K. A. Gumaa. Evaluation of blood glucose lowering activity of three plant diet additives. **Int J Pharmacog** 1991; 29(2): 81–88.

M27518 Swanston-Flatt, S. K., C. Day, P. R. Flatt, B. J. Gould and C. J. Bailey. Glycaemia effects of traditional European plant treatments for diabetes studies in normal and streptozotocin diabetic mice. **Diabetes Res** 1989; 10(2): 69–73.

M27524 Misra, P., N. L. Pal, P. Y. Guru, J. C. Katiyar and J. S. Tandon. Antimalarial activity of traditional plants against erythrocytic stages of *Plasmodium berghei*. **Int J Pharmacog** 1991; 29(1): 19–23.

M27532 Upadhyaya, G. L., A. Kumar and M. C. Pant. Effect of karela as hypoglycemic and cholesterolemic agent. **Jdai** 1983; 25(1): 12–15.

M27682 Palacinchamy, S., E. Amal Bhaskar and S. Nagarajan. Anti-

bacterial activity of *Cassia alata*. **Fitoterapia** 1991; 62(3): 249–252.

M27764 Kumazawa, N., S. Ohta, S. H. Tu, A. Kamogawa amd M. Shinoda. Protective effects of various methanol extracts of crude drugs on experimental hepatic injury induced by Alphanaphthylisothiocyanate in rats. **Yakugaku Zasshi** 1991; 11193): 199–204.

M27766 Han, G. Q., J. X. Pan, C. L. Li and F. Tu. The screening of Chinese traditional drugs by biological assay and the isolation of some active components. **Int J Chinese Med** 1991; 16(1): 1–17.

M27767 Hussain, H. S. N. and Y. Y. Deeni. Plants in Kano Ethnomedicine; screening for antimicrobial activity and alkaloids. **Int J Pharmacog** 1991; 29(1): 51–56.

M27825 Lorenzetti, B. B., G. E. P. Souza, S. J. Sarti, D. S. Filho and S. H. Ferreira. Myrcene mimics the peripheral analgesic activity of lemongrass tea. **J Ethnopharmacol** 1991; 34(1): 43–48.

M27829 Igea, J, M., J. Cuesta, M. Cuevas, L. M. Elias, C. Marcos, M. Lazaro and J. A. Comparied. Adverse reaction to pomegranate ingestion. **Allergy** 1991; 46(6): 472–474.

M28176 Kulkarni, R. R., P. S. Patki, V. P. Jog, S. G. Gandage and B. Patwardhan. Treatment of osteoarthritis with a herbomineral formulation: A double-blind, placebo-controlled, cross0over study. **J Ethnopharmacol** 1991; 33(1/2): 91–95.

M28186 Khanna, A. K., R. Chander and N. K. Kapoor. Hypolipidemic activity of Abana in rats. **Fitoterapia** 1991; 62(3): 271–274.

M28283 Elujoba, A. A., O. O. Ajulo and G. O. Iweibo. Chemical and biological analyses of Nigerian Cassia species for laxative activity.

J Pharm Biomed Anal 1989; 7(12): 1453–1457.

M28316   Ali, M. A., M. Mikage, F. Kiuchi, Y. Tsuda and K. Kondo. Screening of crude drugs used in Bangladesh for nematocidal activity on the larva of *Toxacara canis*. **Shoyakugaku Zasshi** 1991; 45(3): 206–214.

M28471   Caceres, A., O. Cabrera, O. Morales, P. Mollinedo and P. Mendia. Pharmacological properties of Moringa oleifera. 3. Effect of seed extracts in the treatment of experimental Pyodermia. **Fitoterapia** 1991; 62(5): 449–450.

M28491   Joshi, P. Herbal drugs used in Guinea worm disease by the Tribals of southern Rajasthan (India). **Int J Pharmacog** 1991; 29(1): 33–38.

M28758   Ganai, G. N. and G. J. Jha. Immunisuppression due to chronic Lantana camara, L. Toxicity in sheep. **Indian J Exp Biol** 1991; 29(8): 762–766.

M29106   Raja Reddy, K. Folk medicine from Chittoor district, Andhra Pradesh, India, used in the treatment of jaundice. **Int J Crude Res** 1988; 26(3): 127–140.

M29141   Miell, J., M. Papouchado and A. J. Marshall. Anaphylactic reaction after eating a mango. **Brit Med J** 1988; 297(6664): 1639–1640.

M29225   Vadavathy, S. and K. N. Rao. Antipyretic activity of six indigenous medicinal plants of Tirumala Hills, Andhra Pradesh, India. **J Ethnopharmacol** 1991; 33(1/2): 193–196.

M29299   Liu, Y. Pharmaceutical composition containing extracts of fruits and vegetables for treating and preventing diabetes. **Patent-US-4,985-248** 1991; 6 pp.

M29313   Zheng, Y. Z. and N. Zhang. Treatment of 305 cases of infantile diarrhea with kexieding capsule. **Fujian J Traditional Chinese Med** 1988; 19(3): 13,14.

M29342   Chang, I. M., I. C. Guest, J. Lee-Chang, N. W. Paik, and R. Y. Ryun. Assay of potential mutagenicity and antimutagenicity of Chinese herbal drugs by using SOS Chromotes (*E. coli* PQ37) and SOS UMU test (*S. typhimurium* TA1535/PSK 1002). **Proc First Korean-Japan Toxicology Symposium Safety Assessment of Chemicals In Vitro** 1989; 133–145.

M29360   Madulid, D. A., F. J. M. Gaerlan, E. M. Romero and E. M. G. Agoo. Ethnopharmacological study of the Ati tribe in Nagpana, Barotac Viejo, Iloilo. **Acta Manilana** 1989; 38(1): 25–40.

M29782   Kamalu, B. P. and J. C. Agharanya. The effect of a nutritionally-balanced cassava (*Manihot esculenta* Crantz) diet on endocrine function using the dog as a model 2. thyroid. **Brit J Nitr** 1991; 65(3): 373–379.

M29790   Kamalu, B. P. The effect of a Nutritional-balanced cassava (*Manihot esculenta* Crantz) diet on endocrine function using the dog as a model 1. Pancreas. **Brit J Nitr** 1991; 65(3): 365–372.

M29843   Carbajal, D., A. Casaco, L. Arruzazabala, R. Gonzalez and V. Fuentes. Pharmacological screening of plant decoctions commonly used in Cuban folk medicine. **J Ethnopharmacol** 1991; 33(1/2): 21–24.

M29965   Kiuchi, F., N. Nakamura, N. Miyashita, S. Nishizawa, Y. Tsuda and K. Kondo. Nematocidal activity of some anthelmintics, traditional medicines, and spices by a new assay method using larvae of *Toxacara canis*. **Shoyakugaku Zasshi** 1989; 43(4): 279–287.

M29966   Naovi, S. A. H., M. S. Y. Khan and S. B. Vohora. Anti-bacterial, antifungal and anthelmintic investigations on Indian medicinal plants. **Fitoterapia** 1991; 62(3): 221–228.

M29993 Nwodo, O. F. C. and E. O. Alumanah. Studies on *Abrus precatorius* seeds. II. Antidiarrhoeal activity. **J Ethnopharmacol** 1991; 31(3): 395–398.

M30038 Caceres, A. and S. Lopez. Pharmacological properties of *Moringa oleifera*. 3. Effect of seed extracts in the treatment of experimental pyodermia. **Fitoterapia** 1991; 62(5): 449,450.

M30046 Lam, L. K. T. and B. L. Zheng. Effects of essential oils on Glutathione S-Transferase activity in mice. **J Agr Food Chem** 1991; 39(4): 660–662.

M30100 Azuine, M. A. and S. V. Bhide. Chemopreventive effect of turmeric against stomach and skin tumors induced by chemical carcinogenesis in Swiss mice. **Nutr Cancer** 1992; 17(1): 77–83.

M30208 Kobayashi, N. Pharmaceutical compositions containing lemongrass extracts and antioxidants. **Patent - Japan Kokai Tokkyo Koho-01 221,320** : 2 pp. 1989.

M30257 Unander, D. W. and B. S. Blumberg. In Vitro activity of Phyllanthus (Euphorbiaceae) species against the DNA polymerase of Hepatitis viruses. Effects of growing environment and Inter- and intra-specific differences. **Econ Bot** 1991; 45(2): 225–242.

M30497 Ali, M. B., A. H. Mohamed, W. M. Salih and A. H. homeida. Effect of an aqueous extract of *Hibiscus sabdariffa* calyces in the gastrointestinal tract. **Fitoterapia** 1991; 62(6): 475–479.

M30756 Ogunti, E. O., A. J. Aladesanmi and S. A. Adesanya. Antimicrobial activity of *Cassia alata*. **Fitoterapia** 1991; 62(2): 537–539.

M30769 Liu, D. X., X. J. Yin, H. C. Wang, Y. Zhou and Y. H. Zhang. Antimutagenicity screening of water extracts from 102 kinds of Chinese medicinal herbs. **Chung-Kuo Chung Yao Tsa Chi Li** 1990; 15(10): 617–622.

M30962 Palanichamy, S. and S. Nagarajan. Antiinflammatory activity of *Cassia alata* leaf extract and kaempferol 3-0-sophoroside. **Fitoterapia** 1990; 61(1): 44–47.

M30985 Akintonwa, A. and O. L. Tunwashe. Fatal cyanide poisoning from cassava-based meal. **Human Exp Toxicol** 1992; 11(1): 47–49.

M31053 Chauhan, J. S., N. K. Singh and S. V. Singh. Screening of higher plants for specific herbicidal principle active against dodder, Cuscuta reflexa Roxb. **Indian J Exp Biol** 1989; 27(10): 877–884.

M31056 Arias, R. J., G. Schmeda-Hirschmann and A. Falcao. Feeding deterrency and insecticidal effects of plant extracts on *Lutzomyia longipalpis*. **Phytother Res** 1992; 6(2): 64–67.

M31067 Zia-Ul-Haque, A., M. H. Qazi and M. E. Hamdard. Studies on the antifertility properties of active components isolated from the seeds of *Abrus precatorius* Linn. 1. **Pakistan J Zool** 1983; 15(2): 129–139.

M31104 Qureshi, S., A. H. Shah and A. M. Ageel. Toxicity studies on *Alpinia galanga* and *Curcuma longa*. **Planta Med** 1992; 58(2): 124–127.

M31296 Caceres, A., E. Jauregu, D. Herrera and H. Logemann. Plants used in Guatemala for the treatment of dermatomucosal infections. 1. Screening of 38 plant extracts for anticandidal activity. **J Ethnopharmacol** 1991; 33(3): 277–283.

M31549 Hakizamungu, E., L. Van Puyvelde and M. Wery. Screening of Rwandese medicinal plants for anti-trichomonas activity. **J Ethnopharmacol** 1992; 36(2): 143–146.

N00137 Shankar, T. N. and V. S. Murthy. Effect of turmeric (*Curcuma longa*) on the growth of some intestinal bacteria In Vitro. **J Food Sci Technol** 1978; 15: 152.

N00138   Dhar, S. K., S. Gupta and N. Chandhoke. Antifertility studies of some indigenous plants. **Proc XI Ann Conf Indian Pharmacol Soc, New Delhi**. 1978.

N00186   Garg, S. K., V. S. Mathur and R. R. Chaudhury. Screening of Indian plants for antifertility activity. **Indian J Exp Biol** 1978; 16: 1077–1079.

N03109   Gomez, G. A. and J. E. Sokal. Use of vinblastine in the terminal phase of chronic myelocytic leukemia. **Cancer Treat Rep** 1979; 63: 1385–1387.

N11092   Locksley, H. D., M. B. E. Fayez, A. S. Radwan, V. M. Chari, G. A. Cordell and H. Wagner. Constituents of local plants. XXV. Constituents of the antispasmodic principle of *Cymbopogon proximus*. **Planta Med** 1982; 45: 20–22.

N13077   ANON. Avocado pear-MAO inhibitor interaction. **Pharm Int** 1982; 3(4): 122.

N14164   Bansal, R., N. Ahmad and J. R. Kidwai. Effect of oral administration of *Eugenia jambolana* seeds & chloropropamide on blood glucose level & pancreatic cathepsin B in rats. **Indian J Biochem Biophys** 1981; 18: 377.

N15216   Maduagwu, E. N. adn I. B. Umoh. Detoxification of cassava leaves by simple traditional methods. **Toxicol Lett** 1982; 10: 245–248.

N19357   Adolf, W., H. J. Operferkuch and E. Hecker. Irritant Phorbol derivatives from four *Jatropha* species. **Phytochemistry** 1984; 23(1): 129–132.

N19806   Kiso, Y., Y. Suzuki, N. Watanabe, Y. Oshima and H. Hikino. Antihepatotoxic principles of *Curcuma longa* rhizomes. **Planta Med** 1983; 49(3): 185–187.

P00001   Tuntivanich, U., S. Tiwakornpunnarai and C. Dejsupa. Studies of insecticidal activity of organic compounds in *Momordica charantia*

Linn. **Sci Thailand** 1981; 38(3): 750–754.

P00004   Avirutnant, W. and A. Pongpan. The antimicrobial activity of some Thai flowers and plants. **Mahidol Univ J Pharm Sci** 1983; 10(3): 81–86.

P00035   Laohathai, P. and C. Ratanasangwan. Antifungal activity of Thai medicinal plants. **Undergraduate special project report** 1975.

P00044   Avirutnant, W. and A. Pongpan. The antimicrobial activity of some Thai flowers and plants. **Mahidol Univ J Pharm Sci** 1983; 10(3): 81–86.

P00047   Chaiyasothi, T. and V. Rueaksopaa. Antibacterial activity of some medicinal plants. **Undergraduate Special Project Report.** Fac Pharm Mahidol Univ Bangkok 1975; 109 pp.

P00050   Praphapraditchote, K., C. Nookhwan and R. Mekmanee. Hypoglycemic effect of *Momordica charantia* in rabbits. **Abstr 6th Congress of the Pharmacological and Therapeutic Society of Thailand** 1984; 75.

P00083   Achararit, C., W. Panyayong and E. Ruchatakomut. Inhibitory action of some Thai herbs to fungi. **Undergraduate special project report** 1983.

P00089   Soytong, K., V. Rakvidhvasastra and T. Sommartya. Effect of some medicinal plants on growth of fungi and potential in plant disease control. **Abstr 11th Conference of Science and Technology, Bangkok, Thailand** October 24–26, 1985; 361

P00093   Maneelrt, S. and A. Satthampongsa. Antimicrobial activity of *Momordica charantia*. **Undergraduate special project report** 1978; 18 pp.

P00096   Praphaditchote, K. Hypoglycemic effect of *Momordica charantia* Linn. in rabbits. **Master Thesis** 1984; 59 pp.

P00098   Anon. Verasing Mungmum (1982). The use of medicinal herbs for the treatment of kidney stone in the urinary system. **Abstr Seminar on the Development of Drugs from Medicinal Plants, Bangkok, Thailand** 1982; 117.

P00117   Limserimanee, S. and S. Siriratana. Inhibitory actions of some Thai herbs (medicinal plants) to fungi. **Undergraduate special project report** 1983.

P00126   Sankawa, U. Modulators of Arachidonate cascade contained in medicinal plants used in traditional medicine. **Abstr 3rd Congress of the Federation of Asian Oceanian Biochemists**, Bangkok, Thailand 1983; 28.

P00142   Apisariyakul, A. and V. Anantasarn. A Pharmacological study of the Thai medicinal plants used as cathartics and antispasmodics. **Abstr 10th Conference of Science and Technology Thailand Chiengmai Univ Chiengmai Thailand** 1984; 452,453.

R00001   Mokkhasmit, M., K. Swasdimongkol and P. Satrawaha. Study on toxicity of Thai Medicinal Plants. **Bull Dept Med Sci** 1971; 12(2/4): 36–65.

R00050   Kesorn, C. and C. Pawitarapok. Study on medicinal plants used for laxative and antidysentery. **J Assoc Military Surg** 1973; 19(1): 7–16.

T00001   Bhatnagar, S. S., H. Santapau, J. D. H. Desa et al. Biological activity of Indian Medicinal Plants. Part 1. Antibacterial, antitubercular, and antifungal action. **Indian J Med Res** 1961; 49: 799.

T00048   Prakash, V., K. C. Singhal and R. R. Gupta. Anthelmintic activity of *Punica granatum* and *Artemisia siversiana*. **Indian J Pharmacol** 1980; 12: 61A.

T00213   Gopalakrishnan, M. and M. R. Rajasekharasetty. Effect of papaya (*Carica papaya*) on pregnancy and estrous cycle in albino rats of wistar strain. **Indian J Physiol Pharmacol** 1978; 22: 66–70.

T00216   Singh, S. and S. Devi. Teratogenic and embryonic effect of papain in rats. **Indian J Med Res** 1978; 67: 499.

T00295   Chang, C. F., A. Isogai, T. Kamikado, S. Murakoshi, A. Sakurai and S. Tamura. Isolation and structure elucidation of growth inhibitors for silk-worm larvae from avocado leaves. **Agr Biol Chem** 1975; 39: 1167–1168.

T00325   Yun, H. S. and I. M. Chang. Plants with liver protective activities (1). **Korean J Pharmacog** 1977; 8: 125–129.

T00337   Czajka, P., D. Pharm, J. Field, P. Novak and J. Kunnecke. Accidental aphrodisiac ingestion. **J Tenn Med Assoc** 1978; 71: 747.

T00359   Halberstein, R. A. and A. B. Saunders. Traditional medical practices and medicinal plant usage on a Bahamian Island. **Cul Med Psychiat** 1978; 2: 177–203.

T00368   Adam, S. E. I. Toxicity of Indigenous plants and agricultural chemicals in farm animals. **Clin Toxicol** 1978; 13: 269–280.

T00398   Shum, L. K. W., V. E. C. Coi and H. W. Yeung. Effects of *Momordica charantia* seed extract on the rat mid-term placenta. **Abstr International symposium on Chinese Medicinal materials Research Hong Kong** 1984; Abstr-78.

T00435   Nauriyal, M. M. and I. Gupta. Some pharmacological actions of Lantana camara leaves. **Indian J Anim Sci** 1977; 47: 844.

T00440   ANON. Studies on the toxic effects of certain burn escharotic herbs. **Chung-Hua I Hsueh Tsa Chih** (New series) 1978; 4: 388.

T00509   Barrois, V. and N. R. Farnsworth. The value of plants indicated by traditional medicine in cancer therapy. **WHO, Geneva** Nov. 13–17, 1978.

T00511   El-Merzabani, M. M., A. A. El-
           Aaser, A. K. El-Duweini and A.
           M. El-Masry. A Bioassay of anti-
           mitotic alkaloids of *Catharanthus
           roseus*. **Planta Med** 1979; 36:
           87–90.

T00514   El-Merzabani, M. M., A. A. El-
           Aaser, M. A. Attia, A. K. El-
           duweini and A. M. Ghazal.
           Screening system for Egyptian
           plants with potential anti-tumor
           activity. **Planta Med** 1979; 36:
           150–155.

T00549   Bannerjee, A., and S. S. Nigam.
           In Vitro anthelmintic activity of
           the essential oils derived from
           the various species of the genus
           Curcuma Linn. **Sci Cult** 1978;
           44: 503,504.

T00687   Salah Ahmed, M., G. Honda and
           W. Miki. Herb drugs and herbal-
           ists in the Middle East. Institute
           for the study of languages and
           cultures of Asia and Africa.
           Studia Culturae Islamicae No. 8,
           1979; 1–208.

T00693   Weenen, H., M. H. H. Nkunya, D.
           H. Bray, L. B. Mwasumbi, L. S.
           Kinabo and V. A. E. B. Kilimali.
           Antimalarial activity of Tanza-
           nian medicinal plants. **Planta
           Med** 1990; 56(4): 368–370.

T00701   Ayensu, E. S. Medicinal plants
           of the West Indies. **Unpublished
           Manuscript** 1978; 110 pp.

T00706   Devi, S. and S. Singh. Changes
           in placenta of rat fetuses induced
           by maternal administration of
           papain. **Indian J Exp Biol** 1978;
           16: 1256–1260.

T00768   Chauhan, S., S. Agrawal, R.
           Mathur and R. K. Gupta. Phos-
           phatase activity in testis adn pros-
           tate of rats treated with embelin
           and *Vinca rosea* extract. **Experi-
           enta** 1979; 35: 1183–1185.

T00794   Koelz, W. N. Notes on the Eth-
           nobotany of Lahul, a province of
           the Punjab. **Q J Crude Res**
           1979; 17: 1–56.

T00850   Prakash, A. O. Glycogen con-
           tents in the rat uterus. Response

           to *Hibiscus rosa-sinensis* ex-
           tracts. **Experientia** 1979; 35:
           1122,1123.

T00888   Kholkute, S. D. and K. N. Udupa.
           Antiestrogenic activity of *Hibis-
           cus rosa-sinensis* flowers. **Indian
           J Exp Biol** 1976; 14: 175,176.

T01112   Rao, V. S. N., P. Dasaradhan and
           K. S. Krishnaiah. Antifertility
           effect of some indigenous plants.
           Indian J Med Res 1979; 70:
           517–520.

T01199   Woo, W. S., K. H. Shin, I. C.
           Kim and C. K. Lee. A survey of
           the reponse of Korean medicinal
           plants on drug metabolism. **Arch
           Pharm Res** 1978; 1: 13–19.

T01280   Olusi, S. O., O. L. Oke and A.
           Odusote. Effects of cyanogenic
           agents on reproduction and neo-
           natal development in rats. **Biol
           Neonate** 1979; 36: 233–243.

T01287   Gupta, M. P., T. D. Arias, M.
           Correa and S. S. Lamba.
           Ethnopharmacognostic observa-
           tions on Panamanian medicinal
           plants. Part 1. **Q J Crude Drug
           Res** 1979; 17(3/4): 115–130.

T01313   Virmani, O. P., G. N. Srivastava
           and P. Singh. *Catharanthus
           roseus* - The tropical periwinkle.
           Indian Drugs 1978; 15: 231-252.

T01348   Asthana, R. B. and M. K. Misra.
           Orally effective hypoglycemic
           agent from *Vinca rosea*. **Indian J
           Biochem Biophys** 1979; 16: 30.

T01351   Gopakumar, B., B. Ambika and
           V. K. K. Prabhu. Juvenomimetic
           activity in some south Indian
           plants and the probable cause of
           this activity in *Morus alba*.
           Entomol 1977; 2: 259–261.

T01420   Tang, C. S. Macrocyclic piperi-
           dine nad piperideine alkaloids in
           Carica papaya. **Trop Foods
           Chem Nutr** 1979; 1: 55–68.

T01545   Avadhoot, Y. and K. C. Varma.
           Antimicrobial activity of essen-
           tial oil of seeds of Lantana
           camara var. aculeata Linn. **In-
           dian Drugs Pharm Ind** 1978;
           13: 41,42.

T01570   Prakash, A. O. Acid and Alkaline Phosphatase activity in the uterus of rat treated with *Hibiscus rosa-sinensis* Linn. extracts. **Curr Sci** 1979; 48: 501–503.

T01575   Takemoto, D. J., R. Kresie and D. Vaughn. Partial purification and characterization of a guanylate cyclase inhibition with cytotoxic properties from the bitter melon (*Momordica charantia*). **Biochem Biophys Res Commun** 1980; 94: 332–339.

T01640   Prakash, G. Senescence factor and foliar abscission in *Catharanthus roseus*. **Indian J Plant Physiol** 1979; 22: 24–29.

T01650   Misawa, M. Production of natural substances by plant cell cultures described in japanese patents. **Plant Tissue Culture its Bio-Technol Appl Int Cong 1976** 1977; 17–26.

T01655   Issar, R. K. and A. H. Israili. Pharmacognostic studies of the Unani drug "Ghongchi-Safaid" (*Abrus precatorius* Linn. seeds). **J Res Indian Med Yoga Homeopathy** 1978; 13: 34–44.

T01679   Nwude, N. and O. O. Ebong. Some plants used in the treatment of leprosy in Africa. **Leprosy Rev** 1980; 51: 11–18.

T01692   Bhargava, N. C. and O. P. Singh. Fortege, and indigenous drug in common sexual disorders in males. **Mediscope** 1978; 21(6): 140–144.

T01694   Billore, K. V. and K. C. Audichya. Some oral contraceptives—family planning tribal way. **J Res Indian Med Yoga Homeopathy** 1978; 13: 104–109.

T01696   Eshiett, N. O., A. A. Ademosun and T. A. Omole. Effect of feeding cassava root meal on reproduction and growth of rabbits. **J Nutr** 1980; 110: 697–702.

T01727   Chow, S. Y., S. M. Chen and C. M. Yang. Pharmacological studies on Chinese herb medicine. lll. Analgesic effect of 27 Chinese herb medicine. **J Formosa Med Assoc** 1979; 75: 349–357.

T01728   Singh, M. P., S. B. Malla, S. B. Rajbhandari and A. Manandhar. Medicinal plants of Nepal—retrospects and prospects. **Econ Bot** 1979; 33(2): 185–198.

T01745   Farnsworth, N. R. and C. J. Kaas. An approach utilizing information from traditional medicine to identify tumor-inhibiting plants. **J Ethnopharmacol** 1981; 3(1): 85–99.

T01769   Gasperi-Campani, A., L. Barbieri, P. Morelli and F. Stirpe. Seed extracts inhibiting protein synthesis in vitro. **Biochem J** 1980; 186: 439–441.

T01782   Kholkute, S. D. and K. N. Udupa. Biological profile of total benzene extract of *Hibiscus rosa-sinensis* flowers. **J Res Indian Med Yoga Homeopathy** 1978; 13(3): 107–109.

T01802   Singh, N. and R. Nath, A. K. Agarwal and R. P. Kohli. A Pharmacological investigation of some indigenous drugs of plant origin for evaluation of their antipyretic, analgesic and anti-inflammatory activities. **J Res Indian Med Yoga Homeopathy** 1978; 13: 58–62.

T01868   Wilson, R. T. amd W. G. Mariam. Medicine and magic in Central Tigre: A contribution to the ethnobotany of the Ethiopian plateau. **Econ Bot** 1979; 33: 29–34.

T01925   Lal, S. D. and K. Lata. plants used by the Bhat community for regulating fertility. **Econ Bot** 1980; 34: 273–275.

T02040   Gangrade, H., S. H. Mishra and R. Kaushal. Antimicrobial activity of the oil and unsaponifiable matter of red roselle. **Indian Drugs** 1979; 16: 147–148.

T02106   Oliver-Bever, B. Oral hypoglycaemic plants in West Africa. **J Ethnopharmacol** 1980; 2(2): 119–127.

T02110   Anton, R. and M. Haag-Berrurier. Therapeutic use of Natural Anthraquinone for other than laxative actions. **Pharmacology Suppl** 1980; 20: 104–112.

T02114   Das, P. C. Oral contraceptive (Long-acting). **Patent-Brit-1445599** 1976; 11pp.

T02146   Sussman, L. K. Herbal Medicine on Mauritius. **J Ethnopharmacol** 1980; 2(3): 259–278.

T02196   Cantoria, M. Aromatic and Medicinal Herbs of the Philippines. **Q J Crude Drug Res** 1979; 14: 97–128.

T02211   Tyagi, R. K., M. K. Tyagi, H. R. Goyal and K. Sharma. A Clinical study of Krimi Roga. **J Res Indian Med Yoga Homeopathy** 1978; 13: 130–132.

T02279   Wang, D. X. Treatment of generalized scleoderma with combined traditional Chinese and Western medicine. **Chung-Hua l Hsueh Tsa Chih (Engl Ed)** 1979; 92: 427–430.

T02367   Vaidya, R. A., A. R. Sheth, S. D. Aloorkar, N. R. Rege, V. N. Bagadia, P. K. Devi adn L. P. Shah. The inhibitory effect of the Cowage plant *Macuna pruriens* and L-DOPA on chlorpromazine-induced hyperprolactinemia in man. **Neurology (India)** 1978; 26: 177,178.

T02368   Vaidya, R. A., S. D. Aloorkar, A. R. Sheth and S. K. Pandya. Activity of Bromoergocryptine, *Macuna pruriens* and L-DOPA in the control of hyperprolactinemia. **Neurology (India)** 1978; 26: 179–182.

T02434   Babbar, O. P., B. L. Chowdhury, M. P. Singh, et al. Nature of antiviral activity detected in some plant extracts screened in cell cultures infected with vaccina and Ranikhet disease virus. **Indian J Exp Biol** 1970; 8: 304.

T02439   Atal, C. K., U. Zutshi and N. Chandhoke. Role of Trikatu-three acrids of Ayurveda, in the enhancement of drug bioavailability. **Indian J Pharmacol** 1980; 12: 60A.

T02456   Bhavani Shankar, T. N., N. V. Shantha, H. P. Ramesh, I. A. S. Murthy and V. S. Murthy. Toxicity studies in turmeric (*Curcuma longa*). Acute toxicity studies in rats, guinea pigs and monkeys. **Indian J Exp Biol** 1979; 18: 73–75.

T02459   Chang, I. M. and H. S. Yun. Liver-protective activities of *Plantago asiatica* seeds. **Planta Med** 1980; 39: 246A.

T02487   Koelz, W. N. Notes on the Ethnobotany of Lahul, A province of the Punjab. **Q J Crude Drug Res** 1979; 17: 1–56.

T02554   De Oliviera, M. M., M. Santos, and A. C. Coni. Analgesic activity of dimeric proanthocyanidins —preliminary experiments. **ARQ Inst Biol Sao Paulo** 1975; 42: 145–150.

T02572   Kumar, A., G. D. Tiwari and N. D. Pandey. Studies on the antifeeding and insecticidal properties of bitter gourd (*Momordica charantia* L.) against mustard sawfly *Athalia proxima* Klug. **Pestology** 1979; 3(5): 23–25.

T02632   Matthes, H. W. D., B. Luu and G. Ourisson. Chemistry and biochemistry of Chinese drugs. Part VI. Cytotoxic components of *Zingiber zerumbet, Curcuma zedoaria* and *C. domestica*. **Phytochemistry** 1980; 19: 2643–2650.

T02635   Krishnamurthy, V. No easy way to new pill. **Indian Express**, September 17, 1980.

T02650   Prakash, A. O. Protein concentration in rat uterus under the influence of *Hibiscus rosa-sinensis* Linn. ectracts. **Proc Indian Acad Sci Ser** 1979; B 45: 327–331.

T02666   Anon. Antifertility studies on plants. **Annual Report of the Director General - Indian Council of Medical Research** 1979; 71,72.

T02678   Dhawan, B. N., M. P. Dubey, B. N. Mehrotra, R. P. Rastogi and J. S. Tandon. Screening of Indian plants for biological activity. Part IX. **Indian J Exp Biol** 1980; 18: 594–606.

T02688   Das, R. P. Effect of papaya seed on the genital organs and fertility of male rats. **Indian J Exp Biol** 1980; 18: 408–409.

T02699   Holdsworth, D. K., C. L. Hurley and S. E. Rayner. Traditional medicinal plants of New Ireland, Papua New Guinea. **Q J Crude Drug Res** 1980; 18(3): 131–139.

T02717   Eilert, U., S. B. Wolter and A. Nahrstedt. The antibiotic principle of seeds of *Moringa oleifera* and *Moringa stenopetala*. **Planta Med** 1981; 42: 55–61.

T02774   Padmawinata, K. and E. Hoyaranda. The effect of juice of *Averrhoa carambola* fruits and the aqueous extract of *Persea americana* leaves on rat blood pressure. **Abstr 4th Asian Symp Med Plants Spices Bangkok, Thailand**. Sept. 15–19, 1980.

T02963   Benjamin, T. V. Analysis of the volatile constituents of local plants used for skin disease. **J Afr Med Pl**. 1980; 3: 135–139.

T02985   Bhavani Shankar, T. N. and V. S. Murthy. Effect of turmeric (*Curcuma longa*) fractions on the growth of some intestinal and pathogenic bacteria *In vitro*. **Indian J Exp Biol** 1979; 17: 1363–1366.

T02988   Gonzalez, J. Medicinal plants in Colombia. **J Ethnopharmacol** 1980; 2(1): 43–47.

T03008   Sharma, O. P., H. P. Makkar, R. N. Pal and S. S. Negi. Lantadene a content and toxicity of the Lantana plant (*Lantana camara* Linn.) to guinea pigs. **Toxicon** 1980; 18: 485–488.

T03054   Chan Jr, H. T. and C. S. Tang. The Chemistry and biochemistry of papaya. **Trop Foods: Chem Nutr (Proc Int Conf)** 1979; 1979: 33–53.

T03084   Vijayalaxmi. Genetic effects of turmeric and curcumin in mice and rats. **Mutat Res** 1980; 79: 125–132.

T03102   Rao, M. R. R. and S. R. Parakh. Effect of some indigenous drugs on the sexual behavior of male rats. **Indian J Pharm Sci** 1978; 40: 236E.

T03107   Adewunmi, C. O. and V. O. Marquis. Molluscicidal Evaluation ofsome Jatropha species grown in Nigeria. **Q J Crude Drugs Res** 1980; 18: 141–145.

T03115   Jain, J. P., L. S. Bhatnager and M. R. Parsai. Clinical trials of haridra (*Curcuma longa*) in cases of Tamak Swasa & Kasa. **J Res Indian Med Yoga Homeopathy** 1979; 14(2): 110–119.

T03162   El-Sayed, A. and G. A. Cordell. Catharanthus alkaloids. XXXIV. Catharanthamine, a new antitumor bisindole alkaloid from *Catharanthus roseus*. **J Nat Prod** 1981; 44: 289–293.

T03252   Pardanani, D. S., R. J. Delima, R. V. Rao, A. Y. Vaze, P. G. Jayatilak and A. R. Sheth. Study of the effects of Speman on semen quality in oligospermic men. **Indian J Surg** 1976; 38: 34–39.

T03316   Adu-Tutu, M., Y. Afful, K. Asante-Appiah, D. Lieberman, J. B. Hall and M. Elvin-Lewis. Chewing stick usage in Southern Ghana. **Econ Bot** 1979; 33: 320–328.

T03367   Rizvi, S. J. H., D. Mukerji and S. N. Mathur. A new report of some possible source of natural herbicide. **Indian J Exp Biol** 1980; 18: 777–781.

T03389   Khan, M. R., G. Ndaalio, M. H. Nkunya, H. Wevers and A. N. Sawhney. Studies on African Medicinal Plant Part 1. Preliminary screening of medicinal plants for antibacterial actiivty. **Planta Med Suppl** 1980; 40: 91–97.

T03533   Kokate, C. K., H. P. Tipnis, L. X. Gonsalves and J. L. D'Cruz. Anti-insect and juvenile hormone mimicking activities of essential oils if *Adhatoda vasica, Piper longum* and *Cyperus rotundus*. (Abstract). **Abstr 4th Asian Symp Med Plants Spices**, Bangkok, Thailand, 1980; 154.

T03535   Komai, K. and K. Ueki. Plant growth inhibitors in Purple Nutsedge (*Cyperus rotundus* L.). **Zasso Kenkyu** 1980; 25(1): 42-47.

T03554   Shankara, M. R., N. S. N. Murthy and L. N. Shastry. Method of manufacture and clinical efficacy of ramsamanikya mishrana in tamaka shwasa (bronchial asthma). **Indian J Pharm Sci** 1979; 41: 267B.

T03555   Meksongsee, L., Y. Jiamchaisri, P. Sinchaisri and L. Kasamsuksakan. Effects of some Thai medicinal plants and spices on the alkylating activity of ethyl methane sulfonate. **Abstr 4th Asian Sym Med Plants Spices Bangkok, Thailand Sept. 15-19, 1980** 1980; 1980: 118.

T03560   Chang, I. M. and H. S. Yun. Evaluation of medicinal plants with potential hepatonic activities and study on hepatonic activities of Plantago semen. (Abstract). **Abstr 4th Asian Symp Med Plants Spices**, Bangkok, Thailand 1980; 69.

T03591   Sharma, O. P., H. P. S. Makkar, R. K. Dawra and S. S. Negri. Hepatic and renal Baijal, A., R. S. Mathur, M. Wadhwa and A. Bahel. Effect of steroidal fraction of *Abrus precatorius* Linn. on testes of albino rats. **Geobios** 1981; 8(1): 29–31.

T03740   Anon. A Barefoot Doctors's Manual, Revised Edition, Cloudburst Press of America, 2116 Western Ave., Seattle, Washington, USA. (ISBN-0-88930-012-7) **Book** 1977.

T03759   Baijal, A. and R. S. Mathur. Effect of steroidal fraction of *Abrus precatorius* Linn. on the

epididymis of albino rats. **Geobios** 1981; 8(3): 129–131.

T03791   Trivedi, V. P. and K. Shukla. A study of an indigenous compound drug on reproductive physiology. **J Sci Res Pl Med** 1980; 1(3): 41–47.

T03823   Zhung, Y. L., J. R. Yeh, D. J. Lin, J. C. Yuan, R. L. Zhou and P. Q. Wang. Antihypertensive effect of *Hibiscus sabdariffa* **Yao Hsueh T'Ung Pao** 1981; 16(5): 60C.

T03902   Prakesh, A. O., R. B. Gupta and R. Mathur. Effect of oral doses of *Abrus precatorius* Linn. seeds on the oestrus cycle, body weight, uterine weight and cellular structures of uterus in albino rats. **Probe** 1980; 19: 286–292.

T03906   Maheswari, J. K., K. K. Singh and S. Saha. Ethno-Medicinal uses of plantsby the Tharus of Kheri District, U. P. **Bull Med Ethnobot Res** 1980; 1: 318–337.

T03946   Singwi, M. S. and S. B. Lall. Effect of *Hibiscus rosa-sinensis* on testicular lactate dehydrogenases of *Rhinopoma kinneari* Wroughton. (Microchiroptera. Mamalia). **Curr Sci** 1981; 50: 360–362.

T03949   Tiwari, P. V. Preliminary clinical trial on flowers of *Hibiscus rosa-sinensis* as an oral contraceptive agent. **J Res Indian Med Yoga Homeopathy** 1974; 9(4): 96–98.

T04002   Gonsalves, L. X., C. K. Kokate and H. P. Tipnis. Anti-insect and juvenile hormone mimicking activities of *Cyperus rotundus* and *Lantana camara*. **Indian J Pharm Sci** 1979; 41: 250A.

T04005   Singwi, M. S. and S. B. Lall. Effect of flower extract of *Hibiscus rosa-sinensis* on testicular lactate dehydrogenases of a non-scrotal bat *Rhinopoma kinneari* Wroughton. **Indian J Exp Biol** 1981; 19: 359–362.

T04012   Kholkute, S. D. and K. N. Udupa. Antifertility properties of *Hibiscus rosa-sinensis*. **J Res**

Indian Med Yoga Homeopathy
1974; 9(4): 99–102.

T04064   Tezuka, H. and K. Kitabatake. Growth-inhibitory activity in papaya latex against Candida species. **Bull Brew Sci** 1980; 26: 47–49.

T04176   Sofowora, E. A. and C. O. Adewunmi. Preliminary screening of some plant extracts for molluscicidal activity. **Planta Med** 1980; 39: 57–65.

T04205   Chang, I. M. and W. S. Woo. Screening of Korean medicinal plants for antitumor activity. **Arch Pharm Res** 1980; 3(2): 75–78.

T04226   Jayatilak, P. G., A. R. Sheth, P. P. Mugatwala nad D. S. Pardanani. Effect of an indigenous drug (Speman) on human accessory reproductive function. **Inidan J Surg** 1976; 38: 12–15.

T04260   Yasuraoka, K., J. Hashiguchi and B. L. Blas. Laboratory Assessment of the molluscicidal activity of the plant Jatropha curcas against *Oncomelania* snail. **Proc Philippine-Japan Joint Conf on Schistosomiasis Res & Control,** Manila, Japan Int Coop Agency 1980; 110–112.

T04410   Singh, M. P., R. H. Singh and K. N. Udupa. Antifertility activity of a benzene extract of *Hibiscus rosa-sinensis* flowers in female albino rats. **Planta Med** 1982; 44: 171–174.

T04479   Wu, D. Y. Treatment of 136 cases of uterine mycoma with "Kung Ching Tang". **Chung I Tsa Chih** 1981; 22(1): 34,35.

T04521   Rockwell, P. and I. Raw. A mutagenic screening of various herbs, spices, and foood additives. **Nutrition and cancer** 1979; 1: 10–15.

T04564   Singwi, M. S. and S. B. Lall. Cytostatic and cytotoxic effect of flower extract of *Hibiscus rosa-sinensis* on spermatogenically and androgenically active testes of non-scrotal bat *Rhinopoma*

kinneari Wroughton. **Indian J Exp Biol** 1980; 18: 1405–1407.

T04575   Bourdoux, P., F. Delange, M. Gerard, M. Mafuta, A. Hanson and A. M. Ermans. Antithyroid action of cassava in humans. **Int Dev Res Cent Rept IDRC** 1980; 61-8: 167–172.

T04583   Ghosh, R. K. and I. Gupta. Effect of *Vinca roseai* and *Ficus racemososus* on hyperglycaemia in rats. **Indian J Anim Health** 1980; 19: 145–148.

T04621   Medina, F. R. and R. Woodbury. Terrestrial plants molluscicidal to Lymnaeid hosts of *Fasciliasis hepatica* Puerto Rico. **J Agr Univ Puerto Rico** 1979; 63: 366–376.

T04637   Khan, Z. U. Antifertility properties of two indigenous medicinal plants. Paper presented at 5th international congress on hormonal steroids, New Delhi, 29 October to 4 November, 1978; 12 pp.

T04646   El Kheir, Y. M. and M. S. El Tohami. Investigation of molluscicidal activity of certain Sudanese plants used in folk medicine. I. A preliminary biological screening for molluscicidal activity of certain Sudanese plants used in folk medicine. **J Trop Med Hyg** 1979; 82: 237–241.

T04647   Weninger, B., M. Haag-Berrurier and R. Anton. Plants of Haiti used as Antifertility agents. **J Ethnopharmacol** 1982; 6(1): 67–84.

T04688   Woo, W. S., E. B. Lee and I. Chang. Biological evaluation of Korean medicinal plants II. **Yakhak Hoe Chi** 1977; 21: 177–183.

T04748   Commachan, M. and S. S. Khan. Plants in aid of family planning programme. **Sci Life** 1981; 1: 64–66.

T04890   Godhwani, J. L. and J. B. Gupta. Modification of immunological response by garlic, guggal nad turmeric: An experimental study in animals. **Abstr 13th Annu Cinf**

Indian Pharmacol Soc Jammu-tawi India 1980; Abstr-12.

T04893 Takemoto, D. J., C. Dunford and M. M. Mc Murray. The cytotoxic and cytoatatic effects of the bitter melon (*Momordica charantia*) on human lymphocytes. **Toxicon** 1982; 20: 593–599.

T04904 Meyer, B. N., N. R. Ferrigni, J. E. Putnam, L. B. Jacobsen, D. E. Nichols and J. L. Mc Laughlin. Brine shrimp: A convenient general biossay for active plant constituents. **Planta Med** 1982; 45: 31–34.

T05011 Arnason, T., F. Uck, J. Lambert and R. Hebda. Maya Medicinal plants of San Jose Succotz, Belize. **J Ethnopharmacol** 1980; 2(4): 345–364.

T05013 Hussein Ayoub, S. M. and A. Baerheim-Suendsen. Medicinal and aromatic plants in the Sudan. Usage and exploration. **Fitoterapia** 1981; 52: 243–246.

T05018 Kloos, H. Preliminary studies of medicinal plants and plant products in markets of Central Ethiopia. **Ethnomedicine** 1977; 4(1): 63–104.

T05027 Koentjoro-Soehadi, T. and I. G. P. Santa. Perspectives of male contraception with regards to Indonesian traditional drugs. **Proc Second Congress of Indonesian Society of Andrology, Bali Indonesia** 1982; 12 pp.

T05032 Morton, J. F. Caribbean and Latin American folk medicine and its influence in the United States. **Q J Crude Drug Res** 1980; 18(2): 57–75.

T05034 Holdsworth, D. K. Traditional medicinal plants of the North Solomons Province Papau New Guinea. **Q J Crude Drug Res** 1980; 18: 33–44.

T05058 Nguyen, Van Dan. List of simple drugs and medicinal plants of value in Vietnam. **Proc Seminar of the use of Medicinal Plants in Healthcare**, Tokyo 13–17 September 1977, WHO Regional Office Manila. 65–83.

T05121 Meisner, J., M. Weissenberg, D. Palevitch and N. Aharonson. Phagodeterrency induced by leaves and leaf extracts of *Catharanthus roseus* in the larva of *Spodoptera littoralis*. **J Econ Entomol** 1981; 74: 131–135.

T05122 Su, H. C. F., R/ Horvat and G. Jilani. Isolation, purification, and characterization of insect repellents from *Curcuma longa* L. **J Agr Food Chem** 1982; 30: 290–292.

T05133 ANON. Food coloring agents from Hibiscus flowers. Patent - **Japan Kokai Tokkyo Koho-81** 1981; 141,358 5 pp.

T05236 Kedar, P. and C. H. Chakrabarti. Effects of bitter gourd (*Momordica charantia*) seed & glibenclamide in streptozotocin induced diabetes mellitus. **Indian J Exp Biol** 1982; 20: 232–235.

T05377 Sharma, O. P., H. P. S. Makkar and R. K. Dawra. Biochemical effects of the plant *Lantana camara* in guinea pig liver mitochondria. **Toxicon** 1982; 20: 783–786.

T05532 Ramachandran, C., K. V. Peter and P. K. Gopalakrishnan. Drumstick (*Moringa oleifera*). A multipurpose Indian vegetable. **Econ Bot** 1980; 34: 276–283.

T05549 Iwu, M. M. and B. N. Anyanwu. Phytotherapeutic profile of Nigerian Herbs. 1. Antiinflammatory and antiarthritic agents. **J Ethnopharmacol** 1982; 6(3): 263–274.

T05564 Gershbein, L. L. Regeneration of rat liver in the presence of essential oils and their components. **Food Cosmet Toxicol** 1977; 15: 173–182.

T05584 Lim-Sylianco, C. Y. and F. Blanco. Antimutagenic effects of some anticancer agents. **Bull Philipp Biochem Soc** 1981; 4(1): 1–7.

T05602 Komai, K. and K. Ueki. Secondary metabolic compounds in purple nutsedge (*Cyperus rotundus* L.) and their plant growth inhibition. **Shokubutsu No Kagaku Chosetsu** 1981; 16: 32–37.

T05679 Prakash, A. O., R. B. Gupta and R. Mathur. Effect of oral administration of forty-two indigenous plant extracts on early and late pregnancy in albino rats. **Probe** 1978; 17(4): 315–323.

T05765 Zhu, F. Q., W. J. Zhang and J. X. Xu. Experience of treating 42 cases of ectopic pregnancy by the method of combining TCM and Western Medicine. **Zhejiang-Zhongyi Zazhi** 1982; 17: 102.

T05868 Ferrigni, N. I., J. E. Putnam, B. Anderson, L. B. Jacobsen, D. E. Nichols, D. S. Moore, J. L. Mc Laughlin, R. G. Powell and C. R. Smith Jr. Modification and evaluation of the potato disc assay and antitumor screening of Euphorbiaceae seeds. **J Nat Prod** 1982; 45: 679–686.

T05878 Sharma, O. P., P. S. Makkar, R. K. Dawra and S. S. Negi. A review of the toxicity of Lantana camara (Linn.) in animals. **Clin Toxicol** 1981; 18: 1077–1094.

T05879 Chile, S. K., M. Saraf and A. K. Barde. Efficacy of *Vinca rosea* extract against human pathogenic strains of *Trichophyton rubrum* Sab. **Indian Drugs Pharm Ind** 1981; 16(1): 31–33.

T05880 Benjamin, T. V. and A. Lamikanra. Investigations of *Cassia alata*, a plant used on Nigeria in the treatment of skin diseases. **Q J Crude Drug Res** 1981; 19: 93–96.

T05894 Kapoor, S. L. and L. D. Kapoor. Medicinal plant wealth of the Karimnagar District of Andhra Pradesh. **Bull Med Ethnobot Res** 1980; 1: 120–144.

T05943 Hussein Ayoub, S. M. and D. G. I. Kingston. Screening of plants in Sudan folk medicine for anticancer activity. **Fitoterapia** 1982; 53: 119–123.

T05949 Nwodo, O. F. C. and J. H. Botting. Uterotonic activity of extracts of the seeds of *Abrus precatorius*. **Planta Med** 1983; 47(4): 230–233.

T06024 Sukumar, K. and Z. Osmani. Insect sterilants from *Catharanthus roseus*. **Curr Sci** 1981; 50: 552,553.

T06031 Sawhney, A. N., M. R. Khan, G. Ndaalio, M. H. H. Nkunya and H. Wevers. Studies on the rationale of African traditional medicine. Part III. Preliminary screening for antifungal activity. **Pak J Sci Ind Res** 1978; 21: 193–196.

T06061 Hafez, E. S. E. Abortifacients in primitive societies and in experimental animal models. **Contraceptive Delivery Systems** MTP Press, Ltd., Lancaster, England. (ISSN: 0143-6112). 1982; 3(3): 452.

T06174 Rastogi, R. P. and B. N. Dhawan. Research on medicinal plants at the Central Drug Research Institue. Lucknow (India). **Indian J Med Res Suppl** 1982; 76: 27–45.

T06208 Godhwani, J. D., J. B. Gupta and A. P. Dadhich. Modification of immunological response by garlic, guggal and turmeric: An experimental study in albino rats. **Proc Indian Pharmacol Soc** 1980; Abstract-I2.

T06311 Kirti, S., K. Vinod, P. Nigam and P. Srivastava. Effect of *Momordica charantia* (karela) extract on blood and urine sugar in diabetes mellitus—study from a diabetic clinic. **Clinician** 1982; 46(1): 26–29.

T06317 Thyagarajan, S. P., K. Thiruneelakantan, S. Subramanian and T. Sundaravelu. In Vitro inactivation of HBSAg by *Eclipta alba* Hassk. and *Phyllanthus niruri* Linn. **Indian J Med Res Suppl** 1982; 76: 124–130.

T06320   Dabral, P. K. and R. K. Sharma.
          Evaluation of carbohydrates and
          amino acids of some non-culti-
          vated lefuminous seeds. **J In-
          dian Chem Soc** 1981; 58:
          98–100.

T06336   Fuzellier, M. C., F. Mortier and
          P. Lectard. Antifungic activity of
          Cassia alata L. **Ann Pharm Fr**
          1982; 40: 357–363.

T06351   Shah, N. C. Herbal folk medi-
          cine in Northern India. **J
          Ethnopharmacol** 1982; 6(3):
          293–301.

T06352   ANON. Newspaper clipping
          from the Philippines dated June
          6, 1983 concerning a plant con-
          traceptive. **Newspaper (Philip-
          pines)** 1983.

T06358   Prakash, A. O. Effect of *Hibis-
          cus rosa-sinensis* Linn. extracts
          on corpora lutea kof cyclic
          guinea pigs. **Sci Cult** 1980; 46:
          330,331.

T06395   Emeruwa, A. C. Antibacterial
          substance from *Carica papaya*
          fruit extract. **J Nat Prod** 1982;
          45: 123–127.

T06435   Van Den Berghe, D. A., M.
          Ieven, F. Mertens, A. J. Vlietinck
          and E. Lammens. Screening of
          higher plants for biological ac-
          tivities. II. Antiviral activity. **J
          Nat Prod** 1978; 41: 463–467.

T06479   Lal, S. D. and B. K. Yadav. Folk
          medicine of Kurushetra district
          (Haryana), India. **Econ Bot**
          1983; 37(3): 299–305.

T06510   Adesina, S. K. Studies on some
          plants used as anticonvulsants in
          Amerindian and African tradi-
          tional medicine. **Fitoterapia**
          1982; 53: 147–162.

T06535   Yamamoto, H., T. Mizutani and
          H. Nomura. Studies on the mu-
          tagenicity of crude drug extracts.
          I. **Yakugaku Zasshi** 1982; 102:
          596–601.

T06539   Rojas, N. M. and A. Cuellar.
          Catharanthus roseus G. Don. 1.
          Microbiological study of its al-
          kaloids. **First Latinamerican &**

T06540   **Caribbean Sym on Pharmaco-
          logically Active Natural Prod-
          ucts, Cuba 1982 UNESCO**
          1982; 194.
          Sharma, O. P., R. K. Dawra, H. P.
          S. Makkar. Effect of *Lantana
          camara* toxicity on lipid
          peroxidation in guinea pig tissues.
          **Res Commun Chem Pathol
          Pharmacol** 1982; 38: 153–156.

T06579   Tanaka, S., M. Saito and M.
          Tabata. Bioassay of crude drugs
          for hair growth promoting activ-
          ity in mice by a new simple
          method. **Planta Med Suppl**
          1980; 40: 84–90.

T06590   Babbar, O. P., M. N. Joshi and
          A. R. Madan. Evaluation of
          plants for Antiviral Activity. **In-
          dian J Med Res Suppl** 1982;
          76: 54–65.

T06609   Husson, J. Vitamin B12 defi-
          ciency improved by papain.
          Presse Med 1982; 11(48): 3575.

T06638   Banerjee, A. and S. S. Nigam.
          Antifungal efficacy of the essen-
          tial oils derived from the various
          species of the genus Curcuma
          Linn. **J Res Indian Med Yoga
          Homeopathy** 1978; 13(2): 63–70.

T06640   Ross, S. A., N. E. El-Keltawi and
          S. E. Megalla. Antimicrobial ac-
          tivity of some Egyptian aromatic
          plants. **Fitoterapia** 1980; 51:
          201–205.

T06729   Ross, S. A., S. E. Megalla, D. W.
          Bishay and A. H. Awad. Studies
          for determining antibiotic sub-
          stances in some Egyptian plants.
          Part 1. Screening for antimicro-
          bial activity. **Fitoterapia** 1980;
          51: 303–308.

T06756   Hirschhorn, H. H. Botanical rem-
          edies ofthe former Dutch East
          Indies (Indonesia). I: Eumycetes,
          Pteridophyta, Gymnospermae,
          Angiospermae, (Monocotyledons
          only). **J Ethnopharmacol**. 1983;
          7(2): 123–156.

T06766   Farouk, A., A. K. Bashir and A.
          K. M. Salih. Antimicrobial ac-
          tivity of certain Sudanese plants

used in Folkloric medicine. Screening for antibacterial activity (I). **Fitoterapia** 1983; 54(1): 3–7.

T06767 Ikram, M. A review on the medicinal plants. **Hamdard** 1981; 24(1/2): 102–129.

T06787 Tiwari, K. C., R. Majumder and S. Bhattacharjee. Folklore information from Assam for family planning and birth control. **Int J Crude Drug Res** 1982; 20: 133–137.

T06788 Hoelscher, M. Exposure to phytoestrogens may surpass DES residues. **Feedstuffs** 1979; 51: 54–68.

T06797 Niranjan, G. S. and S. K. Katiyar. Chemical examination and biological evaluation of proteins isolated from some wild legumes. **J Indian Chem Soc** 1981; 58: 70–72.

T06809 Chen, C. F., S. M. Chen, S. Y. Chow and P. W. Han. Protective effects of *Carica papaya* Linn. on the exogenous gastric ulcers in rats. **Amer J Chin Med** 1981; 9: 205–212.

T06813 Razzack, H. M. A. The concept of birth control in Unani medical literature. **Unpublished Manuscript of the Author**. 1980; 64 pp.

T06838 Kedar, P. and C. H. Chakrabarti. Effects of Jambolan seed treatment on blood sugar, lipid and urea in streptozotocin induced diabetes in rabbits. **Indian J Physiol Pharmacol** 1983; 27(2): 135–140.

T07026 Verma, O. P., S. Kumar and S. N. Chatterjee. Antifertility effects of common edible *Portulaca oleracea* on the reproductive organs of male albino mice. **Indian J Med Res** 1982; 75: 301–310.

T07075 Sharma, A. K. Bacterial growth inhibition of unsaponifiable matter of fixed oil from *Momordica charantia*. **Indian Drugs Pharm Ind** 1981; 16: 29–30.

T07146 Pong, J. J., W. F. Wang, T. F. Lee and W. Liu. Effect of 28 herbal drugs on the uptake of 86-RU by mouse heart muscle. **Chung Ts'ao Yao** 1981; 12(1): 33,34.

T07170 Morrison, E. Y. S. A. and M. West. Indian medicinal plants on blood sugar levels in the dog. **West Indian Med J** 1982; 31: 194–197.

T07201 Joshi, M. C., M. B. Patel and P. J. Mehta. Some folk medicines of Dangs, Gujarat State. **Bull Med Ethnobot Res** 1980; 1: 8–24.

T07238 Delaveau, P., P. Lallouette and A. M. Tessier. Stimulation of the phagocytic activity of reticuloendothelial system by plant drugs. **Planta Med** 1980; 40: 49–54.

T07240 Morimoto, I., F. Watanabe, T. Osawa, T. Okitsu and T. Kada. Mutagenicity screening of crude drugs with *Bacillus subtilis* Rec-assay and Salmonella/microsome Reversion assay. **Mutat Res** 1982; 97: 81–102.

T07251 Vijayalakshimi, K., S. D. Mishra and S. K. Prasad. Nematicidal properties of some indigenous plant materials against second stage juveniles of *Meloidogyne incognita* (Koffoid and white) Chitwood. **Indian J Entomol** 1979; 41(4): 326–331.

T07369 Holdsworth, D. and B. Wamoi. Medicinal plants of the Admiralty Islands, Papau, New Guinea. Part I. **Int J Crude Drug Res** 1982; 20(4): 169–181.

T07374 Rao, R. R. and N. S. Jamir. Ethnobotanical studies in Nagaland. I. Medicinal plants. **Econ Bot** 1982; 36: 176–181.

T07420 Jilani, G. and H. C. F. Su. Laboratory studies on several plant materials as insect repellents for protection of cereal grains. **J Econ Entomol** 1983; 76(1): 154–157.

T07439 Saxena, R. C. *Cyperus rotundus* in conjunctivitis. **J Res Ayur Siddha** 1980; 1(1): 115–120.

T07449   Wang, K. R., Y. L. Zhao, D. S. Wang and M. L. Zhao. Effects of traditional Chinese herbs, toad tincture and adenosine 3',5' cAmp on Ehrlich ascites tumor cells in mice. **Chin Med J** 1982; 95(7): 527–532.

T07475   Rouquayrol, M. Z., M. C. Fonteles, J. E. Alencar, F. Jose De Abreu and A. A. Craveiro. Molluscicidal activity of essential oils from Northeastern Brazilian plants. **Rev Brasil Pesq Med Biol** 1980; 13: 135–143.

T07620   Bhavani Shankar, T. N., N. V. Shantha, H. P. Ramesh, I. A. S. Murthy and V. S. Murthy. Toxicity studies on turmeric (*Curcuma longa*): Acute toxicity studies in rats, guinea pigs and monkeys. **Indian J Exp Biol** 1980; 18: 73–75.

T07645   Rao, V. S. Pharmacological screening and comparative efficacy of some indigenous anthelmintics. **Abstr 4th Asian Symp Med Plants Spices Bangkok, Thailand** 1980; 1980: 145.

T07660   Vitalyos, D. Phytotherapy in domestic traditional medicine in Matouba-Papaye (Guadeloupe). **Dissertation - Ph.D.- Univ Paris** 1979; 110 pp.

T07722   Okoli, B. E. Wild and cultivated cucurbits in Nigeria. **Econ Bot** 1984; 38(3): 350–357.

T07727   Abraham, S. K. and P. C. Kesavan. Genotoxicity of garlic, turmeric and asafoetida in mice. **Mutat Res** 1984; 136(1): 85–88.

T07731   Pushpangadan, P. and C. K. Atal. Ethno-Medico-Botanical investigations on Kerala 1. Some primitive tribals of western Ghats and their herbal medicine. **J Ethnopharmacol** 1984; 11(1): 59–77.

T07823   Dixit, R. S. and H. C. Pandey. Plants used as folk-medicine in Jhansi and Lalitpur sections of Bundelkhand, Uttar Pradesh. **Int J Crude Drug Res** 1984; 22(1): 47–51.

T07844   Rojas Hernandez, N. M., C. A. Jimienez Misas, A. M. Lopez Abraham and C. Hernandez Suarez. **Rev Cubana Farm** 1981; 15: 139–145.

T07856   Yousif, G., G. M. Iskander and D. El Beit. Investigation of the alkaloidal components in the Sudan flora. III. **Fitoterapia** 1983; 54(6): 269–272.

T07907   Wink, M. Chemical defense of Lupins. Mollusc-repellent properties of quinolizidine alkaloids. **Z Naturforsch Ser C** 1984; 39(6): 553–558.

T07986   Ahmed, E. M., A. K. Bashir and Y. M. El Kheir. Investigations of molluscicidal activity of certain Sudanese plants used in folk-medicine. Part IV. **Planta Med** 1984; 1: 74–77.

T07988   Ungsurungsie, M., O. Suthienkul and C. Paovalo. Mutagenicity screening of popular Thai spices. **Food Chem Toxicol** 1982; 20: 527–530.

T08016   Martinez, M. A. Medicinal plants used in a totonac community of the Sierra Norte De Puebla. Tuzamapan De Galeana, Puebla, Mexico. **J Ethnopharmacol** 1984; 11(2): 203–221.

T08047   Itokawa, H., S. Mihashi, K. Watanabe, H. Natsumoto and T. Hamanaka. Studies on the constituents of crude drugs having inhibitory activity against contraction of the ileum caused by histamine or barium chloride (1). Screening test for the activity of commercially available crude drugs and the related plant materials. **Shoyakugaku Zasshi** 1983; 37(3): 223–228.

T08049   Prakash, A. O. Biological evaluation of some medicinal plant extracts for contraceptive efficacy. **Contraceptive Delivery Systems** 1984; 5(3): 9,10.

T08066   Feroz, H., A. K. Khare and M. C. Srivastava. Review of scientific studies on anthelmintics from plants. **J Sci Res Pl Med** 1982; 3: 6–12.

T08109 Wambebe, C. and S. L. Amosun. Some neuromuscular effects of the crude extracts of the leaves of *Abrus precatorius* **J Ethnopharmacol** 1984; 11(1): 49–58.

T08119 Sharma, O. P., H. P. S. Makkar and R. K. Dawra. Biochemical changes in hepatic microsomes of guinea pig under Lantana toxicity. **Xenobiotica** 1982; 12(4): 265–269.

T08135 Prakash, A. O. and R. Mathur. Effect of oral administration of *Hibiscus rosa-sinensis* Linn. Extract on early and late pregnancy in albino rats. **J Jiwaji Univ** 1976; 4: 79–82.

T08142 El-Shayeb, N. M. A. and S. S. Mabrouk. Utilization of some edible and medicinal plants to inhibit aflatoxin formation. **Nutr Rep Int** 1984; 29(2): 273–282.

T08190 Kiso, Y., Y. Suzuki, C. Konno, H. Hikino, I, Hashimoto and Y. Yagi. Liver-protective drugs. 3: The validity of the oriental medicines. Application of carbon tetrachloride-induced liver lesion in mice for screening of liver protective crude drugs. **Shoyakugaku Zasshi** 1982; 36: 144–238.

T08191 Sabnis, S. D. and S. J. Bedi. Ethnobotanical studies on Dadra-Nagar Haveli and Daman. **Indian J Med Res** 1983; 6(1): 65–69.

T08282 John, D. One hundred useful raw drugs of the Kani Tribes of Trivandrum Forest Division, Kerala, India. **Int J Crude Drug Res** 1984; 22(1): 17–39.

T08288 Lee, C. Y., J. W. Chiou and W. H. Chang. Studies on the antioxidative activities of spices grown in Taiwan. **Chung-Kuo Nung Yeh Hua Hsueh Hui Chih** 1982; 20(1/2): 61–66.

T08384 Kalyanasundaram, M. and C. J. Babu. Biologically active plant extracts as mosquito larvicides. **Indian J Med Res** 1982; 76: 102–106.

T08388 Mulchandani, N. B. and S. A. Hassarajani. 4-methoxy-nor-securinine, a new alkaloid from *Phyllanthus niruri* **Planta Med** 1984; 1: 104,105.

T08396 Karunanayake, E. H., J. Welihinda, S. R. Sirimanne and G. Sinnadorai. Oral hypoglycaemic activity of some medicinal plants of Sri Lanka. **J Ethnopharmacol** 1984; 11(2): 223–231.

T08445 Pandey, D. K., N. N. Tripathi, R. D. Tripathi and S. N. Dixit. Antifungal activity of some seed extracts with special reference to that of Pimpinella diversifolia DC. **Int J Crude Drug Res** 1983; 21(4): 177–182.

T08446 Panigrahi, S., B. J. Francis, L. A. Cano, M. B. Burbage. Toxicity of *Jatropha curcas* seeds from Mexico to rats and mice. **Nutr Rep Int** 1984. 29(5): 1089-1099.

T08478 Balick, M. J. Ethnobotany of palms in the Neotropics. **Advances on Economic Botany in the Neotropics** G. T. Prance and J. A. Kallunki (Eds) New York Botanical Garden, Bronx, N. Y. 1984; 1: 9–23.

T08514 Boukef, K., H. R. Souissi and G. Balansard. Contribution to the study on plants used in traditional medicine in Tunisia. **Plant Med Phytother** 1982; 16(4): 260–279.

T08524 Akbar, S., M. Nisa and M. Tariq. Effects of aqueous extract of *Cyperus rotundus* Linn. on Carrageenin-induced oedema in rats. **Nagarjun** 1982; 25(11): 253–255.

T08527 Uppal, R. P. and B. S. Paul. Haematological changes in Experimental Lantana poisoning in sheep. **Indian Vet J** 1982; 59(1): 18–24.

T08539 Kiuchi, F., M. Shibuya, T. Kinoshita and U. Sankawa. Inhibition of prostaglandin biosynthesis by the constituents of medicinal plants. **Chem Pharm Bull** 1983; 31(10): 3391–3396.

T08589   Lopez Abraham, A. N., N. M. Rojas Hernandez and C. A. Jimenez Misas. Potential antineoplastic activity of Cuban Plants. IV. **Rev Cubana Farm** 1981; 15(1): 71–77.

T08621   Jensen, N. J. Lack of mutagenic effect of turmeric oleoresin and curcumin in the salmonella/mammalian microsome test. **Mutat Res** 1982; 105(6): 393–396.

T08662   Ng, T. B. and H. W. Yeung. Bioactive constituents of Cucurbitaceae plants with special emphasis on *Momordica charantia* and *Trichosanthes kirilowii*. **Proc Fifth Asian Symposium on Medicinal Plants and Spices Seoul Korea** 1984; 5: 183–196.

T08685   Singh, Y. N., T. Ikahihifo, M. Panuve and C. Slatter. Folk Medicine in Tonga. A study of the use of herbal medicines for obstetric and gynaecological conditions and disorders. **J Ethnopharmacol** 1984; 12(3): 305–329.

T08730   Van Den Berg, M. A. Ver-O-Peso: The ethnobotany of an Amazonian market. **Advances in Economic Botany Ethnobotany in the Neotropics**, G. T. Prance and J. A. Kallunki (Eds) New York Botanical Garden, Bronx, New York 1984; 1: 140–149.

T08732   Arnold, H. J. and M. Gulumian. Pharmacopoeia of traditional medicine in Venda. **J Ethnopharmacol** 1984; 12(1): 35–74.

T08733   Singh, N., R. Nath, D. R. Singh, M. L. Gupta and R. P. Kohli. An experimental evaluation of the protective effects of some indigenous drugs on carbon tetrachloride-induced hepatotoxicity in mice and rats. **Q J Crude Drug Res** 1978; 16(1): 8–16.

T08770   Bisset, N. G. and G. Mazars. Arrow poisoning in South Asia part 1. Arrow poison in ancient India. **J Ethnopharmacol** 1984; 12(1): 1–24.

T08771   Cosminsky, S. Knowledge of body concepts of Guatemala wives. Chapter 12. **Anthropology of Human Birth**. 1982; 233–252.

T08806   Kargbo, T. K. Traditional practices affecting the health of women and children in Africa. **Unpublished Manuscript** 1984.

T08817   Goh, S. H., E. Soepadmo, P. Chang, U. Barnerjee et al. Studies on Malaysian medicinal plants. Preliminary results. **Proc Fifth Asian Symposium on Medicinal Plants and Spices South Korea** 1984; August 20–24. 5: 473–483.

T08867   Ishii, R., K. Yoshikawa, H. Minakata, H. Komura and T. Kada. Specificities of Bioantimutagens in plant kingdom. **Agr Biol Chem** 1984; 48(10): 2587–2591.

T08889   Singh, K. V. and R. K. Pathak. Effect of leaves extracts of some higher plants on spore germination of *Ustilago maydes* and *U. nuda*. **Fitoterapia** 1984; 55(5): 318–320.

T08931   Adewunmi, C. O. and V. O. Marquis. A rapid In Vitro screening method for detecting schistosomicidal activity of some Nigerian medicinal plants. **Int J Crude Drug Res** 1983; 21(4): 157–159.

T08932   Chandravadana, M. V. and A. B. Pal. Triterpenoid feeding deterrent of *Raphidopalpa foveicollis* L. (red pumpkin beetles) from *Momordica charantia* L. **Curr Sci** 1983; 52(2): 87–89.

T08985   Takemoto, D. J., C. Jilka, S. Rockenbach and J. V. Hughes. Purification and characterization of an cystostatic factor with antiviral activity from the bitter melon. **Prep Biochem** 1983; 13(5): 397–421.

T09033   Sircar, N. N. Pharmaco-Thera-peutics of Dasemani Drugs. **Ancient Sci Life** 1984; 3(3): 132–135.

T09046   Calixto, J. B., R. A. Yunes, A. S. O. Neto, R. M. R. Valle and G. A. Rae. Antispasmodic effects of an alkaloid extracted from *Phyllanthus sellowianus*. A comparative study with Papavarine. **Brazil J Med Biol Res** 1984; 17: 313–321.

T09049   Tripathi, R. K. R. and R. N. Tripathi. Reduction in bean common Mosaic Virus (BCMV) infectivity vis-a-vis crude leaf extract of some higher plants. **Experientia** 1982; 38(3): 349.

T09137   Jilka, C., B. Strifler, G. W. Fortner, E. F. Hays and D. J. Takemoto. In vivo antitumor activity of the bitter melon (*Momordica charantia*). **Cancer Res** 1983; 43(11): 5151–5155.

T09230   Deka, L., R. Majumdar and A. M. Dutta. Some Ayurvedic important plants from district Kamrup (Assam). **Ancient Sci Life** 1983; 3(2): 108–115.

T09302   Hemadri, K. and S. Sasibhushana Rao. Antifertility, abortifacient nd fertility promoting drugs from Dandakaranya. **Ancient Sci Life** 1983; 3(2): 103–107.

T09361   Rukachaisirikul, N., L. Benchapornkullanij, V. Rukachaisirikul, S. Permkan, P. Dampawan and P. Wiriyachitra. Extraction of substances toxic *Spodoptera litura* Fabr. from some readily available plants. **Warasan Songkhia nakkharin** 1983; 5(4): 359–362.

T09366   Sircar, N. N. Pharmaco-therapeutics of Dasemani Drugs. **Ancient Sci Life** 1984; 3(3): 132–135.

T09390   Jain, S. P. and H. S. Puri. Ethnomedical plants of Jaunsar-Bawar Hills, Uttar Pradesh, India. **J Ethnopharmacol** 1984; 12(2): 213–222.

T09391   Pei, S. J. Preliminary study of ethnobotany in Xishuang Banna, People's Republic of China. **J Ethnopharmacol** 1985; 13(2): 121–137.

T09394   Arseculeratne, S. N., A. A. L. Gunatilaka and R. G. Panabokke. Studies on medicinal plants of Sri Lanka. Part 14. Toxicity of some traditional medicineal herbs. **J Ethnopharmacol** 1985; 13(3): 323–335.

T09486   Sebastian, M. K. and M. M. Bhandari. Medico-Ethno botany of mount Abu, Rajasthan, Indian. **J Ethnopharmacol** 1984; 12(2): 223–230.

T09505   Barde, A. K. and S. M. Singh. Activity of plant extracts against *Scytalidium anamorph* of *Hendersonula toruloidea* causing skin and nail diseases in man. **Indian Drugs** 1983; 20(9): 362–364.

T09507   May, G. and G. Willuhn. Antiviral activity of aqueous extracts from medicinal plants in tissue cultures. **Arzneim-Forsch** 1978; 28(1): 1–7.

T09530   Petiard, V. Antimitotic activities of *Catharanthus roseus* Tissue cultures. **J Med** 1981; 447–469.

T09546   Kosuge, T., H. Ishida, H. Yamazaki and M. Ishii. Studies on active substances in the herbs used for oketsu blood coagulation, in Chinese medicine. 1: On anticoagulative activities of the herbs for oketsu. **Yakugaku Zasshi** 1984; 104(4): 1050–1053.

T09552   Choi, S. Y. and I. M. Chang. Plants with liver protective activities. **Ann Rep Nat Prod Res Inst Seoul Natl Univ** 1982; 21: 49–53.

T09553   Whistler, W. A. Traditional and herbal medicine in Cook Islands. **J Ethnopharmacol** 1985; 13(3): 239–280.

T09622   Kosuge, T., H. Ishida and H. Yamazaki. Studies on active substances in the herbs used for oketsu ("stagnant blood") in Chinese medicine 111: On the anticoagulative principles in *Curcumae rhizoma*. **Chem Pharm Bull** 1985; 33(4): 1499–1502.

T09667   Aynehchi, Y., M. H. Salehi Sormaghi, M. Shirudi and E. Souri. Screening of Iranian plants for antimicrobial activity. **Acta Pharm Suecica** 1982; 19(4): 303–308.

T09672   Browner, C. H. Plants used for reproductive health in Oaxaca, Mexico. **Econ Bot** 1985; 39(4): 482–504.

T09679   Macfoy, C. A. and A. M. Sama. Medicinal plants in Pujehun District of Sierra Leone. **J Ethnopharmacol** 1983; 8(2): 215–223.

T09735   Dominguez, X. A. and J. B. Alcorn. Screening of medicinal plants used by Huastec Mayans of Northeastern Mexico. **J Ethnopharmacol** 1985; 13(2): 139–156.

T09739   Laurens, A., S. Mboup, M. Tignokpa, O. Sylla and J. Masquelier. Antimicrobial activity of some medicinal species of Dakar markets. **Pharmazie** 1985; 40(7): 482–485.

T09858   Thompson, W. A. R. Herbs that heal. **J Roy Coll Gen Pract** 1976; 26: 365–370.

T09869   Pal, A. K., K. Bhattacharya, S. N. Kabir and A. Pakrashi. Flowers of *Hibiscus rosa-sinensis*, a potential source of contragestative agent. II. Possible mode of action with reference to anti-implantation effect of the benzene extract. **Contraception** 1985; 32(5): 517–529.

T09888   Todd, S., T. Miyase, H. Arichi, H. Tanizawa and Y. Takino. Natural antioxidative components isolated form rhizome of *Curcuma longa* L. **Chem Pharm Bull** 1985; 33(4): 1725–728.

T09890   Kalyanasundaram, M. and P. K. Das. Larvicidal and Synergistic activity of plant extracts for mosquito control. **Indian J Med Res** 1985; 82(1): 19–23.

T09977   Memon, A. R. and M. U. Dahot. Investigation of Phospholipase B activity in *Moringa oleifera* seeds. **J Chem Soc Pak** 1985; 7(1): 7–15.

T09984   Said, M. Potential of herbal medicines in modern medical therapy. **Ancient Sci Life** 1984; 4(1): 36–47.

T10064   Jain, S. P. and D. M. Verma. Medicinal plants in the Folk-lore of Northern Circle Dehradun Up India. **Nat Acad Sci Lett (India)** 1981; 4(7): 269–271.

T10072   Yeung, H. W., W. W. Li, L. K. Law and W. Y Chan. Purification and partial characterization of momorcharins, abortifacient proteins from the Chinese drug, Kuguazi (*Momordica charantia*) seeds. **Advances in Chinese Medicinal Materials Research, World Scientific Press, Philadelphia, Pa** 1984; 311–318.

T10116   Velazco, E. A. Herbal and traditional practices related to material and child health care. **Rural Reconstruction Review** 1980; 35–39.

T10126   Aswal, B. S., D. S. Bhakuni, A. K. Goel, K. Kar, B. N. Mehrotra and K. C. Mukherjee. Screening of Indian Plants for Biological activity. Part X. **Indian J Exp Biol** 1984; 22(6): 312–332.

T10128   Chinoy, N. J., R. J. Verma, M. G. Sam and O. M. D'Souza. Reversible antifertility effects of papaya seed extract in male rodents. **J Androl 6 2: Abstr-M10** 1985.

T10130   Bhattacharya, K., S. N. Kabir, A. K. Pal and A. Pakrashi. Effect of benzene extract okf *Hibiscus rosa-sinensis* flowers in facultative delayed implantation and uterine uptake of estrogen in mice. **IRCS Med Sci** 1984; 12(9): 841–842.

T10133 Sahu, T. R. Less known uses of weeds as medicinal plants. **Ancient Sci Life** 1984; 3(4): 245–249.

T10183 Jaysweera, D. M. A. Medicinal plants (Indigenous and exotic) used in Ceylon. Part II. Cactaceae-Fagaceae. National Science Council of Sri Lanka, Colombo, 1980; 160 pp.

T10290 Woo, W. S., E. B. Lee, K. H. Shin, S. S. Kang and H. J. Chi. A Review of research on plants for fertility regulation in Korea. **Korean J Pharmacog** 1981; 12(3): 153–170.

T10321 Tiwari, K. C., R. Majumder and S. Bhattacharjee. Folklore medicines from Assam and Arunachal Pradesh (District Tirap). **Int J Crude Res** 1979; 17(2): 61–67.

T10348 Mossa, J. S. A study on the crude antidiabetic drugs used in Arabian folk medicine. **Int J Crude Drug Res** 1985; 23(3): 137–145.

T10354 Khan, M. R., G. Ndaalio, M. H. H. Nkunya, H. Wevers. Studies on the rationale of African traditional medicine. Part II. Preliminary screening of medicinal plants for anti-gonoccoci activity. **Pak J Sci Ind Res** 1978; 27(5/6): 189–192.

T10387 Namba, T., M. Tsunezaku, Y. Takehana, S. Nunome et al., Studies on dental caries prevention by traditional chinese medicines. IV. Screening of crude drugs for anti-plaque action and effects on *Artemisia capillaris* spikes on adherence of *Streptococcus mutans* to smooth surfaces and synthesis of glucan. **Shoyakugaku Zasshi** 1984; 38(3): 253–263.

T10448 Chakraborty, D., P. K. Mahapatra and A. K. Nag Chaudhuri. A Neurospsychopharmacological study of *Syzygium cumini*. **Planta Med** 1986; 2: 139–143.

T10453 Shin, K. H. and W. S. Woo. A survey of the response of medici-nal plants on drug metabolism. **Korean J Pharmacog** 1980; 11: 109–122.

T10567 Singh, J. D. The teratogenic effect of dietary cassava on the pregnant albino rat: A preliminary report. **Teratology** 1981; 24: 289–291.

T10568 Chang, I. M. and H. S. Yun. Plants with liver-protective activities, Pharmacology and toxicology of aucubin. **Advances in Chinese Medicinal Materials Research** World Scientific Press, Philadelphia, PA. 1984; 269–285.

T10623 De Ribeiro, R., M. M. R. Fiuza De Melo, F. De Barros, C. Gomes and G. Trolin. Acute antihypertensive effect in conscious rats produced by some medicinal plants used in the State of Sao Paulo. **J Ethnopharmacol** 1986; 15(3): 261–269.

T10632 Singh, Y. N. Traditional medicine in Fiji. Some herbal folk cures used by Fiji Indians. **J Ethnopharmacol**. 1986; 15(1): 57–88.

T10633 Almagboul, A. Z., A. K. Bashir, A. Farouk and A. K. M. Salih. Antimicrobial activity of certain Sudanese plants used in folkloric medicine. Screening for antibacterial activity (IV). **Fitoterapia** 1985; 56(6): 331–337.

T10651 Sharma, O. P., H. P. S. Makkar, R. K. Dawra and S. S. Negi. Changes in blood constituents of guinea pigs in Lantana toxicity. **Toxicol Lett** 1982; 11: 73–76.

T10776 Maruyama, Y., H. Matsuda, R. Matsuda, M. Kubo, T. Hatano and T. Okuda. Study on *Psidium guajava* L. (1). Antidiabetic effect and effective components of the leaf of *Psidium guajava* L. (Part 1). **Shoyakugaku Zasshi** 1985; 39(4): 261–269.

T10822 Tripathi, A. K. and S. M. A. Rizvi. Antifeedant activity of indigenous plants against *Diacrisia obliqua* Walker. **Curr Sci** 1985; 54(13): 630,631.

T10823　Gundidza, M. Screening of extracts from Zimbabwean higher plants II: Antifungal properties. **Fitoterapia** 1986; 57(2): 111–113.

T10824　Saigopal, D. V. R., V. S. Prasad and P. Sreenivasulu. Antiviral activity in extracts of *Phyllanthus fraternus* Webst. (*P. niruri*). **Curr Sci** 1986; 55(5): 264–265.

T10828　Hedberg, I., O. Hedberg, P. J. Madati, K. E. Mshigeni, E. N. Mshiu and G. Samuelsson. Inventory of plants used in traditional medicine in Tanzania. Part III. Plants of the families Papilionaceae-Vitaceae. **J Ethnopharmacol** 1983; 9(2/3): 237–260.

T10907　Hershman, J. M., A. E. Pekary, M. Sugawara, M. Adler, L. Turner, J. A. Demetriou and J. D. Hershman. Cassava is not a goitrogen in mice. **Proc Soc Exp Biol Med** 1985; 180(1): 72–78.

T10928　Darias, V., L. Bravo, E. Barquin, D. M. Herrera and C. Fraile. Contribution to the Ethnopharmacological study of the Canary Islands. **J Ethnopharmacol** 1986; 15(2): 169–193.

T11017　Trivedi, V. P. and K. Shukla. A study of effects of an indigenous compound drug on reproductive physiology. **J Sci Res Pl Med** 1980; 1(3/4): 41,47.

T11055　Franzblau, S. G. and C. Cross. Comparative in vitro antimicrobial activity of Chinese medicinal herbs. **J Ethnopharmacol** 1986; 15(3): 279-288.

T11107　Singh, S., N. K. Dube, S. C. Tripathi and S. K. Singh. Fungitoxicity of some essential oils against *Aspergillus flavus*. **Indian Perfum** 1984; 28(3/4): 164–166.

T11177　Prakash, A. O. Potentialities of some indigenous plants for anti-fertility activity. **Int J Crude Drug Res** 1986; 24(1): 19–24.

T11178　Wong, C. M., T. B. Ng and H. W. Yeung. Screening of *Trichosanthes kirilowii, Momordica charantia* and *Cucurbitas maxima* (Family Cucurbitaceae) for compounds with antilipolytic activity. **J Ethnopharmacol** 1985; 13(3): 313–321.

T11208　Venkataraghavan, S. and T. P. Sundaresan. A short note on contraceptive in Ayurveda. **J Sci Res Pl Med** 1981; 2(1/2): 39.

T11226　Onawunmi, G. O. and E. O. Ogunlana. A Study of the antibacterial activity of the essential oil of lemon grass (*Cymbopogon citratus* (DC.) Stapf). **Int J Crude Drug Res** 1986; 24(2): 64–68.

T11229　Bambhole, V. D. and G. G. Jiddewar. Evaluation of *Cyperus rotundus* in the management of obesity and high blood pressure of human subjects. **Nagarjun** 1984; 27(5): 110–113.

T11279　Prakesh, A. O., S. Shukla, S. Mathur, V. Saxena and R. Mathur. Evaluation of some indigenous plants for anti-implantation activity in rats. **Probe** 1986; 25(2): 151–155.

T11371　Anderson, E. F. Ethnobotany of Hill Tribes of Northern Thailand. 1. Medicinal plants of Akha. **Econ Bot** 1986; 40(1): 38–53.

T11438　Jadon, A. and R. Mathur. Effects of *Abrus precatorius* Linn. seed extract on biochemical constituents of male mice. **J Jiwaji Univ** 1984; 9(1): 100–103.

T11525　Sristava, S. L., V. K. Kediyal and R. C. Sundriyal. Screening of floral extract of some flowering plants for antifungal activities against Bipolaris oryzae. **J Environ Biol** 1984; 5(4): 217–221.

T11569　Jain, H. C. Indian plants with oral hypoglycaemic activity. **Abstr Internat Res Cong Nat Prod Coll Pharm Univ N Carolina**, Chapel Hill, NC. July 7–12, 1985. Abstr. 152.

T11593　Syamasundar, K. V., B. Singh, R. S. Thakur, A. Husain, Y. Kiso and H. Hikino. Antihepatotoxic principles of *Phyllanthus niruri* herbs. **J Ethnopharmacol** 1985; 14(1): 41–44.

T11767 Yun, H. S. and I. M. Chang. Liver protective activities of Korean Medicinal plants. **Korean J Pharmacog** 1980; 11: 149–152.

T11789 Namba, T., M. Tsunezuka, N. Kakiuchi, D. M. R. B. Dissanayake, U. Pilapitiya, K. Saito and M. Hattori. Studies on dental caries prevention by traditional medicines (Part V11). Screening of Ayurvedic medicines for anti-plaque action. **Shoyakugaku Zasshi** 1985; 39(2): 146–153.

T11794 Saksena, N. and H. H. S. Tripathi. Plant volatiles in relation to fungistasis. **Fitoterapia** 1985; 56(4): 243,244.

T12027 Anderson, E. F. Ethnobotany of Hill tribes of Northern Thailand. II. Lahu Medicinal Plants. **Econ Bot** 1986; 40(4): 442–450.

T12033 Rojas, M. C. N. and M. C. A. Cuellar. Comparative microbiological studies of the alkaloids of *Catharanthus roseus* and other related compounds. **Rev Cubana Farm** 1981; 15(2): 131–138.

T12054 Liu, X. L. Twelve cases of aplastic anemia treated mainly by ready made Chinese drugs. **Chung l Tsa Chih** 1984; 25(10): 759–760.

T12072 Singhal, K. C. Anthelmintic activity of *Punica granatum* and *Artemisia siversiana* against experimental infections in mice. **Indian J Pharmacol** 1984; 15(2): 119–122.

T12086 Datta, S. C., T. Das and R. K. Bhatak. Inhibitors in leaves of road-side trees during various seasons. **Sci Cult** 1985; 51(9): 313–315.

T12115 Rao, Y. S. Experimental production of liver damage and its protection with *Phyllanthus niruri* and *Capparis spinosa* (both ingredients of LIV.52) in white albino rats. **Probe** 1985; 117–119.

T12126 Prakash, A. O., S. Shukla, R. Mathur. *Hibiscus rosa-sinensis* Linn. its effect on Beta-Glucuronidase in the uterus of ovariectomized rats. **Curr Sci** 1985; 54(15): 734–736.

T12135 Meir, P. and Z. Yaniv. An In Vitro study on the effect of *Momordica charantia* glucose uptake and glucose metabolism in rats. **Plantsa Med** 1985; 1: 12–16.

T12145 Tignokpa, M., A. Laurens, S. Mboup and O. Sylla. Popular medicinal plants of the markets of Dakar (Senegal). **Int J Crude Drug Res** 1986; 24(2): 75–80.

T12164 Chaudhury, R. Controversies and challenges in the clinical evaluation of antifertility plants. **J Vivekananda Inst Med Sci** 1984; 3(1): 6–12.

T12220 Chakraborty, T. and G. Poddar. Herbal drugs in diabetes - Part 1. Hypoglycaemic activity of indigenous plants in streptozotocin (STZ) induced diabetic rats. **J Inst Chem (India)** 1984; 56(1): 20–22.

T12438 Bille, N., J. C. Larsen, E. V. Hansen and G. Wurtzen. Subchronic oral toxicity of turmeric oleoresin in pigs. **Food Chem Toxicol** 1985; 23(11): 967–973.

T12445 Leite, J. R., M. L. D. V. Seabra, E. Maluf, K. Assolant et al., Pharmacology of lemongrass (*Cymbopogon citratus* Stapf). 111. Assessment of eventual toxic, hypnotic and anxiolytic effects on humans. **J Ethnopharmacol** 1986; 17(1): 75–83.

T12460 Wanjari, D. G. Antihemorrhagic actiivty of *Lantana camara*. **Nagarjun** 1983; 27(2): 40,41.

T12546 Shashikanth, K. N. and A. Hosono. In vitro mutagenicity of tropical spices to streptomycin dependent strains of *Salmonella typhimurium* TA98. **Agr Biol Chem** 1986; 50(11): 2947,2948.

T12554   Kinoshita, G., F. Nakamura and
          T. Maruyama. Immunological
          studies on polysaccharide frac-
          tions from crude drugs.
          Shoyakugaku Zasshi 1986;
          40(3): 325–332.

T12574   Souza Formigoni, M. L. O., H. M.
          Lodder, O. G. Filho, T. M. S.
          Ferriera and E. A. Carlini. **J Ethno-**
          pharmacol 1986; 17(1): 65–74.

T12612   Holdsworth, D., B. Pilokos and
          P. Lambes. Traditional medici-
          nal plants of New Ireland, Papau
          New Guinea. **Int J Crude Drug**
          Res 1983; 21(4): 161–168.

T12686   Leatherdale, B. A., R. K.
          Panesar, G. Singh, T. W. Atkins,
          C. J. Bailey and A. H. C. Bignell.
          Brit Med J 1981; 282(6279):
          1823,1824.

T12703   Welihinda, J. and E. H.
          Karunanayake. Extra-pancreatic
          effects of *Momordica charantia*
          in rats. **J Ethnopharmacol**
          1986; 17(3): 247–255.

T12706   Welihinda, J., E. H.
          Karunanayake, M. H. R. Sheriff
          and K. S. A. Jayasinghe. Effect
          of *Momordica charantia* on the
          glucose tolerance in maturity on-
          set diabetes. **J Ethnopharmacol**
          1986; 17(3): 277–282.

T12725   Guerin, J. C. and H. P. Reveillere.
          Antifungal activity of plant ex-
          tracts used in therapy. l. Study of
          41 plant extracts against 9 fungi
          species. **Ann Pharm Fr** 1984;
          42(6): 553–559.

T12794   Madaan, S. Speman in oligosper-
          mia. **Probe** 1985; 115–117.

T12861   Takemoto, D. J., C. Dunford, D.
          Vaughn, K. J. Kramer, A. Smith
          and R. G. Powell. Guanylate cy-
          clase activity in Human Leuke-
          mic and normal lymphocytes.
          Enzyme 1982; 27: 179–188.

T12882   Pakrashi, A., K. Bhattacharya, S.
          N. Kabir and A. K. Pal. Flowers
          of *Hibiscus rosa-sinensis*, a
          potential source of contra-
          gestative agent. III. Interceptive
          effect of benzene extract in

          mouse. **Contraception** 1986;
          34(5): 523–536.

T13374   Parry, O., F. K. Okwuasaba and
          C. Ejike. Skeletal muscle relax-
          ant action of an aqueous extract
          of *Portulaca oleracea* in the rat.
          J Ethnopharmacol 1987; 19(3):
          247–253.

T13391   Chile, S. K., K. M. Vyas and R. K.
          Chourasia. Anti-respiratory activ-
          ity of *Vinca rosea* against human
          pathogenic strains of *Trichophy-*
          ton rubrum. **Hindustan Antibiot**
          Bull 1984; 26(1/2): 33–37.

T13392   Chile, S. K. and K. M. Vyas. Ef-
          ficacy of *Vinca rosea* extracts
          against protease from human
          pathogenic strains of *Trichophy-*
          ton rubrum. **Hindustan Antibiot**
          Bull 1984; 26(3/4): 114–116.

T13678   Das, P. C., A. K. Sarkar and S.
          Thakur. Studies on animals of a
          Herbo-Mineral compound for
          long acting contraction. **Fito-**
          terapia 1987; 58(4): 257–261.

T13699   Polasa, K. and C. Rukmini. Mu-
          tagenicity tests of cashewnut shell
          liquid, rice-bran oil and other veg-
          etable oils using the Salmonella
          typhimurium/microsome system.
          Food Chem Toxicol 1987;
          25(10): 763–766.

T13791   Lee, J. H., S. K. Kang, and B. Z.
          Ahn. Antineoplastic natural
          products and the analogues. X1.
          Cytotoxic activity against L1210
          cell of some raw drugs from the
          Oriental medicine and folklore.
          Korean J Pharmacog 1986;
          17(4): 286–291.

T13846   Weniger, B., M. Rouzier, R.
          Daguilh, D. Henrys, J. H. Henrys
          and R. Anthon. Popular medicine
          of the Plateau of Haiti. 2. Ethno-
          pharmacological inventory. **J**
          Ethnopharmacol 1986; 17(1):
          13–30.

T13856   Hemadri, K. and S. S. Rao. Jaun-
          dice: Tribal Medicine. **Ancient**
          Sci Life 1984; 3(4): 209–212.

T13890   Bali, H. S., S. Singh and S. C.
          Pati. Preliminary screening of

some plants for molluscicidal activity against two snail species. **Indian J Anim Sci** 1985; 55(5): 338–340.

T13893 Ojha, J. H., V. V. Prasad and B. Singh. A preliminary clinical trial of Vijayasara compound in cases of insulin-independent diabetes. **Nagarjun** 1983; 27(2): 37–39.

T13897 Ng, T. B., C. M. Wong, W. W. Li and H. W. Yeung. Acid-ethanol extractable compounds from fruits and seeds of the bitter gourd *Momordica charantia*: Effects on lipid metabolism in isolated rat adipocytes. **Amer J Chin Med** 1987; 15(1/2): 31–42.

T13960 Mukerjee, T., N. Bhalla, G. Singh Aulakh and H. C. Jain. Herbal drugs for urinary stones. Literature appraisal. **Indian Drugs** 1984; 21(6): 224–228.

T14020 Thomas, K. D. nd B. Ajani. Antisickling agent in an extract of unripe pawpaw fruit (*Carica papaya*). **Trans Roy Soc Trop Med Hyg** 1987; 81(3): 510,511.

T14094 Jain, A. K., H. Tezuka, T. Kada and I. Tomita. Evaluation of genotoxic effects of turmeric in mice. **Curr Sci** 1987; 56(19): 1005,1006.

T14117 Shukla, S., S. Mathur, R. Mathur and A. O. Prakash. Fertility regulation through indigenous plants and their mode of action. **Planta Med** 1986; 6: 552-B.

T14146 Okwuasaba, F., C. Ejike and O. Parry. Skeletal muscle relaxant properties of the aqueous extract of *Portulaca oleracea*. **J Ethnopharmacol** 1986; 17(2): 139–160.

T14170 Boum, B., L. Kamdem, P. Mbganga, N. Atangana and Y. Sabry. Contribution to the pharmacologic study of two plants used in traditional medicine against worms. **Rev Sci Technol (Health Sci Ser)** 1985; 2(3/4): 83–86.

T14178 Kloss, H., F. W. Thiongo, J. H. Ouma and A. E. Butterworth. Preliminary evaluation of some wild and cultivated plants from snail control in Machakos District, Kenya. **J Trop Med Hyg** 1987; 90(4): 197–204.

T14221 Siang, S. T. Use of combined traditional Chinese and Western medicine in the management of burns. **Panminerva Med** 1983; 25(3): 197–202.

T14330 Sharma, V. K. and S. Kaur. Contact dermatitis due to plants in Chandigarh. **Indian J Dermatol Venereol Leprol** 1987; 53(1): 26–30.

T14342 Ohta, S., N. Sakurai, T. Inoue and M. Shinoda. Studies on chemical protectors against radiation. XXV. Radioprotective activities of various crude drugs. **Yakugaku Zasshi** 1987; 107(1): 70–75.

T14473 Zaidi, Z. B., V. P. Gupta, A. Samad and Q. A. Naqvi. Inhibition of spinach mosaic virus by extracts of some medicinal plants. **Curr Sci** 1988; 57(3): 151,152.

T14489 Lama, S. and S. C. Santra. Development of Tibetan Plant Medicine. **Sci Cult** 1979; 45: 262–265.

T14492 Shukla, S., R. Mathur and A. O. Prakash. Anti-implantation efficacy of *Moringa oleifera* Lam. and *Moringa concanensis* Nimmo in rats. **Int J Crude Drug Res** 1988; 26(1): 29–32.

T14569 Shukla, S., R. Mathur and A. O. Prakash. Antifertility profile of the aqueous extract of *Moringa oleifera* roots. **J Ethnopharmacol** 1988; 22(1): 51–62.

T14570 Nisteswar, K. Review of certain indigenous antifertility agents. **Deerghayu International** 1988; 4(1): 4–7.

T14676 Kulakkattolickal, A. Piscicidal plants of Nepal. Preliminary toxicity screening using grass carp (*Ctenopharyngodon idella*) fingerlings. **J Ethnopharmacol** 1987; 21(1): 1–9.

T14745 Okwuasaba, F., C. Ejike and O. Parry. Comparison of the skeletal muscle relaxant properties of *Portulaca oleracea* extracts with dantrolene sodium and methoxy-verapamil. **J Ethnopharmacol** 1987; 20(2): 85–100.

T14750 Pasricha, J. S. and A. Puri. Contact dermatitis due to eucalyptus oil. **Indian J Dermatol Venereol Leprol** 1986; 52(4): 201,202.

T14752 Le Grand, A., P. A. Wondergem, R. Verpoorte and J. L. Pousset. Anti-infectious phytotherapies of the tree-savannah of Senegal (West Africa). II. Antimicrobial activity of 33 species. **J Ethno-phmarmacol** 1988; 22(1): 25–31.

T14756 Verpoorte, R. and P. P. Dihal. Medicinal plants of Surinam. IV. Antimicrobial activity of some medicinal plants. **J Ethno-pharmacol** 1987; 21(3): 315–318.

T14776 Carlini, E. A., J. D. D. P. Contar, A. R. Silva-Filho, N. G. Solveira-Filho, M. L. Frochtengarten and O. F. A. Bueno. Pharmacology of lemon grass (*Cymbopogon citratus* Stapf). Effects of teas prepared from the leaves on laboratory animals. **J Ethnopharmacol** 1986; 17(1): 37–64.

T14776 Carlini, E. A., J. D. D. R. Contar, A. R. Silva-Fillho et al. Pharmacology of lemongrass *(Cymbo-pogon citratus)*: I. Effect of teas prepared from the leaves on laboratory animals. **Pharmacol** 1986; 17(1): 37–64.

T14891 Kamboj, V. P. A Review of Indian Medicinal Plants with Interceptive Activity. **Indian J Med Res** 1988; 4: 336–355.

T14959 Srivastava, Y., H. Venkatakrishna-Bhatt, Y. Verma and A. S. Perm. Retardation of retinopathy by *Momordica charantia* L. (bitter gourd) fruit extract in alloxan diabetic rats. **Indian J Exp Biol** 1987; 25(8): 571–572.

T14966 Dubey, D. K., A. R. Biswas, J. S. Bapna and S. C. Pradhan. Hypo-glycaemia and antihyperglycaemic effects of *Momordica charantia* seed extracts in albino rats. **Fitoterapia** 1987; 58(6): 387–394.

T14976 El-Keltawi, N. E. M., S. E. Megalla and S. A. Ross. Antimicrobial activity of some Egyptian aromatic plants. **Herba Pol** 1980; 26(4): 245–250.

T14998 Umarani, D., T. Devaki, P. Govindaraju and K. R. Shanmugasundaram. Ethanol induced metabolic alterations and the effect of *Phyllanthus niruri* in their reversal. **Ancient Sci Life** 1985; 4(3): 174–180.

T14999 Yang, L. L., K. Y. Yen, Y. Kiso and H. Kikino. Antihepatotoxic Actions of Formosan Plant Drugs. **J Ethnopharmacol** 1987; 19(1): 103–110.

T15019 Namba, T., M. Tsunezuka, K. H. Bae and M. Hattori. Studies on dental caries prevention by traditional Chinese medicines Part 1. Screening of crude drugs for antibacterial action against *Streptococcus mutans*. **Shoyakugaku Zasshi** 1981; 35(4): 295–302.

T15029 Jacobson, M., M. M. Crystal, and R. Kleiman. Effectiveness of several polyunsaturated seed oils as boll weevil feeding deterrents. **J Amer Oil Chem Soc** 1981; 58(11): 982,983.

T15054 Parry, O., F. Okuasaba and C. Ejike. Effect of an aqueous extract of *Portulaca oleracea* leaves on smooth muscle and rat blood pressure. **J Ethno-pharmacol** 1988; 22(1): 33–44.

T15123 Conner, D. E. and L. R. Beuchat. Inhibitory effects of plant oleo-resins on yeasts. **Interact Food Proc Int IUMS-ICFMH Symp.**, 12th 1983; 1984: 447–451.

T15148 Sinha, P. and S. K. Saxena. Effect of treating tomatoes with leaf extract of *Lantana camara* on development of fruit rot caused by *Aspergillus niger* in the presence of *Drosophila busckii*. **Indian J Exp Biol** 1987; 25(2): 143–144.

T15220 Kapoor, R. K. Diabetes mellitus. **Indian J Homoeopath Med** 1984; 19(3): 114–120.

T15244 Nagabhushan, M., U. J. Nair, A. J. Amonkar, A. V. D'Souza and S. V. Bhide. Curcumins as inhibitors of nitrosation In vitro. **Mutat Res** 1988; 202(1): 163–169.

T15267 Prakash, A. O. Ovarian response to aqueous extract of *Moringa oleifera* during early pregnancy in rats. **Fitoterapia** 1988; 59(2): 89–96.

T15276 Zheng, M. S. An experimental study of antiviral action of 472 herbs on Herpes Simplex Virus. **J Trad Chin Med** 1988; 8(3): 203–206.

T15279 Koshimizu, K., H. Ohigashi, H. Tokuda, A. Kondo and K. Yamaguchi. Screening of edible plants against possible anti-tumor promoting activity. **Cancer Lett** 1988; 39(3): 247–257.

T15295 Caceres, A., L. M. Giron and A. M. Martinez. Diuretic activity of plants used for treatment of urinary aliments in Guatemala. **J Ethnopharmacol** 1987; 19(3): 233–245.

T15296 Chen, C. P., C. C. Lin and T. Namba. Development of natural crude drug resources from Taiwan. (Vl). In vitro studies of the inhibitory effect on 12 microorganisms. **Shoyakugaku Zasshi** 1987; 41(3): 215–225.

T15323 Ramirez, V. R., L. J. Mostacero, A. E. Garcia, C. F. Mejia, P. F. Pelaez, C. D. Medina and C. H. Miranda. Vegetales empleados en medicina tradicional Noreruana. **Banco Agrario Del Peru & NACL Univ Trujillo**, Trujillo, Peru, June 1988; 54pp.

T15327 Kone-Bamba, D., Y. Pelissier, Z. F. Ozoukou and D. Kouao. Hemostatic activity of 216 plants used in traditional medicine in the Ivory Coast. **Plant Med Phytother** 1987; 21(2): 122–130.

T15330 Wee, Y. C., P. Gopalakrishnakone and A, Chan. Poisonous plants in Singapore—a colour chart for identification with symptoms and signs of poisoning. **Toxicon** 1988; 26(1): 47.

T15375 Gonzalez, F and M. Silva. A survey of plants with antifertility properties described in the South American folk medicine. **Abstr Princess Congress 1** Thailand, Dec. 1987; 20 pp.

T15445 Caceres, A., L. M. Giron, S. R. Alvarado, and M. F. Torres. Screening of Antimicrobial Activity of plants popularly used in Guatemala for the treatment of Dermatomucosal diseases. **J Ethnopharmacol** 1987; 20(3): 223–237.

T15466 Okwuasaba, F., O. Parry and C. Ejike. Investigation into the mechanism of action of extracts of *Portulaca oleracea*. **J Ethnopharmacol** 1987; 21(1): 91–97.

T15467 Okwuasaba, F., O. Parry and C. Ejike. Effects of extracts of *Portulaca oleracea*.on skeletal muscle in vitro. **J Ethnopharmacol** 1987; 21(1): 55–63.

T15468 Okwuasaba, F., O. Parry and C. Ejike. Preliminary clinical investigation into the muscle relaxant actions of an aqueous extract of *Portulaca oleracea* applied topically. **J Ethnopharmacol** 1987; 21(1): 99–106.

T15475 Singh, V. P., S. K. Sharma, and V. S. Khare. Medicinal plants from Ujjain District Madhya Pradesh. Part II. **Indian Drugs Pharm Ind** 1980; 5: 7–12.

T15561 Wadhwani, C. and T. N. Bhardwaja. Effect of *Lantana camara* L. extract on fern spore germination. **Experienta** 1981; 37(3): 245,246.

T15609 Mampane, K. J., P. H. Joubert and I. T. Hay. Jatropha curcas:

Use as a traditional Tswana Medicine and its role as a cause of acute poisoning. **Phytother Res** 1987; 1(1): 50,51.

T15661   Shukla, S., R. Mathur and A. O. Prakash. Histoarchitecture of the genital tract of ovariectomized rats treated with an aqueous extract of *Moringa oleifera* roots. **J Ethnopharmacol** 1989; 25(3): 249–261.

T15693   Srivastava, K. C. Extracts from two frequently consumes spices —cumin (*Cuminum cyminum*) and turmeric (*Curcuma longa*)— inhibit platelaet aggregation and alter eicosanoid biosynthesis in human blood platelets. **Prostaglandis Leukotrienes Essent Fatty Acids** 1989; 37(1): 57–64.

T15727   Sakai, K., N. Oshima, T. Kutsuna, Y. Miyazaki, H. Nakajima, T. Muraoka, K. Okuma and T. Nishino. Pharmaceutical studies on crude drugs. 1. Effect of the Zingiberaceae crude extracts on sulfaguanidine absorption from rat small intestine. **Yakugaku Zasshi** 1986; 106(10): 947–950.

T15786   Maikere-Faniyo, R., L. Van Puyvelde, A. Mutwewingabo and F. X. Habiyaremye. Study on Rwandese medicinal plants used in the treatment of diarrhea 1. **J Ethnopharmacol** 1989; 26(2): 101–109.

T15876   Costa, M., L. C. Di Stasi, M. Kirizawa, S. L. J. Mendacolli, C. Gomes and G. Trolin. Screening in mice of some medicinal plants used for analgesic purposes in the state of Sao Paulo. **J Ethnopharmacol** 1989; 27(1/2): 25–33.

T15879   Spring, M. A. Ethnopharmacological analysis of medicinal plants used by laotian Hmong refugees in Minnesota. **J Ethnopharmacol** 1989; 26(1): 65–91.

T15880   Darias, V., L. Brando, R. Rabanal, C. Sanchez Mateo, R. M. Gonzalez Luis and A. M. Hernandez Perez. New contribu-

tion to the Ethnopharmacological study of the Canary Islands. **J Ethnopharmacol** 1989; 25(1): 77–92.

T15892   Sinha, R. Post-testicular antifertility effects of *Abrus precatorius* seed extract in albino rats. **J Ethnopharmacol** 1990; 28(2): 173–181.

T15904   Murugavel, T., A. Ruknudin, S. Thangavelu and M. A. Akbarsha. Antifertility effect of *Vinca rosea* (Linn.) leaf extract on male albino mice—a sperm parametric study. **Curr Sci** 1989; 58(19): 1102–1103.

T15923   Palanichamy, S. and S. Nagarajan. Analgesic activity of *Cassia alata* leaf extract and kaempferol 3-0-sophoroside. **J Ethnopharmacol** 1990; 29(1): 73–78.

T15943   Rathore, H. S. and V. Saraswat. Protection of mouse testes, epididymis and adrenals with Speman against cadmium intoxication. **Probe** 1986; 25: 257–268.

T15944   Mukherjee, S., T. K. Ghosh and D. De. Effect of Speman on prostatism-A clinical study. **Probe** 1986; 25: 237–240.

T15956   Fernando, R. Plant poisoning in Sri Lanka. **Toxicon** 1988; 26(1): 20.

T15975   Hirschmann, G. S. and A. Rojas De Arias. A survey of medicinal plants of Minas Gerais, Brazil. **J Ethnopharmacol** 1990; 29(2): 159–172.

T15987   Palanichamy, S. and S. Nagarajan. Antifungal activity of *Cassia alata* leaf extract. **J Ethnopharmacol** 1990; 29(3): 337–340.

T16092   Karunanayake, E. H., S. Jeevathayaparan and K. H. Tennekoon. Effect of *Momordica charantia* fruit juice on streptozotocin-induced diaberes in rats. **J Ethnopharmacol** 1990; 30(2): 199–204.

T16122   Shanmugasundaram, E. R. B., U. Subramaniam, R. Santhini and K.

R. Shanmugasundaram. Studies on brain structure and neurological function in alcoholic rats controlled by an Indian medicinal formula (SKV). **J Ethnopharmacol** 1986; 17(3): 225–245.

T16133   Gupta, A., C. O. Wambebe and D. L. Parsons. Central and cardiovascular effects of the alcoholis extract of the leaves of *Carica papaya*. **Int J Crude Drug Res** 1990; 28(4): 257–266.

T16158   Boye, G. L. Studies on antimalarial action of *Cryptolepis sanguinolenta* extract. **Proc Int Symp on East-West Med, Seoul, Korea** 1989; 243–251.

T16172   Shanmugasundaram, E. R. B. and K. Radah Shanmugasundar. An Indian herbal formula (SKV) for controlling voluntary ethanol intake in rats with chronic alcoholism. **J Ethnopharmacol** 1986; 17(2): 171–182.

T16181   Chabra, S. C., R. L. A. Mahunnah and E. N. Mshiu. Plants used in traditional medicine in Eastern Tanzania. I. Pteridophytes and Angiosperms (Acanthaceae to Canellaceae). **J Ethnopharmacol** 1987; 21(3): 253–277.

T16185   Mishra, A. K. and N. K. Dubey. Fungitoxicity of essential oil of *Amomum subulatum* against *Aspergillus flavus*. **Econ Bot** 1990; 44(4): 530–532.

T16238   Guerin, J. C. and H. P. Reveillere. Antifungal activity of plant extracts used in therapy. l. Study of 41 plant extracts against 9 fungi species. **Ann Pharm Fr** 1984; 42(6): 553–559.

T16239   Kumar, D. S. and Y. S. Prabhakar. On the Ethnomedical significance of the Arjun tree, *Terminalia arjuna* (Roxb.) Wight & Arnot. **Indian J Homoeopath Med** 1984; 19(3): 114–120.

T16253   Macrae, W. D., J. B. Hudson and G. H. N. Towers. Studies on the pharmacological activity of Ama-

T16262   zonian Euphorbiaceae. **J Ethnopharmacol** 1988; 22(2): 143–172.

Misas, C. A. J., N. I. M. R. Hernandez and A. M. L. Abraham. Contribution to the biological evaluation of Cuban plants. V. **Rev Cub Med Trop** 1979; 31: 37–43.

T16330   Misas, C. A. J., N. M. R. Hernandez and A. N. L. Abraham. Contribution to the biological evaluation of Cuban plants. II. **Rev Cub Med Trop** 1979; 31: 13–19.

T16358   Renu. Fungitoxicity of leaf extracts ofsome higher plants against *Rhizoctonia solani* Kuehn. **Nat Acad Sci Lett** 1983; 6(8): 245,246.

T16362   Sharma, O. P. Lantana camara toxicity, control and utilization. **Biol Mem** 1984; 9(2): 204–209.

T16366   Cliff, J., P. Lundquist, H. Rosling, B. Sorbo and L. Wide. Thyroid function in a cassava-eating population affected by epidemic spastic paraparesis. **Acta Endocrinol** 1986; 113(4): 523–528.

T16412   Kausalya, S., L. Padmanabhan and S. Durairajan. **Clinician** 1984; 48(12): 460–464.

T16453   Sreejayan and M. N. A. Rao. Oxygen free radical scavenging activity of the juice of *Momordica charantia* fruits. **Fitoterapia** 1991; 62(4): 344–346.

T16468   Sivaswamy, S. N., B. Balchandran, S. Balanehru and V. M. Sivaramakrishnan. Mutagenic activity okf South Indian food items. **Indian J Exp Biol** 1991; 29(8): 730–737.

T16478   Vedavathy, S., K. N. Rao, M. Rajaiah and N. Nagaraju. Folklore information from Rayalaseema region, Andhra Pradesh for family planning and birth control. **Int J Pharmacog** 1991; 29(2): 113–116.

T16493   Palanichamy, S., E. Amala Bhaskar, R. Bakthavathsalam and S. Nagarajan. Wound healing activity of *Cassia alata*. **Fitoterapia** 1991; 62(2): 153–156.

T16506 Zia-Ul-Haque, A., M. H. Qazi and M. E. Hamdard. Studies on the antifertility properties of active components isolated from the seeds of *Abrus precatorius* Linn. 11. **Pak J Zool** 1983; 15(2): 141–146.

T16521 Thamlikitkul, V., T. Dechatiwongse, C. Chantrakul, S. Nimitnon, W. Punkrut, S. Wongkonkatape, N. Boontaeng, S. Taechaiya, A. Riewpaiboon, S. Timsard, et al., Randomized double-blind study of *Curcuma domestica* Val. for dyspepsia. **J Med Assoc Thailand** 1989; 72(11): 613–620.

T16531 Nwodo, O. F. C. Studies on *Abrus precatorius* seeds. 1. Uterotonic activity of seed oil. **J Ethnopharmacol** 1991; 31(3): 391–394.

T16555 Ratnasooriya, W. D., A. S. Amarasekera, N. S. D. Perera and G. A. S. Premakumara. Sperm antimotility properties of a seed extract of *Abrus precatorius*. **J Ethnopharmacol** 1991; 33(1/2): 85–90.

T16608 Polasa, K., B. Sesikaran, T. P. Krishna and K. Krishnaswamy. Turmeric (*Curcuma longa*)—induced reduction in urinary mutagens. **Food Chem Toxicol** 1991; 29(10): 699–706.

T16624 Murugavel, T. and M. A. Akbarsha. Anti-spermatogenic effect of *Vinca rosea* Linn. **Indian J Exp Biol** 1991; 29(9): 810–812.

T16652 Lee, E. B. and Y. S. Lee. The screening of biologically active plants in Korea using isolated organ preparations (V). Anticholinergic and oxytoxic actions in rat's ileum and uterus. **Korean J Pharmacog** 1991; 22(4): 246–248.

T16664 Chattopadhyay, R. R., S. K. Sankar, S. Ganguly, B. N. Banerjee and T. K. Basu. **Indian J Physiol Pharmacol** 1991; 35(3): 145–151.

T16711 Panthong, A., D. Kanjanapothi and W. C. Taylor. ethnobotanical review of medicinal plants from Thai traditional books, Part 1. Plants with antiinflammatory, anti-asthmatic and antihypertensive properties. **J Ethnopharmacol** 1986; 18(3): 213–228.

T16714 Sethi, N., D. Nath and R. K. Singh. Teratological aspects of *Abrus precatorius* seeds in rats. **Fitoterapia** 1990; 61(1): 61–63.

T16715 Lokar, L. C. and L. Poldini. Herbal remedies in the traditional medicine of the Venezia Guilia Region (Northeast Italy). **J Ethnopharmacol** 1988; 22(3): 231–239.

T16726 Abraham, Z., S. D. Bhakuni, H. S. Garg, A. K. Goel, B. N. Mehrotra and G. K. Patnaik. **Indian J Exp Biol** 1986; 24: 48–68.

T16785 Rao, V. S. N., A. M. S. Menezes and M. G. T. Gadelha. Antifertility screening of some indigenous plants of Brazil. **Fitoterapia** 1988; 59(1): 17–20.

T16952 Ohta, S., N. Sato, S. H. Tu and M. Shinoda. Protective effects of Taiwan crude drugs on experimental liver injuries. **Yakugaku Zasshi** 1992; 113(12): 870–880.

TI4342 Ohta, S., N. Sakurai, T. Inoue and M. Shinoda. Studies on chemical protectors against radiation. XXV. Radioprotective activities of various crude drugs. **Yakugaku Zasshi** 1987; 107(1): 70–75.

T03294 Vaidya, A. B., T. G. Rajagopalan, N. A. Mankodi, D. S. Antarkar, P. S. Tathed, A. V. Purohit and N. H. Wadia. Treatment of Parkinson's disease with Cowhage plant—*Macuna pruriens* Bak. **Neurology** (India) 1978; 26: 171–176.

T04225 Solepure, A. B., N. M. Joshi, B. V. Deshkar, S. R. Muzumdar and

C. D. Shirole. The effect of 'Speman' on quality of semen in relation to magnesium concentration. **Indian Practitioner** 1979; 32: 663–668.

T06167   Nath, C., G. P. Gupta, K. P. Bhargava, V. Lakshmi, S. Singh and S. P. Popli. Study of antiparkinsonian activity of seeds of *Macuna prurita* Hook. **Indian J Pharmacol** 1981; 13: 94–95.

W00002   Chopra, R. N., R. L. Badhwar and S. Ghosh. Poisonous plants of India. Manager of Publications, Government of India Press, Calcutta. Volume 1, 1949.

W00006   Garg, S. K. and G. P. Garg. A preliminary report on the smooth muscle stimulating property of some indigenous plants on isolated rat uterus. **Bull P. G. I.** 1970: 4: 162.

W00015   Rangaswami, S. and S. Sankarasubramanian. Chemical components of the flowers of *Moringa pterygosperma*. **Curr Sci** 1946; 15: 316–317.

W00025   Khurana, S. M. P. and K. S. Bhargava. Effect of plant extracts on the activity of three papaya viruses. **J Gen Appl Microbiol** 1970; 16: 225–230.

W00088   Sen Gupta, K. P., N. C. Ganguli and B. Battacharjee. Bacteriological and Pharmacological studies of a vibriocidal drug derived from an indigenous source. **Antiseptic** 1956; 53: 287.

W00113   Ayensu, E. S. Medicinal plants of West Africa. Reference Publications, Inc, 1978.

W00128   Orataliza, I. C., I. F. Del Rosario, M. Minda Caedo and A. P. Alcaraz. The availability of carotene in some Philippine vegetables. **Philippine J Sci** 1969; 98: 123.

W00135   Dixit, R. S., S. L. Perti and R. N. Agarwal. New repellents. **Labdev** 1965; 3: 273.

W00138   Chang, S. Y., D. Y. Mao and P. Hsu. The antitumor action and toxicity of the alkaloidal fraction AC-875 from *Vinca roseus*. **Yao Hsueh Hsueh Pao** 1965; 12: 772–777.

W00232   Ray, P. G. and S. K. Majumdar. Antimicrobial activity of some Indian plants. **Econ Bot** 1976; 30: 317–320.

W00276   Kulkarni, R. D. and B. B. Gaitonde. Potentiation of tolbutamice action by jasad bhasma and karela *(Momordica charantia)*. **Indian J Med Res** 1962; 50: 715–719.

W00298   Mourgue, M., J. Delphaut, R. Baret and R. Kassab. Study of toxicity and localization of the toxalbumin (curcin) of the seeds of Jatropha curcas. **Bull Soc Chim Biol** 1961; 43: 517.

W00332   Garg, S. K. and G. P. Garg. Effect of *Areca catechu* and *Carica papaya* on fertility in female albino rats. **Bull P. G. I.** 1970; 4: 150.

W00335   Garg, S. K. effect of *Curcuma longa* on fertility in female albino rats. **Bull P. G. I.** 1971; 5: 178.

W00346   Lee, E. B., H. S. Yun and W. S. Woo. Plants and animals used for fertility regulation in Korea. **Korean J Pharmacog** 1977; 8: 81–87.

W00374   Dhawan, B. N., G. K. Patnaik, R. P. Rastogi, K. K. Singh and J. S. Tandon. Screening of Indian plants for biological activity. VI. **Indian J Exp Biol** 1977; 15: 208–219.

W00384   Sharma, L. D., H. S. Bahga and P. S. Srivastava. In vitro anthelmintic screening of indigenous medicinal plants against Haemonchus contortus (Rudolphi, 1803) Cobbold, 1898 of sheep and goats. **Indian J Anim Res** 1971; 5(1): 33–38.

W00408   Friese, F. W. Certain little-known anthelmintics from Brazil. **Apoth ZTG** 1929; 44: 180.

W00456   Kim, N. D. Anthelmintics in crude drugs on the drugs for tapeworms. **Yakhak Hoe Chi** 1974; 19: 87.

W00486 Jayatilak, P. G., D. S. Pardanani, B. D. Murty and A. R. Sheth. Effect of an indigenous drug (Speman) on accessory reproductive functions of mice. **Indian J Exp Biol** 1976; 14: 170.

W00500 Silva, M. J. M., M. Pinheiro De Sousa and M. Z. Rouquayrol. Molluscicidal activity of plants from Northeastern Brazil. **Rev Brasil Farm** 1971; 52: 117–123.

W00534 Kobayashi, J. Early Hawaiian uses of medicinal plants in pregnancy and childbirth. **J Trop Pediatr Environ Child Health** 1976; 22: 260.

W00667 Caius, J. F. and K. S. Mhaskar. The correlation between the chemical composition of anthelmintics and their therapeutic value in connection with the hookworm inquiry in the Madras presidency. XIX. Drugs allied to thyme. **Indian J Med Res** 1923; 11: 353.

W00673 Ricardo, M. S. Investigation of Quinine in *Phyllanthus niruri*. **Anales Univ Santo Domingo** 1944; 8: 295.

W00678 Lotlikar, M. M. and M. R. Rajarama Rao. Pharmacology of a hypoglycaemic principle isolated from the fruits of *Momordica charantia*. **Indian J Pharmacy** 1966; 28: 129.

W00799 Kerharo, J. Historic and Ethnopharmacognostic review on the belief and traditional practices in the treatment of sleeping sickness in West Africa. **Bull Soc Med Afr Noire Lang Fr** 1974; 19: 400.

W00903 Oakes, A. J. and M. P. Morris. The West Indian Weedwoman of the United States Virgin Islands. **Bull Hist Med** 1958; 32: 164.

W01047 Collier, W. A. and L. Van De Piji. The antibiotic action of plants, especially the higher plants, with results with indonesian plants. **Chron Nat** 1949; 105: 8.

W01074 Frisbey, A., J. M. Roberts, J. C. Jennings, R. Y. Gottshall and E. H. Lucas. The occurrence of antifungal substances in seed plants with special reference to *Mycobacterium tuberculosis* (third report). **Mich State Univ Agr Appl Sci Quart Bull.** 1953; 35: 392–404.

W01145 Krishnamurti, G. V. and T. R. Seshadri. The bitter principle of *Phyllanthus niruri*. **Proc Indian Acad Sci Ser** 1946; A 24: 357–364.

W01223 Nene, Y. L., P. N. Thapliyal and K. Kumar. Screening of some plant extracts for antifungal properties. **Labdev J Sci Tech** 1968; 6B(4): 226–228.

W01244 Casey, R. C. D. Alleged antifertility plants of India. **Indian J Med Sci** 1960; 14: 590–601.

W01267 Hodge, W. H. and D. Taylor. The ethnobotany of the island Caribes of Dominica. **WEBBIA** 1956; 12: 513–644.

W01270 Asprey, G. F. and P. Thornton. Medicinal Plants of Jamaica. IV. **West Indian Med J** 1955; 4: 145–165.

W01280 Logan, M. H. Digestive disorders and plant medicine in Highland Guatemala. **Anthropos** 1973; 68: 537–543.

W01284 Simpson, G. E. Folk Medicine in Trinidad. **J Amer Folklore** 1962; 75: 326–340.

W01316 Asprey, G. F. and P. Thornton. Medicinal Plants of Jamaica. III. **West Indian Med** 1955; J4: 69–82.

W01362 Prakash, A. O. and R. Mathur. Screening of Indian plants for antifertility activity. **Indian J Exp Biol** 1976; 14: 623–626.

W01378 Gupta, M. L., T. K. Gupta and K. P. Bhargava. A study of antifertility effects of some indigenous drugs. **J Res Indian Med** 1971; 6: 112–116.

W01586 Stanislas, E., R. Rouffiac and J. J. Foyard. Phyllanthus niruri alkaloids, flavonoids, and lignans. **Plant Med Phytother** 1967; 1: 136–141.

W01662 Gallo, P. and H. Valeri. The Antibiotic activity of the seed of avocado pear (*Persea americana*). **Rev Med Vet Parasitol** 1953; 12: 125–129.

W01723 Abbott, B. J., J. Leiter, J. L. Hartwell, M. E. Caldwell, J. L. Beal, R. E. Perdue Jr. and S. A. Schepartz. **Cancer Res** 1966; 26: 761–935.

W01791 Pan. P. C. The application of Chinese traditional medicine in the treatment of vaginal cancer. **Chin J Obstet Gynecol** 1960; 8: 156–162.

W01792 Mueller-Oerlinghausen, B., W. Ngamwathana and P. Kanchanapee. Investigation into Thai medicinal plants said to cure diabetes. **J Med Assoc Thailand** 1971; 54: 105–111.

W01818 Malcolm, S. A. and E. A. Sofowora. Antimicrobial activity of selected Nigerian folk remedies and their constituent plants. **Lloydia** 1969; 32: 512–517.

W01996 Peng, M. T., H. C. Lee and H. S. Lin. Effect of Psidium root on the reproductive organs of rats and mice. **Tohoku J Exp Med** 1955; 62: 287–297.

W02033 Roca-Garcia, H. Weeds: A link with the past. **Arnoldia** (Boston) 1970; 30(3): 114–115.

W02043 Shukla, O. P. and C. R. Krishna Murti. Bacteriolytic activity of plants latices. **J Sci Ind Res** 1961; C 20: 225–226.

W02108 Stepka, W., K. E. Wilson and G. E. Madge. Antifertility investigation on Momordica. **Lloydia** 1974; 37: 645C.

W02263 Soundararajan, R. Studies on the keeping quality of ghee. 1. Influence of common flavouring materials. **Indian J Dairy Sci** 1958; 11: 96–100.

W02290 Dragendorff, G. Die Heilpflanzen Der Verschiedenen Volker Und Zeiten, F. Enke, Stuttgart, 1898; 885 pp.

W02402 Shivpuri, D. N. and K. L. Dua. Allergy to papaya tree (*Carica papaya*). **Ann Allergy** 1963; 21: 139–144.

W02435 Devadatta, S. C. and R. C. Appanna. Availability of calcium in some of the leafy vegetables. **Proc Indian Acad Sci Ser B** 1954; 39: 236–242.

W02459 Wang, V. F. In Vitro antibacterial activity of some common Chinese herbs on *Mycobacteria tuberculosis*. **Chung-Hua I Hsueh Tsa Chih** (Engl Ed) 1950; 68: 169–172.

W02493 Schultes, R. E. De plantis toxicariis a mundo novo tropicale commentationes. IV. **Bot Mus Leafl Harv Univ** 1969; 22(4): 133–164.

W02544 Rathore, J. S. and S. K. Mishra. Inhibition of root elongation by some plant extracts. **Indian J Biochem Biophys** 1971; 9: 523,524.

W02604 Kholkute, S. D., S. Chatterjee, D. N. Srivas Ava and K. N. Udupa. Antifertility effect of the alcoholic extract of Japa (*Hibiscus rosa-sinensis*). **J Res Indian Med** 1972; 7: 72,73.

W02781 Anon. Pharmacological investigations with antibiotics and chemotherapeutics. **Annu Rev Biochem & Allied Res In India** 1954; 25: 112–118.

W02855 Roig Y Mesa, J. T. Plantas Medicinales, Aromaticas O Venenosas De Cuba. Ministerio De Agricultura, Republica De Cuba, Havana, 1945; 872 pp.

W02856 Li, F. K. Problems concerning artificial abortion through oral administration of traditional drugs. **Ha- Erh-Pin Chung-I** 1965; 1: 11–14.

W02949 Pinheiro De Sousa, M. and M. Z. Rouquayrol. Molluscicidal activity of plants from Northeast Brazil. **Rev Bras Fpesq Med Biol** 1974; 7(4): 389–394.

W03029 ANON. More secret remedies. What they cost and what they contain, 1912; 185–209.

W03044   Ueki, H., M. Kaibara, M. Sakagawa and S. Hayashi. Antitumor activity of plant constituents. 1. **Yakugaku Zasshi** 1961; 81: 1641–1644.

W03071   Nayar, S. L. Poisonous seeds of India. **J Bombay Nat Hist Soc** 1954; 52: 1–18.

W03073   Singh, A. and J. D. Kohli. A plea for research into indigenous drug employed in Veterinary practice. **Indian Vet J** 1956; 32: 271–280.

W03088   Bhandari, P. R. and B. Mukerji. *Lochnera rosea* Linn Reichb. **Gauhati Ayurvedic Coll Mag** 1959; 8: 1–4.

W03093   Pachauri, S. P. and S. K. Makherjee. Effect of *Curcuma longa* (Haridra) and *Curcuma amada* (Amragandhi) on the cholesterol level in experimental hypercholesterolemia of rabbits. **J Res Indian Med** 1970; 5: 27–31.

W03295   Shukla, G. S. and V. K. Upadhyaya. Studies on the food preference of *Mylabris pustulata* Thunb. (Coleoptera. Meloidae). **Zool Beitra** 1973; 19(1): 9–12.

W03363   Gazit, S. and A. Blumenfeld. Inhibitor and auxin activity in the avocado fruit. **Physiol Plant** 1972; 27: 77–82.

W03405   Heal, R. E., E. F. Rogers, R. T. Wallace and O. Starnes. A survey of plants for insecticidal activity. **Lloydia** 1950; 13: 89–162.

W03417   Nayar, S. L. Vegetable insecticides. **Bull Natl Inst Sci India** 1955; 4: 137–145.

W03487   Chopra, R. N. Indigenous drugs of India. Their medical and economic aspects. The art press, Calcutta, India, 1933; 550 pp.

W03491   Attia, M. S., S. Ahmad, S. A. H. Zaidi and Z. Ahmed. Studies on the bacteriostatic properties of wild medicinal plants of Karachi (Pakistan) Region 1. **Pak J Sci Ind Res** 1972; 15: 199–207.

W03518   Indira, M., M. Sirsi, S. Randomir and S. Dev. Occurrence of estrogenic substances in plants. I. Estrogenic activity of *Cyperus rotundus*. **J Sci Ind Res** 1956; 15C: 202–204.

W03527   Radomir, S., S. Devi and M. Sirsi. Chemistry and Antibacterial activity of Nut Grass. **Curr Sci (India)** 1956; 25: 118–119.

W03671   Belkin, M. and D. B. Fitzgerald. Tumor-damaging capacity of plant materials. 1. Plants used as cathartics. **J Nat Cancer Inst** 1952; 13: 139–155.

W03693   George, M. and K. M. Pandalai. Investigations on plant antibiotics. Part IV. Further search for antibiotic substances in Indian medicinal plants. **Indian J Med Res** 1949; 37: 169–181.

W03711   Sirsi, M. In Vitro study of the inhibitory action of some chemotherapeutic agents on a freshly isolated strain of *Cryptococcus neoformans*. **Hibdustan Antibiot Bull** 1963; 6(2): 39,40.

W03791   Osman, H. G. and E. W. Jwanny. Serological and chemical investigation on the agglutinins of *Phaseolus montcalm.* **J Chem U A R** 1963; 6(2): 191–204.

W03804   Wasuwat, S. A list of Thai medicinal plants, Asrct, Bangkok, Report No. 1 on Res. Project. 17. **A.S.R.C.T. Bangkok Thailand** 1967; 17: 22 pp.

W03885   Sharaf, A. and M. Naguib. A Pharmacological study of the Egyptian plant, *Lantana camara*. **Egypt Pharm Bull** 1959; 41(6): 93–97.

W03968   ANON. The herbalist. Hammond book company, Hammond Indiana, 1931; 400 pp.

W04017   Kerhado, J. Nebreday (*Moringa oleifera*), A popular Senegalese remedy. Therapeutic use on African chemistry and pharmacology. **Plant Med Phytother** 1969; 3: 214–219.

W04097   Uppal, R. P. and B. S. Paul. Preliminary studies with crude Lantadene, toxic principle of Lantana camara in albino rats.

Haryana Agr Univ J Res 1971; 1(2): 98–102.

W04173   Dwivedi, S. K., G. A. Shivnani and H. C. Joshi. Clinical and biochemical studies in Lantana poisoning in Ruminants. **Indian J Anim Sci** 1971; 41(10): 948–953.

W04174   Hunt, S. E. and P. J. Mc Cosker. Serum adenosine deaminase activity in experimentally produced liver diseases of cattle and sheep. Yellow-wood, Lantana, carbon tetrachloride, and chronic copper poisoning. **Brit Vet J** 1970; 126(2): 74–81.

W04179   Miles, S. B. The countries and tribes of the Persian Gulf. Frank Cass & Co. Ltd., London, 1966; 390–399.

W04249   Lee, H. K. and Y. S. Chung. Antifungal activities of medicinal plants in Korea. **Kisul Yon'guso Pogo** 1963; 2: 76–78.

W04255   Heim, F and Rullier. The toxic principles of the seed and oil of the Physic-nut tree (Jatropha curcas L.). **Bull Del Office Colonial** 1919; 12: 96–110.

W04271   Hunt, S. E. and P. J. Mc Cosker. Correlation between K1 and K2 in the fractional clearance of bromosulphthalein in cattle and sheep suffering from different hepatotoxic diseases. **Experientia** 1969; 25: 588,589.

W04316   Meghal, S. K. and M. C. Nath. Effect of spice diet on the intestinal synthesis of thiamine in rats. **Ann Biochem Exp Med** 1962; 22: 99–104.

W04510   Jamwal, K. S. and K. K. Anand. Preliminary screening of some reputed abortifacient indigenous plants. **Indian J Pharm** 1962; 24: 218–220.

W04546   Jelliffe, D. B., G. Bras and K. L. Stuart. The clinical picture of veno-occlusive disease of the liver in Jamaican children. **Ann Trop Med Parasitol** 1954; 48: 386–396.

W04570   Kubas, J. Investigations on known or potential antitumoral plants by means of microbiological tests. Part 111. Biological activity of some cultivated plant species in *Neurospora crassa* test. **Acta Biol Cracov Ser Bot** 1972; 15: 87–100.

W04573   Krupe, M., W. Wirth, D. Nies and A. Ensgraber. Studies on the "Mitogenic" effect of hemoglutinating extracts of various plants on the human small lymphocytes in peripheral blood cultured in vitro. **Z Immunitatsforsch Allerg Klin Immunol** 1968; 135(1): 19–42.

W04602   Garg, S. K. and G. P. Garg. A preliminary report on the smooth muscle stimulating property of some indigenous plants on isolated rat uterus. **Bull Postgrad Ins Med Educ Res Chandigarh** 1970; 4(4): 162–164.

W3022A   Mokkhasmit, M., K. Swasdimongkol, W. Ngarmwathana and U. Permphiphat. Study on toxicity of Thai medicinal plants. (Continued). **J Med Assoc Thailand** 1971; 54(7): 490–504.

X00001   ANON. Unpublished data, National Cancer Institute. National Cancer Inst. Central Files 1976.

X00003   Kong, Y. C. Plants used for rheumatism, arthritis and related conditions in Chinese traditional medicine. **Personal Communication** 1977.

X00012   Popli, S. P. Screening of Indian indigenous plants for antifertility activity. Progress report on project 74219 (WHO), Dec. 20, 1977.

About the Author

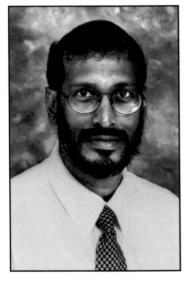 A native of Guyana, Ivan A. Ross is a biologist at the United States Food and Drug Administration. At the age of seventeen he was awarded a scholarship by the United States Agency for International Development to study agriculture at Tuskegee University. After completing his studies he returned to Guyana and was appointed to the Guyana Ministry of Agriculture. During this tour of duty, most of his time was spent in the isolated communities of the Aborigines population, incorporating modern agriculture and health care methods with the traditional system. Dr. Ross' interest in traditional medicine originated at this time. He later entered the University of Maryland, College Park, where he studied animal science and biochemistry. In 1987 he joined the United States Department of Health and Human Services, Food and Drug Administration, as a biologist in the Division of Toxicological Research. He is an active investigator and has published several research articles, primarily dealing with food safety. Other areas of his wide-ranging experience include Lecturer of Agricultural and Rural Development at Gambia College, Gambia, West Africa, and seminars throughout Gambia on food safety, health awareness, and agricultural techniques. When not in the laboratory, Dr. Ross is either farming or writing.